Carcinogenic Mind

About this book

The role of the psyche in the genesis of cancer has been discussed by scientists for several hundred years. This book presents about 2000 studies that prove that our mind is the main source of cancer.

The author, one of the leading psycho-oncologists of Ukraine, physician, psychotherapist, molecular biologist, and Buddhist practitioner, uses an interdisciplinary and integrative approach, involving data from psychology, oncology, psychoneuroimmunology, philosophy, epigenetics, and other branches of knowledge. Step by step, Dr. Matrenitsky uncovers the inseparable connection of psychological, social, spiritual, and physical mechanisms of cancer. It is explored throughout the whole continuum of illness, starting with a predisposition in the womb and childhood.

A tumor is just the tip of the iceberg. Its unseen root is inability to cope with the problems of life, psychological traumas and intrapersonal conflicts, arising from unmet needs. This leads to chronic psycho-physiological stress, which suppresses the immune system and other systems providing anti-cancer protection. The result is an existential crisis, leading to the loss of the will to live, initiating a program of unconscious self-destruction.

Overcoming the crisis, achievement of post-traumatic growth, and spiritual awakening can revive the natural healing powers of the body, support the medical treatment, and bring the patient to stable remission or complete healing.

The book is written in the popular-science format to build a 'mind-body' bridge between medical doctors and psychologists, as well as to provide a comprehensive guide for public health professionals and students. It is supplemented with a detailed glossary and offers a holistic roadmap to understanding the personal causes that have contributed to one's development of the disease, in order to find new ways to cure it.

An alternative to the standard biomedical approach to preventing cancer, the book shows how new 'anticancer' mindsets and lifestyle will help us to get and stay healthy.

Carcinogenic Mind

The Psychosomatic Mechanisms of Cancer

Contribution of chronic stress and emotional attitudes to the onset and recurrence of disease, how to prevent it and help the treatment

Vladislav Matrenitsky, M.D., Ph.D.

Foreword by Bernie Siegel, M.D.

Anticancer.Help Publishing

Visit author web-site at www.carcinogenic-mind.com.

Cover design by Julia Kolesnik.
Literary editor Louise Larchbourne.
ISBN-978-617-628-087-3.

Anticancer.Help Publishing,
a division of the Center for Psychotherapy, Psychosomatics and Psycho-oncology Expio
67 Vyshgorodska Str.,
Kyiv 04114, Ukraine.

I dedicate this book:

- to my family, who are constantly supporting me with their love;

- to my teachers, thanks to whom I became who I am today: Vladimir Frolkis, Vladimir Stepanov, Nikolay Oorzhak, Jorg Barthel, Namkai Norbu Rinpoche, Dmitry Androshchuk;

- to the pioneers of psycho-oncology, who showed us the way of discovering the true causes of cancer: Claus Bahnson, George Bykhovsky, Lydia Temoshok, Carl and Stephanie Simonton, Bernie Siegel, Lawrence LeShan, Jimmie Holland, Tom Laughlin;

- to my patients, who inspired me to write this book.

Acknowledgments

I express my deep gratitude to my reviewers, colleagues, and friends who have made valuable comments and suggestions while reading the manuscript: Dr. Galina Pilyagina, Dr. Alexander Weiserman, Dr. Viktor Priymak, Dr. Mikhail Mylnikov, Vitor Rodrigues, Ph.D., Serge Beddington-Behrens, Ph.D., Gennady Melnik.

Testimonials

This book should be read by every physician-oncologist and every cancer patient. It sheds light on those aspects of cancer that are virtually unknown in this country, and convincingly proves the importance of the use of psychotherapy in oncology.

Moreover, the book helps patients understand what can be done to improve health after completing the course of traditional special treatment.

Viktor V. Priymak, M.D., Ph.D., surgeon-oncologist,
Head of the Department of Abdominal and Retroperitoneal Tumors of the National Cancer Institute, Kiev, Ukraine

* * *

This monograph presents a deep analysis of the influence of psychological problems on the development of cancer. The author has thoroughly reviewed modern scientific data on one of the most problematic areas of medicine. He has reasonably showed that in the treatment of oncological diseases, in addition to the surgical-pharmacological approach prevailing in this country, the participation of psychotherapists and psychologists is mandatory.

"The carcinogenic mind" is the way of being of which cancer becomes the natural result. Therefore, adequate and timely psycho-correction can be an effective aid for patients confronting a life-threatening illness.

Galina Y. Pilyagina, M.D., Ph.D., Dr. Med. Sci., psychiatrist, psychotherapist,
Professor, Head of the Department of Psychiatry, Psychotherapy and Medical Psychology of the National Medical Academy of Postgraduate Education after P.L. Shupik, Kiev, Ukraine

* * *

The book has a clear logic, contains a huge array of information from different areas of modern psychology and biomedicine. At the same time, it is written in quite accessible language and is not overloaded with specific terminology. When the author has to discuss the mechanisms that determine the complex processes in the body, he explains it simply and intelligibly.

Therefore, the book can be recommended not only for a narrow circle of specialists, but also for people who do not have special education but are interested in the theoretical and practical issues of cancer set forth in it.

Alexander M. Vaiserman, M.D., Ph.D., Dr. Med. Sci., molecular biologist,
Head of the Laboratory of Epigenetics of the Institute of Gerontology of the National Academy of Medical Sciences of Ukraine, Kiev

Foreword

It is a pleasure to read the work that Dr. Matrenitsky has put together. It is sad that the medical profession still has not included what his book reveals as a part of medical education. Over fifty years ago when I wrote my book *Love, Medicine & Miracles*, I was called a controversial person who was blaming his patients for getting cancer. What I was doing was teaching them how to heal and cure their disease, but I was a surgeon, and so made other doctors who were not aware of mind-body unity confused and unable to understand that I was empowering my patients and not making them feel guilty. You don't have to fight a war and empower your enemy, the cancer. You have to work on healing and curing your life and body.

Jungian therapist Elida Evans, in the 1920s wrote in her book, *A Psychological Study of Cancer*, "cancer is growth gone wrong, a message to take a new road in your life." The poet W. H. Auden in his poem "Miss Gee," wrote about cancer:

Childless women get it.
And men when they retire;
It's as if there had to be an outlet
For their foiled creative fire.

Doctors years ago yelled at me, "Just because it rhymes doesn't make it true." Today we can see it is true.

I started an organization called ECaP; Exceptional Cancer Patients. These people outlived expectations, participated in their experience of cancer, and were not victims. When I wrote articles for medical journals they were returned with the comment, "interesting but inappropriate for our journal." When I sent it to psychiatry journals they sent it back too with this comment: "appropriate but not interesting. We know all this." My articles were about mind-body interaction and how dreams and drawings revealed what was happening in the body.

Century ago Jung diagnosed a brain tumor from a dream and many Jungian therapists have helped me to see what information lies within a patient's dream or drawing. My book *The Art of Healing* contains many examples, as do many other books written by Jungians; but because they didn't know anatomy, as doctors do, they did not see what I was able to see. I used this knowledge to diagnose and help me decide whether to operate or not.

Dr. Matrenitsky uses a term that I do not accept; "spontaneous healing." Why do I not? Because this healing isn't spontaneous. That is what his book is telling us. Solzhenitsyn's book *The Cancer Ward* has a beautiful explanation—and I must say here, fiction writers write the truth because they observe life and turn it into fiction through the characters they create.

Solzhenitsyn has one of the men on the cancer ward say, "I found this book in the hospital library. It says here there are cases of "self-induced healing", not recovery through treatment, but actual healing, see." It was as though self-induced healing fluttered out of the great open book like a RAINBOW-COLORED BUTTERFLY and they all held up their foreheads and cheeks for its healing touch as it flew past.

The rainbow coloring is your life in order and harmony. How does that happen? You burst out of your cocoon and become your beautiful authentic self. I learned to ask patients why they didn't die when they were expected to and they all had a story to tell me. They did not deny their mortality but started living their authentic lives. New jobs, new locations, adopting pets, finding a home on the ocean, leaving their troubles to God, or telling God what they needed—and He better respond.

I'll conclude with one example. A patient was expected to die within two months. He moved to Colorado to die in the beautiful mountains. I told the family to call me for the funeral. A year later, no call, so I called the family to criticize them for ignoring me. That patient answered the phone and said "It was so beautiful here I forgot to die."

A letter I received said, "I bought a dog, put in a backyard wildlife site," and much more; and then ended, "I didn't die and now I am so busy I'm killing myself. Help, where do I go from here?" I told her to take a nap. Physical fatigue is not a threat, as emotional fatigue is. Monday morning we have more heart attacks, strokes, and illnesses of all sorts. The problem is people, not Monday. So read this book and learn how to induce a life and body you can love and which will do its best to keep you alive and healthy.

Bernie Siegel, M.D.,
Author of *Love, Medicine & Miracles*, *Peace, Love & Healing*, and *The Art of Healing*

Contents

Introduction

Understanding how much you can participate
in your health or illness
is a significant first step in getting well.
For many of our patients,
it is the most critically important step.
It may well be for you, too.
Carl and Stephanie Simonton,
Getting Well Again

"Why me?" along with paralyzing fear and denial—these are typical of the responses triggered by a cancer diagnosis. It is probably because what we all fear most is the unknown and the unexpected. For cancer, despite certain medical achievements in its diagnostics and treatment, remains one of the most enigmatic diseases. This is not because we know too little about its biological mechanisms (today, they are perhaps studied better than those of any other disease), but because the logic behind cancer's choosing a particular victim remains inexplicable. Given two people living in the same place, with a similar state of health, age, lifestyle, and occupation, why does one develop cancer while the other does not? After all, the carcinogens around them are the same.

Why is the fight against cancer still unsuccessful, despite the massive financial injections into scientific research throughout many countries? In 1971, Richard Nixon, the president of the richest country in the world, the United States, declared a war on cancer, and, respectively, the national law on cancer was approved. However, after forty-five years had passed, another president—Barack Obama—declared in 2016 the new plans to defeat cancer, which will be another "flight to the Moon" for the United States. A new national mission was being created, headed by the US Vice President. Obviously, this has occurred because of a lack of any significant progress in the field of oncology.

The problem of cancer worsens every year. The increase in morbidity and the severe complications of chemo- and radiotherapy prompt us to think whether or not this is the time to begin paying attention to other possibilities, which, for certain reasons (which will be discussed below), are not focused on by conventional medicine. Could it be that the issue is that we are "flying" in the wrong direction?

The achievements of molecular biology, notably the detection of new oncogenes and signaling pathways for their activation and blocking, each time give rise to the hope that the proper target for effective treatment has been found. Much was expected from the development of gene therapy methods. However, although more than 100 oncogenes and fifteen genes suppressing tumor growth were discovered about ten years ago, we are still far from targeted therapy (Soto A. M., Sonnenschein C., 2005).

As it seems to me, the problem is that we have forgotten about the entire human body itself while looking deeper and deeper into molecules, for the whole is always more than the arithmetical sum of its constituent parts. The famous Russian physician, naturopath, and gerontologist Abraham Zalmanov (1997) explained the failure of scientists in the fight against cancer:

> The reason is very simple: the cancer cell was studied separately. They did not bother to explore the cancer patient, with all his endless reactions. And when they confine themselves to studying one cell or one tissue as an isolated part, there is always a necrology and never a biology ... Attempts to find an antidote to cancer remain fruitless, because the strategic key is the cancer cell, the cancerous tissue, and not the person affected by cancer.

As we know, it is the mind that makes a human being; perhaps in more convenient terms, it can be referred to as the psyche. Unfortunately, modern "conventional" medicine still regards the psyche as something separate from the body and diseases, rarely seeking to utilize its possibilities in treatment. Meanwhile, folk medicine around the world has recognized the importance of interaction between the mind, spirit, and body a long time ago. Both traditional Chinese medicine and Indian Ayurveda, which originated 3,000 to 6,000 years ago, usually correlate the state of organs and the occurrence of diseases with certain mental and emotional states. For example, the ancient Indian physician Bhaskare Bhatte believed that anguish, anger, sadness, and fright are "the first steps on the ladder to any illness" (Uryvaev Y. V., Babenkov G. I., 1981). These medical traditions seek to return a person to the balance of the mind, body, and spirit in order that they should heal as naturally as possible.

In ancient Greek and Roman cultures, a similar opinion was prevalent. Aristotle, in the third century BC, said that there is a relationship between mood and health: "Souls and body, I suggest, react sympathetically upon each other." Socrates wrote that it is not possible to "produce health of the body apart from the health of the soul." Plato assured his readers that the treatment of many diseases is unknown to doctors, because they ignore the whole, which must also be studied. Parts can not feel good, if the whole does not feel good. Cicero, in the first century BC, expressed the idea of the impact of grief and worries on human health, and recognized the occurrence of bodily diseases due to mental suffering.

Hippocrates, the famous ancient Greek physician who is known in history as the "father of medicine," and after him, the Roman physician of the second century AD, Galen, developed the doctrine of the four temperaments—sanguine, choleric, melancholic, and phlegmatic. They found them related to certain diseases: sanguine to circulatory disorders, choleric and phlegmatic to hepatic diseases, and melancholic to psychic disorders. Isaac the Syrian (1998), the famous theologian and mystic of the sixth century, wrote that "Passions are the ailment of the soul, something accidental, that has entered into the nature of the soul and driven the person away of their natural health."

The Australian doctor Jan Gawler, who cured himself of cancer and on the basis of his experience wrote the best-selling book *You can conquer cancer* (1997), convinces that a healthy organism cannot get cancer. He suggests we reflect on this statement and understand that it is self-evident: a healthy body cannot at the same time be sick. Cancer is treated as a local disease, as if the problem is only in the tumor, assuming that otherwise the patient is perfectly healthy. The new approach, according to Gawler, is to treat the body as a whole. If we manage to restore the normal, healthy state of the organism, then, in response to it, all malignant tumors will be eliminated, wherever they may be.

By sharing such an approach to health, progressive scientists and medical doctors in the 1990s established the foundations of integrative medicine, as a prototype of future medicine. Integrative medicine treats a person as a whole system, where the body, energy, mind, and spirituality are all seen as equal partners and not separate from one another. This integrative approach distinguishes *holistic*[1] medicine from the traditional (conventional) kind, which regards a person as a kind of biological mechanism in which it is enough to "repair" an unhealthy organ or system. Isolated treatment of a particular organ, typically using only pharmacological medicine, is often accompanied by the side effects of drugs on other organs.

The aim of integrative medicine, on the contrary, is to treat the whole person, not the disease, and to apply different methods to different people. Since the disease appears in the person, and not only in the cell or body, then during treatment it is necessary to take into account interpersonal relationships, because the emotions created by them are always associated with the ailment. As one of the pioneers of psychosomatic medicine, Victor von Weizsäcker (1947), said, "the disease is situated between people and is a consequence of their relationships and the nature of conflicts." Therefore, addressing the patient's personal, spiritual, and social harmony is vitally important for successful therapy.

An integrative approach in modern medicine was initially formed on the basis of the biopsychosocial model of ailments proposed by George Engel in 1977. According to this model, the disease not only results from organic, bodily injuries, but also reflects a violation of the functioning of the personality's psychological structures, caused by various factors—external, social, and internal

---

[1] The terms in italics are explained in the Glossary at the end of the book.

(Engel G. L., 1977). The foundations of such a trinity were laid in the works of one of the founders of psychosomatic medicine, Franz Alexander, as early as 1939. Thirty years later, another dimension was added to this model—the spiritual dimension (not limited to religiosity), including elements of transcendence, the meaning and purpose of life, love, and *transpersonal* interrelations, thereby expanding the paradigm to one that is biopsychosocial-spiritual (Barnum B. S., 1996; Sulmasy D., 2002). As a result, modern medicine is gradually approaching that understanding of the unity of the body, the psyche, and the spirit which developed in oriental medicine, especially traditional Indian and Chinese, since ancient times.

The advantage of this approach is a patient-centered, holistic attitude toward patients, that takes into account the individual characteristics of each person and, especially, his/her psychological and spiritual needs. As a result, for example, by the early 1990s, more than a third of the population of the USA had already used relaxation techniques, visualization, hypnosis, and biofeedback, and more than 50% had resorted to prayer as a complementary therapy (Eisenberg et al., 1993). Under pressure from the public and not without resistance from representatives of "conventional medicine," in 1992, the National Center for Complementary and Alternative Medicine (NCCAM) was established at the US Institute of Health. Over time, it became the world's leading research center in this industry. The amount of funding for the center started from $2 million, and in 2008 reached $120 million. In 2005, NCCAM subsidized over 1,200 research projects in 260 organizations.

The basic principles of Integrative Medicine include:
- the synthesis of modern, alternative, and traditional medicine, that brings a new qualitative level of integrity to conventional therapy;
- the necessity to treat the person, not the disease;
- owing to the body's powerful and natural ability for self-diagnosis, self-healing, regeneration, and recovery, in any disease, it is necessary first of all to maintain and activate this internal potential;
- most diseases have psychosomatic origins.

Psychosomatic pathology (from the Greek psyche—the soul and soma—the body) in its standard sense is a disorder of the functions of internal organs and systems originally associated with acute or chronic psychological trauma, and the specifics of an individual's emotional response. Without psychological assistance, temporary pathophysiological disorders develop into psychosomatic diseases. It often happens that the medical examination does not reveal the physical or organic cause of the illness. Therefore, if the unhealthy state is the result of stresses and emotions such as, for example, anger, anxiety, depression, and guilt, we are talking about the psychogenic origin of the disease, and it can be classified as psychosomatic. This is confirmed by the successful elimination of pathologies of this kind using methods that normalize the state of mind, such as psychotherapy, hypnosis, meditation, etc.

Studies by G. Rosen et al. (1982) in the United States and England show that 50% to 75% of all problems for which people go to doctors are basically emotional, social, or family-connected, despite the fact that they manifest themselves as a pain syndrome or disease. In former Soviet Union medicine, this was well understood also. At the beginning of the twentieth century, the famous doctors Vasiliy Obraztsov and Nikolay Strazhesko, speaking about angina pectoris, paid attention to the fact that painful attacks would often occur in patients who were either physically tense or experiencing some kind of negative emotional state. Later, the psychosomatic approach to the origin and treatment of cardiovascular diseases was developed by academicians of the Academy of Medical Sciences of the USSR, doctors Georgiy Lang and Alexander Myasnikov. In the same period, in 1936, the Psychosomatic Society was established in the United States, and since 1939 it has been publishing the journal *Psychosomatic Medicine*.

Dr. Oakley Rey (2004), Honorary Professor of Psychology, Psychiatry and Pharmacology at Vanderbilt University in Nashville, TN, USA, believes that according to the current biopsychosocial, or "mind-body," paradigm, there is no real separation between the mind and the body, in light of the revealed wide interaction between the brain and nervous, endocrine, and immune systems. This model surpasses the old biomedical model: the basis for this conclusion are the experimental and clinical data provided by actively developing scientific directions—*epigenetics*, psychoneuroimmunology, and psychoneuroendocrinology. More and more research is being done to confirm this, which I shall cover in the upcoming chapters.

This situation in science is also reflected in oncology, manifested in two main opinions about the origin of malignant diseases. According to the traditional biomedical model, cancer is the result of a carcinogenic effect of a person's environment, often combined with bad habits (for example, smoking) and heredity, where psychological factors are secondary consequences of the disease. According to the new biopsychosocial model, most cases of cancer can be of a psychogenic nature, and physical factors can exert their carcinogenic effect only if the organism is in a psychophysiological imbalance.

As a result, a new, modern direction of psychology was born—psycho-oncology (in the territory of the former USSR, the term onco-psychology is in more common usage), which studies the influence of psychological factors on the onset and progress of cancer. Its main task is to study the psychology of oncological patients, their different responses to the disease, development of diagnostic methods, psychotherapy and rehabilitation of patients, ways to cope with this crisis situation, activate the patients' own healing resources, and help their family members and caregivers. Psycho-oncology is based on the hypothesis that oncological disease is related to a biopsychosocial conflict in the individual, and must be considered as a combination of biological, psychological, and social problems.

It is natural that psycho-oncology should have become one of the most important components of integrative oncology—the modern part of integrative medicine, which links together the efforts of oncologists, psychologists, and specialists in alternative medicine in order to create an individual program for each particular patient in accordance with the nature and stage of their disease.

By involving experts from these areas, integrative oncology can work with a person in a much more complete way. This has an important influence on the course of the treatment process and extends the life of the patient. As we will see later, particularly effective are combined programs that unite intensive patient education with self-regulation methods, psychotherapy, diet, physical activity, and spiritual practices. Progress in this direction is promoted by the establishing of the international Society for Integrative Oncology (www.integrativeonc.org), which publishes its own journal.

The integrative and psychosocial approach has proved to be very effective: Dr. David Betty, Executive Director of the National Cancer Institute of Canada, noted at the end of the last century that the most notable results in the treatment of cancer over the past decade have been achieved in the field of psychosocial therapy (Holland J. C., Bultz B. D., 2007).

The integrative approach is also the basis of this book. Having started my psychotherapeutic practice with cancer patients and studying the literature on oncology and psychology, I could not help but pay attention to the colossal gap between the positions and knowledge of practical oncologists and psychotherapists, especially in the post-Soviet states. I share the opinion of the pioneers of psycho-oncology Carl and Stephanie Simonton (1978), who noticed that the price which has to be paid for the narrow specialization of most doctors is that it hinders the exchange of information between representatives of different disciplines, all working on curing cancer. Since each discipline develops its own language and system of analysis, important data often get lost in obscurity.

My qualification in this regard was quite wide in scope, because over the years of my professional activity I have studied many branches of knowledge about human beings. I have been interested in the riddles of the psyche, aging, and diseases since my youth, so I decided to study medicine. But after graduating from university and working for several years as a general practitioner, I realized that that kind of medical practice was not for me, since it only temporarily relieves the symptoms of diseases. I wanted to understand the true causes of health disorders. Expecting to find them at the molecular level, I entered a postgraduate course at the Institute of Gerontology of the Academy of Medical

Sciences of the USSR, where I studied the physiology and molecular biology of the stress mechanisms active in aging.

However, by the time I presented my Ph.D. dissertation, I realized that the secrets of life, illness, aging, and death did not lie only in the plane of physical existence; so as a result, I embarked on a spiritual quest. I studied hermetic alchemy, visited Sufi teachers in Turkey and Cyprus, studied the methods of folk medicine of Siberian shamans and the practices of Chinese qigong, immersed myself in Buddhism. Gradually, I came to the understanding that the basis of all human misfortunes, whether health-related or social, was spiritual and psychological in nature. Our problems are caused by what Buddhism calls the ignorance of our true nature, or, to put it simply, by a non-harmonious state of mind. Therefore, I expanded my profession to psychotherapy and eventually came to specialization in transpersonal psychotherapy and psychosomatic medicine. When life began sending me cancer patients, I treated them using the newest scientific biopsychosocial-spiritual approach to pathology. Actually it was not something new to me—I had arrived at these ideas even before I learned about them.

As I was exploring the discipline, I was shocked by the glaring illiteracy of clinical oncologists in the field of psycho-oncology and the lack of this service in Ukraine. So, the idea was born of a book that would consider the total development of cancer—from its predisposition, through the emergence and progression of the disease, to its outcome—simultaneously on four levels: biological, psychological, social, and spiritual. As far as I know, this is the first attempt of its kind in this branch of knowledge.

Although this task is quite complex, I wanted this book to be accessible to the understanding of both medical doctors and psychologists, a kind of "bridge" between the biological and psychological visions of this disease—which, in essence, is the psychosomatic approach to medicine. So I have written it as simply as possible, trying to avoid many special professional terms. I also considered it appropriate to supplement the academic scientific data with practical observations not only from medical doctors and psychologists, but also from well-known healers working with cancer patients, whose experience does not become any less valuable simply because of their lack of a specialized education. In all other aspects, this is a full-fledged research monograph, where all the statements are confirmed by references to the corresponding authors, presented in the list of references. Many topics are illustrated by examples from my own practice. The book also has a terminological dictionary, in the hope that an educated and curious reader will be able to understand the material, as its ultimate goal is to explain to the patient, directly or through professionals who read it, that cancer is a psychosomatic disease, and its source is an erroneous mind set.

A lot of good books explain the psychological sources of illnesses. However, people tend to have their doubts: is this the author's fantasies? Is he mistaken? Does this concern me? I hope that the large amount of scientific data presented here on each of the topics will convince the reader that our psyches are both capable of both giving rise to an oncological disease and curing it. By exploring these data, the reader can ascertain that this book is not only the theoretical reasoning of the author, but an analysis of the factual material accumulated by science, so the reader can check for him/herself the validity of my conclusions. In addition, I complement my reflections by citations from many other authors who share my approach.

Most people have formed the opinion that cancer attacks a person from the "outside," and it is impossible to fight it. Therefore, the origin of the disease is often associated with negative external forces, curses, fate, punishments of God, etc. Ignorant of the true causes of cancer, falling under the spell of statistics and medical prognosis, often not finding psychological and spiritual support from physicians, the patient can be demoralized by fear, helplessness, and hopelessness, which suppress the healing capabilities of the body. My hope is that this book will help the patient understand the origins of the disease, revive his hope, enhance his ability to control what is happening, and so actively fight for his health. This is exactly the case when knowledge really is power.

The information presented in the book is able to answers the paramount questions of cancer patients:
  - "Why me" and "Why this disease?"
  - How do the adversities of childhood lay the foundation of this disease?
  - What features of our character weaken the defenses of the body?
  - How does the suppression of negative emotions lead to the accumulation of "mental poisons" that create imbalance in body and mind?
  - How can distress lead to a precancerous condition within the body?
  - Is cancer an unconscious desire for death?
  - Do depression, hopelessness, and loss of meaning in life promote the disease?
  - Why does the lack of psychological help increase the likelihood of both the occurrence and relapse of the disease?
  - How can we help ourself get the most positive effect from a conventional treatment?
  - How can we reduce the side effects of medical therapy?
  - How can we prevent the relapse of a tumor?
  - How can we fully recover from the disease?
  - How can we rekindle our desire to live?

This book gives a kind of "road map" of oncological diseases to both physicians and psychologists. It will assist them to analyze not only what factors led to the disease's occurring in this particular patient, but also how these factors can be affected, how to prevent their reappearance in the future, how to resurrect a patient's will to live and increase the resources needed for their healing.

The central ideas of this book are as follows:

- Oncological pathology is a psycho-social-spiritual-somatic disease. Its source is the lack of love in our life, untreated (often from childhood) mental traumas, and unmet, suppressed needs. The most important of these needs are to express our feelings, to be a unique personality and to live as our soul wants.

- The above factors lead to a dissatisfaction with our lives, deep intrapersonal conflicts, psycho-spiritual crisis, and chronic physiological stress in the body. The results is an unconscious desire for death and the emergence of the oncodominant—the psychophysiological root of tumors (explained in Chapter 16).

- Carcinogens in the environment only become able to provoke an ailment when chronic stress reaches the level of oncogenic distress. When that occurs, it destroys the immunity and other systems of anti-cancer protection of the body.

- Cancer treatment should not be limited to removing or affecting the tumor. The tumor is only a local symptom of systemic imbalance of the organism, based on the oncogenic distress.

- Disease is not a life sentence. The path to health lies through the resolution of the crisis, the cure of chronic psychic traumas and conflicts, and finding ways to satisfy a patient's deep needs. Discovering the new meaning in our lives and opening up those areas where we are closed down awaken the colossal healing reserves of the organism and lead to a stable remission or even a complete healing.

Albert Einstein said that if we want to change something small in life, we need to change our attitude, but if we need big changes, we have to change our thinking. I will continue this thought: if we want to be healed, that is, to change our health—we first have to change our life!

Part I

Stress, Psychosomatics, and Psycho-Oncology

Chapter 1

The History of Psycho-Oncology

Modern medicine will become really scientific
only when physicians and their patients have learned to manage
the forces of the body and the mind
that operate in the healing power of nature.
René Dubos,
well-known microbiologist and writer

1.1. Domestic Observations

The folk healers of the Kievan Rus (predecessor of Ukraine, ninth to twelfth centuries) already noted that the unifying element among the causes of the appearance of a tumor, or "thickening," is that "painful privations occupied a significant place in the life of the patient" (Bogoyavlenskiy N. A., 1955). Russian doctors of the late seventeenth century were clearly aware of the connection between mental overstrain and bodily ailments: "If you want to be healthy, stop worrying all the time and do not carry grief like a burden." They linked cancer to the state of mind and emphasized that the tumor "is full of melancholic poison." Doctors of the mid-eighteenth century believed that "the deep seated cause of cancer is a long period of grief" (Prussak A. V., 1956).

In the nineteenth century, the outstanding therapist and honorary member of the Imperial St. Petersburg Academy of Sciences, Professor Grigory Zakharin, stated: "The two main signs of cancer are age and grief, and after inception, their progress is rapid ... One can diagnose without even seeing the patient, just by listening to the story. What the connection is between grief and cancer, I do not know—nobody knows, but it undoubtedly exists. The percentage of cancer based in grief is as great as the percentage of amyelotrophy based in syphilis" (Rudnitsky I., 1930). Famous Russian clinicians Fyodor Inozemtsev (1845) and Nikolay Pirogov (1854), in the middle of the nineteenth century, noted the importance of mental factors in the occurrence of breast tumors.

In 1904, doctors M. N. Diterikhs and N. A. Velyaminov described so-called hysterical breast tumors, recorded in medical literature since 1678, which arise in women with a hysterical character under the effect of emotional distress. The authors noted that these tumors can manifest "in an infinite number of forms" and therefore can easily be mistaken for organic disease. However, they can progress into malignant neoplasms. (In our time, they are defined as dyshormonal focal diseases of the mammary gland (mastopathy) and are considered as psychosomatic. These tumors occur in neurotic women experiencing psychological distress with a prevalence of negative emotions, often based on personality and behavioral disorders—Vorobiev V. V., 2008).

Professor Sergey Fedorov (1928) discussed in his clinical lectures the onset of cancer after a nervous shock, and, in the same period, the connection of negative mental experiences with the development of uterine cancer was observed in Prof. Winter's clinic (Rudnitskiy I., 1930). Professor Georgy Bykhovskiy, the founder of a network of cancer clinics in Ukraine, reported in 1928 on cases when cancer patients explained the appearance of their illness as result of distressing life experiences. He also drew attention to his observations that at the end of the first World War and during the civil war in Russia, which was followed by devastation, the number of cancer patients increased, and the disease "became younger" (in that the average patient age decreased). It is interesting that, during this time, the psychiatrist A. M. Rosenstein noted that "nervousness became mass-dispersed" in what had become a "nervous era", and suggested classifying neurotic disorders as social diseases (Aleksandrovsky Yu., 2008).

Under the guidance of Professor G. Bykhovskiy, Dr. Fyodor Milrud (1930) in the Kiev Clinical Institute in 1927–9 interviewed 133 patients who had either cancer or other general illnesses, and found a strong connection with traumatic life experiences preceding the onset of the disease. These experiences were detected in 30.8% of cancer patients compared with 14% of others. Based on the study, the author recommended that all physicians should conduct a similar survey of newly admitted cancer patients.

Considering the numerous facts accumulated by that time about the connection of "mental tension" and the tumor process, the first All-Ukrainian congress of surgeons, held in 1926, recommended the following actions to combat cancer: "Along with surgical and radiological treatment, the congress considers it necessary to pay special attention to the prevention of cancer, in particular, prevention of fatigue and straining one's nervous system" (Trudy, 1927). Dr. Igor Rudnitskiy in the article "Mental experiences and cancer," published in 1930, states: "It has already been firmly established that grief and affliction take the first place in the etiology of cancer." Later on, Soviet clinicians A. N. Gorevaya and colleagues (1974) reported painful mental experiences or strong nervous tension occurring in many patients prior to the onset of breast cancer.

As for experimental studies, few know today that it was in the laboratory of the famous Soviet physiologist Ivan Pavlov that the study of the psychic factors in the development of malignant tumors took place for the first time in science. As is known, Pavlov (1966) developed the theory of experimental *neuroses* on the dog model for the application of the data obtained in the treatment of human beings, for which he won the Nobel Prize in Medicine and Physiology in 1904. In his experiments, a "collision" of conditioned reflexes, e.g. food and defensive reflexes, was applied. This led to a breakdown in higher nervous activity and to the appearance in the animals experimented on of a state analogous to human neuroses. This itself can be considered a model of internal psychological conflict.

In the 1940s, Maria Petrova, the closest student and colleague of Ivan Pavlov, in the course of further research on dogs modeled a state of chronic neurosis. This was achieved by the application of repeated electric shock or other traumatic stimuli purposefully to overload the nervous system. As the neurosis became chronic, various pathological processes developed in the animals. Petrova believed that its cause was the functional weakening and depletion of the cerebral cortex, which is the condition that today we call chronic stress today.

One of the results of these experiments was that "spontaneous" tumors would emerge, which prompted researchers to explore this phenomenon by itself. Based on the data obtained from neurotic dogs, the scientist concluded that there is undoubtedly a leading role for the central nervous system (mainly the brain) in the origin of malignant and benign neoplasms. Petrova (1946) states: "According to the many years of our experience, the phenomena associated with a decrease in the tone of the whole organism, the root cause of which is psychic trauma, seem to be most significant as a predisposition toward all sorts of diseases, up to and including cancer." In subsequent experiments, where mice that were subjected to prolonged (four–six months) neurotic stress by electricity, their sensitivity to a carcinogenic substance was increased, thus accelerating the development of neoplasms (Melikhova E. F., 1956).

These studies largely determined the direction of Soviet experimental oncology of that period, whereby the role of the nervous system and stress in the development of malignant neoplasms was confirmed in various research institutes and universities (Yurmin E. A., 1954; Vodakova E. I., Serdyukova O. A., 1955; Ukolova M. A., 1963; Kozhevnikova E. P., 1953; Arkhipov G. N., 1971), including in the Institute of Physiology of the Academy of Sciences of the Ukraine (Samunjan E. N., 1954), where the laboratory of compensatory and protective functions of the body was headed by academician Rostislav Kavetskiy, the future founder of Ukrainian oncology.

In 1955, he wrote: "... Outstanding domestic clinicians and pathologists have long pointed out the link between the development of malignant neoplasms and mental trauma," but "... the role of the central nervous system in the pathogenesis of neoplastic disease is still poorly understood." (Kavetskiy R. E., 1955). This later became one of the leading directions in the Ukrainian Research Institute of Experimental and Clinical Oncology of the Ministry of Health of the Ukrainian SSR, established in 1960 and headed by Kavetskiy.

The laboratories of the Institute have received convincing data that chronic stress, especially when combined with a hopeless conflictual situation, can become a pathogenetic basis for oncological and cardiovascular diseases. The damaging effect of excessive stress on the *endothelium* (inner layer) of the blood vessels has been established, which can cause a significant stimulation of the process of metastasis. It was also found that in the case of tumor development under conditions of excessive stress, the protective mechanisms of the brain are not able to limit the stress response, so the stress becomes anomalous, causing even more damage to the body. Hence, the task was to develop new medicines to counter the destructive effects of stress, in order to achieve a significant reduction of its pathological effects at the level of target organs, and to inhibit the process of metastasis (Balitskiy K. P., Shmalko Y. P., 1987).

Following on the progress in the study of oncogenic stress, in 1984 the Institute held the fifth Symposium of the European Working Group on Psychosomatic Cancer Research (EUPSYCA). Unfortunately, at that point, the development of this direction in Ukrainian science was interrupted. With the change of the scientific generation, the priority of the new heads of the institute has become, in line with the times, the development of pharmaceutical methods of cancer treatment. Psychosomatic approaches to the subject were forgotten, and presently there is not even a mention of them on the Institute's website. Perhaps because this direction cannot match the level of income generated by antitumor drug production? Also to be noted is that experiments have shown that radiation therapy and surgical operations cause a progressive deterioration in the activity of the sympathoadrenal and hypothalamic-pituitary-adrenal systems, reduce antitumor immunity, activate metastasis, and contribute to postoperative complications (Balitskiy K., Shmalko Y. P., 1987). In view of the close cooperation of the Institute of Experimental Oncology with the Clinical Institute of Oncology, which is now separated from the former, it is not surprising that this direction was not further supported.

Meanwhile, experimental studies of the role of stress in oncogenesis are actively developing in the West, while in the post-Soviet region, such research is currently almost not being conducted.

1.2. Observations Made in Other Countries

In ancient medicine, cancer was considered a disease of melancholy ("black bile"), and its occurrence was associated with negative emotions. The Roman doctor Galen (first century AD) came to the conclusion that frequently depressed women overflow with melancholy and develop cancer more often than cheerful women (Kühn K. G., 1821–1833). The same observation was made by the Greek philosopher and physician of the second century AD, Alexander Aphrodisiensis (1841): "The so-called melancholic juice causes rheumatic disease and tumor growth." It is interesting that the ancient Greek word onkos, root of the word 'oncology', means not only mass, bulk, a physical burden or load, but also metaphorical weight, trouble, and an unwieldy tragic mask, which denoted the psychic load weighing down its wearer (Mukherjee S., 2010), and this link is not a superficial connection. Michael Psellos (1841), a Byzantine philosopher and scholar of the eleventh century AD wrote, "A terrible melancholic fluid causes indurations that, if not dissolved, give birth to many monsters—gangrene, cancer, and numerous tumors."

Traditional Chinese medicine holds that cancer affects the entire body, and that the cause of the disease is the dysfunction of internal organs provoked by emotional stress. The resulting imbalance of the internal environment allows various pathogenic factors to block energy meridians, and the tumor develops owing to a stagnation of vital energy and blood. According to the ancient Indian text *Yoga-Vasishtha*, cancer is a consequence of an imbalance in the body caused by a person's inability to control his/her mind (Amritanshuram R. et al., 2013).

Despite the fact that oncological diseases have been known about since time immemorial, the frequency of their occurrence is directly related to the development of our civilization and the accompanying stresses.

The well-known writer and medical missionary Dr. Albert Schweitzer (1957), a Nobel laureate, wrote that when he arrived in the Gabon in 1913, he was amazed at not being able to find a single case of cancer. In the following years, oncological diseases began to appear more and more often, and he concluded that it was due to the fact that local people were living more and more in the manner of the whites.

The famous anthropologist and explorer of the Arctic Vilhjalmur Stefansson noted in his book *Cancer: Disease of Civilization?* (1960), that there was no cancer in the Eskimo people soon after his arrival in the Arctic and that the subsequent increase in its incidence was associated with closer contact with white civilization. In his study, Stefansson also refers to the observations of Dr. L. A. White, who practiced in Alaska for about seventeen years. His work led him to the following conclusions: (1) there are practically no hypertensive and atherosclerotic diseases among indigenous peoples; (2) diabetes is extremely rare; (3) malignant diseases were also extremely rare (he saw only one proven case). Dr. White had not observed any strokes and no coronary heart disease.

A similar observation was published in 1912 by Dr. Samuel King Hutton. In the course of extensive and thorough studies of the Labrador Eskimos' health, he noticed that they have none of the diseases that occur in Europe—primarily cancer. During the same period Dr. Eugene Payne, who examined about 60,000

Indians of Brazil and Ecuador for twenty-five years, also found no occurrence of cancer (Berglas A., 1957).

At first glance, these observations confirm that the incidence of cancer grows in parallel with the increase in environmental pollution, the accumulation of industrial carcinogens, the effects of smoking, etc. However, a lot of evidence suggests that there is another existing reason, more important than external cancer-inducing elements.

In the history of Western medicine since the eighteenth century, there has been an increasing understanding of the relationship between cancer and the emotional state of the patient. Many of these observations were made in the UK.

Doctor M. Deshaies-Gendron (1701), considering the nature and causes of cancer, noted its relationship with life tragedies, grief, and major troubles, and their resulting severe anxiety and depression. In 1783, J. Burrows wrote that cancer is caused by the unpleasant experiences of the soul, anxious flashes of consciousness that have troubled the patient for many years.

Dr. Nunn, in 1822, wrote the book *Cancer of the Breast*, which gives examples of the influence of emotional factors on the appearance of cancer. In particular, one of his female patients, after having undergone a nervous shock due to the death of her husband, soon discovered a growing tumor, from which she eventually died. Dr. Walter Walshe, in *The Nature and Treatment of Cancer*, published in 1846, reported that emotions cause such a degree of disruption in innervation that they distort the process of feeding tissues, and this in turn leads to the formation of cancer. Dr. Walshe personally observed cases in which this connection was evident, but he doubted its reality and believed he was mistaken in what he saw, regardless of the evidence.

Surgeon Willard Parker (1885) concluded, that grief is especially associated with this disease [cancer]. G. Snow, in the book *Cancer and the Cancer Process* (1893), came to the conclusion that of all the possible causes that result in various forms of cancer, the most powerful are the neurotic. The most frequent among them, he claims, are negative emotional experiences, followed by extreme poverty and exhausting labor. These causes have a serious impact on the development of other factors contributing to this disease. Dr. Snow also found that cancer of the uterus and breasts might appear after an "antecedent emotion of depressive character."

In France, the connection between the state of a person's psyche and cancer was also observed. Surgeon Claude Chapuys in 1607 described the appearance of cancer after "sadness, boredom, anger and wrath." Jean-Baptiste Doyen (1816) published the *Dissertation on cancer, considered as a disease of the nervous system*, where examples of patients who had developed the disease after long periods of sorrow were presented. Dr. J. Amussat (1854) found that "the effect of grief is ... the most common cause of cancer."

Dr. Samuel Koval in 1955 conducted an analysis of research on the psychology of cancer that was performed in the eighteenth and nineteenth centuries. Published in the prestigious journal of the American Psychoanalytic Association, *Psychoanalytic Review*, and entitled "Emotions as the Cause of Cancer," this work singled out the following most common psychological aspects of cancer patients:

- Loss of a significant person (parent, child, spouse, etc.) as a result of death or separation,

- A state of *frustration* because of the failure of important life events or goals,

- A tendency to feel despair, helplessness, and grief when experiencing stress, frustration, and / or loss.

An outstanding oncologist of the early twentieth century, Eli Jones published a book in 1911 titled *Cancer—Its Causes, Symptoms and Treatment*. He wrote:

> Worrying weakens the nervous system, lowers the 'nerve power' and thus opens the way for the invasion of cancer. In all countries where you find insanity on the increase you will find cancer a close second. In Chicago, where insanity has increased the fastest in the world, cancer has increased 812% from 1861 to the present time.

In 1926, Elaida Evans, a student of Carl Jung, one of the leading figures in modern psychology, published the fundamental work, *A Psychological Study of Cancer*. Her conclusion was that cancer, like most diseases, is a symbol of something not being right in the patient's life, a warning that he should choose a different path.

1.3. The Paradox of Oncology

If the connection between cancer and psycho-traumatic events was already "firmly established" by the beginning of the twentieth century, then it would seem that the rapid development of medical science, like the entire intellectual progress of the century, should lead to further discoveries in the field of cancer psychology and the development of new methods to address underlying psychological problems and traumas. However, medicine and psychology moved in different directions, and the technical perfection of medicine ended up poorly serving the patients: by removing the consequences of cancer (tumor), physicians ignored the cause (psyche).

In this regard, the well-known psycho-oncologists Carl Simonton and Stephanie Simonton (with James Creighton, 1978) wrote about a completely unjustified situation in medicine. Though the development of psychiatry and psychology finally led to the emergence of diagnostic methods that allowed scientists to investigate the relationship of cancer to mental states, and therapeutic methods were developed that could help resolve emotional difficulties, it was at this point that the medical establishment lost all interest in this problem.

How can we explain this? On the one hand, the rapture of technical progress in the twentieth century pushed the importance of understanding the human soul into the background. The organism seemed to be a machine that simply required the repair of broken parts. On the other hand, the physicians of past centuries, not having had the sophisticated diagnostic equipment we have today, would listen to and examine their patients for much longer, and this allowed them to understand their life situation, emotional state, and how it related with the disease. Today, the teaching of psychology in medical universities is allocated an unacceptably short time. Most practitioners learn nothing about the latest research results in the fields of psychosomatics and psychoneuroimmunology.

Moreover, in this era of "global commerce," the pharmaceutical and medical industry is not really interested in developing a psychotherapeutic approach, because this cannot be patented, put on a conveyor belt and, like pills, sold in millions of copies. Hospitals, pharmacies, medical staff, pharmaceutical companies, manufacturers, and sellers of medical equipment are much more interested in the process of diagnosis and treatment, as opposed to a rapid cure. No one has the incentive to reduce the cost or length of treatment. The industry is benefit-oriented, so more and more new drugs are continually being prescribed.

Over the past fifty years, advertising has firmly embedded in our minds the notion that medicines are the only way to escape from disease; that illnesses only derives from outside sources, and that our inner world has nothing to do with them. This position has become the public's world view—i.e., a generally accepted outlook, shared not only by patients, but also by doctors. Bruce Lipton, author of the bestseller *Biology of Belief* (2005), writes: "Pharmaceutical corporations have turned us into the real drug addicts with all the consequences that follow." At the same time, in the US alone, approximately 6.5% of all hospital admissions are the result of a misuse of drugs (Pirmohamed M. et al., 2004), and about 225,000 people die each year from this misuse (Madeira S. et al., 2007).

In fact, a sick person goes to the physician not for health, but in order to get rid of the pain and trouble caused by the illness. "The doctor's attempts to change the patient's outlook, and persuade him to make any efforts for his own recovery, inevitably encounter resistance," complains Russian psycho-oncologist Alexander Danilin (2011)—"For the doctor, in turn, it is much easier just to prescribe medicine, paying no attention to the patient's attitude toward life, as this requires a much lower expenditure of mental strength and incommensurably less time to examine the patient. Moreover, 'time is money'. The process of prescribing pills is much more cost-efficient. The wishes of the doctor and the patient coincide. Everything remains the same."

As a result of this approach, usually, only symptoms are treated—external manifestations of the disease, while its causes remain in the *subconscious* and continue their pathogenic action. According to Dr. A. F. Buzunov (2010), a researcher of psychosomatics, in many cases the effect of such primitive symptomatic therapy is reduced only to the temporary elimination of external manifestations of the illness. In his words, all medical art is often limited to the conscious formation of drug dependence, to the joy and income of pharmaceutical manufacturers.

The world-famous healer Jose Silva also says that our human ability to make ourselves sick is exploited as much as possible. Hospitals and pharmaceutical industry are thriving business, since the costs of treatment are huge both for individuals and states. However another our human ability—to make ourselves healthy—is an almost untouched field of activity that is only starting to be recognized (Stone R. B., Silva J., 1992).

Fortunately, slow as it may be, the truth is making itself known, and the reason for this is the accumulation of new data on the psychosocial nature of most diseases, including cancer.

1.4. Clinical Development of Psycho-Oncology

The first psycho-oncology service was created in 1950 at the Sloan-Kettering Memorial Center for Cancer Research in New York City, and later developed into the Department of Integrative Medicine. In 1967, the Psychological Service was organized at the Hospice of St. Christopher in London, and in 1983 the British Society for Psychosocial Oncology was established (www.bpos.org). In the same period, similar societies and associations arose in Italy (www.siponazionale.it), Canada (www.capo.ca), France (www.sfpo.fr) and the USA (www.apos-society.org), followed by the International Psycho-Oncology Society (www.ipos-society.org). Thanks to the efforts of the latter, societies of psycho-oncology were organized in many countries of all continents, carrying out research and educational work in this field. A *Journal of Psychosocial Oncology*, *Journal of Psycho-Oncology* and *Journal of Psychosocial Oncology Research & Practice* were established.

In accordance with the "mind-body" paradigm, the ideas of the practical impact of the psyche on the tumor have been introduced. In 1959, Dr. Eugene Pendergrass, president of the American Cancer Society, said at its gathering:

> There is solid evidence that the course of disease in general is affected by emotional distress ... Thus, we as doctors may begin to emphasize treatment of the patient as a whole as well as the disease from which the patient is suffering. We may learn how to influence general body systems and through them modify the neoplasm which resides within the body (Pendergrass E. P., 1961).

This was practically realized in the late 1970s by American oncologist Carl Simonton and his wife, psychologist Stephanie Matthews-Simonton. They used guided imagery techniques to assist terminal cancer patients whose life expectancy was about a year. The result at that time was incredible: out of 159 patients, 19% completely got rid of the disease, 22% had a slowed illness development, and the rest of the patients lived on average twice as long as expected. The Simontons' book *Getting Well Again* (with James Creighton, 1978) has become an international bestseller, and their methods are still actively used today in psycho-oncology.

Skeptical of the Simontons' data, Professor of Psychiatry at Stanford University David Spiegel organized a one-year program in the form of weekly sessions for women with advanced breast cancer. Apart from the standard medical therapy, the program included group psychotherapy, hypnosis, and relaxation exercises. Women from the control group received only conventional medical therapy. To his astonishment, Dr. Spiegel found that women who passed through the program lived an average of eighteen months longer (Spiegel D. et al., 1989).

Since that time, similar programs have become the object of serious experimental attention from scientists who have demonstrated their effectiveness in treating cancer and increasing the life expectancy of patients. For example, in the department of breast oncology of the Essen-Mitte Clinic in Germany, which is the academic study base of the University of Duisburg-Essen, more than 1,500 patients took part in a special therapy program, based on the development of mindfulness. During the eleven-week program, at six hours per session, specially trained instructors instructed patients in the principles of meditation, integrative nutrition, exercises (walking, yoga, qigong); helped them develop self-help strategies (massage, hydrotherapy); and provided group support (Dobos G. J. et al., 2012).

In one of the largest centers of integrative oncology in the USA, the MD Anderson Center, in addition to conventional oncology, the following areas are also considered important: acupuncture, holistic medicine, information technology, massage, psychotherapy, body-oriented therapy, music therapy, dietology, and spiritual help on a multi-confessional basis.

Gradually, the understanding of the causes of cancer among the general population is changing. For example, a survey of almost three thousand cancer patients in Australia revealed that stress comes as the key factor of disease in people's understanding, followed by heredity factors, with smoking coming only in third place (Willcox S. J. et al., 2011). In another study, it was found that 60% of healthy people believe that the psyche is associated with the appearance of tumors and 71% that it is associated with their progression, while among the cancer patients, 85% associated the development of cancer with the state of mind (Lemon J. et al., 2004). In the study of Russian researchers, 50% to 71% of oncological patients, regardless of the location of their tumors, identified psychological factors as the main factor in the development of their disease (Bukhtoyarov O., Arkhangelskiy A., 2008).

Therefore it is not surprising that cancer patients are increasingly using complementary and alternative medicine. Between 30% and 70% of cancer patients use one or more treatments that fall under the definition of alternative medicine, and specifically up to 75% of women with breast cancer use these methods (Astin J. A., 2006).

According to statistics provided by the American Cancer Recovery Foundation, conventional medical therapy (surgery, radiation, and chemotherapy) constitutes only about 15% of the total volume of activities undertaken by surviving patients, who share an integrative approach. Oncologists and health authorities in the USA (Committee of the Institute of Medicine) and in Europe (Central European Cooperation Group) have officially recommended treating the psychological distress of cancer patients (Adler N. E., Page A. E., 2008; Beslija S. E. et al., 2003). The American Society of Clinical Oncology, in conjunction with the National Comprehensive Cancer Network (www.nccn.org), has developed a directive on the diagnosis of distress, which states that all patients should be examined for distress on their first visit to the clinic, [later] at appropriate intervals, and according to clinical indications.

This attitude to stress has not only medical, but also economic importance, as psychological help significantly reduces the cost of treating patients. For example, the California community of physicians, Kaiser Permanente, determined that psychotherapeutic assistance reduces the average length of stay in hospital by 77.9%, reduces the hospitalization rate by 66.7%, the frequency of visiting doctors in the outpatient clinics by 47.1%, and the frequency of emergency calls by 45.3% (Sobel D. S., 2000).

1.5. The Spiritual Dimension of Integrative Medicine and Oncology

Issues around spirituality become very real for a sick person as well as for members of their families. Suffering, pain, loss of loved ones, disability, loss of social status, the threat of losing one's life—all this raises deep questions about the meaning of life, illness, and death. If such stressors are ignored by the patient or by their family, it can cause additional mental suffering and even worsen the course of the disease. Sadly, the majority of medical institutions have become so bureaucratized, overregulated, commercialized, and limited in terms of the time that can be assigned to patients, that health care has been turned into a conveyor belt where the average doctor has no opportunity or appropriate skills to pay attention to the spiritual and psychological state of the patients.

Spirituality, generally understood to be a person's search for his or her sense, place, and purpose in the world, is an integral part of our life and largely determines its quality. Spirituality is not equivalent to religiosity; a spiritually oriented person does not need to be in the framework of any confession in order to learn and improve him- or herself and the world. Spirituality is defined as an unlimited set of personal motivations, norms of behavior, experience, values, and attitudes based on the search for *existential* understanding, meaning, purpose, and transcendence. But, religiosity is defined as a set of norms of behavior, values, and attitudes that are based on a previously recorded religious doctrine and an institutionalized organization (DeCicco T., 2007).

According to V. D. Troshin (2011),

> Man's spiritual activity is an evolutionarily and genetically conditioned process, the goal of which is to achieve the optimal mode of vital activity of the organism in the constantly changing conditions of the external environment. Spiritual activity is considered as a synthesis of the spiritual and psychic activity of man in general, where the brain, psyche, and spirit are integrative systems interacting with society, nature, and the universe.

The World Health Organization recognized the need to consider spiritual health as an important element of health in general. In 1997, at the WHO Assembly, it was noted that it was erroneous not to include the fourth (*spiritual— V. M.)* measurement of health in its definition. The WHO Executive Board's special group proposed the following changes to the preamble of the WHO Constitution: "Health is a dynamic state of complete physical, mental, spiritual, and social well-being and not merely the absence of disease or infirmity" (WHO, 1997). At the 58th UN General Assembly on Health in 2005, it was stated that the scientific link between religion, spirituality, and health was too often a "forgotten" subject, avoided because of irrational, emotional, or "political" considerations. They suggested that it was time for the scientific community to integrate the religious and spiritual factors that guided human behavior throughout the centuries into health and the humanities (Stuckelberger A., 2005).

Conventional, illness-oriented "biomedicine" seems to overlook the fact that the patient is a human being, where the body is just one of the components, and that everyone depends entirely on spiritual and social relationships with the surrounding world. Therefore, in the origin and development of the disease, psycho-spiritual and social components are as important as biological ones, which currently dominate our general understanding of the etiology and pathogenesis of the disease. As E. N. Apanel (2012) notes, in traditional medical publications the concept of "spirituality" is given a very modest place, apparently considered chiefly as something of "high and remote abstract matter, detached from everyday real life," whereas in essence spirituality is the basic and inalienable component of human health. The well-known Austrian psychiatrist, psychologist, and creator of logotherapy Viktor Frankl (1984), wrote that "Man lives in three dimensions: the somatic, the mental, and the spiritual. The spiritual dimension cannot be ignored, for it is what makes us human."

The aspect of spirituality is therefore of great importance in oncology, where a serious threat of death can often lead the patients to a deep spiritual crisis, loss of meaning of life and of self-identity (Jim H. S. et al., 2006; Edwards A. et al., 2010). On the other hand, being supported by physicians or psychologists allows the patient to find in his sufferings the meaning that will allow him to perk up, gain a new vision of his situation, and so find the strength to fight the disease. A spiritual orientation therefore becomes an important factor in helping the patient cope with the stress of the disease, and activates their own healing resources (we will discuss this more fully in Chapter 33.2).

This holistic approach based on the biopsychosocial-spiritual model of medicine and returns to the historically formed understanding of unity of the body, psyche, and soul. It sets new tasks for health care—to help the patient not only physically, but also psychologically, socially, and spiritually (Barnum B. S., 1996; Sulmasy D., 2002), where all four dimensions are equally important in understanding the origin of the disease and for the restoration of a person's health and well-being.

Applying a biopsychosocial-spiritual approach can contribute to the significant success of therapy (Ben-Arye E. et al., 2006). According to Dr. A. A. Misyak (2002) of Kiev's Institute of Experimental Pathology, Oncology and Radiobiology, the spiritual level is the main one to be addressed in the rehabilitation of cancer patients, as it enables all the other levels. Without attending to it, it is impossible to effectively restore the patient's social significance. Belarusian psycho-oncologist K. V. Yatskevich (2007) believes that a spiritual approach to oncology is the most important practical way to help and support a patient in expressing, forming, and strengthening their intention to change themselves and get rid of the disease.

It is gratifying that the urgency and necessity of such changes in medicine is now advocated by an increasing number of scientists and physicians (Hutchison E. D., 2008; Sinha A., Kumar S., 2014; Hatala A. R., 2013; Lake J. et al., 2012; Dyer A., 2011; Puchalski C. M., 2013; Polischuk Yu. L., 2010; Zalevskiy G. V. et al., 2009; Troshin V. D., 2011). A search for the keywords "spirituality and health" in the largest medical research database PubMed, produces over 6,400 topical scientific articles for October 2018, while in the database of Google Scholar—more than 700,000 sources in English and more than 20,000 in Russian.

The Canadian Association of Psychosocial Oncology in 2010 developed standards for psychosocial assistance to the population. It states that "psychosocial health services are psychological, social, and spiritual care services and interventions that enable patients, their families, and health care providers to   optimize   biomedical   health   care   and   to   manage   the psychological/behavioural, social and spiritual aspects of illness and its consequences so as to promote better health" (www.capo.ca). This is a modern, broader approach to patient-centered oncological care (Motenko J. S., 2012) that often leads to *post-traumatic growth*, which positively transforms one's personality, health, and life.

From the biopsychosocial-spiritual point of view, a patient's initial spiritual level can be an important etiological factor in cancer development. For example, in their *synergetic* biopsychosocial-spiritual approach to oncological diseases, P. I. Sidorov and E. P. Sovershaeva (2015) observe the disturbances of the animogenesis process in cancer patients—their ontogenetic (*ontogenesis*) spiritual and moral development. In a similar model, S. A. Kulakov (2009a) draws attention to the *existential vacuum* or frustration in the spiritual sphere of cancer patients.

Noting its special importance, I will exclusively devote Chapter 18 to this issue.

Chapter 2

Is Cancer a Psychosomatic Disease?

It is not possible to produce health of the body
apart from the health of the soul.
Socrates

Supporting the clinical observations of the past, an impressive amount of scientific data has currently been accumulated indicating that psychological problems are closely related to the onset of oncological illness. This gives grounds for an increasing number of authors to believe that cancer is basically a psychosomatic disease (Grinker R. R., 1966; Brémond A. et al., 1986; Meneghetti A., 1977; Kulakov S. A., 2009; Vasyutin A., 2011; Hamer R. G., 2000; Malkina-Pykh I., 2013; Sidorov P. I., Sovershaeva E. P., 2015). However, the cited works lack a comprehensive analysis of the issue not only in psychology, but also in epigenetics, stressology, spirituality, philosophy, psychoneuroimmunology, and psychoneuroendocrinology. Only by such an interdisciplinary, integrative approach can we understand whether cancer really develops according to the laws common to all psychosomatic illnesses.

2.1. The General Psychological Mechanisms of Somatic Diseases

Let us begin our analysis of the problem with a definition of psychosomatic pathology. This health problem arises from the process of *somatization*—the tendency of a person to experience psychological stress at the physiological level, in other words, the "embodiment" of negative emotions. This leads first to the appearance of uncomfortable sensations, and then, with their long existence, to various structural disturbances and dysfunctions of internal organs. Therefore, psychosomatics is considered as a bodily reflection of a person's psychic life, where the body acts as a kind of screen where symbolic messages of the subconscious are projected (Barsky A. J., Klerman J. L., 1983; Kholmogorova A. B., Garanyan N. G., 2000; Sandomirsky M. E., 2005).

Somatization can be acute, when it is caused by acute stress (for example, the loss of a loved one), or chronic (i.e. persistent and/or current), reflecting prolonged psychological problems. It can last a lifetime (Lipowski Z. J., 1986), turning into a psychosomatic disease. Such a disease testifies to a violation of a person's integrity, reflected in the lack of harmony between the mental, social, spiritual, and physical levels of their being, and therefore it can be called "aholistic" (Starostin O. A., 2013).

In this context, Alexander Mitscherlich (1954) formulated the concept of two-phase *psychological defense*. If the intrapsychic conflict that underlies the traumatic experience is not resolved, then the first phase of defense is developed—the mental one. Here, owing to the action of various forms of psychological defense, neurotic symptoms associated with emotional and behavioral disorders begin to arise. If these methods of defense prove ineffective, the second phase begins—the bodily phase, during which somatic disorders start developing.

This point of view is shared by one of the creators of psychosomatic medicine, Austrian psychoanalyst Felix Deutsch (1933), who noted that "neurosis on a small scale is played out in every organic disease." The prominent Soviet physiologist and student of Ivan Pavlov, Konstantin Bykov, wrote that neuroses are the beginning of any disease, whatever its cause (cited in Svyadosch A. M., 1971).

From another point of view, the process of somatization is regarded as an imperfect, primitive mechanism of psychological defense. When overwhelmingly intense psychotraumatic experiences are not allowed to emerge into consciousness in order to protect one's mental balance, they are repressed into the *subconscious*. But as they still need to be discharged or released, they are therefore "channeled"—or manifested—at a bodily level.

In developing this approach, psychoanalyst Clemens de Boor (1965) contraposed psychopathic and psychoneurotic behaviors that emerge on account of unresolved conflict to a psychosomatic disorder. When psychopathic or psychoneurotic responses to frustration are suppressed in one's behavior and do not find a discharge, then they are replaced by bodily reactions, which, owing to their intensity and duration, we call diseases. People around the patient respond to somatic illness with care and sympathy, whereas the psychopathic forms of behavior are perceived with indignation or emotional irritation, notes de Boor.

Thus, in some people the so-called mental way of processing an intrapersonal conflict or a psychotraumatic situation will predominate. Then the consequences of both acute and chronic stress will come out as *neurotic* symptoms, ranging from psychological to psychopathological manifestations (this process is called psychogenesis). Others have a predominantly somatic way of processing psychological problems. It is more associated with the chronic impact of frustration and involves psychosomatic disorders, so this process called somatogenesis (Topolyanskiy V. D., Strukovskaya M. V., 1986, Janca A. et al., 1995). On the whole, such individuals do not permit themselves to experience a neurotic reaction, avoid showing their anxiety or fear to other people, and therefore turn away from their feelings (Rotenberg V. S., Arshavskiy V. V., 1984).

Mental or somatic modes of stress processing are generally associated with different types of personality and differ in the regulation of autonomic functions (digestion, circulation, respiration, and metabolism) that ensure the effectiveness of adaptive reactions. As a consequence, such people's state of health and energy reserve are different (Soldatova O. G. et al., 2007). The other reasons leading to an unconscious choice by the personality of the psychic or somatic mode of conflict processing will be analyzed in more detail in Chapters 8 and 12.

The formation of a psychosomatic disorder begins with a single psychosomatic reaction. The symptoms disappear when the stressful situation that caused these reactions changes. If the situation persists, then a functional psychosomatic syndrome arises—the so-called organ's neurosis (without structural changes), characterized by recurring somatic symptoms. Finally, a psychosomatic disease (psychosomatosis) develops with morphological (structural) changes in the organs (Baykova I. A., 1999).

The most important factor that determines how this process unfolds is the duration of the existence of a psychotraumatic factor (conflict) that causes chronic emotional stress. This gradually depletes a person's adaptive capacity, disrupts the barrier of psychic adaptation (see Chapter 12.2), and renders the disorder of the internal organs chronic (Aleksandrovskiy Y. A., 1976). In other words, the deeper the chronic psychophysiological stress, the more intensively the somatization process shifts toward morphological changes.

New horizons in psychosomatic medicine are being opened by achievements of *epigenetics* (from the Greek επί —upon). This relatively young science studies the *expression* (change in activity) of genes, when the structure of DNA, unlike *mutations*, remains unchanged, and where these changes can be reversible and inheritable. Epigenetics shifts the emphasis from the conservative structure of the *genome* to the mechanisms of its response to signals from the external environment. It shows that gene expression depends on such external factors as the quality and quantity of food and water, air pollution, physical activity, and psycho-emotional reactions. They act as regulators, or "switchers," of the genes' activity, forcing them to produce certain substances (mainly proteins) that are necessary for the adaptation and survival of the organism. In other words, epigenetics acts as a mechanism for the evolution of living systems. Alterations in the epigenetic regulation of genes are associated with a variety of human diseases, in particular cardiovascular, pulmonary, neurodegenerative, and cancer (Santos-Reboucas C. B., Pimentel M. M., 2007). We will discuss these phenomena in more detail below. The well-known English biologist, the Nobel laureate Peter Medawar (1983), has commented on these discoveries: "Genetics proposes; epigenetics disposes."

In recent years, there have been rapid developments in a new direction: behavioral epigenetics. It explores how social interactions, particularly those causing stress, through specific biological pathways lead to functional modifications of the genome. It helps us to understand how traumatic events in early periods of our lives impact on the psyche and human behavior, and bring about a predisposition or vulnerability to various illnesses, including psychosomatic ones, that comes to the surface later under the influence of life's psychotraumatic problems (Rozanov V. A., 2012).

Of relevance here is the work of the Italian Professor Antonio Meneghetti, who developed a new direction in psychology—ontopsychology. Describing the mechanisms of psychosomatics, he largely anticipated discoveries in the field of epigenetics and psychoneuroimmunology. His clinical experience allowed him to claim that a mental action is able to alter the biology of the body on the molecular level. The psyche, affecting the "building" genes, is able to materialize the [mental] impulse and formalize it into appropriate structures, coordinated from within the immune system (Meneghetti A., 1977).

When psychosomatics first began, it included only seven diseases: bronchial asthma, hypertension, rheumatoid arthritis, peptic and duodenal ulcers, ulcerative colitis, thyrotoxicosis, and neurodermatitis (the so-called "Holy Seven"). Later on, myocardial infarction, angina pectoris, osteochondrosis, eczema, psoriasis, zoster, diabetes, mastopathy, and others were added to this list.

Walter Bräutigam with his co-authors (1997), who represented psychosomatic medicine in Germany, suggested that psychosomatics shows a clear tendency to include groups of diseases that have traditionally been seen as being internal, infectious, neurological, and mental illnesses. From the point of view of the biopsychosocial-spiritual paradigm of medicine, this is quite natural; since the influence of psychological factors can be found in development of any disease, the psychosomatic approach can be applied to all of them (Novikova I. A., Soloviev A. G., 2001, Selhub E. M., 2002). This was first noted by Novalis (Friedrich von Hartenberg) back in the nineteenth century (Bräutigam W. et al., 1997).

The great American psychologist Abraham Maslow (1993) believed that placing in a common space all of the diseases that the psychiatrists and physicians are dealing with, as well as all of the violations that provide food for thought to existentialists, philosophers, religious thinkers, and social reformers, gives us enormous theoretical advantages.

This position is increasingly supported by scientists who recommend avoiding the division of diseases into categories of psychosomatic and somatic.

In other words, there is a greater need to study the influence of psychosocial-spiritual factors on the occurrence and course of any somatic diseases, as well as taking into account these factors in the diagnosis, prevention, treatment, and rehabilitation of patients. "A harmony of personality development is only possible if the spiritual, neuro-psychic and physical are all unified, and this reflected in harmony of health," says Professor V. D. Troshin (2009), head of the Department of Neurology, Neurosurgery and Medical Genetics of the Nizhny Novgorod State Medical Academy (Russia).—"Psychosomatics is like the head and heart of health care. Psychosomatics now affirms the interconnection between spiritual, psychological, and medical factors in any illnesses, and proclaims a spiritual and biological view on both diagnosis and treatment. The psychosomatic approach to human pathology and its prevention is mandatory in the practice of any medical doctor."

In my opinion, only in this way can we talk about the medicine of the future. As we will see later, the achievements of modern epigenetics, psychoneuroimmunology, and psychoneuroendocrinology actually obviate the sense of the division of human pathology into the bodily and the psychic. E. V. Sadalskaya and co-authors (2001) argue that "... perhaps a radical revolution in medicine will be associated with the transition from the concept of psychosomatic diseases as a special group of diseases to a common psychosomatic approach to all diseases in the clinic of internal diseases." From these positions, cancer is no exception. According to Antonio Meneghetti (1977), cancer should also be seen from the perspective of psychosomatics; and since the cause of its occurrence lies exclusively in the psyche, all other views of the study of this disease, assert ontopsychologists, are simply useless.

2.2. Biopsychosocial–Spiritual Characteristics of Psychosomatic Patients

According to the biopsychosocial-spiritual model, there are four components that make up psychosomatic pathology:

1. Biological, determined by heredity, type of temperament, constitution, and previous diseases that have weakened the body.

2. Psychological, formed by personal characteristics (including the prevailing types of psychological defense), psycho-traumatic experiences, conflict experiences, and ways of coping with stress.

3. Social, determined by the degree of dysfunction of the family unit, cultural and religious conditioning, and the effectiveness of interaction with the micro- and macrosocial environments (the actual family, co-workers, society).

4. Spiritual, determined by the presence or absence of an *existential vacuum* (to be explained in Chapter 11.2), moral and ethical values, awareness of the

meaning and purpose of one's life, the strength of death anxiety, religious beliefs, and the capacity for self-realization and transcendental experiences.

Considering the ontogenesis of psychosomatic patients in this perspective, we start off by observing that in childhood they had often experienced problems and dysfunctions in the family unit. In particular, there were many stressful events: diseases, alcoholism, violence and/or early deaths of parents or close relatives, fights and violence, together with a high level of criticism directed at children (Kholmogorova A. B. et al., 2011; Kholmogorova A. B., Garanyan N. G., 2008). As a result, these patients never completely get over the situations of loneliness experienced in early childhood and triggered by similar situations in later life. At an early age, they already had to suppress feelings that were regarded negatively by authority figures, so they did not learn how to use their emotions fully in their struggle to adapt to difficult situations (Bastiaans J., 1982; Pilipenko G. N. et al., 2009). Owing to having had their fundamental needs infringed upon in childhood, especially with regard to their human dignity, the psychological wound is present in all psychosomatic personalities in some degree (Rusina N. A., 2011).

Subsequently, such people often demonstrate fixed forms of behavior—obsession, an adherence to stereotypes, stubbornness, and pedantry, all of which speak of a rejection of the requirements of the external world. They are highly likely to develop *neuroticism* (traits of emotional instability, anxiety, and low self-esteem), *alexithymia* (the inability to comprehend and express one's own emotions and understand the feelings of others), and introversion (a tendency to retreat into one's own inner world). Such people also avoid showing their anxiety or fear to others and suppress their feelings. All this is fraught with development of reactive anxiety or reactive depression, leading to excessively strong emotional responses to stressful situations (Kosenkov N. I., 1997; Rotenberg V. S., Arshavskiy V. V., 1984).

For example, in a comprehensive study by the Russian-German team of the Moscow Research Institute of Psychiatry and the Department of Psychosomatic Medicine and Psychotherapy of the University of Freiburg, it has been shown that psychosomatic patients have not only a high level of alexithymia but also an internal ban on expressing their feelings, especially those of fear. They also have a narrow emotional vocabulary range, are fixed on negative experiences while aspiring to appear successful. In addition, they lack support from those around them, because they do not trust other people and therefore cannot establish deep and ongoing relationships with them (Kholmogorova A. et al., 2011).

The fact that psychosomatic patients are ashamed to show their emotions, especially if they are aggressive, is noted by most researchers in the field of psychosomatics. This aspect, as we shall see later, is especially important in terms of their being predisposed toward oncological diseases. Such individuals are often very emotionally controlling, hiding in this way their own needs, frustrations, anger, and hostile feelings toward themselves, as well as being unaware of their helplessness and dependence. Many have a strong sense of responsibility and duty, a hypertrophied commitment to moral and ethical ideas. They express ambitions, display straightforwardness, and reject compromises. There is a narrowing of their range of interests, a distortion in their value system, limited goals and needs, which are reflected in the inadequacy of the claims regarding their life purpose. These people also find it difficult to adapt to new life situations, are vulnerable and oversensitive, and often feel anxiety in situations of real or imagined threat or failure. Facing a challenge or threat, they behave in a passive-defensive way (Malatesta C. Z. et al., 1987; Crawford J. S., 1981; Siegman A. W. et al., 1998; Starshenbaum G. V., 2015; Rusina N. A., 2011).

They also show a pragmatic and concrete type of thinking, a limited ability to fantasize, dependence on a significant other (Bräutigam W. et al., 1997), concern about other people's expectations and evaluations of them, together with little confidence in their own ability to achieve results. Therefore, when making important decisions, they tend to rely on other people's judgments. They usually have a low opinion of themselves and of life in general, along with an inability to be independent and resist social pressure (Shevelenkova T. D., Fesenko P. P., 2005).

Often, these people have neurotic and infantile personality structure, showing passivity, suppressed aggression, and exaggerated claims (Karvasarskiy B. D., 2002; Byilkina N. D., 1997). Their psychological infantilism, based on maladaptive "childish" thinking, can lead to situations whereby they believe other people's points of view are their own, and as a result are vulnerable to external influences owing to incorporated beliefs and parental attitudes (introjection). Hence, many psychosomatic patients do not have their own point of view, but express hypertrophied conformism and dependence on others, a desire to shift responsibility onto other people, while their self-identity is disrupted. They have a tendency to consider their point of view as erroneous and, accordingly, punish themselves, to the point of expressed self-aggression (Sandomirskiy M. E., 2005; Mendelevich V. D, Solovieva S. L., 2002).

The majority of psychosomatic patients live in dysfunctional families, where significant marital dissatisfaction is double that of harmonious families (Kulakov S. A., 2003). The behavioral tendency of such personalities to avoid conflict as much as possible, to live by all means in accordance with generally accepted norms, causes a huge intrapsychic tension. This leads to the dysfunction of organs and systems, especially if this tension cannot be diverted or expressed through verbalization, facial expressions, gestures, and psychomotor strategies. The result of such a repressed expression of feelings and blocked communication is somatization (Bastiaans J., 1982).

There is also a lack of spirituality (understood according to the definition given in Chapter 1.4) in psychosomatic patients—a low level and abstract nature of the meaningfulness of life, i.e. they have little sense of meaning and what they do is indeterminate (Shevelenkova T. D., Fesenko P. P., 2005). They usually unable to manifest full creativity and self-giving, have a mental-energetic basic defect, which leads to a decrease in psychic energy, needed to establish emotional ties (Bastiaans J., 1982; Shtrakhova A. V., Kulikova E. V., 2012). The constant orientation toward "significant others" blocks their own development (Kulakov S., 2009), provokes a kind of "spiritual defeat," breaks the unity of the mental and physical, and violates their harmonious, integral psychosomatic functioning (Starostin O. A., 2013). The absence of an external symbolic support of spirituality—constructive life goals and the existential meaning of life—serves to prevent the psychological adaptation of the personality in psychosomatic disease (Sandomirsky M. E., 2005).

In the opinion of I. V. Semenov (2005), psychosomatic pathology is spiritual in origin, and at its heart is a moral error or a deliberate choice to feel imprisoned as opposed to feeling free. This allows the author to argue that it is our individual human consciousness that is both the source of the spiritual-psychosomatic pathology and as the way to eliminate it. Since spirituality is the regulator of neuro-psychic and somatic human activities (Troshin V. D., 2009), then in addition to biological, psychological, and social factors, it plays an important and often pivotal role in the occurrence and progression of psychosomatic disorders (Starostin O. A., 2013). This is confirmed by the growing number of studies that we will be considering.

Another important source of psychosomatic disorders is stressful, emotionally significant events—not only acutely stressful events, such as the death of a close relative, divorce, job loss, etc., but also intra- and interpersonal conflicts and negative events that take up a significant length of time. This kind of pathogenic effect on future psychosomatic patients is produced by these events and conflicts for several reasons. First, these patients are usually fully identified with a significant object. When this object is another person, then they seem to exist with his/her help, and so the loss of this person destroys the potential patient's world. Secondly, they are not able to adequately process the bereavement. Therefore, it remains unresolved, does not lose its subjective significance, and leads to chronic stress and depression, thus causing somatization (Topolyansky V. D., Strukovsky M. V., 1986; Smulevich A. B., 1997; Mendelevich V. D., Solovieva S. I., 2002; Kulakov S. A., 2003, Rusina N. A., 2011).

I have included only the basic, most common characteristics of psychosomatic patients. Each pathology has its own specific features (Bräutigam W. et al., 1997; Malkina-Pykh I., 2013). However, even from this brief review what is obvious is that stress is an independent risk factor for the development of all diseases that are psychosomatic in nature (Kamenetskiy D. A., 2001). To paraphrase Mark Sandomirsky (2005), psychosomatic disorders can be rightfully called "diseases of unreacted stress." Since psychological imbalance and stressful events occur throughout life for both "classic" psychosomatics and cancer patients, we need to understand the ways in which stress exerts its devastating impact, whether or not it actually has an oncogenic effect, and to what extent biopsychosocial-spiritual characteristics of psychosomatic patients correspond to those of patients with cancer. This will give us the possibility of finally understanding whether the cancer is indeed a psychosomatic illness.

2.3. The Biomedical Model of Origin and Development of Oncological Diseases

To explore the relationship between the psychological and biological aspects of cancer, it is necessary to understand the basic biological mechanisms of the oncological process.

In modern oncology, cancer is understood not only as a malignant neoplasm (tumor) in a particular organ or tissue, but as a complex disease of the whole organism involving many of its systems. The tumor is considered as a specific tissue, where a constant interaction between tumor cells and their *microenvironment* is occurring. The tumor can secrete signal molecules that affect both specific local targets and the organism as a whole, therefore contributing to the further progress of the disease (Fidler, I. J., 1995; Szlosarek P. et al., 2006).

In the emergence and development of cancer, conventional biomedical science identifies the following phases:

1. A predisposition to cancer. First of all, it is hereditary genetic defects which cause various oncogenic syndromes; then, advanced age, constitutional features (in particular, early puberty in women or obesity), endocrine and eating disorders, and bad habits such as smoking and alcohol abuse.

2. A precancerous state. This is manifested by the emergence of diseases, mainly chronic, characterized by a prolonged course of inflammatory and dystrophic (*dystrophy*) processes. This includes benign neoplasms, which have a tendency to malignant transformation.

3. Malignization: the initial period of malignant transformation of cells in normal tissues and benign tumors.

4. The manifested clinical picture of illness. This is determined by the type of cancer process, its localization, the diagnosed stage, the presence of metastases, and complications.

5. Relapse: the recurrence of the disease after a certain period of clinical well-being after the therapy. From the perspective of conventional medicine, this depends on the stage of the tumor at the time of the beginning of the treatment; its localization, the form of its growth and histological structure; the nature and extent of the therapy; and the age of the patient.

6. The outcome of the disease: remission (temporary weakening or disappearance of the symptoms of the disease), recovery, or death due to complications caused by tumor growth.

Regarding the etiology (cause of origin) of cancer, conventional medicine still focuses on "material" carcinogenic factors—physical (traumatic, thermal, and radiation damage), chemical, and biological (viruses)—provoking pre-cancer diseases. Great importance is also attributed to immunodeficient states and diseases of DNA repair (restoration). Only recently has the attention of medical science (and so far only a limited attention of practical medicine) been attracted by psychosocial factors, which, as I discuss in this book, should take a much more prominent role.

With regard to the pathogenesis of cancer, or the sequence of processes and mechanisms of malignancy of the cell, there are three main stages:

1. Initiation (the more correct, but less common term is initialization). This occurs when the cell is first affected by the carcinogen and potentially dangerous changes start to appear in the functions of special cellular genes, called proto-oncogenes. These are regular genes, usually responsible for the synthesis of proteins that regulate cell growth, reproduction, and differentiation (the obtaining by a cell of a specified function during maturation). A proto-oncogene can become an oncogene owing to mutations or epigenetic modifications, thus gaining excessive activity and triggering the formation of a tumor. At the initiation stage, unauthorized deactivation of suppressor genes, whose actions are opposite to those of proto-oncogenes, also occurs. In addition, the suppression or the blocking of genes causing apoptosis ("suicide") of damaged or mutated cells and the activation of genes that inhibit apoptosis is observed. This stage alone does not lead to the development of the disease.

2. Promotion or the beginning of the process of tumor cell transformation. This occurs with repeated exposure to the cell of the same carcinogenic factor that triggered the initiation, or another one. The activation of oncogenes and the initiation of the mechanism of cell transformation can also be caused by other factors—promoters—that were not originally carcinogens. As the example can be considered the *transcription factor*: a complex of the stress hormone cortisol with its *receptor*, which regulates the activity of many genes. An important feature of malignant transformation is the ability of tumor cells to not differentiate. Their maturation is suspended, and as a result they remain "eternally young." Continually multiplying, the cells accumulate and create a tumor.

3. Tumor progression. Transformed cells increase their rate of division and multiplication. They develop their own substances that suppress the ability of the immune system to destroy them. Also, these altered cells activate special angiogenic factors (from the Greek ἀγγεῖον—vessel, and γένεσις—origin, occurrence) causing the formation of blood vessels to enhance the nutrition of the tumor. Gradually, the tumor cells germinate into the blood and lymphatic

vessels, from where they spread throughout the body and create the secondary focus of tumor growth: metastases.

Fortunately, our body is not unarmed against the impact of carcinogenic agents. Throughout the course of evolution, we have developed various defensive mechanisms that protect us against dangerous factors within our internal and external environments. These mechanisms create so-called anticancer (antiblastoma) resistance, or antitumor defenses. These include the body's ability to counteract the penetration of carcinogenic agents into the cell, repair genome damages, suppress the activity of oncogenes, detect and destroy tumor cells, and inhibit their reproduction—in other words, "restrain" the development of cancer.

According to the theory of containment, the atypical cells with the potential of malignant reproduction appear from time to time in the body of every person. The cause of this can be both external carcinogenic factors, and internal errors in the reproduction of cells, that is, mutations, leading to the activation of oncogenes. Scientists have calculated that in normal mammalian cells, more than 100,000 DNA lesions occur daily (Barnes D. E., Lindahl T., 2004). As a rule, they are effectively corrected by intracellular reparation systems, but a number of cells still become mutated. However, this is not yet a death sentence for the cell. It is believed that out of every ten mutant cells, only one undergoes a malignant transformation (Kozlov V. A., 1982). Therefore, exposure of the body to carcinogens, and even the appearance of the first tumor cells, does not always lead to the development of a tumor.

Even the emergence of an initial tumor is not always followed by cancerous disease. There are research data (discussed in detail in Chapter 10) demonstrating that throughout life, as a reaction to distress, all of us periodically develop different tumors in the initial stage. When the body as a whole is in a state of harmonious health, these initial stage tumors recede by themselves, or stop in their development without even being noticed. This phenomenon (spontaneous regression) is directly related to the psychosocial-spiritual state of a person and, in all likelihood, is based on epigenetic regulatory mechanisms. But, if the protective anticancer system weakens, then, as confirmed by clinical observations, tumors will occur ten times more often than with normal protection.

2.4. The Concept of The Biopsychosocial– Spiritual Origin of Cancer

The synergetic biopsychosocial-spiritual concept of oncological diseases is, in my opinion, the most grounded one. It is being developed in parallel by an academician of the Russian Academy of Sciences, Prof. Piotr Sidorov and his colleague E. P. Sovershaeva (2015), from the Northern State Medical University in Arkhangelsk, as well as Sergey Kulakov (2009), professor of the Department of Clinical Psychology of the State Pedagogic University in St. Petersburg. This doctrine corresponds to the assumptions discussed in the previous chapters.

In accordance with this concept, the formation of oncological disease is considered in two vectors, allowing us to analyze simultaneously both temporal and qualitative characteristics of the system or organism. The first vector is dynamic (temporal) and includes fractals (development intervals, or phases) of the disease from its predisposition to the outcome. The second vector is ontogenetic; it embraces the four levels of human existence: the body, the psychic, the social, and the spiritual. Accordingly, each phase of the disease is determined by a unique combination of processes occurring at the intersection of these vectors.

Accepting this concept as a basis, I have embedded into it certain modifications. They reflect the analysis of existing scientific data on the onset and development of cancer from the standpoint of psychology, stressology, oncology, physiology and molecular biology, and spirituality and philosophy, taking into account my own practical experience. Some stages are changed, while most phases and levels are filled with additional or new content, which I will formulate and argue in this book.

In the following chapters, the process of occurrence and course of oncological diseases will be analyzed at the following conditional stages: predisposition, provocation, precancerous state, initialization, promotion and progression, outcome and consequences of the disease. The results of my research will be summarized in the final conclusion in the form of a "road map," reflecting the hypothesis of a six-step biopsychosocial-spiritual mechanism of cancer development.

This will also allow me to support and expand the integrative synergetic concept of the origins of cancer, and coordinate it with the official biological theory of carcinogenesis. The main focus in my research emphasizes the imbalance of the mind and spirit, which creates a state of chronic emotional stress and psycho-spiritual crisis. Therefore, we need to start out by considering the research data, which demonstrate that it is chronic stress, caused by psycho-emotional imbalances, that leads to a critical weakening of the body's anticancer protective system.

Chapter 3

Stress: Acute, Chronic, and Oncogenic

My life has been full of terrible misfortunes,
most of which never happened.
Mark Twain

3.1. The Psychophysiology of Acute Stress and Distress

To understand how our emotional reactions lead first to acute and then to chronic stress, and how these psychological processes are associated with cancer, we need to take a short excursion into psychophysiology. This science explores emotional and mental processes in the form of physiological reactions within the organism.

We can conditionally describe the following contour in man:

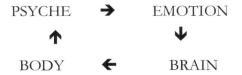

The psyches of all living beings are systems for processing internal and external information and creating on this basis a subjective internal image of the world, with the aim of orienting themselves in it, managing their states and behaviors, as well as meeting their needs. The highest form of the psyche is the human mind, which includes consciousness (based on self-awareness, or the ability to perceive ourselves), and the subconscious (the mental processes that take place without manifesting in consciousness and are usually inaccessible to conscious control).

The work of the psyche is largely determined by the social attitudes, programs, and beliefs that are "loaded" into it from early childhood and/or are developed in the process of our life experiences. Our emotions are the tool by which we receive feedback on how successfully our beliefs and image of the world are helping us achieve goals. In the words of Russian academician Piotr Simonov (1987), a well-known psychophysiologist, biophysicist, and psychologist, "Emotions are the reflection by a human's (and animals') brain of an actual need (its quality and magnitude) and the probability (possibility) of its satisfaction, which the brain evaluates on the basis of genetic and previously acquired experience." The body perceives emotions in the form of chemicals, which are released by the nervous, endocrine, and immune systems, and which then induce it to act. Lastly, the psyche evaluates these actions as being effective or ineffective—the circle is a closed one. If the evaluation has a high significance for us, we will feel strong negative or positive emotions, to the degree that we experience the state of mental overstrain known as stress.

Stress is an unspecified (general) reaction of the body to any demand presented to it, be it physical or psychological, that perturbs the consistency of its homeostatic state. The law of maintaining the consistency of the internal environment of the body is therefore a fundamental principle of preserving the health and survival of living beings. A stressor is any suddenness, any new life situation that serves to break this consistency or potentially threaten it, and disturbs the habitual course of life. Hans Selye, the creator of the "stress concept," showed that the physiological response to stressors is a universal model of protective reaction, the same for humans and animals, aimed at preserving the integrity of the body. Stress is an integral part of our life, and just like life itself it cannot be avoided. Selye (1975) said that "stress creates the aroma and taste of life." However, if the stressful impact exceeds the adaptive capabilities of the body, then a stage of uncompensated stress occurs (distress), leading to the malfunction of organs and systems, which progress to disease.

Usually, stress is classified in terms of its duration—short-term (acute), long-term (chronic), and by origin—physiological and psychological.

Physiological stress can result from strong physical activity, respiratory failure, excessively high or low body temperature, an active inflammatory process, significant blood-pressure disorders, allergic reactions, various pain symptoms, etc.

Psychological stress can be informational and emotional; one tends not to exist without the other. Informational stress mainly occurs due to an overload of information, when a person cannot cope with a task or problem, comprehend something, or find an adequate solution. Such a state occurs periodically in many students, operators, and dispatchers. Today, emotional stress is the most common type of stress we find. It is usually generated by negative emotions in the face of threats, danger, fear, resentment, etc., in response to information coming from the outside world. In its extreme forms, it becomes the cause of psycho-traumatic experiences. Its main sources include hardship, loss, and conflict, which can be both external or internal.

However, positive emotions can cause the same nonspecific stressful physiological reaction as negative emotions, producing a mobilizing and stimulating effect. In this case the situation is called "eustress." In other words, an organism initially responds to enormous joy and great grief with the same physiological changes. According to Selye (1975), everything pleasant and unpleasant which accelerates the rhythms of life can lead to stress. A painful blow or a passionate kiss can both be the cause. Eustress therefore is a factor in evolution; it helps us to evolve—by improving our concentration, raising the desire to achieve goals, creating a positive emotional color for the work process, and assisting the body to act more intensively, as well as to develop skills to adapt to new circumstances, thus increasing our psychological and biological endurance.

Any living being reacts to a stressful situation in one of three ways (or their combinations): fight, flight, or freeze (immobilizing, when the first two options are impossible). We can see a lot of "freezing" in today's society, when in response to psychological stress a person finds they cannot react and express their emotions.

Under the influence of stressful stimuli, the body develops complex changes referred to by Hans Selye as a "general adaptation syndrome." In other words, this is a set of nonspecific adaptive reactions that arise in response to the stressor and are directed at overcoming its adverse health effects.

How we react to stress depends on the following main factors:

1. Intensity, duration, and frequency of the stressor;

2. Adaptive potential of the organism; that is, its adaptive capabilities, which in turn are determined by:

- heredity, which sets the type of constitution and physiological response of the organism to stimuli,

- early experience in life, mainly in childhood, affecting our ability to cope with adversity,

- personality traits: emotional, intellectual, and behavioral, which define the type of psychological defense we will manifest, together with the kind of strategy we will be inclined to use in order to survive.

How does emotion, a creation of the mind, affect the physiology of the body? Any strong emotion arising from any impact on us: psychological shock, trauma, pain, illness, etc., is accompanied by a chain reaction, beginning in the cerebral cortex and ending in our genes and molecules. "When the breath of stress sweeps along the body, the internal environment rebuilds (adapts) its composition—

physical, chemical, and biological properties—providing the body with the most favorable conditions in the fight against danger," wrote Professor G. N. Kassil (1983), director of the Laboratory of Neurohumoral Regulations Institute of Physiology of the Academy of Sciences of the USSR.

What happens in our body at the time of acute stress? Let us take a typical situation, associated with a certain health threat: a slight traffic accident, resulting in damage to the bumper of our car. At the moment of the collision, we have an intense experience of danger, and often a surge of fear. According to Hans Selye's classification, this is the stage of anxiety. There is an operative mobilization of the protective resources of the organism with parallel suppression of functions that, under the action of this stressor, have less significance for the survival of the organism—for example, digestion, regeneration, growth, lactation, reproductive functions. Thus the body responds to the stressing factor, and if an organism's reserves are sufficient, then, as a result of the activation of the functions of different systems, the adaptation quickly develops.

The physiological and biochemical details of what happens next in the body are needed here in order to clearly understand in the following chapters how this mechanism is disturbed by oncogenic stress.

Our mind classifies the situation as a danger and sends signals to the brain—in particular, to the *limbic* system. This is a brain region united anatomically and functionally—the hypothalamus, hippocampus, *amygdala*, reticular formation, and some others—that are involved in the management of emotional and instinctive behavior; that is why this area is also called the "emotional brain." It activates the sympathetic branch of the peripheral nervous system, injecting into the main organs and systems an operative stock of "emergency" hormones: catecholamines (epinephrine and norepinephrine). As a result, the heart rate increases and intensifies, the vessels of the heart and skeletal muscles expand, the strength of the skeletal muscles increases, the bronchi dilate, the abdominal arteries narrow, and our metabolism speeds up. In this way our organism starts the mechanism of the timely reaction to danger that has been factored into us by evolution.

If the collision did not happen, and everything was limited by an emergent deceleration, the stress response would have ended at the first stage, and changes in the body described would quickly return to normal. However, the accident is estimated by our mind as a much more serious stress factor, especially in the case of a conflictual situation.

Our sympathetic nervous system is now unable to fully cope with the increased requirements of the brain and body, and therefore the second stage of stress reaction unfolds. The hypothalamus activates the hypophysis (the central regulator of our endocrine system), which then generates ACTH (adrenocorticotropic hormone), which affects the adrenal glands, resulting in the release of additional doses of epinephrine and norepinephrine from its medulla and glucocorticoid hormones (cortisol and corticosterone) from the cortex. Also, other hormones are produced, but so far they are not that important for us. The catecholamine content can increase more than tenfold within a few seconds, leading to significant changes in the state of the body.

Epinephrine boosts our blood pressure. The heart beats even more strongly, the excitation of our nervous system increases, sweating starts, and the serum level of cholesterol, glucose, and triglycerides (energy resources) increases. The influx of epinephrine stops digestion, as the blood drains from the stomach and intestines and flows to the muscles. The pituitary gland affects the thyroid and other endocrine glands, the intestine is activated, breathing is quickened to provide more oxygen—the body is preparing to fight the danger or flee from it.

This normal bodily response to life's circumstances is the very same "general adaptation syndrome," since it contributes to our daily survival. All these biochemical changes in the body provide an optimal solution to dangerous situations and do not harm the person. However, after stress the body needs to recover. Therefore, after the completion of the situation, we generally feel fatigue-exhausted—the body wants to relax and recuperate its nervous and endocrine systems. The parasympathetic branch of the nervous system, which controls energy and resources, activates, as well as the GABAergic[1] and antioxidant systems. Endogenous opiates and *prostaglandins* are released. All this reduces the mobilizing effect of stress. After a while we calm down.

However, what will happen if we are to blame for the accident, if the damage to other car is serious, and if we did not renew our insurance? Our mind rushes to build a picture of the challenges ahead. This image of the future and the expectation of troubles ahead—a creation of the mind—again leads to the activation of the mechanisms behind the stress reaction. Although it is usually not as expressed as strongly as before, all its physiological mechanisms work in a similar way: heart palpitations, sweating, and the release of hormones.

This image of the anticipated danger can be called an illusory stressor, because it is based solely on our anxiety about an imagined future. But why do we feel imaginary stressors in the same way as we do a genuinely occurring event? Why does the mother, waiting for her teenage son to come home late, experience the physiological manifestations of stress just by imagining that he's gotten into trouble? Why does this teenager, going home by night bus after watching an erotic film with a friend and recalling the bright scenes, feels the physiological phenomenon of an erection? Why is the girl, who will be going to visit the dentist tomorrow, covered in a cold sweat simply from remembering the image of a drill? Waking up at night because of a nightmare, where we are chased by a wild

---

[1] γ(gamma)-aminobutyric acid (GABA) is the main inhibitory *neurotransmitter* in the adult brain. Working in tandem with the glutamate (excitatory neurotransmitter), GABA provides the inhibitory-excitatory balance required for proper brain function.

beast or bandit, why do we find our body in the same state of excitement as if this was really happening, even though we only saw the images in a dream, that is a product of our mind?

The reason is that our brain is not able to distinguish a real situation from an imaginary one. It reacts in the same way to images coming from the mind as to images coming from our eyes and other senses. As early as the 1930s, Edmund Jacobsen conducted research into muscle physiology at Harvard University and the University of Chicago. He discovered similarities in recording electrical signals from the muscles of people doing physical exercise and signals from the same muscles in people who only imagined they were doing it (Jacobsen E., 1962). Recent neuroscience studies have shown that when we are imagining motion and making real movements, the corresponding neurons in the brain are excited at the same intensity (Rizzolatti G., Craighero L., 2004).

Thus, we experience stress not only at the moment when it happens—in the example above, at an accident—but every time we remember it or imagine its consequences for the future. This "virtual" stress and the resulting actual strain on the body can significantly suppress the body's natural defenses. There is a specific physiological mechanism for it: our emotional memory depends largely on the function of the amygdala of the limbic system, while the long-term memory is implemented by the hippocampus. As was discovered at the University of Minnesota, after the impact of any stressful event on the brain, every reminder of it will continue to activate the synthesis of stress hormones and cause the amygdala and hippocampus to spread the reaction to the whole organism. In this way, the initial imprint of stress will gain in strength (Bloom F. E., Lazerson A., 2000).

These data is very important in understanding how our negative thoughts and the emotions caused by them—especially fear and anxiety—strengthen and prolong those daily stresses that we actually experience.

Since the lives of many people are almost daily filled with various problems and negative emotions, this creates a chronic overload for the adaptive mechanisms in our bodies, as well as producing a cumulative effect of systemic disturbances. In general, our body has a long-term capability to resist stress, which depends on heredity and the adversities of childhood (this will be discussed in the next part). According to Hans Selye's classification, this is the second stage of the stress reaction: the stage of resistance (sustainability). It is characterized by the restructuring of the body's defense systems and its adaptation to the action of stressors.

If a negative experience is very intense and prolonged, for example, during disaster or the death of a loved one, then ordinary stress can achieve damaging properties and turn into destructive stress, or distress. It becomes very severe and produces a deeply negative impact on a person's psyche, body, and behavior. Its key characteristic, according to Hans Selye, is to do us harm.

When the degree or intensity of current stress that is in the stage of resistance decreases, the hormonal changes in the body and the metabolic shifts accompanying them gradually normalize without pathological consequences. If stress persists, it creates a cumulative effect, whereby the adaptive capabilities of the body becomes ineffective and stress hormones cause pathological reactions instead of the normal physiological ones. The result is that stress often progresses to a chronic stage, causing an inability to resist and to adapt, and eventually, after a time, forms the third and final stage of the general adaptation syndrome: that of exhaustion. It is characterized by an oppression of all the person's protective processes and low resistance to any stressor. At this stage, pathological changes appear and various diseases develop, which are often irreversible and can lead to death.

Chronic stress is the most favorable condition for the development of precancerous changes, so we will consider this in more detail.

3.2. Chronic Stress, Emotions, and Health

> There is nothing more permanent
> than the unexpected ...
> *Paul Valery,*
> *French poet and philosopher*

When our life is in a state of chronic emotional imbalance, the content of stress hormones is increased almost all the time, because even several hours after a stressful event the levels of epinephrine and cortisol remain high. These hormones are very slowly deactivated, as most of us do not engage in physical activity which might burn them up. Therefore, the body remains tense and the result is disturbed and inadequate sleep that does not give us enough rest.

A long-term increase in stress hormones in the blood often has dangerous consequences: high blood pressure and an increased heart rate, high levels of cholesterol and triglycerides (fatty acids) and glucose (sugar). There is also a risk of obesity. Over time, coagulability increases, which in turn creates a risk of blood clots. This increases the load on the thyroid gland, bone tissue depletes, and osteoporosis develops. The work of the muscular and immune systems is disrupted and inflammatory processes occur. In addition, the structure and function of the brain suffers, especially in the hippocampus and amygdala areas, followed by disruption of cognitive and emotional abilities, memory disorders, anxiety, and depression.

An excess of epinephrine and cortisol in the blood corrodes our body, in much the same way as rust eats up metal. In fact, the body destroys itself, beginning with the central link: the hypothalamic-pituitary-adrenal system. Pathophysiologists call this "metabolic syndrome," and in the modern classification of diseases it corresponds to the diagnosis of an adaptation disorder. The cumulative impact of all these factors results in diseases such as atherosclerosis and coronary heart disease, hypertension, ulcers, colitis, eczema, diabetes, rheumatism, various kinds of allergy, and other psychosomatic disorders. But the main danger one faces is the emergence of a predisposition to cancer (Pothiwala P. et al., 2009; Russo A. et al., 2008).

Recent studies have shown that, at the molecular level, many of the pathogenic effects of stress occur by epigenetic mechanisms. To date, the methylation mechanism of the epigenetic control of genome expression has been the most studied. Methylation happens when a special chemical label—a methyl group (formed from one carbon atom and three hydrogen atoms)—attaches to the cytosine bases of DNA. This reduces the activity of the appropriate gene, since access to it becomes difficult. The other two detected epigenetic regulators are the processes of modification of *histones*, chromosomal (see *chromosomes*) proteins (which are acetylation, methylation, phosphorylation, ribosylation, etc.), and the synthesis of non-coding *micro-RNA*, which limit gene expression (Romani M. et al., 2015). Knowing all these mechanisms will help us further to better understand how stress and cancer are linked.

Epigenetic modifications of the genome are particularly noticeable as a result of stress and are associated with changes in memory processes. This leads to subsequent behavioral disorders—anxiety, *post-traumatic stress disorder (PTSD)*, depression, as well as to metabolic imbalances. Most of these effects are associated with the influence of the hormone cortisol and its *receptor* (Banerjee T., Chakravarti D., 2011; Hunter R. G., 2011), which, when combined, form a transcription factor. For example, in experiments with rats, the chronic stress that develops when the rodents are kept near a predator is similar in consequences to post-traumatic stress disorder in humans. It entails significant and diverse changes in the methylation of the gene of the *nerve tissue growth factor* BDNF in different regions of the hippocampus, thereby distorting the brain function (Roth T. L. et al., 2011). In addition, under the effect of cortisol on DNA during stress, the epigenetic changes alter the synthesis by immune cells of *pro-inflammatory agents—cytokines-interleukins* (Mifsud K. R. et al., 2011).

Recently the discovery was made of the important role, in generating and maintaining stress and its pathological consequences, played by another neurotransmitter—glutamate, as well as its receptors (Marsden W., 2011; Peterlik D. et al, 2016). Also called glutamic acid, glutamate is one of the most common amino acids in the human body. In normal quantities, it participates in the brain's implementation of cognitive functions, memory, and learning processes, ensures the functioning of muscles and bones, and is involved in the mechanisms of immunity and pain. Excess of glutamate leads to neurological and mental illnesses, in particular depression, epilepsy, Alzheimer's disease, and other neurodegenerative diseases. For the sake of brevity, the glutamatergic system will not be considered in this book.

There comes a time with chronic stress when the cortisol content begins to fall and reaches below-normal levels (Bergen A. W. et al., 2012, Juster R.-P. et al., 2011). This may reflect the body's attempt to compensate for the impact of a long-term elevated level of this hormone (Kudielka B. M. et al., 2009). At this stage, a decrease in the concentration of cortisol also has a pathogenic effect, since the hormone ceases to adequately suppress the action of pro-inflammatory cytokines, which, for example, contributes to a rise in inflammation and fatigue in cancer patients (Bower J. E. et al., 2007; Schrepf A. et al., 2013). Similar data have been found for the catecholamines epinephrine and norepinephrine in the brain: their levels decrease as a result of chronic stress (Roth K. A. et al., 1982), as well as the content of epinephrine in the adrenal glands (Nakagawa K., Kuriyama K., 1975). According to Selye, all this may indicate a syndrome of depletion of the adrenal glands, and, in general, correspond to the third stage of the stress reaction, namely, exhaustion of the organism's adaptive resources.

3.2.1. Chronic Stress: The Epidemic of the Twenty-First Century

Science has accumulated a large amount of data on the negative effects of chronic stress on our health and quality of life. Since most organs are subject to the negative long-term effects of glucocorticoids and catecholamines (Antoni M. H. et al., 2006), many of the most common diseases are believed to be due to chronic stress (Segerstrom S. C., Miller G. E., 2004). Some scientists even believe that stress lies behind about ten thousand diseases and more than a hundred thousand painful symptoms (Tigranyan R. A., 1988). Research done in the 1960s found that more than a third of patients with serious physical illnesses experienced an unusually high level of stress in the years preceding the disease (Rahe R. H. et al., 1964).

Professor Paul Rosch (1991), director of the American Institute of Stress, argues that 75% to 90% of all primary calls to doctors are associated with stress disorders. An analysis of the medical records of patients repeatedly and long treated for coronary heart disease, chronic pneumonia, and bronchial asthma, shows that as stress increases, the disease progresses, whereas actions taken to overcome stress have very positive results (Sokolova G. B., Tsarkova M. Yu, 1987). It has been found that 30% of women who experience chronic stress cannot become pregnant (Lynch C. D. et al., 2014).

A large-scale medical epidemiological study of British civil servants, known as the Whitehall analysis, shows that lower-level employees with less autonomy and greater stress are twice as likely to develop a metabolic syndrome—a precursor of heart disease, diabetes, and cancer—as employees at a higher job level, and have a greater propensity to die prematurely (Chandola T. et al., 2006). A *meta-analysis* of existing studies shows us that having negative social relationships (which is the main source of psychological stress) is comparable to the health risk caused by the use of tobacco and alcohol, obesity, or lack of physical activity (Holt-Lunstad J. et al., 2010).

Even an inferior socio-economic situation (a consequence of low-quality education, less prestigious work, and therefore a lower income) is a significant stress factor, leading to a risk of cardiovascular disease and premature death (Stowe R. P. et al., 2010). In cases of divorce, losing a loved one, and other psychic traumas leading to depression, sleep impairments, and post-traumatic stress disorder, there are significant disruptions in the activity of the peripheral nervous system and the hypothalamic-pituitary-adrenal system (McEwen B. S., 2000; Kiecolt-Glaser J. K. et al., 2002), which are the basis for the subsequent development of many serious diseases.

Therefore, in the second half of the twentieth century, the stressful causes of diseases were arranged under separate headings in the International Classification of Diseases (ICD-10). For example, "stress-related and somatoform disorders" (i.e., disorders for which no organic basis can be found), as well as professional stress and its variety—"professional burnout," occurs when people do not consider their physiological capabilities and do not pay attention to signals the body sends in the form of ailments and fatigue. Employees are less likely to claim insurance for a temporary disability, and as a result, their morbidity increases—first come neuroses, then depression, and afterward severe illnesses with fatal outcomes follow. Sadly, this is the price we pay for of ambition and only "focusing on results."

Somatoform disorders are the first bodily signals of intolerance to stress, and are precursors of more serious diseases. According to the report of the working group of the European College of Neuropsychopharmacology (ECNP), these disorders today predominate over everything else. On average, almost a fifth of the population of Europe suffer from them for over a year, and the expenses associated with their treatment have become a first priority (Wittchen H. U., Jacobi F., 2005).

Regular and frequent activation of the stress hormonal system results in our no longer needing a specific additional stimulus, as it does not rest even for a minute. Many of us live like runners, ever ready for the "Warning!" signal, forgetting to relax and "unclench," and thereby causing major damage to our health. The stress modern man experiences has changed from our being "physically conditioned" by life threats to our being "socially conditioned" by relationships, and the state of the organism is its indicator. Unfortunately, very few people realize that their ailments are caused by stress. We are so used to periodic headaches, bad sleep, digestive disorders, colds, fatigue, irritability, the need for external stimulants (coffee, nicotine) and relaxants (alcohol, tranquilizers), that we consider this to be almost normal, claiming to have a kind of "vegetative-vascular dystonia"[1] and not thinking about the real reasons why we feel bad.

Moreover, we can also "infect" each other with stress. As scientists from the Brain Institute in Germany have discovered, stress manifests as a contact disease. We have a "primary carrier," and he or she "infects" others who store stress in themselves until it explodes, "infecting" others around them (Engert V. et al., 2014). It may well be that this "explosion" lies behind our epidemics of flu and colds. Indeed, an analysis conducted at the Carnegie Mellon University revealed a direct and reproducible relationship between stress, infections, and influenza (Cohen S. et al., 1991). Even the creator of psychoanalysis, Sigmund Freud, noted that strong emotions could weaken one's resistance or increase one's susceptibility to infectious diseases (Freud S., 1905).

In regard to stress, a human is a unique being, because out in nature, in the animal world, there is no situation of chronic stress. As I have already mentioned, there are only the normal physiological stress reactions such as "fight, flight, or freeze," usually short-lived and not repeated too often. It is only we human beings, with our tendencies to suppress emotions owing to conditioning via a large number of social rules and regulations, who do not react properly to stress. Most of the time, we never allow ourselves to "fight" or "flee" from what is happening and "freeze" psychologically, and so negative consequences begin to accumulate in our bodies. As a result, we are at risk of various diseases, both somatic and psychiatric (Berry D. S., Pennebaker J. W., 1993; Kendler K. S., Karkowski-Shuman L., 1997).

Unlike us, an animal under natural conditions: a) reacts fully to danger; b) does not fuel its body with stress from the thoughts that this situation might happen again; and c) has time to fully recover from the danger. However, in captivity, animals placed in stressful situations demonstrate the same physiological symptoms of stress as we humans do. For example, if a sheep is placed next to a cage where a wolf is sitting, a severe stress reaction will begin to develop in its body, and after a few days it may even die from heart failure. In dogs that have experienced severe fear, all sort of ailments can develop, such as diseases of the gastrointestinal tract and heart, allergies, refusal to take food, and a gradual deterioration of the general condition (Reinhardt C., Nagel M., 2003). Female monkeys can develop a very "human" type of subordination stress owing to their being in a subordinate relationship with another monkey. This leads to cellular changes in the endometrium (internal mucosa of the uterus) and a high

---

[1]Vegetative-vascular dystonia, and similarly, neuro-circulatory dysfunction, is a stress-induced disorder of the autonomic nervous system, which may result in headaches, weakness, fatigue, low efficiency, sleep disorders, fainting, decreased sexual activity, dizziness, and panic attacks. It often has cardial, respiratory or dyspeptic accentuation.

risk of malignant transformation (Shively C. A. et al., 2004). It is due to the ability of animals to develop a state of chronic stress in captivity that scientists, as we will see further, can experimentally confirm the relationship of this type of stress with cancer.

3.2.2. Emotional Mechanisms of Chronic Stress

The primary and most destructive source of chronic stress in a human being is suppressed or repressed negative emotions. Psychology defines the suppression of emotions as an erroneous defense mechanism—the conscious avoidance of disturbing negative feelings or information, in order to maintain a positive self-image. This is achieved mainly through the replacement of these emotions with distracting thoughts or actions, and often associated with the need for the individual to keep everything under control. Unlike suppression which is intentional, the repression of emotions occurs unconsciously; as a result of our social attitudes and norms, we believe that certain negative emotions are unacceptable and so we force them out of our consciousness into the unconscious (subconscious), where they continue to "live," exercising a "polluting" effect in both our psyches and our bodies.

Most of us who experience chronic stress have no idea how many negative emotions are hidden inside us, as we push them out of consciousness. We think we are tired or upset, but in reality we may be experiencing forms of repressed anger. Mental tension, fear, the experience of danger, feelings of failure and a lack of self-regulation create the effect of accumulation of background anger and hostility. But, if we always perceive the world as a threatening and dangerous place, our ability to adapt and solve our problems will start to decline and our biological reserves will be depleted. This, in turn, leads to imbalances in many of our organs and systems, creating conditions conducive for diseases to show up.

Eighty years ago, Franz Alexander (1939) argued that suppressed emotions find a way out in the disorder of *vegetative functions*. Later, it was established that people who suppress their anger are prone to the development of various psychosomatic diseases, including cancer (Malatesta C. Z. et al., 1987; Crawford, J. S., 1981; Siegman A. W. et al., 1998; Kune G. A. et al., 1991; Thomas S. P. et al., 2000). Biochemically, suppressed anger leads to an increase in epinephrine level (Funkenstein D. H. et al., 1957), thus intensifying the initial stress state. If one is inclined to anger and does not have sufficient social support, then under stress, more interleukin-6 (a protein substance which causes inflammation) is synthesized (Puterman E. et al., 2013), which by itself, as we will learn further, is a risk factor for cancer.

However, this does not mean that, instead of suppressing our negative emotions, we need to spill them out willingly on surrounding people! This is another extreme which also has significant negative consequences. For example, even an ordinary family quarrel results in a lowered immune system response in spouses; their physical wounds will heal more slowly, and the pro-inflammatory interleukins will accumulate. These changes will persist as long as twenty-four hours after the quarrel. Moreover, the higher the level of hostility and the stronger the negative emotions, the more interleukins are released, and the longer the wounds will take to heal (Kiecolt-Glaser J. K. et al., 2005). Other scientists found that with people exhibiting greater hostility and anger during family quarrels, their level of the stress hormone cortisol was higher in these moments, and that the function of protective immune cells is lower than with people who are calm (Miller G. E. et al., 1999).

A study of 1623 patients with uncomplicated myocardial infarction revealed that the risk of developing a heart attack increases by a factor of 2.3 within two hours of having experienced intense anger. Such an infarction can often be caused by a family quarrel or a conflict at work (Mittleman M. A. et al., 1995). If we are constantly angry, the consequences will be even worse. For example, in those teachers who are unable to control themselves and who therefore take their anger out on their students, the level of cortisol becomes chronically elevated (Steptoe A. et al., 2000). It has also been found that those who care for elderly people with Alzheimer's disease, and who are often angry with them and have poor control over their anger, show a decrease in the ability of their lymphocytes to protect them from pathogenic agents (Scanlan J. M. et al., 2001). As a consequence of this kind of chronic stress, an inflammatory process will develop within their bodies, their wound healing mechanism will become compromised, and their susceptibility to infectious diseases increase (Gouin J. P. et al., 2011).

In view of what I have just said, it appears that the angrier we are with others, the more we destroy ourselves? This sounds almost like a scientifically based biblical sermon! But the fact remains that very consistently angry people experience more complications after an operation and have to stay in the hospital longer (Stengrevics S. et al., 1996; Sharma A. et al., 2008). On the contrary, if someone is able to relax well, especially before surgery, the outcome of their operation will be much more favorable (Montgomery G. H. et al., 2002). Further, we will see that suppressed or repressed anger becomes one of the leading psychophysiological mechanisms of cancer.

Hence it follows that we need to take responsibility for owning our emotions, and be able to express them in a proper way. Such an approach can bring effective help: awareness and written description of traumatic events of life and expression of associated emotions have a positive effect on physical and mental health, normalizing the functions of the autonomic nervous and endocrine systems (Pennebaker J. W., 1999).

Which deep psychological causes create a protracted emotional imbalance and chronic stress will be explained in Part III.

3.2.3. The Immune System—The Main "Victim" of Chronic Stress

> Our immune cells are constantly
> eavesdropping on our internal dialogue.
> *Deepak Chopra,*
> *Ignite Your Immune System*

Since our immune system is the main means whereby our body protects itself against newly emerged cancer cells (and we will often be referring to this fact throughout the book), we need to understand what happens to it under chronic stress. To do this, let us briefly recall how the immune system is organized. It incorporates a whole complex of cells, organs, and tissues that interact with one another, including the central organs such as bone marrow and thymus, and peripheral organs such as the spleen, lymph nodes, and lymphoid tissue.

In the bone marrow there is hematopoietic tissue, where the leukocytes (white blood cells) are produced. They play a major role in protecting the body from various external and internal damaging agents. Penetrating the walls of capillaries into tissues, leukocytes absorb and digest harmful substances and biological aggressors, and when carrying out this function are called phagocytes. In injuries or infectious diseases, phagocytes die in the process of fighting, forming pus and local inflammation.

There are also stem cells (undifferentiated, generic) in the red bone marrow, which migrate to the thymus (the gland located behind the sternum). Here, they mature and differentiate, turning into specialized leukocytes: T, B, and NK lymphocytes, whose goal is the recognition and destruction of foreign cells. The T-lymphocyte family include T-helpers cells, whose main task is to enhance the immune response, and T-killers—lymphocytes, whose main function is the elimination of those of our body cells that become defective owing to attacks by both viruses and bacteria, as well as to mutations (including tumor cells). B-lymphocytes are responsible for the production of antibodies: special molecules that determine and neutralize external objects (mainly extracellular pathogens), this process followed by the destruction of the latter by phagocytes. NK-lymphocytes ("natural killers") are large specialized cells that have a particular toxicity in relation to tumor cells and virus-infected cells.

So many varieties of immune cells are needed for the body to respond flexibly to the emergence of constantly changing, mutating strange agents. Lymphocytes and some phagocytes also produce cytokines (including interleukins)—small protein molecules that regulate intercellular and intersystem interactions. They control the growth, activity, and destruction (apoptosis) of cells, the process of inflammation, and also coordinate the interaction between the nervous, immune, and endocrine systems.

These systems relate together both anatomically and biochemically. For example, the neurons of one of the most important parts of the brain, the hypothalamus (the "command post" of the body's response to stress), are connected through the sympathetic nervous system with neurons regulating the activity of spleen and lymph nodes, as well as the red bone marrow and thymus. In one of the lateral regions of the hypothalamus there are special neurons that release regulatory neuropeptides (a kind of protein), called orexins. They participate in stress mechanisms and are able to directly affect the immune system, enhancing the function of the spleen's NK cells (Wrona D., Trojniar W., 2003; Wenner M. et al., 2000).

The discovery of the direct influence of the immune system on the brain was very unexpected. Various pathogenic stimuli of the environment, antigens (substances that cause the body's immune response), are able to activate certain brain structures that are responsible, in particular, for the regulation of eating, the sleep/wake cycle, the water–salt metabolism, stress reactions, etc. This leads to a change in many functions of the body (Korneva E. A., Perekrest S. V., 2013). In addition, it was discovered by Professor Candace Pert (1999) at the University of Georgetown that lymphocytes are capable of producing neuropeptides that affect our mind, memory, and ability to think. The author commented that the more she observed the immune cells, the more they reminded her of mobile brain cells. Later, other scientists established that both immune and nerve cells release cytokine regulators capable of cross-influencing each other (Besedovsky H. O., del Rey A., 2007). In recent decades, the participation of the immune system in the formation of mental and neurological diseases has also been confirmed (Kerr D. et al., 2005).

The effects of the brain and stress on the immune system are studied today in psychoneuroimmunology, an interdisciplinary science designed to investigate the relationships between psychological, behavioral, neuroendocrine processes, and immunology.

The foundations of this science were laid in the 1970s, when Robert Ader, professor of the medical center at the University of Rochester in the United States, made another fundamental discovery about the relationship between the brain and the immune system. He based his studies on the same principle as Ivan Pavlov, who, as is known, was the first to establish that information taken in from the external environment through the brain can affect the functions of internal organs. Many people who have taken a biology class can recall that Pavlov and his colleagues studied conditioned reflexes in dogs, in which saliva could be transported to the cheek from outside the oral cavity through a fistula (artificial canal). In 1902, researchers found that the secretion of saliva in experimental dogs began not only in response to the food they actually received, but also just after they were placed in an experimental chamber where they were usually fed, prior to feeding.

Pavlov called this phenomenon "psychic salivation" and it formed the basis of his fundamental doctrine of higher nervous activity. This is another example of how the image (of the chamber in this case) affects the functions of the body according to information stored in memory. In the works of Pavlov that I mentioned earlier, he and his team, in fact, laid the foundations for the study of stress (at that time the scientist called it a breakdown in higher nervous activity): by subjecting dogs to an electric current, their conditioned reflex in response to food was violated. Pavlov regarded this as a model of experimental neurosis.

Professor Ader similarly studied whether it is possible to develop a conditioned reflex in the immune system. He gave rats water sweetened with saccharin, along with an injection of a chemical (cyclophosphamide) that had an inhibitory function on immunity. After some time, rats were given only sweetened water. It turned out that their immune functions were reduced in the same way they would have been if cyclophosphamide have been injected (Ader R., Cohen N., 1975). This was evidence that the brain is able to directly affect the immune system, otherwise how else could rats learn to influence their immunity?

Later, it was confirmed that people are also capable of similar reactions. A group of scientists from the Medical College of Cornell University in New York studied the immune reactions of women who were prescribed chemotherapy for ovarian cancer. Analyses were taken several days before the start of treatment and also on the day it began just before the drug was to be administered. By this time, the immune response of leukocytes (their ability to reproduce in response to the introduction of a provocative stimulator of T-cell division) was decreasing, and women already began feeling nauseous, despite the fact that there was no medicine in their bodies (Bovbjerg D. H. et al., 1990). It is obvious that such changes in the organism were created by an emotion of fear based on information about the effects of chemotherapy that these women held in their memory. Fortunately, our minds can also create the opposite effect; and one well-proven way to increase the effectiveness of immunity, especially in the fight against cancer, is to work with visualization, in particular, imagining immune cells destroying cancer cells (Simonton-Atchley S., 1993; Gruzelier J. H., 2002).

Studying the effect of stress on the immune system, scientists have also discovered that acute short-term stress can increase the effectiveness of the immune response (Dhabhar F. S. et al., 2010). From an evolutionary viewpoint, such a reaction is necessary to help infected wounds heal when animals fight each other, in order to survive. However, when stress becomes chronic, the effectiveness of immunity decreases, and this was first mentioned by Hans Selye. Since then, a lot of research has emerged to validate this finding. According to *meta-analyses*, thirty-six scientific works came out between 1977 and 1991 (Herbert T. B., Cohen S., 1993), and about 300 studies by 2004, all of which focused on the relationship between stress and the immune system. These studies have proven that the longer stress lasts, the more the functions of the immune system are suppressed at its various levels, so while a stress starts out by being positive and adaptive, it ends up by becoming a pathogenic process (Segerstrom S. C., Miller G. E., 2004).

In particular, chronic stress in mice leads to atrophy of the thymus, which, as I noted above, is one of the main organs responsible for the immune response (Hasegawa H., Saiki I., 2002). In this state, the activity of NK lymphocytes decreases and they lose the ability to reproduce and develop protective immunity (Cohen S. et al., 2001). For example, chronic stress significantly reduces the ability of our immune system to create protective antibodies when vaccinated against influenza (Segerstrom S. C., Miller G. E., 2004), while the severity of an infectious disease is determined by the degree of stress-impairment of the immune system (Peterson P. K. et al., 1991). Sadly, our stress, as a rule, is skillfully supported by hysteria in the mass media, which likes to frighten us with being infected by flu and therefore requires us to stock up with drugs or immediately vaccinate. Guess who pays for these campaigns? A similar relationship with stress is demonstrated by the herpes virus: the higher our stress, the more often attacks occur, the herpes infection becomes more active and more enduring (Glaser R., Kiecolt-Glaser J. K., 1994).

Both chronic and "academic" (caused by pressure of exams) stress, as well as painful bereavements, divorces, depression, and other significant negative events in our lives, reduce the functions of the immune system and make us more vulnerable to various diseases (Ader R. et al., 2000; Quan N. et al., 2001; Kiecolt-Glaser J. K. et al., 2002). The longer the stress caused by a severe loss lasts, the more strongly the protective function of NK lymphocytes is suppressed (Herbert T., Cohen S., 1993). Stress and negative self-esteem are directly related to a reduction in the number of protective NK lymphocytes and T-helpers in AIDS patients and carriers of the immunodeficiency virus HIV (Evans D. L. et al., 1995; Ventegodt S. et al., 2004b). Disruptions of the function of the immune system under stress can also lead to situations whereby it begins to attack its own organism. This results in autoimmune diseases, such as rheumatoid arthritis, psoriasis, and multiple sclerosis (Jacobs G. D., 2001).

In the mechanism of the negative effects of stress on immunity, a big role is played by stress hormones. Evidence shows that an increase in cortisol levels caused by chronic stress is related to immunosuppression both in animals and in humans (Sheridan J. F. et al., 1998; Kiecolt-Glaser J. K. et al., 1998). This is because the cells of the nervous system, leukocytes and lymphocytes, have on their surface receptors for epinephrine, norepinephrine, and cortisol, and increased levels of these hormones can lead the protective properties of immune cells to become inhibited; when this happens, they remain passive instead of attacking viruses that have penetrated the body, or the cancer cells that have developed in it. The effect is realized at the level of chromosomes; in the following sections, we will learn how stress hormones change the activity of the genome, and what it leads to.

A group of scientists from the University of British Columbia in Canada and the National University of Ireland found receptors in immune cells capable of responding to both neurotransmitters and medicines, possessing the properties of tranquilizers (Song C., Leonard B. E., 2000). That is, immune cells respond to the same signals as brain cells. Both immune and nerve cells produce another class of regulatory substances: endogenous opiates, or our "internal narcotic drugs." These play an important role in our behavioral responses, our emotional motivation, responses to stress and pain, and immune reactions (Narayan P. et al., 2001). All these data once again confirm the correctness of Professor Candace Pert's conclusions regarding the affinity between immune and brain cells.

From this perspective, we can quite understand the results of studies which found that bad moods and negative emotions are associated with a decrease in the number of T-lymphocytes and the ability of the immune system to produce antibodies, while good moods and positive emotions are associated with an increase in the number of T-lymphocytes and an improvement in the immune response (Stone A. A., 1987; Futterman A. D. et al., 1994). Anger can also lead to a gradual decrease in the immune defenses of the body during the six hours after it is experienced, while the emotion of joy brings an immediate increase in the content of immunoglobulin A, which is an indicator of the state of immunity (Rein G. et al., 1995).

At the Department of Psychiatry at Ohio State University (USA), scientists carried out extensive long-term studies on the impact of negative emotions on immunity. In the initial experiments conducted on healthy newlyweds, it was found that those who showed more negative emotions and hostility during family disputes demonstrated a greater decline of protective properties of NK-lymphocytes, an effect that would persist for twenty-four hours (Kiecolt-Glaser J. K. et al., 1993). In addition, the levels of epinephrine, norepinephrine, growth hormone, and ACTH (corticotropin, a pituitary hormone), would increase in their blood. ACTH, in turn, would stimulate the synthesis of the second major type of stress hormone: corticosteroids (Malarkey W. B. et al., 1994). After two years of marriage, in people who are undergoing chronic marital stress, the state of cellular immunity that protects the body from various pathogens was significantly worse, unlike its condition in those who were not stressed. This deterioration in immunity creates conditions for the development of diseases (Jaremka L. M. et al., 2013).

Further, the objects of study were married couples who had lived together for twelve years or more. Scientists have shown that the stress that they develop during a half-hour dispute suppresses the body's ability to heal itself. The experimental wounds (a puncture of the skin with a blister, as when taking blood from a finger for analysis), if inflicted on each of the spouses before they started "sorting things out," would take a day longer to heal than they would if the two were in a state of emotional balance. Moreover, in couples with increased aggressiveness toward each other in a dispute, the healing of wounds would occur twice as slowly and the content of the pro-inflammatory cytokine in their blood would increase (Kiecolt-Glaser J. K. et al., 2005). Therefore, it is natural that the increase in the inflammatory state of the body is the key mechanism by which family stress worsens health (Black P. H., 2006). It was interesting that those spouses who used the so-called cognitive approach to a dispute, that is, who showed conscious attention to their partners and tried to understand their arguments and would discuss them, manifested less growth in the amount of inflammatory cytokines over the course of twenty-four hours than did those who would just spill out their negative emotions on each other (Graham J. E. et al., 2009).

Unfortunately, for most people, very little changes throughout their lives, and if they possess negative traits, those tend to be retained until old age. A further study under this program was performed on people of average age of sixty-seven, who had been married for about forty-two years. Although the average frequency of conflict in these families was 31% lower than in young couples, nonetheless, the immune system was much more disturbed because of dispute among those who showed greater aggressiveness and dissatisfaction with their marriage. With women, in addition, the balance of stress hormones ACTH, cortisol, and norepinephrine was also in disorder (Kiecolt-Glaser J. K. et al., 1997).

All these data enable us to understand that our immune and nervous systems are constantly in contact and react to each other through changes in our emotional state. That is, our words and thoughts can affect the immune system in the same way as the conditioning stimuli do in animals studied by Pavlov and Ader. I emphasize once more that the stressful situations in themselves do not necessarily lead to a drop in immunity—what is the central is the way in which we cope with them.

"The way we evaluate the problem affects the state of immunity more than stress in itself," says Susan Bauer-Wu (2002), director of the research center at the Dana-Farber Cancer Institute in Boston. —"People with a high level of stress, but who can cope with it, will retain a healthy immune system. At the same time, people experiencing low stress, but who are unable to control it, demonstrate a decrease in immune system activity and a raised susceptibility to disease." This is especially important with cancer patients. For example, when studying patients with breast and lung cancer, scientists found that stress-related disorders of the natural diurnal fluctuations in corticosteroid hormones, the so-called circadian cycle, were a negative prognostic sign and that such patients would tend to die earlier (Sephton S. E. et al., 2000, 2012).

Now we can understand why, in accordance with the theory of cancer containment, the immune system of a person in a state of chronic stress is not able to effectively protect them from carcinogens and mutations. The problem is that most people do nothing to reduce the destructive effect of chronic stress on their bodies. In the following chapters, we will consider studies directly confirming a decrease of immunity in the precancerous state.

3.2.4. Mind, the Creator of Stress

> People do not care about the events themselves,
> but their opinion about these events.
> Epictetus,
> *ancient Greek philosopher*

At this point in our study many of readers will probably agree that stress only seemingly comes from the outside world—one's job, finances, the family, etc. It becomes clear that the true source of stress is the mind, which decides if something is stressful or not. Modern man is no longer being met with life-threatening situations provoking useful "fight or flight" reactions. Today, our stresses are mostly psychological, but the organism reacts in the same way as our ancestors did tens of thousands of years ago. Therefore, being ill-prepared for an exam can cause the release of the same stress hormones into the bloodstream as would occur if we were to encounter a predator. The physiological stress response in human beings, unlike animals, depends not so much on the immediate presence of a stress agent, but on its psychological impact on the individual, its subjective significance.

A follower of Hans Selye, Richard Lazarus (1966) wrote that psychological stress can be defined as a phenomenon of awareness arising from comparing the requirements imposed on the individual with his or her ability to cope with these demands. In other words, how the level of intensity of stress is all about the attitudes of the person experiencing it. If we overestimate the threat emanating from the stress factor, and underestimate our own capabilities to handle it, then the damaging effect of the stressor will be substantial. Therefore, the stress researcher George Everly (1981) came to the conclusion that it is our emotional and mental evaluation of stimuli, both external or internal, that determines whether or not they become sources of stressors. If the irritant is not interpreted by consciousness as a threat, then no stress reaction develops. Consequently, Everly believes, most of the stressful reactions that we experience are actually created by us ourselves and will continue for as long as we allow them to.

The same opinion was held by H. Basowitz and his colleagues (1955): we should not consider stress as a factor imposed on the body. It should be regarded as a reaction of the organism to internal and external processes, reaching those threshold levels where physiological and psychological integrative features of the body are strained to the limit and beyond. The well-known Russian psychologist and psychiatrist, Professor F. B. Berezin and his team were even more definite: "The center of gravity in assessing mental stress cannot be transferred to the features of the environment. Stress is not a collection of environmental influences, but an internal state of the organism, in which the execution of its integrative functions is complicated" (Sokolova E. D. et al., 1996).

For example, if we look at some different types of psychological stress, we will find:

- professional stress (arising in manual workers, businessmen, etc.);
- family stress;
- interpersonal stress (arising in problems with communication, conflicts, fears, etc.);
- personal stress (for example, if a person's life does not correspond with what they believe should be their social role);
- intrapersonal stress (occurs with unrealized needs, comes from a sense of purposelessness of existence, etc.).

Based on this classification, there is no doubt that these types of stress are associated with the various social roles that we perform, together with the functioning of certain rules and guidelines in our mind that are associated with these roles. When, for various reasons, these beliefs do not work, acute or chronic emotional imbalance develops. However, since our beliefs are the derivatives of our mind, we are responsible for the consequences to which these feelings lead.

Psycho-oncoloogists C. and S. Simonton, together with J. Creighton (1978), noted that the most important thing is to remember that we ourselves determine the significance of the events occurring in our life. For instance, a person who chooses to take the position of a victim will affect his life by giving heightened significance to events that confirm the hopelessness of his particular situation. Each of us chooses, though not always consciously, how to respond to various events. The magnitude of stress we experience is determined, according to the authors, first by the value that we give to it, and secondly, by the rules that we ourselves once worked out and that indicate acceptable ways of getting out of a stressful situation.

Since what happens in our mind is reflected in the brain, and then in the body, we can arrive at a well-founded conclusion that stress, too, is created by our mind, that is, by our attitude to life. This conclusion is by no means new. For two and a half thousand years, Buddhism has taught people that the better we know our minds, the more we realize that all our experiences, especially negative ones, based on affection, aversion, stress, anxiety, fear, or anguish, are products of our mind. Today, there are scientific confirmations for this ancient teaching.

Research at the University of Pennsylvania shows that the way we both see and react to events in our lives today predicts our chronic diseases for the next ten years, regardless of our current state of health and our future stresses (Piazza J. R. et al., 2013). Manager of this research project David Almeida, a professor at the department of human development and family studies, in an interview with *Medical News Today* said: "For example, if you have a lot of work to do today and you are really grumpy because of it, then you are more likely to suffer negative health consequences ten years from now than someone who also has a lot of work to do today, but doesn't let it bother them." This study of 2,000 people was quite strict and included eight consecutive daily interviews and four saliva tests for cortisol content during these eight days. The test was repeated with each accessible participant ten years later to determine whether there were any changes in their responses to stress, and to assess their health. The results were obvious: those who coped better with stress had fewer health problems, especially with regard to chronic joint pain and cardiovascular problems.

A Tibetan proverb comes to mind: "If you want to know what happened— look at your body, if you want to know what will happen—look at your mind."

These studies remind us that the stressful events themselves are not the real problem, but our perception of them is, and the results can be quite serious. For example, women who are prone to overestimating the seriousness of their life's vicissitudes are at higher risk of developing breast tumors than those who assess problems more realistically (Cooper C. L., Faragher E. B., 1993). Dr. Gawler (1984) notes that the main factor with cancer patients is not the very problem they face, but the reaction they have to it. Many of them are unable to cope with a serious problem, especially if it is associated with abrupt changes in their lives. Inability to respond correctly to a challenging situation, to find a way out and to ease the mind, altogether leads to those shifts in the body's biochemistry known as stress. This weakens the immune system and, thereby, adds another powerful ingredient to those forces that cause cancer.

This position is shared by scientists from the laboratory of neuroendocrinology at Rockefeller University in the United States. Our brain, they argue, is the key organ responsible for stress, because it determines what constitutes a threat, and therefore creates a physiological and behavioral response. This response can be either adaptive or damaging, up to disruption of the shape and size of nerve cells and structural changes in certain areas of the brain, associated with our emotions, such as the hippocampus, amygdala, and prefrontal cortical areas. Bruce McEwen, the head of this laboratory and one of the world's leading authorities in psychoneuroimmunology, created the concept of allostatic load. The term "allostasis" comes from the Greek words allos, meaning different, and stasis, meaning stability—it literally means "achieving stability through change." However, in response to long-term stress ("load"), damaging changes accumulate in the body due to the extremely long-term effects of neuronal, endocrine, and immune mediators (stress agents) on various organs and systems (McEwen B. S., Gianaros P. J., 2010).

To paraphrase a popular proverb, we can say that "stress is not so black as our mind likes to paint it." Rather, it is our ability to understand our reactions to stress and manage them that determines the reactions of our immune system to stress. This conclusion is confirmed by a study showing that mental processes, such as our motivation or a semantic interpretation of what is happening, are more important for managing stress than emotional reactions (Maier K. J. et al., 2003). Greg Anderson, who overcame his metastatic lung cancer and afterward created the Cancer Recovery Foundation in the USA, wrote in his book *The Cancer Conqueror* (1990) that we can and should develop a positive, workable approach to stress management:

> The perfect no-stress environment is the grave. When we change our perception we gain control. Stress becomes a challenge, not a threat. When we commit to action, to actually doing something rather than feeling trapped by events, the stress in our life becomes manageable.

My vision of the central role of the mind in generating stress and coping with it, and its role in the occurrence of cancer, is key to this book and will be supported with plenty of evidence.

3.3. Oncogenic Distress

We have so far considered only a small amount of data on the mechanisms of the carcinogenic effects of chronic stress. In the following chapters, the results of many studies will be presented, demonstrating its effects at various levels including the intracellular and genomic, as well as the hormonal- and immune-system, levels. But even previously mentioned materials reveal that chronic stress can, over time, create a state of oncogenic distress in the body, which provokes the development of cancer. It was already noted by the Simontons in the 1970s that the physical state, described by Selye as a result of stress, practically coincides with the conditions in which atypical cells can multiply and turn into a dangerous malignant tumor. At the second conference on the psychophysiological aspects of cancer conducted by the New York Academy of Sciences (1968), it was pointed out that stress-related issues such as insufficient emotional discharge (especially from anger), severe suffering due to loss of a loved one, as well as despair and hopelessness play an important role in the development of cancer.

Continuing the observations of the doctors of the past, modern researchers also confirm the connection between stress and the onset of cancer, by using wider social and epidemiological studies of the population (Antoni M. et al., 2006; Chida Y. et al., 2008). In particular, the meta-analysis of available research demonstrates that the psychosocial factors that cause stress correspond to a higher incidence of all types of cancer in initially healthy people, worsen the survival rate of cancer patients, and increase the mortality rate in society (Chida Y. et al., 2008).

Thirty years of monitoring of almost seven thousand employees in a West Scotland company in the UK, revealed the relationship between the experience of daily average level stress with that of the development of breast and prostate cancer (Metcalfe C. et al., 2007). Researchers from the University of New York found that in men with a high level of stress and a lack of satisfying relationships with their families and friends, the PSA antigen content (a specific risk factor for prostate cancer) increased two to three times (Stone A. A. et al., 1999). Excessive stress and a lack of social support in women's lives was also seen to increase the incidence of breast cancer by nine times (Price M. A. et al., 2001).

In a cancer center in Athens, 1,088 women with the same diagnosis were observed for four and a half years. In 813 cases, a link was found between the disease and chronic stress, which had developed as a result of: the death of a loved one; negative behavior of spouses; unexpected changes in lifestyle; constant conflicts in the family; financial problems; an unsatisfactory sexual life; psychiatric problems, and allergies. Less important, but also statistically significant were the following factors: disappointment in relationships; a lowering of one's standard of living; a family history of breast cancer; arterial hypertension; late onset of the first menstruation, and the occurrence of menopause (Ioannidou-Mouzaka L. et al., 1986).

In Finland, in the oncology unit at the Medical Faculty in the University of Tampere, the history of stressful events (not related to the diagnosis) in the lives of patients with newly diagnosed prostate, breast, and melanoma cancers was studied. The experience of significant stresses was found in 80% of those examined. Of these, one-third of the events were associated with acute loss (death of a loved one or loss of social status), while others had a variety of chronic stressful situations (Lehto U. S. et al., 2008).

In a similar study by the Russian scientist R. A. Akhmerov (2013), out of a group of cancer patients a total of 450 precipitating life experiences were revealed. The patients attributed 22.44% of these to unpleasant and stressful events, whereas in the control group (non-oncological patients), only 4.22% of such events had occurred. Another study of seventy-three women with cervical cancer showed a significant presence of negative stress events in their lives for six months prior to diagnosis (Goodkin K. et al., 1986).

Italian scientists found that in the lives of men with lung cancer and women with breast cancer, the number of distresses (especially related to the death of relatives and problems at work) in the two years before the tumor was diagnosed was more than twice as many as in the life of patients with hepatitis, used as a control group (Cotrufo P., Galiani R., 2014). Researchers from the universities of Rochester and Texas in the United States found many strong psychotraumatic, stressful, and emotional events in the lives of cancer patients, in contrast to events in the lives of people who did not have cancer (Smith W. R., Sebastian H., 1976; Palesh O. et al., 2007).

According to V. V. Ogorenko (2011) from the Dnipropetrovsk Medical Academy (Ukraine), significant stressful events occurred before the onset of the disease in patients with brain cancer. In 51.2% of those surveyed, there was stress associated with the death of close relatives (spouses, children, parents), or the patients had witnessed the sudden deaths of other people. Forty-nine point eight percent of cases showed stress connected with their own or their parents' divorce, and/or their children having an unsuccessful family life. The third most common group of stresses (38.4% of patients) was associated with economic need and loss of professional status due to retirement or compelled change of job.

A study conducted at the Kuban State University (Russia) found that the number of stressful situations reached a critical level in the last two years before diagnosis in patients with thyroid cancer (Egikyan M. A., 2014). Norwegian researchers studying a large group (14,231 women) showed that the incidence of rectal cancer in widows increased twofold. After divorce, there was a 17% increase in the incidence of breast, lung, and cervical cancer (Kvikstad A. et al., 1995).

Psychiatrists from St. Petersburg (Russia) studied the relationship between emotional and psychological disorders caused by stress, and the subsequent onset of cancer. This relationship was clearly seen in 79% of cases and would develop from a moment of a psychic trauma, over a three-month to a three- to five-year period (Gnezdilov A. V., 1996). Professor Theodore R. Miller (1977) of the Sloan-Kettering Cancer Center (USA) claimed that in his clinical practice, he observed more than a thousand cases of cancer in a husband or wife after suffering stress related to the same disease or the death of a spouse.

The following chapters will also present data from numerous studies linking the origin of cancer to specific psychosocial-spiritual causes, such as a dysfunctional family, the stress of loss, unresolved psychological conflicts, or some kind of existential crisis.

Experiments on animals confirm the oncogenic effect of stress. I have already cited data on pioneering research conducted in the laboratory of Ivan Pavlov. Following on from it, researchers from different countries used a variety of methods to evoke stress in animals in order to produce a carcinogenic effect. This included electric stimulation, living in crowded cages, immobilization, rotational stress, abdominal incision probing, flashing light, intense cooling, and fluorescent lighting.

For example, in the experiments of Kiev's Institute of Experimental and Clinical Oncology, conducted under the leadership of R. E. Kavetskiy in the 1950s and 1960s, stress-inducing electroconvulsive effects provoked breast cancer in mice and rats (Turkevich N. M., 1955; Hayetskiy I. K., 1965). Scientists from the Johns Hopkins Cancer Research Center have found that chronic stress can provoke the onset of cancer in animals with a strong predisposition to this disease. In this study, mice were exposed to carcinogenic skin irradiation with ultraviolet light. For those who were previously exposed to chronic stress, skin cancer developed 50% faster than in mice that were not stressed (Parker J. et al., 2004). In other experiments, the mice were stressed for four months every other day, after which they were given the carcinogen urethane. As a result, the incidence of lung tumors was higher in this group than in control rodents which were given urethane but were not stressed (Adachi S. et al., 1993).

When female mice are kept socially isolated, they suffer chronic stress, accompanied by an increase in the level of corticosterone and the activation of genes involved in tumor growth mechanisms. Consequently, breast tumors in these animals appeared more active and were larger than in animals not subjected to stress (Hermes G. L. et al., 2009). Similar results in mice were also brought about by chronic acoustic stress and a prolonged restriction of mobility: in these rodents the content of corticosteroids would grow, immunity would decrease, and pancreatic tumor growth activity would appear (Partecke L. I. et al., 2016). In studies on female monkeys subjected to stress due to their having a subordinate position in their group, a higher incidence of uterine and breast cancer would be found (Shively C. A. et al., 2004). According to Professor Carol Shively, the head of the group of scientists at the Medical Center of Wake Forest University, these results reinforced the importance of more thoroughly studying the influence of stress and socioeconomic situation on the risk in women of developing breast and endometrial cancer. Similar studies on animals have accumulated since the middle of the last century (Balitskiy K. P., Shmalko Y. P., 1987; Antoni M. et al., 2006).

Although most researchers have detected stimulation of cancer development in animals under the influence of repeated stress stimuli, it was found that stress can also inhibit the development of tumors. The outcome depends on the type of tumor and the stage of the tumor process, the type and intensity of the stressor, and the state of the animal's organism (see reviews in Balitskiy K. P., Shmalko U. P., 1987, Justice A., 1985). In the cases of tumor inhibition, mostly moderate, short-term physical stressors were used, which we can probably regard as producing the eustress described by Selye. The mechanism of this inhibitory effect can be associated with the stimulating effect of such stress on the immune system (Zorrilla E. P. et al., 2001). A similar effect, in particular, may be seen in physical exercise; According to some studies, it improves the survival rate of cancer patients (Sanchis-Gomar F. et al., 2012).

As evident from all the data presented, chronic stress, whatever its origin, contributes to the development of cancer. Therefore, we need further to analyze and define the specific psychosocial causes that create a state of chronic oncogenic distress in the human body.

Part II

Predisposition to Cancer: Disorders of Individual Development

Chapter 4

Diathesis–Stress Model of Diseases

> In each person continues to live a frightened,
> fearful child, ardently desiring to be loved.
> *Sandor Ferenczi, psychoanalyst*

Why do life's stresses cause disease in some people, but not in others, and why does the disease take on one form or another? This question was also of interest to the creator of psychoanalysis, Sigmund Freud (cited in Sadock B. J., Sadock V. A., 2007). He placed great importance upon the human *constitution* and believed that depending on its type, stressful experiences cause different fixations, a fixation being an unconscious process of focusing attention on a psychological trauma, resulting in delays and disturbances in one's mental development, the suppression of pathogenic material from the consciousness, and the onset of a neurosis.

However, the constitution is only one of the factors predisposing the body to increased vulnerability to external and internal pathogenic influences. In general, predisposition to any disease is a function of a complex form of interaction of the organism with the environment. Physicians often use the term "diathesis" (from the Greek διαθεσις– inclination), or "biological diathesis," which refers to the constitutional (biological) predisposition of the organism to certain diseases owing to inherited, congenital, or acquired properties and physiological characteristics that lead the bodily functions to a long-term unstable equilibrium. This results in a disorder of adaptation and inadequate responses to ordinary impacts, as well as the development of pathological reactions to external hazards, and renders existing diseases more severe as they progress (Davydovskiy I., 1962).

The following question is undoubtedly of interest: is there a specific predisposition to cancer?

Doctor Thomas Watson, to the best of my knowledge, was the first who mention the importance of predisposition in the development of cancer. He wrote back in 1871: "Great mental stress has been assigned as influential in hastening the development of cancerous disease in persons already predisposed."

In the beginning of the 20th century, the outstanding Ukrainian pathophysiologist, academician Alexander Bogomolets, introduced the concept of "cancer diathesis." In one of his books (1926) he wrote: "In order for the germ of a cancerous tumor that has arisen in the body to turn into a malignant neoplasm and cause a clinical cancer, a number of conditions are needed. They form the concept of cancer diathesis, i.e., the organism's predisposition to develop a cancerous tumor." Giving his main attention at the time to the protective functions of the *reticuloendothelial system*, Bogomolets also considered neuro-humoral relationships important in the development of cancer (Balitskiy K. P., Veksler I. G., 1975)—in fact, what is being studied by modern psychoneuroendocrinology.

A known Soviet endocrinologist, gerontologist, and oncologist, Professor Vladimir Dilman (1986) created the concept of "cancrophilia" (from the Latin cancris—cancer and the Greek philia—affection), meaning a set of metabolic conditions that increase the likelihood of a malignant transformation of the cell. This syndrome, according to Dilman, is especially characteristic in the process of normal aging after middle age, although its occurrence can be accelerated at an earlier age under the influence of specific external and internal factors. These are: acute and chronic stress, mental depression, excessive nutrition, obesity, type 2 diabetes mellitus, atherosclerosis, pregnancy, the mechanism of accelerated development of the body, as well as the syndrome of carcinogenic aging.

Undoubtedly, an important factor is the hereditary predisposition to cancer. Thus, genetically caused disorders of the ability to repair DNA, associated with low activity of the corresponding enzymes, markedly increase the frequency of point mutations and chromosomal distortions, enhancing the risk of malignant tumors and leukemia (Belitskiy G., 2006). However, epigenetics indicates that it is not only mutations, but also stress that can affect the activity of genes (without changing the structure of DNA), and set these changes so that they are inherited (McEwen B. S., 2007). Therefore, in the next chapter we will analyze the data to establish the most appropriate form to use in talking about hereditary oncopathology.

When discussing the psychosomatic nature of cancer, it is also necessary to understand what is connected with the predispositions to psychosomatic diseases. Of these, Franz Alexander (1939) considered the constitutional insufficiency of certain organs; that is, an individually weak and highly vulnerable part of the body that receives the main blow of negative emotions. Following Alexander, George Engel (1977), founder of the biopsychosocial model of medicine, distinguishes resolving and delaying predisposing factors in the development of diseases. In his opinion, predisposition is a specific readiness, both congenital and (under certain conditions) acquired, that because of the traumatic situation resulted in an organic or neurotic disease.

This relationship between readiness (predisposition) and a stressful situation allows the scientists to form the model of diathesis–stress development of pathology that is central to this book. According to this concept, the combination of two main factors is necessary for the emergence of any disease: first, the biological diathesis (vulnerability, predisposition) already present, and secondly, the additional impact of stressors—in particular, unfavorable socio-psychological factors (Meehl P. E., 1962; Holmogorova A. B., Garanyan N. G., 1999; Tukaev R. D., 2012). At the same time, the "psycho-soma" union does not act as an alliance of separate parts, but as two sides of a single whole, and the level of biological diathesis is often determined by the frequency and intensity of previous stressful events.

Some scientists also distinguish psychosomatic diathesis, a disorganization of the mental adaptation of the individual to the external environment, which is the borderline state. Under the impact of external (in particular, stressful) and internal (genetically determined) causes, a disorder of adaptation can go into somatoform disorders, and then into psychosomatic disorders (Sidorov P. I., Novikova I. A., 2010; Ovsyannikov S. A., Tsygankov B. D., 2001). A. P. Kotsyubinskiy and colleagues (2013) talk about a specific category of people with a constitutionally determined vulnerability to psychosomatic diseases, which is understood as the clinically undetectable decrease in the resistance of certain somatic systems to stressful effects. According to S. A. Ovsyannikov and B. D. Tsygankov (2001), psychosomatic diathesis is a result of the combination of a "weak" type of the nervous system (expressed in a melancholic temperament against the background of sensitivity and a passive life position) and a general lowering of the biological energy in the organism.

As the name implies, psychosomatic diathesis includes mental diathesis, that is, a psychological predisposition to diseases. Its causes can be considered as (Gurvich I. N., 2000):

- macrosocial (social) factors that form the stress of the environment;

- intrapsychic (actual psychological) factors that create a perception of the social environment as threatening, or stressful, based on memory, thinking, and the characteristics of the motivational sphere of the individual;

- behavioral (outward, or externalized) factors, able to modify the nearest social environment in the direction of increasing or decreasing its stressogenicity. This can be also an ability to cope with stress;

- somatopsychic factors—the influence of the existing bodily pathology on the human psyche, distorting the self-perception and perception of the social environment.

As we shall see later, almost all of the above features of psychosomatic diathesis are also characteristic of cancer patients. In particular, S. A. Kulakov (2009a) and P. I. Sidorov and E. P. Sovershaeva (2015) mention the following factors of predisposition to oncological diseases in their synergistic biopsychosocial-spiritual model:

- in the somatogenic vector—hereditary burden;

- in the psychogenic—the premorbid features of the personality (character accentuation, personality disorder) plus psychophysiological features, that presuppose the presence of specific inherent characteristics, contributing to the development of the disease;

- in the sociogenic vector—family dysfunction, which forms the so-called "oncogenic family," where violations of family relationships and distribution of roles affecting the upbringing of the child in the family are noted;

- in the *noo-/animogenesis* vector—peculiarities of the self-concept (a set of personal representations of oneself) and spiritual–moral disharmony, arising due to deficit in or ambivalence of family relations, that create an either aware or unaware psycho-emotional tension.

German researchers H. J. F. Baltrusch and M. Waltz (1985) claim:

> Environmental stressors, as well as mediating variables at the cognitive, affective, behavioural and physiological levels of adaptation, are suggested as major components of a model of multidimensional pathology [of cancer].

All the above suggests that the diathesis–stress model of carcinogenesis, proposed by the prominent English psychologist Hans Eysenck and his German colleague Ronald Grossarth-Maticek (Grossarth-Maticek R. et al., 1994), is legitimate. In fact, it is based on the concept of psychosomatic diathesis.

It is interesting that as early as 1928 Georgy Bykhovskiy, a professor at Kiev's Clinical Institute mentioned in Chapter 1.2 as the inspirer of the first Ukrainian psycho-oncological study, wrote:

> For the development of cancer, a combination of several factors is necessary. Among the factors of paramount importance involved in the formation of cancer there are constitution and associated heredity, as well as the influence of various external stimuli. The constitution is in close connection with the endocrine glands. The system of endocrine glands, in turn, depends on the central nervous system. In this way, a connection is established between manifestations of tumors and the influence of the central nervous system.

Thus, the Ukrainian surgeon anticipated not only the diathesis–stress idea, but also the basic concept of modern psychoneuroendocrinology.

Among macrosocial factors of psychosomatic diathesis, it is necessary to single out disorders in children's attachment to parents and children's psychological traumas, which becomes the basis of dysontogenesis (in a broad sense, understood as a disorder of individual development of a person, from embryogenesis to childhood). Its consequences are inadequate functions of the neuro-endocrine-immune system, distortion of emotional and adaptive reactions in later life, and cognitive diathesis. The latter is explained as negative basic beliefs arising from distortion of thinking and manifested in cognitive mistakes: arbitrary reasoning, overgeneralization, polarized ("black and white") thinking, etc. (Beck A. T., 1979).

It is dysontogenesis, as follows from the large amount of data accumulated by science (both animal experiments and human observations), that creates a basic predisposition to cancer. Therefore, in this part, I focus on the consideration of disorders occurring during the individual development of the organism. There are two main periods of ontogeny:

1. Perinatal[1], which includes three stages:

- antenatal (or prenatal)–here predisposition is created by stresses and illnesses experienced by the mother during pregnancy;

- intranatal (from Latin intra—inside, during the actual delivery process)— predisposition is caused by complications of this process;

- neonatal (from Latin neo—new, occurring within 28 days after birth)— predisposition is due to separation from the mother, poor maternal care, eating disorders, and stresses and illnesses experienced by the mother.

2. Postnatal,[2] where the predisposition is created by stress caused by the same factors as in the neonatal period, as well as by disorders deriving from disturbances in the attachment to parents, childhood psychological traumas, and living conditions.

Such stressful events, especially during critical periods of early development, can lead to epigenetic changes in gene expression and various neuro-endocrine-immunological disorders. These changes, in later life, affect the protective functions of the body and its physical and mental development, and also lead to stress and disease susceptibility (Borghol N. et al., 2011; Lucassen P. et al., 2013).

Next we will consider what role epigenetic heredity, determined by the stresses experienced by parents, plays in the predisposition to cancer.

---

[1] Perinatal: occurring in the period around a birth.
[2] Postnatal: includes the early stage (up to a year) and the later stage (after a year).

Chapter 5

The Role of Heredity

> Do not teach your children,
> they will still be like you.
> Teach yourself.
> *English proverb*

From modern oncology it is known that tumors, regardless of location, can be both hereditary and non-hereditary—in other words, occur at random. Of all cases of cancer, hereditary forms constitute only 5%–10% of specific localizations (Belyalova N. S., Belyalov F. I., 2005).

At the heart of the development of any hereditary disease (including cancer) is a mutation, i.e. a change in the genes at different parts of the DNA or in chromosomes (in Chapter 19.5 we will look at the causes that cause mutations and make sure that their accumulation is largely related to acute and chronic stress). When parents pass their genetic information to their child at conception, they can also transmit mutated genes that can trigger the development of malignant tumors.

Such genetic information can accumulate in families, which leads to the emergence of the phenomenon of "family cancer." According to medical observations, about 18% of healthy people have two or more relatives with cancer (Akulenko L., 2004). At the same time, those who had cancer in the first line of kinship: parents and siblings, and in the second line: grandmothers, grandfathers, aunts, uncles, and cousins, are generally considered a risk group. The closer the degree of kinship with the cancer-stricken person, the higher the relative's risk of the disease—although until the time of the onset of cancer, this person is in this respect considered absolutely healthy. However, in fact, their body is already weakened; for example, in women who had cancer-stricken relatives in the first and second lines of kinship, protective immune functions were weakened, even taking into account the stress they underwent (Bovbjerg D. H., Valdimarsdottir H., 1993).

However, as early as 1928, the German professor Karl Bauer, who developed the mutational theory of tumor formation, prophetically stated: "There is no hereditary cancer transmission in the exact sense of this expression. ... It's about inheriting the tendency of tissues to form tumors under certain external conditions." It is interesting that in the same year in Ukraine, Professor Georgy Bykhovskiy recommended: "When collecting anamnesis in patients with malignant neoplasms, along with questions about heredity, it is necessary to raise the question of the mental experiences preceding the onset of this disease."

But, only recently medical genetics began to agree with Bauer's point of view, saying that in cases of "family cancer" there is no inheritance of the disease, but inheritance of an extremely high risk of oncological pathology, that is, "hereditary predisposition" (Gorbunova V. N., Imianitov E. N., 2007). (A similar opinion now extends to many basic somatic diseases, such as cardiovascular, endocrine, autoimmune, etc. Today they can rightfully be considered psychosomatic). The genetic component of the etiology and pathogenesis of such diseases is formed not by chromosomal or gene disorders (mutations), but by the individual features of the hereditary constitution. These features acquire a pathogenic manifestation only when combined with unfavorable environmental factors (Gorbunova V. N., Imyanitov E. N., 2007; Belyalova N. S., Belyalov F. I., 2005), which gives us the right to consider them from the point of view of the diathesis–stress model.

The illustration is the studies of W. A. Greene and S. N. Swisher (1969) on identical twins, one of whom in each pair was sick with leukemia. It was found that the sick siblings experienced frustration or loss before the onset of the disease, while those who did not fall ill had no such experience.

The data of Vernon Riley (1975) of the University of Washington are also indicative. During his experiments, he subjected a group of mice who were genetically predisposed to cancer to strong stress, while the control group of the same mice line was placed in the most comfortable conditions. As a result of experiments, 92% of stressed rodents got cancer, and only 7% of those who did not undergo stress did. Consequently, although both groups of mice had a genetic predisposition to cancer, stress significantly increased the frequency of its development. This suggests that the presence of even defective genes is not enough to get sick—one needs the influence of social factors.

To understand how these factors work, epigenetics will help us. This science, as we already know, involves the study of the influence of environmental factors, including stress, on the expression of genes. In the context of this chapter, it is especially important that epigenetic changes in gene activity, which occur under the influence of the environment (and in particular behavioral patterns), can be fixed in the genome and remain there for the rest of one's life. Moreover, they can be inherited by succeeding generations. Therefore, the inheritance of acquired characteristics, as claimed by Jean-Baptiste Lamarck as early as the beginning of the 19th century (he was criticized up to the mid-20th century for his "reactionary" anti-Darwin doctrine), actually exists. Thus, our health and even the health of our children and grandchildren largely depends on what has happened in the lives of our parents and ancestors. The potentially dangerous epigenetic changes, inherited by us, can "sleep" to a certain point and be fully activated both in childhood and in adulthood—we will discover the origin of these reasons.

These pathophysiological epigenetic effects, mediated by DNA methylation, histone modification, and the synthesis of microRNA, can occur even in the prenatal period of human life. It becomes obvious that there is a transgenerational memory of the fetal experience, which can be transmitted over several generations (Matthews S. G., Phillips D. I., 2010). Also epigenetic modifications accumulate throughout the stressful life of a person, especially in childhood. This can largely explain the mechanisms of hereditary transmission of a predisposition to cancer. Since DNA methylation, for example, plays a leading role in inhibiting the activity of proto-oncogenes (Gattoni S. et al., 1982, Feinberg A. P., Vogelstein B., 1983), so that in healthy cells oncogenes "sleep." Accordingly, a decrease in the level of DNA methylation and subsequent deactivation of tumor suppressor genes promote the conversion of proto-oncogenes into oncogenes (Daura-Oller E. et al., 2009; Stepanenko A. A., Kavsan V. M., 2012). This, as I have already noted, occurs at the stages of initiation and promotion of tumor growth. Therefore, it is natural that people who are predisposed to oncological diseases show a highly significant correspondence between the reduction of methylation of certain DNA loci and the expression of key cancer genes (Heyn H. et al., 2014). The same changes in methylation have been found in many human tumors: the stomach, kidney, rectum, liver, pancreas, lungs, and cervix (Feinberg A. P., Tycko B., 2004).

A new step in understanding the mechanism of carcinogenesis was the discovery that genetic mutations in normal cells are actually preceded by epigenetic changes. After conducting research on the matter, American scientists from the Center for Epigenetics at Johns Hopkins University and Howard Hughes Medical Institute, together with Swedish researchers from Uppsala University, concluded that cancer develops in three stages. Initially, under the influence of epigenetic factors, the normal regulation of the cell genome is disrupted, which gives rise to a predisposition in the cells to cancer transformation. Only then, at the second stage, a mutation occurs in these epigenetically changed cells, which was previously considered as the beginning of the development of cancer. In the next stage, the so-called genome instability is formed, which leads to tumor growth (Feinberg A. P. et al., 2006). This conclusion was supported by the research of other scientists (Karpinets T. V., Foy B. D., 2005; Tao Y. et al., 2011).

Epigenetic changes in cells undergoing stress are very similar to those found in both precancerous cells and cells in early stages of cancer. In particular, many studies have shown an epigenetic suppression of the activity of genes responsible for stopping cell division and their apoptosis (self-destruction). Early reduction in gene methylation is associated with the effect of transcription factors involved in cell proliferation, in particular c-myc and c-fos factors (see Chapter 19) (Karpinets T. V., Foy B. D., 2005). In the following chapters, we will see that stresses and psychological traumas, experienced throughout life, leave epigenetic traces in the human genome and complicate the way a body responds to subsequent stresses (accumulation effect).

From these positions, analyzing which unfavorable epigenetic information is transmitted by inheritance and creates a predisposition to cancer, it can be concluded that these are the imprints of stresses and psychic traumas experienced by parents. This conclusion is supported by the following studies carried out by psychologists and related specialists.

English psychoanalyst John Bowlby and his followers Mary Ainsworth and Mary Main, in the middle of the twentieth century, developed the theory of attachment. They considered the need for close emotional relations as the central link in the development of the personality from the beginning to the end of life. As a result of their research, it is convincingly proven that disturbance of the attachment of children to the mother has a psychotraumatic effect and distorts the child's ability to regulate distress and interactions with other people. Authors have identified such basic types of attachment as secure and insecure, and among the latter type are avoidant, ambivalent, and disorganized styles, which we will discuss in more detail below (Ainsworth M. D. S., Bowlby J., 1991, Bowlby J., 1984; Main M., 1995). At the moment it is important for us to understand that secure attachment arises from sensitive and responsive upbringing and establishes the child's sense of safety and the perception of other people as caring and reliable, and him- or herself as worthy of love and care. On the contrary, insecure attachment arises in children who were rejected or ignored, so as a result they consider the world dangerous, others not caring and unreliable, and themselves unattractive and unworthy.

In the context of this chapter, it is significant that children who have had complex and psychotraumatic relationships with their parents (in other words, insecure attachments of a disorganized style) have a high chance of maintaining such a disorganized state even in adulthood, unless they get a chance to properly cure and resolve their traumas. Consequently, they are very likely to create disorganized relationships with their own children. For example, scientists at the Oregon Social Research Center in the United States found that if a woman suffered severe physical abuse as a child and retains the unresolved emotional memory of this violence, the likelihood of her abusing her own children is very high (Pears K. C., Capaldi D. M., 2001).

A mother's unresolved psychic trauma, especially with an insecure attachment style, prevents her from reacting sensitively to the child. This, in turn, contributes to the development of insecure attachment in the child of such mother (Iyengar U. et al., 2014). Psychiatrists from Boston, MA, found that post-traumatic stress disorder (PTSD) in a mother having a child around 6 months old leads to the formation of this child's insecure attachment by the age of 13 months. In later life, insecure attachment in these children also leads to an increased risk of developing PTSD (Enlow M. et al., 2014).

Thus, the types of attachment and the nature of the response to stress can be transferred from one generation to another. Studies have shown that in 70% of cases there is a correspondence between the type of attachment of parents and the type of attachment of their children (secure, avoiding, ambivalent). This correlation becomes even more significant (75%) when only such categories of attachment as "secure" and "insecure" are compared (van IJzendoorn M., 1995). Research conducted in University of Quebec shows that the majority (83%) of infants of abused and neglected mothers were classified as insecure, and a significant proportion (44%) manifested attachment disorganization. There was a strong correlation between mother and child attachment, indicative of intergenerational transmission of attachment (Berthelot N. et al., 2015).

One of the biological routes by which insecure patterns of attachment are transmitted from one generation to another is disruptions of the hypothalamic-pituitary-adrenal (HPA) axis and of cortisol production by early experiences of children having an insecure attachment to mother (Ben-Dat Fisher D. et al., 2007; Yehuda R., LeDoux J., 2007).

Also according to the theory of family systems, specific basic ways of relating between mother, father, and child actually reproduce the history of family relationships of past generations, and are highly likely to be reproduced in future generations. Therefore, many behavioral patterns, in particular alcoholism, incest, physical symptoms, violence, and suicides, are repeated from generation to generation (Varga A. Y., Khamitova I. Yu., 2005). The Soviet scientist A. I. Zakharov (1982), studying neuroses in children and adolescents, came to the conclusion that these distortions are usually a clinical and psychological reflection of the family's problems even in three generations: grandparents, parents, and children. The same picture is also noted for bodily dysfunctions; for example, when studying the psychovegetative syndrome, it is found that the child's organism essentially "copies" the illnesses and disorders of the parents, most often of the mother or relatives along the maternal line (Gindikin V. Y., 2000).

This is true for cancer patients, as well. In particular, women with breast cancer, whose relationships with their mothers were characterized by excessive self-sacrifice against the background of repressed aggression, also manifested such self-sacrificing behavior and overreaction to their children, especially daughters, thus forming in them, already in the third generation, a high degree of dependence on the mother (Cutler M., 1954). These data is confirmed by O.

D. Rozhkova (2015)—in female patients, she most often found a closed family system, where the accumulating anxiety circulated inside and was not released outside. This weakens the individual's *self* and potentiates the processes of extreme co-dependence in the family. Therefore, often in several generations of a family of cancer patients, the author could observe a mechanism for transferring a template of co-dependent relationships. One of the pioneers of psycho-oncology, Lawrence LeShan (1989), who has been working in this field for more than fifty years, believes that the emergence of cancer in several generations of one family is associated more with a constantly increasing emotional burden than with genetic manifestations.

Another outstanding psycho-oncologist, surgeon, and oncologist Bernie Siegel (1998) writes:

> …negative conditioning is all too common. Over the years I've found that my patients tend to get the same diseases as their parents and to die at the same age. I think conditioning is at least as much a factor as genetic predisposition (I call it 'psychological genetics'). … Psychological 'genes' can be as helpful or as damaging as physical genes. I often see this when I have drawings from a parent and child who have each developed cancer. How incredible it is to see the similarity. One is often a duplicate of the other, although they were made years apart—neither patient having seen the other's drawing. A hopeless, helpless parent produces a hopeless, helpless child.

Modern research indicates that the transfer of psychological heredity occurs not only after the birth of the child, owing to conditioning, or, in psychological terms, the imprinting on the child of its parents' behavior, but also by the transmission of epigenetic information in the process of conception.

For example, an analysis of the methylation of specific promoter regions of the genome (from which gene expression begins) of immune T-cells in adult men with a history of experiencing chronic physical aggression between the ages of 6 and 15 years concluded that 448 promoters of genes associated with aggressive behavior had a pattern of methylation different from the control group of men without traumatic childhoods (Provencal N. et al., 2014). There is every reason to believe that this methylation pattern will be transmitted to these men's children, as another study found a changed character of gene methylation in adults whose parents experienced a high level of stress in their early childhood (Essex M. et al., 2013).

According to scientists from the Donders Institute for Brain, Cognition and Behaviour (The Netherlands), approximately half of the people examined have an epigenetic modification of α2b-adrenergic *receptors*, which causes their amygdalas to respond more actively to emotional stimuli. Thus parents, by passing the imprints of their stresses to their children, fixed in the state of gene regulation, make their children more prone to experiencing distress (Cousijn H. et al., 2010).

The noted cell biologist and science popularizer Bruce Lipton (2016) reflects on this connection that parents act as genetic engineers for their children in the months before conception:

> In the final stages of egg and sperm maturation, a process called genomic imprinting adjusts the activity of specific groups of genes that will shape the character of the child yet to be conceived. Research suggests that what is going on in the lives of the parents during the process of genomic imprinting has a profound influence on the mind and body of their child—a scary thought, given how unprepared most people are to have a baby.

In animal experiments, it has been also confirmed that the behavioral characteristics of both mothers and fathers can be epigenetically transmitted from generation to generation.

For example, Israeli scientists subjected female rats to chronic stress and afterwards crossbred them with unstressed males. It was found that the synthesis of specific *messenger RNA* in the brain and ovicells of female rats increased. (Through the system of hormone mediators—corticoliberin and adrenocorticotropic hormone—this messenger regulates the level of one of the most important stress hormones: cortisol). However, in the progeny of the stressed females, an increase in the synthesis of this RNA is observed already at birth, together with behavioral disorders, such as anxiety and learning disabilities. Thus, the stress of mothers was transmitted epigenetically (Zaidan H. et al., 2013).

But fathers, as it turned out, also transmit their stress to children. Katharine Gapp and her colleagues from the Institute for Brain Research in Zurich (2014) modeled chronic stress for the offspring of mice. When they grew up, their behavior showed signs of depression, as well as impaired glucose metabolism. If these mice were crossed with ordinary mice, their offspring (not only children but also grandchildren) also showed signs of depression, and also had problems with glucose metabolism. Thus, changes in the behavior and metabolism of the fathers were inherited. Epigenetic transmitters in this case are regulatory *micro-RNA* from the spermatozoa of the fathers. On the other hand, researchers from the Institute of Medical Sciences in Delhi found that oxidative intracellular stress (also takes place during psychological stress—see Chapter 19), which occurs in the spermatozoa of the fathers, causes DNA damage and changes in its methylation. This activates proto-oncogenes and contributes to the occurrence of cancer in the children of such fathers (Dada R. et al., 2015).

These experiments allow a better understanding of the results of studies conducted in the National Charrette Oncology Institute in Israel. They demonstrated that women with breast cancer whose parents survived genocide during the Second World War react much more strongly to the distress of having the disease, to the extent of developing psychological pathologies, than women whose parents did not experience genocide (Baider L. et al., 2014). In general, scientists note today that most recent investigations into cancer etiology have identified a key role played by epigenetics (Wu Y. et al., 2015).

Does this mean that a person is doomed to get cancer before even being conceived in a given family, if his or her future parents are experiencing a high level of stress? Fortunately, no. Epigenetic heredity is only one of the bricks that form the basis of predisposition to cancer. For this predisposition to gain "full power," it is necessary for its other components (which we will talk about in the following sections) to be present, especially psychotraumatic factors in early childhood.

Chapter 6

Pregnancy (The Prenatal Period)

B ernie Siegel (1998) writes:
    Psychologists are now learning that infants are far more perceptive than previously imagined, and I wouldn't be surprised if cancer in early childhood was linked to messages of parental conflict or disapproval perceived in the womb.

Research in recent decades has confirmed the validity of Dr. Siegel's assumption, expressed by him for the first time in 1986. For example, studies on identical twins, conserved blood from newborns, and blood from the umbilical cord taken at birth, showed that chromosomal translocations (rearrangements in chromosomes that cause mutations) that precede childhood leukemia occur while the fetus is developing in the uterus. Subsequent genetic disorders, usually caused by a distorted immune response to infection, are secondary factors in the development of this disease (Greaves M., 2005, 2006). In 2010, in an article published in the journal *Future of Oncology*, Dr. Logan Spector of the Department of Pediatrics at the University of Minnesota stated: "We now strongly suspect that most cases of childhood cancer are initiated some time prior to birth."

The growing amount of scientific evidence suggests that the sources of increased susceptibility for many common and complex diseases can be traced to the prenatal period of life. This contributed to the formulation of the theory of the "prenatal origin of non-hereditary pathologies of functional systems" (Barker D. J. P. et al., 1998) and the concept of "biological imprinting"—the formation of health and predisposition to diseases in early ontogenesis (Hertzman C., 1999). In the 1980s, the International Association of Prenatal and Perinatal Psychology and Medicine was established to study the patterns of human development during and after pregnancy and childbirth, as well as their impact on the entire life (www.birthpsychology.com).

The developing fetus is very sensitive to changes in the internal (maternal) and external environment, occurring during important periods of cellular reproduction, differentiation, and maturation. If a pregnant woman is under stress, endotoxicosis occurs in her body, and the parameters of the electroencephalogram, immune systems, hemostasis, and lipid peroxidation are significantly disturbed (Malgina G. B., 2003), which undoubtedly affects the fetus. In animal experiments, an elevated level of maternal stress hormones during pregnancy results in impaired immune system development in monkeys (Coe C. L. et al., 1996) and causes oxidative damage to mitochondrial DNA in the hippocampus of newborn rats, together with impaired cognitive functions (Song L. et al., 2009). Such changes can lead to functional and/or structural disturbances in the functioning of the hypothalamic-pituitary-adrenal and reproductive systems; GABAergic and opioid regulatory systems in the corresponding cells; and tissues and organs of the fetus. This determines the subsequent state of health and susceptibility to disease in adulthood (Gluckman P. D., Hanson M. A., 2004; Reznikov A. G. et al., 2004; Shonkoff J. P. et al., 2009).

A mother's stress during pregnancy, especially associated with fears, affects the development of the fetus and subsequently alters the excitability of the infant, as well as leading to the weakening of his ability to control behavior (Rieger M. et al., 2004). Chronic maternal anxiety can cause an increased stillbirth rate, fetal growth retardation, and altered placental morphology (Relier J. P., 2001). A study of the experience of pregnancy in women whose adolescent children suffered from psychogenic disorders ranging from somatoform autonomic dysfunctions to psychosomatic disorders (experimental group) was conducted in Kirov's Regional Children Hospital (Russia). In comparison with the mothers of healthy adolescents (control), researchers revealed up to a twofold prevalence of various negative perinatal factors in the mothers of adolescents in the experimental group. They were: toxicosis during pregnancy, the threat of abortion, traumatic experiences and stresses, unwanted pregnancy, and unfavorable prenatal factors (Marincheva L. P. et al., 2012).

More and more data demonstrate that the stress that occurs during pregnancy has long-term effects on health and human behavior owing to changes in the epigenome (Bernal A. J., Jirtle R. L, 2010; Bock J. et al., 2015). For instance, the work of scientists from the University of Constance (Germany) revealed that in adolescents between ten and nineteen years of age whose mothers experienced stress during pregnancy owing to violent actions by their husbands or partners, the methylation level of the cortisol receptor gene was changed, which affected the concentration of this stress hormone in the body (Radtke K. M. et al., 2011). Anxiety in the mother during late pregnancy leads to an increased content of saliva cortisol in their children at ten years of age (O'Connor T. G. et al., 2005).

Studies conducted in the Department of Pediatrics at the University of California by Dr. Sonja Entringer and co-workers (2011), found that young people whose mothers experienced severe stress during pregnancy have a significant decrease in the length of chromosomal *telomeres*, a factor more pronounced in girls. Scientists also found that young people who perceived maternal stress had a reduced sensitivity to insulin and increased level of C-protein, indicating the inflammatory process (Entringer S. et al., 2010). A similar increased level of C-protein was detected by other researchers in people aged twenty-five whose mothers suffered from depression during pregnancy (Plant D. T. et al., 2013). Also, depression and excessive anxiety in pregnant women lead to increased cortisol in the urine of their children at the age of fifteen (O'Donnell K. J. et al., 2013). As we shall expand upon later, the shortening of telomeres, metabolic and immune disorders, and the inflammatory process are predictive signs of the risk of cancer and premature death, as well as aging.

As a result of these and other studies, Dr. S. Entringer and co-workers formed a hypothesis of the developmental origins of health and disease (DOHAD). According to this approach, an increased risk of diseases in adulthood is due to an unfavorable environment in early fetal and infant development. It reprograms the epigenome, alters cellular and tissue responses to normal physiological signals, and increases the susceptibility of the organism to diseases (Swanson J. M. et al., 2009). Scientists believe that such reprogramming, occurring during the development of the organism, creates the risk of cardiovascular, metabolic, and oncological diseases. In particular, the impact of damaging factors, such as stress hormones, during critical developmental periods can alter the course of gene expression in tissues later in life and makes them more susceptible to carcinogenic agents (Walker C. L., Ho S. M., 2012).

It is especially important that a child in the womb can experience not only the reflected stress of the mother, arising from external psycho-traumatic events, but also to experience his own psycho-emotional stress, when sensing a negative attitude from the mother and others, or the mother's thoughts about abortion. The research of G. I. Brekhman (2011) in the interdisciplinary clinical center of the University of Haifa (Israel) showed that such stress in the fetus can distort its mental and physical development. The perceived and recorded emotional experiences of the mother can leave a deep imprint on the unconscious memory of the fetus and be introjected as its own. After birth, in the process of the child's growth, this psychic trauma can control his thinking, emotions, and behavior and manifest in the form of various psychological and psychosomatic problems.

Graham Gorman (1997), examining people's perinatal memories about their mothers' experiences of illnesses, accidents, anxiety, or disasters during pregnancy, indicates that the fetus is capable of experiencing the horror of extinction. This trauma is imprinted in the mind of the embryo and remains forever, as a kind of warning. When an event in later life unconsciously reminds a person of this trauma, a defensive reaction arises, as well as anxious states, low self-esteem, and reduced immunity to various diseases.

These results are confirmed by the Greek psychiatrist Athanassios Kafkalides (1980), who used the psychedelic LSD to uncover the unconscious of his patients. He compared the information he obtained with the patients' mothers' stories. During the sessions, these people had access to the suffering they had experienced in their mother's womb, and began to understand that these emotions are a memory of the mother's feelings. Particularly difficult experiences arose in patients who were unwanted, rejected by their mother, which they had not considered before the sessions. Passage through such experiences produced a powerful therapeutic effect. Similar results were obtained by the British psychiatrist Frank Lake (1980), who believed that the most important thing for the subsequent mental health of a person is how his parents perceive the fact of pregnancy and what happens in its first trimester.

The case of my patient K., who suffered from depressive and psychosomatic disorders, illustrates these observations. In the process of trance therapy, he experienced a presence of himself in a limited space, like a mother's womb, with a strong fear and a vision of the color red around him. In a frank conversation with his mother some time after the session (the conversation went with great difficulty, as he spent all his life inexplicably distancing himself from her), it turned out that in the first month of pregnancy she had tried to give herself an abortion. As a result, his twin sibling had died, while he had survived.

The combination of psychogenic symptoms arising from the influence of negative emotions, thoughts, and behavior of the mother during pregnancy is called prenatal syndrome. It determines the formation of specific characteristics of the personality and the initial level of its self-regulation and stress-resistance (Rozhkova O. D., Druzhkova E. A., 2003). The average psychological portrait of an unwanted child includes such characteristics as decreased self-esteem and cheerfulness, high dependency, increased sensitivity, malevolence, poorly formed feelings of attachment and responsiveness, latent depression, increased need for recognition, neuroses, and psychopathic traits (Brekhman G. I, 2011). As evident, these personality traits largely correspond to the features of psychosomatic patients in general, and, as will be noted later, cancer patients in particular.

Thus, under the influence of early stressful effects perceived by the fetus, a neurobiological pattern of increased reactivity to stress is established for a lifetime—in other words, stress-vulnerability. This is a diathesis, mentioned above, which forms a predisposition to psychosomatic diseases, and, consequently, to cancer. There are now confirmations of this conclusion both in animal experiments and in epidemiological studies in humans.

For example, in the Oncology Research Institute in St. Petersburg (Russia), rats were exposed to lighting stress during pregnancy and feeding periods (they were kept for twenty-four hours in a lighted room and afterwards were transferred to their usual regime), and simultaneously treated with carcinogen N-nitrosoethylurea. It was found that even a short-term exposure to constant light stimulated the growth of tumors in the nervous system and kidneys in the offspring of rats that underwent stress, compared to the offspring of rats kept under standard conditions (Beniashvili D. S. et al., 2001). Experiments at the medical center of Georgetown University in the USA on mice, genetically predisposed to cancer, demonstrated that the stress of pregnant females, caused by injections and other surgical manipulations, as well as the direct administration of stress hormones (glucocorticoids), leads to a twofold increase in the incidence of *neuroblastoma* in mouse cubs after birth, compared to the offspring of females not exposed to stress (Hong S. H. et al., 2015).

The large-scale work carried out by Justo Bermejo, together with colleagues from Sweden, at the German Cancer Research Center in Heidelberg involved an analysis of the Swedish national database of families with cancer. Among 11.5 million people there were two identified groups: 1.2 million cancer patients, 39,000 of whose mothers had suffered the death of a parent during pregnancy. This degree of prenatal maternal stress led to a significant increase in the incidence of cancer in the children in later life. In particular, 217 people of an average age of twenty-two years had tumors of various localizations: thirty-one children of an average age of six years developed acute leukemia, twenty people became ill with Hodgkin's *lymphoma* with the group's average age at twenty years, etc. The trimester of pregnancy when the death of the parent occurred did not significantly affect the specificity of the appearance of cancer in children. The authors suggest that at least in cases of leukemia and lymphoma, a decrease in immunity in mothers caused by severe stress can activate carcinogenic viruses in them and initiate cancer development in children (Bermejo J. L. et al., 2007).

In a similar study performed in Denmark, 9,795 cancer patients were identified among 6 million children. It was found that the children of mothers who had undergone severe stress (the loss of a husband or another child during pregnancy, or in the first year of their child's life) had an average 30% higher risk of developing cancer of various localizations, with a predominance of non-Hodgkin's lymphoma, liver, and testicular cancer (Li J. et al., 2012).

Chapter 7

The Process of Childbirth

Childbirth affects a person's future life. Even if a child is lucky enough to have a favorable intrauterine period, the process of delivery becomes the first serious stress experienced by every person.

The suffering experienced by the child at the time of birth was known even by the doctors of antiquity. Gampopa, an outstanding Tibetan lama, philosopher, and doctor of the eleventh century, wrote in his work, *Ornament of Precious Liberation*: "At birth it feels like a cow that is flayed alive, and as if stung by a wasp" (Clifford T., 1996).

A student of Sigmund Freud, Otto Rank, in his book *The Trauma of Birth* (2010, first published in 1924) wrote that a newborn baby, appearing outside the mother's womb, is experiencing the most severe shock of his entire life. Having lost the "paradise situation," where all his needs were satisfied immediately and without effort, he, as he grows, will also experience separation in the future as a very painful and frightening adversity. In Rank's opinion, the entire psychological life of a person is determined by primary anxiety and primary suppression, conditioned by birth trauma, so most of the events perceived by him as traumatic become pathogenic owing to their similarity to biological birth.

An important contribution to understanding how the conditions of intrauterine development and the process of birth are reflected in the psyche has been made by the outstanding psychotherapist, one of the founders of transpersonal psychology, Stanislav Grof (1985, 1996). He created the concept of perinatal matrices: the deep structures of the unconscious psyche, which contain information about the experiences and sensations of the body from the moment of conception to the completion of birth. Under normal circumstances, a person is not aware of this information, but it is able to determine his worldview, his disposition toward other people, the ratio in him of optimism and pessimism, his trust in himself, his ability to cope with problems, and even his strategy for life. In altered, trance states of consciousness, a person can recall and re-experience his intrauterine sensations and memories of birth complications and traumas. These sensations can lead to a curative effect, for psychosomatic diseases as well. Grof made many of his discoveries while working with cancer patients during sessions using the psychoactive drug LSD-25, which he later replaced with a special trance technique "holotropic breathing."

Each of the perinatal matrices refers to a specific period of the fetus's stay in the uterus and its experiences. For example, the first basic perinatal matrix (BPM-1) corresponds to the period from the moment of conception to the beginning of labor (prenatal). When the course of a pregnancy is favorable and the mother experiences no serious stresses and illnesses, feelings of comfort, satisfaction, tranquility, security, and unity with the mother and the world remain in the person's subconscious and, accordingly, are projected onto his or her later life. Unfavorable pregnancy—in Grof's terms, "bad womb"—can be accompanied by feelings of isolation, fear, alertness, paranoia, hatred, and can result in biological disorders, including those precancerous ones described in the previous chapter.

Of special interest to us is BMP-2, which is formed at the very beginning of labor, when the fetus is periodically compressed by uterine contractions, but the cervix is closed and there is no way out. The aggravations of this period depends on its duration, intensity, and complications (excess fetal size and/or abnormal position, the mother's pelvis being too narrow, insufficient intensity of labor). If also the mother's attitude to the unborn child or to the process of labor is distinctly negative or ambivalent, then the fear and confusion of the inexperienced mother could mean the fetus feels insecurity, anxiety, impending danger, aggression, fear for its life, horror, unbearable feelings and hopelessness. In the future, this could lead to an inclination to anxiety disorder, despair, depression, lack of initiative, inability to enjoy life and a loss of interest in it, and to the suppression of sexual desires.

On the somatic level, BPM-2 can lead to general motor retardation, sensations of constriction and limitation, tension, pressure and suffocation, headaches, heart disorders, constipation, and loss of interest in food and sex. This matrix reflects a highly stressful situation, which, according to Grof, forms in the sufferer a stereotypical psychological reaction of "no escape." It creates the basis for unpleasant life situations, when irresistible and destructive forces press on a passive individual who also feels helpless, to combine in his or her subconscious to form a *system of condensed experience*. BMP-2 in transpersonal experiences can manifest itself in one's memories of helplessness in the case of psychological frustrations, feelings of abandonment, emotional rejection or isolation, threatening events, and situations of repression in a closed family. As we will note further, such experiences are characteristic of oncological patients.

The third perinatal matrix corresponds to the stage of biological birth when uterine contractions continue, but the cervix has already been opened, which allows the child to move along the birth canal. If this period is excessively long or pathologically severe, accompanied by a strong mechanical squeezing, approaching choking, the fetus goes through a desperate struggle for survival. It accumulates a huge tension and aggressiveness, waiting for an ensuing release. This reservoir of delayed emotions can subsequently become the basis not only of primary aggression and violent manifestations, but also of various psychopathological abnormalities. On the physical level, it causes tremors, convulsions, hypertension, and bronchial asthma. At the same time, during BMP-3, the situation no longer seems as hopeless as that of BMP-2, as the child takes an active part in what is happening, and feels that her suffering has a certain direction and purpose. This becomes for her the first experience of conscious passage of the path, the experience of struggle, movement, and progress.

BPM-4 is associated with separation from the mother and the completion of the child's delivery, when the movement through the labor canal reaches its apex, and the painful process of the struggle for birth is over. The peak of excitement, aggression, pain, and tension is followed by unexpected relief and relaxation. According to Grof, this is the phase of experiencing death and rebirth. Depending on the complexity of the course of this stage, people can recall during therapy the feelings of liberation, acceptance, love, salvation and redemption of sins, as well as feelings of resentment, bewilderment, rejection, collapse, emotional death, defeat, and eternal damnation. In general, the fourth matrix determines the future experience of situations characterized by a sense of escape from danger.

Currently, the process of birth is considered one of the factors in the regulation of the epigenome. H. G. Dahlen and colleagues (2013) proposed the hypothesis of the epigenetic impact of childbirth (EPIIC). According to this, adverse events during the labor period (the use of antibiotics, synthetic oxytocin used to stimulate labor, and caesarean section) can modulate the processes of epigenetic regulation and affect health in later life. The authors suggest that the changes (both increase and decrease) in epinephrine, cortisol, and oxytocin levels throughout the process of birth can cause abnormal epigenetic reprogramming, which in turn leads to a failure in the expression of genes in later life.

Also, there has recently been greater scientific attention paid to the negative consequences of caesarean sections. The usage of this method has been increasing dramatically throughout the world. Children born via this operation may have brain function changes that result in sensory impairments, and difficulties in learning and interaction with the mother (Huang X. et al., 2004). Their immune functions are disrupted and the risk of a number of diseases such as asthma, allergy, type 1 diabetes, obesity, gastroenteritis, *celiac disease*, multiple sclerosis, leukemia, and testicular cancer increases (Dahlen H. G. et al., 2013). The study of stem cells from the umbilical cords of babies born by caesarean section showed that in comparison with natural-born children, epigenetic regulation of about 350 DNA regions, including genes known for their participation in the processes that control metabolism and immune defense, is altered (Almgren M. et al., 2014).

At the same time, it must be understood that the heavy emotions and bodily sensations experienced in the process of psychological birth trauma create only a new layer of predisposition, another potential source of mental and bodily problems. Whether a specific pathology will develop, and how serious it will be, are determined by already existing epigenetic heredity, the degree of dysfunction in prenatal development, and the child's future life.

Chapter 8

The Postpartum Period (Postnatal)

The trajectory of later development is shaped fundamentally
by the ways in which the child first learns
(or fails to learn) to manage emotions.
Attachment relationships are the school
in which this emotional learning originally occurs.
Dr. Peter Costello,
Attachment-Based Psychotherapy

The epoch-defining works of Sigmund Freud have proved the crucial importance of developmental conditions in early childhood, as well as showing how motivations and needs influence the formation of a person's character. Thanks to Freud, psychologists began to understand the extreme vulnerability of our psyche in early childhood and the importance of early experiences, especially negative ones, that form the basic structure of the personality.

Our knowledge in this area has expanded on another important discovery of Stanislav Grof (1985, 1996)—a demonstration of how, on the basis of perinatal matrices, the so-called systems of condensed experience (COEX) are subsequently formed. Grof found that the emotionally important events of a person's life are imprinted in his memory, forming specific groups that accumulate a similar experience. That is, memories related to different periods of life, but with similar acting factors, and especially with similar emotional content, are concentrated in closely related clots in the subconscious. This is how COEX emerges.

In accordance with their emotional content, Grof identified two types of COEX. Positive systems are associated with pleasant experiences. People in whom they predominate are in a state of emotional well-being, act in an optimal way, and are able to enjoy themselves and the world. Negative systems unite unpleasant and psychotraumatic memories, and people in whom these predominate perceive themselves and the world from a pessimistic point of view. Such people often remain in a state of depression, anxiety, or are under the influence of a certain emotional distress, depending on the nature and content of the current COEX. The resulting system of condensed experience is not a fixed, rigid structure, but it is capable of changing the way of functioning under the influence of various psychological or physiological influences.

The concept of negative COEX explains coherently how and why intrauterine and psychotraumatic stresses become the nucleus around which the personality of the psychosomatic type eventually forms. According to Stanislav Grof (1996), life brings a lot of emotional experiences, and some of them, one way or another, resemble the central experience. Thanks to the analytical and synthetic work of memory, these experiences are included in the COEX on the basis of identical components or common similarities:

> In the earliest stages of development, the child is a more or less passive victim of the environment and usually has no active role in the core experiences that would be worth consideration. Later on, this situation changes, and the individual gradually becomes more and more instrumental in structuring his interpersonal relations and his general life experiences. Once the foundations of a COEX system are laid, they seem to influence the subject in regard to his perception of the environment, his experiencing of the world, his attitudes, and his behavior.

Thus, if a child experiences stress after birth, especially in addition to pregnancy or labor suffering, the content of his negative COEX will accumulate, while the health deteriorates. Even at the age of one, children are able to "mirror" maternal stress, just as in the womb; when the mother returns to the child in a negative emotional state after a stressful situation, which is reflected in her rapid heartbeat, within a few minutes the baby also develops a rapid heart rate, in proportion to the magnitude of maternal stress (Waters S. F. et al., 2014). In addition, a severely negative state in the mother affects the neuroendocrine system of the infant, weakening the diurnal rhythm of cortisol fluctuations and disrupting the symmetry of the electroencephalogram. Such dependence can exist up to the seventh year of a child's life (Brooker R. J. et al., 2015).

Stressful situations in the family at the time of a child's birth are created by many factors. The main ones are prolonged family conflict, frequent quarrels or domestic violence; the death of a parent, sibling, family member or a close friend; divorce of parents or their decision to live separately; chronic family poverty; a mother with a low level of education; severe and average severity of perinatal complications; low birth weight; genetic disorders and delays in child development; psychopathology or asociality of parents; their negative experience in parenting or its complete absence; and low intellectual development of the parents and their "difficult" temperament.

Other sources of stress for the child are:

- long separation in the first year of life with the mother or the main person caring for the child,
- the birth of a younger sibling sooner than two years after the birth of this child,
- severe or chronic physical illness of the child,
- a somatic or mental illness of one of the parents,
- alcohol or drug addiction of one of the parents,
- a brother or sister with a disability or serious impairment of behavior and learning,
- the absence of a father,
- the repeated marriage of the parent and the appearance of a stepfather or stepmother,
- change of residence, especially placement in a foster family or shelter,
- loss of work or lack of permanent work for parents,
- pregnancy in adolescence (Barrett H., 2003; Archakova T. O., 2009).

In the national epidemiological studies of the population, conducted in the United States during the years 1990–1992 and 2001–2003, it was found that from 53.4% to 74.4% of the respondents experienced at least one stressful event in childhood (under 18). Among the total, 23.2% of people reported only one stress, 16.1% reported two, and 35% reported three or more stressful events (Kessler R. C. et al., 1997).

The combination of several stresses enhances their damaging effects. The repeated and often unexpected stress forms an appropriate COEX and a state of increased "readiness for fight or flight" in the child's body, that is, the physiological picture of chronic stress that I described in Chapter 3.2. Studies at the University of Florida found that if three or more serious stressful events occur in early childhood, children have then a sixfold increase in the likelihood of their developing mental or physical disorders and learning difficulties (Bright M. A. et al., 2014). One of the reasons for this is an increased level of the stress hormone cortisol in the bodies of children in such families, which drastically inhibits their immune responses (Carlsson E. et al., 2014). At the psychological level, these negative experiences lead to the emerging of "accumulated trauma," manifested in the loss of the child's confidence in himself, others, and life, as well as a hidden, deeply ingrained sense of inadequacy and inequality (Lourie J. B., 1996).

8.1. The Role of Disorders of Parent–Child Relationships in Pathology

The main source of stress for the child, first and foremost, is his parents. The prominent American psychoanalyst, physician, and psychologist Karen Horney

(1994) writes that "the main evil" in the development of the child is a lack of genuine warmth and affection, arising from the inability of parents to demonstrate love due to their own neuroses. Freud's follower, renowned English child psychiatrist and psychoanalyst Donald Winnicott (1953), in his studies discovered the importance of the mother and the child's educators in developing his ability to respond to stress. In particular, the failure of the mother at the earliest stages of a child's growth can lead to subsequent severe mental disorders, while a "good-enough mother," who listens to the needs of the child and provides support to him, forms the child's ability to fight the frustrations of adulthood.

Material presented earlier mentioned the elaborations of the English psychoanalyst John Bowlby and his followers in the field of disorders of children's attachment. Today, this direction is getting increasing attention from psychologists. Child psychiatrists, who use this theory in practice, argue that it is the experience of parent–child relationships of the first year of life (which creates a specific type of attachment) that determines the psychological, social, and personal development of the child throughout his later life. During this period, the sense of existential (basic, connected not with some concrete life events, but with the very essence of a person, the meaning of his life) safety is either fixed or broken, the same occurs with the skills of solving difficult situations, and for infants this is the core process of survival and the formation of primary relations. This becomes the basis of the mental health of the developing personality (Pilyagina G. Y., Dubrovskaya E. V., 2007). Fixed attachment distortions (insecure type), as a rule, remain for life, influencing the character and attitude of a person toward himself and others. For example, researchers from the University of New York established that insecure attachment in childhood predicted mental health outcomes, reflected in increased stress-reactivity, anxiety, depression, and lower levels of self-esteem in these people thirty years later (Widom C. S. et al., 2017).

It is important to understand that attachment also functions beyond childhood. It is necessary for an adult to have a harmonious existence, and it is often actualized in family relationships. In fact, any relationship that affects the sense of security and causes positive emotions, and especially those that a person needs during stress, can be called attachment; the childhood experience determines how a person can create such relationships.

Disharmonious relationships with the mother can give the child a negative image of surrounding people—an attitude that they cannot be trusted, that they are unreliable, unpredictable partners; or a negative image of himself (since he as a child is rejected and not accepted by his mother, then he does not deserve the love and attention of others). This kind of a relationship with one's parents at an early age directly affects one's family relationships in adulthood, as well as one's professional achievements and ways of communicating with people, reflecting one's capability of social adaptation.

Attachment disorders and pathological relationships with parents lead to a decrease in the ability of children to cope with stress, neurotic and personality disorders, leading in turn to a variety of physical disorders, and therefore an increased incidence of diseases. For example, a sample survey of children and adolescents in a general hospital revealed that in 53.2% of cases, somatic disorders appear to be caused by mental disorders, including depressive disorders (Antropov Y., 1997). This tendency persists or increases in adulthood owing to greater exposure to stresses and disrupted ability to cope with them (Maunder R. G., Hunter J. J., 2001; Pilyagina G. Y., Dubrovskaya E. V., 2007).

"Psychological shaping in the formative years plays a large part in determining who will develop a serious illness," notes Bernie Siegel (1998). —"Its effects are even more specific, however. It often determines what disease will occur, and when and where it will appear. ... I would estimate that 80 percent of my patients were unwanted or treated indifferently as children. ... Such messages lead to a lifelong feeling of unworthiness. Then an illness is something patient deserves, and treatment becomes undeserved."

Observations of students, conducted at Harvard University over a thirty-five-year period after their graduation, found that only 25% of people who believed that their parents showed a high level of love and care got serious diseases: cardiovascular, asthma, and cancer. Among the students who negatively assessed the quality of their parents' care and had an anxious type of response, the morbidity in the middle of their lives reached 87% (Russek L. G., Schwartz G. E., 1997). Based on such studies, scientists even introduced the concept of a "psychosomatogenic family." In this type of family unit, there is disorder in the main spheres of its life, which becomes the source of mental trauma for a growing and developing child. As a result, a personality prone to psychosomatic diseases is formed (Eidemiller E. G., 1999). This situation is aggravated also by the fact that in such a family, free expression of feelings and negative emotions is not accepted, and an open reaction to psychological pain is not encouraged. This forms a stereotype of patient behavior: suppression of negative emotions, and, as a consequence, their manifestation through the body—somatization.

In a psychosomatogenic family, parents, and especially mothers, are usually not able to timely recognize the bodily conditions and needs of the child, to constructively resolve problems and protect the child from family conflicts. As a result, the child learns the "behavior of the ill person," when the attention, support, and love of the parent can be obtained only by showing bodily symptoms (Sidorov P. I, Novikova I. A, 2007). From studies investigating the psychological characteristics of psychosomatic mothers, they appear as the following: authoritativeness, insistence, obtrusiveness, over-care, domination, open anxiety, and latent hostility (Moore B. E., Fine B. D., 1990).

Such mothers often have had their own unhappy childhood, coming out of it with significant unconscious conflicts. To solve them, they tend to establish symbiotic relationships with their children. As a consequence, the children's attempts to gain independence, self-sufficiency, and to separate from such a mother are unconsciously rejected by her. The father in the psychosomatic family, as a rule, is weak, cannot resist the dominant and authoritarian mother, and has little effect on the child. The psychosomatic mother also either does not know how, or is not able, to teach the child how to translate emotional experiences from the sphere of the physiological into the symbolic sphere. Altogether, these are important sources of the psychological predisposition to somatic diseases (Fusu M. N., 2013). This is confirmed by studies showing that psychosomatic disorders in adolescents occur three times more often where the mother is indulgently hyperprotective, and five times more often where she is dominantly hyperprotective (Marincheva L. P. et al., 2012). A direct relationship between childhood psychic trauma and somatic morbidity in adulthood has also been found (Felitti V. J. et al., 1998).

The American psychoanalyst Heinz Kohut (2000), founder of self-psychology, believes that the development of somatic diseases is based on a disruption in the development of a coherent, stable, and unique "self" due to the lack or insufficiency of an emotionally responsive parental environment. Because of this deficiency, it is difficult in adulthood to maintain a sense of integrity and self-esteem, hence psychosomatic symptoms emerge. Infringements of early-age attachment also contribute to self-destructive behavior, manifested in chemical and non-chemical dependencies, and other forms of autoaggressive behavior, which can lead even to suicide (Pilyagina G. Y., Dubrovskaya E. V., 2007). As we will see in Chapter 12.1, one of the forms of autoaggression can be considered a state of the psyche, leading to cancer.

Galina Pilyagina (2013), a professor at the Ukrainian National Medical Academy of Postgraduate Education, explored the disproportionalities in the psychological development of the personality, resulting from chronic childhood attachment disorders, non-harmonious relationships with parents, or significant psychotraumatic events. She found that, depending on their depth, severity, and irreversibility, such disproportionalities can manifest in a range from imbalance to a deficit of cognitive–emotional functioning. This refers to the lack of either cognitive abilities (including the processes of attention, memory, logical thinking, and imagination), or the ability to recognize and express emotions. In addition, there may be a disbalance between these two functions of the psyche. Having emerged in the child, these disproportionalities are fixed in the adult, over time distorting her character, dramatically increasing her vulnerability to stress agents, and potentiating the development of psychopathological and psychosomatic disorders.

I have already mentioned that some people have a mental way of processing internal conflict or psychic trauma, and others a somatic one (through bodily disorders). The research of Dr. Pilyagina helps in better understanding the origin of such a difference. She has established that cognitive–emotional imbalance or deficiency (CEID) can also manifest itself in two main variants, which the author metaphorically calls "mind-free feelings" or "feeling-free mind," depending on what the prevailing type of attachment disorder was toward the mother.

To better understand the mechanisms of attachment disorders, and this is necessary for our further analysis of the psychology of cancer, let us turn to the classic work of John Bowlby's student and follower, Mary Ainsworth, and her colleagues (1987). If the main style of the mother's parental behavior becomes inconsistent emotionality, with impulsive, unpredictable, and unexplained (for the child) intermittent behavior jumping between punishment and encouragement, he acquires an ambivalent (also known as anxious and preoccupied) or, in its extreme manifestations, a disorganized type of attachment disorder. Then, the behavior of the child varies from anxiety and self-doubt to becoming frozen with fear at the sight of a cruel parent. Such a child, and subsequently an adult, will perceive each impact from the outside that does not meet his expectations as stressful and frustrating, with the corresponding intense emotional reactions.

However, this emotional experience often does not have an external expression in such people, although they experience it deeply internally. At the same time, this personality cannot adequately process the incoming cognitive information. According to G. Y. Pilyagina (2013), this is a regressive-emotional version of CEID with an extreme level of internal frustrating tension, aggression, existential anxiety, and an unmet need for acceptance and meaningfulness. In stressful circumstances, such people quickly develop a disorder of adaptation with a deviation of emotions and behavior, up to emergence of a variety of personality disorders, chemical or behavioral dependence, and impulsive self-destructive actions. Apparently, this imbalance is more conducive to the psychological kind of processing of psychic trauma.

On the other hand, as Mary Ainsworth and coworkers (1987) found, if the mother's behavior was characterized by insensitivity to the emotional state and needs of the child, prolonged rejection and even hostility, with periodic "educational" intrusions and restrictions, then the child develops an avoidant type of attachment disorder. This is a kind of protective behavior, by which he tries to forget about his need for a mother, to suppress excessive negative experiences of abandonment and defenselessness. The child learns a restrained and indifferent manner of behavior, because either his emotional needs are ignored or their expression is forbidden.

Emotional indifference or, conversely, violence in childhood, often leads to the development of dissociative states in the psyche, because a child, who is naturally attached to those closest to him—his parents, and expects from them warmth and support, senses fear, aggression, alienation, or numbness instead. The result is disorders that manifest in alteration or disturbances of certain mental functions, such as consciousness, memory, and a sense of personal identity. Forcibly staying in a stressful stance within the family, the child experiences a tensed anxiety, caused by conflicting feelings of attachment and fear, love and hate, balancing on the edge of depression. Because of this, he does not properly develop such natural manifestations as mourning, caring, guilt, and mature protective mechanisms. Such children, and then adults, tend not to notice traumatic experiences, because in their psyche the processes of repression and denial are dominant. Instead of being expressed externally, unpleasant and unbearable emotions (anger, hatred, etc.) dissociate—in a way split off from the main personality—and exist independently and outside consciousness (Loffler-Stastka H. et al., 2009). Therefore, the emotional part of the child's personality is blocked in its development, and an internal ban on spontaneous expression of feelings is formed.

But the mental, cognitive part progresses faster, reflecting the need to adapt to chronic traumatic conditions and somehow reduce the excessive level of anxiety and helplessness. In this way, a hypercognitive variant of CEID develops. Its distinguishing features are an excessive desire to analyze and control, correctness in one's own and others' actions, on top of "heroic patience" and suppression or repression of emotions, especially aggressive ones. This behavior, which G. Pilyagina (2013) considers one of the forms of self-destruction, quickly leads to depletion of adaptive resources, pathologization of mental activity (in particular, neurasthenia and depression), chronic fatigue syndrome, and the development of various somatization disorders. These data is consistent with the results of the already quoted Russian–German study, which found a negative cognitive pattern associated with emotional life in patients with somatoform disorders. In such patients, there is practically a cult of restraint: complaining is beneath their dignity, anxiety and uncertainty in communication should be carefully concealed, and open expressions of anger and irritation are absolutely unacceptable (Kholmogorova A. B. et al., 2011).

The type of attachment disorder and CEID, formed in childhood, therefore determines the character of the person and the peculiarities of his relationship with others. The modern researcher of attachment disorders Patricia Crittenden, a student of John Bowlby and Mary Ainsworth, and her co-author Andrea Landini (2011) describe insecure types in adult age:

> The Type A pattern (*avoiding*—*V. M.*) in adulthood refers to both dismissing the perspective, intentions, and feelings of the self and also preoccupation with the perspectives, desires, and feelings of others. The source of information regarding others' perspectives is temporal consequences tied to behavior of the self. Type A individuals behave as if following the rule: Do the right thing—from the perspective of other people and without regard to your own feelings or desires.

The Type C pattern (*anxious-preoccupied*—*V. M.*) in adulthood refers to a preoccupation with the perspective of the self and justification of the self, and also dismissing of others, both as valued people and as sources of valid information. The source of information regarding the perspective of the self is one's feelings or one's arousal (i.e., affect). The strategy can be thought of as fitting the following dictum: Stay true to your feelings and do not negotiate, compromise, or delay gratification in ways that favor the perspectives of others.

It is natural that the type of attachment affects the ability to cope with stress in adulthood. This is confirmed by studies of how the youth of Israel reacted to the situation of military operations (artillery shelling) during the conflict with Iraq. While ambivalent-anxious people openly (perhaps excessively) displayed emotional distress, avoiding individuals repressed their anxiety and depression and manifested distress through growing somatization (Mikulincer M. et al., 1993).

According to the research of American scientists, an average of about 35%–40% of the population have insecure types of attachment (Mickelson K. D. et al., 1997), which indicates deep problems in the upbringing of children.

8.2. Attachment Disorders and Alexithymia

Apparently, the emergence of a hypercognitive variant of a child's CEID leads to a lack of development of the emotional intelligence of an adult person: of his ability to effectively comprehend the emotional sphere of life, to distinguish between his own and others' feelings, to understand emotions and their constituent parts in relationships, to use his emotions correctly to resolve tasks related to behavior and motivation. This is how alexithymia emerges, which includes the inability to exhibit the above-mentioned features of emotional intelligence (or difficulty in doing so), excessive attention to external events to the detriment of the internal, and a difficulty in distinguishing between feelings and bodily sensations. This complex of symptoms is especially characteristic of patients with psychosomatic disorders (Taylor G. J., 1984) and also, as we will see below, of cancer patients.

V. V. Kovalev (1979) believes that alexithymia indicates the prevalence of adjustment mechanisms over coping mechanisms in the adaptation of the child to the environment. This is reflected in the form of a psychosomatic response, which is phylo- and ontogenetically older and more rigid than the neurotic, which is more young and flexible. According to A. V. Semenovich (2002), in psychosomatic diseases, the unconsciousness of negative emotions has a primary-dysontogenetic and neuro-psychological nature, such that emotions are not realized because of the lack of formation and deficiency of interhemispheric connections—hence they simply cannot be named.

D. Berenbaum and T. James (1994) consider that alexithymia arises from the imprint of parental behavior, in the form of early learning from a mother who is also alexithymic. In the studies of these authors, the high level of alexithymia of the subjects correlated with the information they gave about decreased emotional expressiveness and predominance of negative emotions in their parental family. A similar opinion is expressed by Walter Brautigam and colleagues (1997):

> Emotional ignorance or a lack of 'emotional education' in psychosomatic patients can be rooted in early childhood or have an inheritable origin. As a result, the psychosomatic patient speaks and operates with 'bodily' formulations, manifesting through somatic agitation, in the language of organs' psychosomatic symptom formation.

It is natural that the less developed one's emotional intelligence, the higher the degree of alexithymia. This inverse relationship is revealed in studies of patients with breast cancer conducted at the St. Petersburg Medical University (Russia). Women examined who have a high level of alexithymia talk about the emotional side of their life as "a control, constant containment, and non-expression of their current emotions" (Kuper E. R., Korneva T. V., 2013). At the University of Bari, Italy, it was found that in women with precancerous cervical lesions, the degree of alexithymia is almost twice as high as in a control group, and the immunity activity (determined by the number of lymphocytes) is lower (Todarello O. et al., 1997).

Similar data was received by psychologists at Obninsk University, Russia: among patients with *lymphogranulomatosis*, alexithymia occurs with a frequency of 66% of cases, while among healthy individuals, it is 32%. This leads to a dysadaptive type of response to the disease with intrapsychic and interpsychic tendencies (Kashenkova M. M., 2009). On the other hand, scientists from the London Institute of Psychiatry found that high rates of the personal characteristics "rationality and antiemotionality" (*this clearly corresponds to the hypercognitive variant of CEID—V. M.*) increase the risk of cancer 40-fold compared to individuals in which indicators of this characteristic are low (Grossarth-Maticek R. et al., 1985).

The conclusion to be drawn from the data above is that the avoidant type of attachment disorder, progressing over time to a hypercognitive variant of cognitive-emotional personality deficiency and alexithymia, results in an erroneous behavioral strategy of coping with the distresses of life, and leads to a somatic manner of processing psychological trauma. Subsequently, it can become the basis for the development of the oncological form of the psychosomatic type of personality—the so-called "C" type, which we will discuss in more detail below.

8.3. How Parents Create Limiting Beliefs and a Distorted Image of a Child's "Self"

As noted earlier, attachment disorders lead to a cognitive diathesis in a child—negative beliefs due to distortion of thinking. This kind of diathesis also forms an attributive style of thinking, ascribing the origin of negative life events to external sources that are, in fact, stable and global. This leads the affected individual to draw negative conclusions about himself and forces him to see the consequences of negative life events as excessively horrible. Because of cognitive diathesis, a depressed and helpless worldview can transpire (Metalsky G. I, Joiner T. E., 1992).

Thinking of this kind distorts the psychological adaptation of the individual and promotes low self-esteem and increased self-criticism, perfectionism, an inferiority complex, feelings of helplessness, and self-doubt, leading to frustration and psychosomatic reactions (Sandomirskiy M. E., 2005). Similar cognitive errors, dysfunctional beliefs and attitudes, according to the researches of N. G. Garanyan and colleagues (2003), are among the causes of the development of diseases, along with macrosocial, family, microsocial, and other factors.

Cognitive diathesis in children is also the result of negative programming by parents, who embed in their childrens' subconscious a negative self-image and defective rules that guide their behavior. Dysadaptive family rules, rigid slogans, and instructions are imprinted in the child and form the basis of her life philosophy and behavior scenarios, distorting her perception of what is happening and preventing effective decisions. Frequent dissatisfaction with the child, constant rebukes, severe restrictions of the child's natural "childlike" activity, threats of punishment, statements such as "you are stupid," "you're mediocre," "you will end up in prison," etc., turn into ties forming a subordinate ego. The known healer and best-selling author Louise Hay (1991), who defeated her cancer[1], argued the following:

> The beliefs that you learned when you were little are still inside the child. If your parents had rigid ideas, and you're very hard on yourself or tend to build walls, your child is probably still following your parents' rules. If you continue to pick on yourself for every mistake, it must be very scary for your inner child to wake up in the morning. "What is she or he going to yell at me about today?"

---

[1] There are doubts about the practical benefits of the healing methods proposed by Louise Hay and even whether she really had cancer. Leaving the solution of the first question to each individual's experience, I believe that Louise was really a cancer patient, for her description of her experience and psychological traits largely corresponds to that of most patients.

In this way, the child forms a negative image of herself as incapable and defective, and this largely determines her inability to cope with life stresses in the future. Negative beliefs about oneself and the world around become a kind of filter, which a person uses to interpret the events in his life in an unhealthy way, and this can lead to emotional and behavioral disturbances. In fact, parents transmit their personality type by inheritance, which together with epigenetic programs creates a predisposition to certain diseases. Often this image of oneself becomes so rigid (and this is typical for psychosomatic patients) that only under the threat of a fatal disease is a person able to change it. Psycho-oncologist Laurence LeShan (1977) often noticed that because of the negative experiences of childhood, the future cancer patient sees the world as indifferent and unconcerned about him. He has the impression that he is pursued by an evil fate, that regardless of his efforts, his life is predetermined, joyless, and doomed.

American naturopath Andreas Moritz (2008), who observed thousands of cancer patients over a period of three decades, writes:

> I began to recognize a certain pattern of thinking, believing, and feeling that was common to most of them. To be more specific, I have yet to meet a cancer patient who does not feel burdened by some poor self-image, unresolved conflict and worries, or past emotional conflict/trauma that still lingers in his subconscious mind and cellular memories. I believe that cancer, the physical disease, cannot occur unless there is a strong undercurrent of emotional uneasiness and deep-seated frustration.

8.4. Physiological and Epigenetic Mechanisms of Attachment Disorders Creating Psychosomatic Predisposition

The main problem here is how the suffering of a child will resonate in adulthood. In general, insecure types of attachment affect health in three directions: they distort physiological reactions to stress, encourage the use of external regulators of emotions (food, tobacco, alcohol, drugs), and contribute to forming a behavioral style unfavorable to health (lack of physical activity, neglect of danger, aggression or submission in relationships, etc.).

People who experience stress in the early period of life have a greater risk of pathophysiological changes in the central nervous system. With age, this increases their vulnerability to stress and predisposes them to mental and physical disorders. Researchers at Emory University in the United States found that the impact of stress during critical periods of a child's development leads to a persistent hyperactive response to stress; in other words, it develops the habit of overreacting to stressful situations (Neigh G. N. et al., 2009).

Accordingly, in a study of the association of attachment disorders and cortisol levels, adults who suffered the loss of a parent as a child, or who had unsatisfactory family relationships, synthesized more cortisol in response to a stressful situation than people in the control group who did not have this kind of stress during childhood (Leuckin L., 1998, 2000). In fact, the mother (or whoever replaces her) becomes an external regulator of the immature nervous and endocrine systems of the child, and therefore inadequate care of the child and the traumas he experiences leads to a functional distortion of the stress response system.

In particular, factors such as the age at which abuse was experienced and its variety, parental responsiveness, the specificity of subsequent stresses, the type of attachment disruption that emerges, and the form of psychopathology or behavioral disorders in the child can define the intensity and features of the hypothalamic-pituitary-adrenal (HPA) system disorder, the health itself and the frequency of diseases (Ciechanowski P. S. et al., 2002; Van Voorhees E., Scarpa A., 2004). According to G. E. Vaillant (1974), the nature of one's relations with parents up to the age of twenty determines the formation of personality traits, such as trust, autonomy, and initiative, and predetermines the individual's health at the age of fifty. A large-scale study conducted in the USA on 9,508 patients found that psychological, physical, or sexual abuse experienced in childhood, being a witness to incidents of mistreatment of the mother, or the presence of a mentally ill, chemically dependent, suicidal, or imprisoned family member leads to serious consequences in adulthood; these are: ischemic heart disease, cancer, chronic lung disease, and liver and musculoskeletal disorders (Felitti V. J. et al., 1998).

Among the reasons for such health problems, as presented by scientists from Trinity College Institute of Neuroscience in Ireland, are disorders of the structure and function of the brain. After examining patients with depression at ages from eighteen to sixty-five, psychiatrists analyzed the conditions of their life, their childhood history of disorders of the psyche, and carried out magnetic resonance imaging of certain areas of the brain. Comparing the results with a control group, the researchers found that childhood stress, parental emotional neglect, and family violence cause significant changes in the structure of the brain, particularly in the hippocampus and prefrontal gray matter (cortex), and contribute to the development of chronic depression in adult life (Frodl T. et al., 2010). Early emotional abuse and alienation experienced by the child also lead to a reduction in both the total brain volume and the volume of the corpus callosum (a band of nerve fibers through which information is exchanged between the hemispheres). This melds the integration of cognitive processes and information processing between the hemispheres into a single whole. As a result, mental and adaptive mechanisms can alter in such a way that they will limit a person's ability to respond flexibly to environmental conditions and stresses in the future (Teicher M., 2002; De Bellis M. D. et al., 1999).

The more psychotraumatic events that happen in childhood—for example, the combination of aggressive behavior of family members, parental alcoholism, rape, problems with physical health, etc.—the stronger the development of diathesis and the more pronounced the vulnerability of the body to stresses in adulthood (Amaral A. P., Vaz Serra A., 2009), up to outcomes in the form of suicide (Borges G. et al., 2008) and cancer (Kelly-Irving M. et al., 2013).

Similar data was received by Ukrainian scientists: the frequency of negative life events that occurred before the period of adulthood affects the stressful load in later life of a person and even the specificity of his attitude to life and death, increasing the likelihood of suicide. Psychological traumas of early periods of development, in terms of the authors, embed an "incubated trauma" which is activated later, under the influence of experienced life problems (Rozanov V. A. et al., 2011), which is in accordance with Grof's concept of the systems of condensed experience. If the abilities for coping with stress are not developed, the foundation is built for frustration experiences, helplessness, and hopelessness. In accordance with the law of forming the COEX, similar experiences will follow in adulthood, when a person will again face serious trials. For example, childhood psychiatric trauma has been shown to increase the risk of post-traumatic stress disorder in adulthood (Fairbank J. A. et al., 2007). This, as shown by scientists from the Institute of Psychiatry in Germany, is associated with a significant change in DNA methylation and gene expression, especially those associated with the development of the nervous and immune systems (Mehta D. et al., 2013).

Even in experiments on rodents, it was found that the quality of maternal care at an early age becomes an important aspect of emotional reactivity of animals in their subsequent periods of life, and determines the level of stress hormonal response. Proper maternal behavior contributes to the development of a calm animal, more prone to exploring new environments. In new and stressful situations, they produce a lower and therefore stable level of corticosteroid hormones. Poor maternal care leads to the development of "cautious" animals that are less likely to explore new situations and have a more expressed emotional and hormonal response to stress. Activation of these two factors leads to early impairments in the cognitive functions of the brain and increases the likelihood of premature death (McEwen B. S., 2007). Experiments based on the early separation of baby monkeys from their mothers demonstrated a subsequent impairment of the immune system function in the infants as they developed (Coe C. L. et al., 1985; Reite M. et al., 1981). The four-hour-long daily separation of three-week-old mouse pups form their mother led to the outcome that under the influence of a carcinogen in these mice, breast cancer was 33% more actively developed than in mice not subjected to separation (Boyd A. L. et al., 2010).

Other epigenetic mechanisms, by which stress in children is reflected in their *genotype*, physiology, and behavior, have also been found. In the University of Wisconsin (USA), it was discovered that this kind of stress leads to an increase in the methylation of the NR3C1 gene, which inhibits the synthesis of receptors for cortisol. As a consequence, cortisol loses its ability to bind to receptors to the fullest and its concentration in the blood increases, causing an overreaction to subsequent stress (Romens S. E. et al., 2015). Researchers from the Douglas Hospital in Montreal, Canada, also found that depending on the maternal style of behavior, the gene encoding the glucocorticoid receptor in rat hippocampi is methylated differently and the histones in the *chromatin* of their brain cells are acetylated in another way. Such differences arose in the early stages of development and persisted throughout the animals' lives (Weaver I. C. et al., 2004).

In a joint study between Yale University (USA) and the Vavilov Institute of Genetics (Russia), there was a comparison between Russian children in orphanages and those living in normal families. It turned out that methylation of DNA in blood cells of orphan children is much higher than in children from stable family units, especially in the areas of genes responsible for the development and functioning of the brain, in particular, interneuronal communication. Separation from parents and being in an orphanage becomes a powerful stressor, significantly altering the work of the epigenome and increasing the vulnerability of such children to future stresses (Yu O. et al., 2012). Understanding this factor is especially important for foster parents, who should raise these children with increased sensitivity and care.

Another consequence of childhood stresses, according to G. E. Miller and co-authors (2011), is the formation of the so-called "pro-inflammatory *phenotype*" of an organism, characterized by an excessive response of the immune system to provoking agents and reduced sensitivity to suppressing hormonal signals, due to disturbances in the activity of endocrine systems. Supportive results of the study of adults, who were inadequately cared for in childhood, were presented by L. Carpenter and his colleagues at Brown University, USA (2010): in response to the standard stress situation in the body, an increased response of systemic inflammation, detected by the content of interleukin-6, was noted. Similar data using the analysis of C-reactive protein was received at the University of Princeton (Danese A. et al., 2007). This corresponds to studies showing that insecure attachment in children promotes the development of diseases associated with inflammatory processes in adulthood (Puig J. et al., 2013). This sort of pro-inflammatory phenotype in women who had psycho-traumatic experiences in childhood and developed breast cancer as adults persisted even after a year past the completion of the primary course of treatment (Crosswell A. D. et al., 2014), which may contribute to their poor survival and greater risk of disease recurrence.

Also, children who had experienced inadequate care were noted to have genetic changes associated with pro-inflammatory reactions that promote the development of depression in adulthood (Cohen-Woods S. et al., 2017). In addition, adult women who developed an avoidant attachment type in childhood have less active protective immune killer cells (Picardi A. et al., 2007), and in conflict situations they produce more cortisol (Powers S. I. et al., 2006). All these disorders in the body, as will be shown below, contribute to the onset of cancer.

8.5. Psychological Traumas and Attachment Disorders in Childhood and their Contribution to the Development of Cancer in Adulthood

What does "attachment disorder" mean when translated from scientific jargon into layman's terms? The answer is very simple: the lack or distortion within the manifestations of parental love.

Donald Winnicott (1994) found that many mothers do not love their own children at the time they gave birth to them. They feel terrible, as if they were stepmothers, trying to pretend that they love, but they simply cannot, writes Winnicott. It is clear that the children of such mothers are unlikely to have a safe attachment to them. This situation is often characteristic of childhood cancer patients.

A retrospective analysis of early childhood adversities found that repeated losses and difficulties in relationships with parents are a common factor for cancer patients (Mandal J. M. et al., 1992; Nair L. et al., 1993). Such patients remember their parents as cold, not involved in their lives, and not responding to their emotional needs (Roe A., Siegelman M., 1963). A very similar observation of women with breast cancer was made by German psychiatrists: "These patients describe an emotionally cold atmosphere in their families along with a pronounced absence of basic trust" (Becker H., 1979). Even the lack of breastfeeding of a female child causes alterations in her organism, contributing to an increased risk of breast cancer around the time before she is set to begin menopause (Potischman N., Troisi R., 1999).

Many cancer patients have unresolved emotional conflicts or psychotraumatic frustration in their relationship with the mother. Reflecting on the prevalence of an attachment disorder in children, we see their life history as characterized by a desperate need to maintain control over their object of love (Pernin G. M, Pierce I. R, 1959). Research carried out at the University of Lisbon revealed the insecure attachment schemes, dysfunctional anger regulation strategies, and a lack of psychophysiological activation in patients with breast cancer (Eusebio S. E., Torrado M., 2017).

Dr. Caroline Thomas, whose foundations for identifying the oncological type of personality study will be considered in the next chapter, observed students who contracted cancer. They showed a lack of warmth, comfort, and mutual understanding in their relationship with their parents. The latter were often unpredictable and kept a distance in their relationships with their children, resulting in dislike, and a hostile attitude toward parents (Thomas C. B. et al., 1979), which, from the position of attachment theory, corresponds to the avoidance type of such disorders. This was later confirmed by a similar study conducted by John Shaffer and colleagues at the Johns Hopkins University in Baltimore (1987).

P. I. Sidorov and E. P. Sovershaeva (2015) indicate that disharmony in the childhood of cancer patients can result from disorders of one or several aspects of family relationships: psychological (openness, trust, mutual moral and emotional support, caring for one another), psychophysiological (sexual relations), social (financial dependence, distribution of roles, authority, leadership), and cultural (national and religious traditions and customs).

One of my cancer patients, after a session of *regressive therapy*, said:

Much of the past surfaced and became clearer. I touched the feelings of my childhood: loneliness, the desire to be close to my parents, and feeling unloved. I understood how my mother influenced me by her hesitations, domination, and poorly disguised anger. I remembered compulsion, a fear of attack, and especially humiliation, if I defended my position, and when I could not have my space without feelings of guilt and shame—as a result, my will and anger turned against me. All this is now manifested in my present relations ...

Bernie Siegel (1998) supports this: "I feel that all disease is ultimately related to a lack of love, or to love that is only conditional, for the exhaustion and depression of the immune system thus created leads to physical vulnerability. I also feel that all healing is related to the ability to give and accept unconditional love."

The Institute of Physiology at the University of Ferrara in Italy conducted a study on the psychological characteristics of seventy-two women with suspected cancer. After the diagnosis, it turned out that those who had a malignant breast tumor noted a lack of maternal openness and of good relations with the mother, whereas patients with bladder cancer spoke of a lack of openness and of good relations with both parents and the father in particular (Grassi L., Molinari S., 1986). Similar results were obtained in the study of childhood memories in patients with various forms of gynecological cancer; in comparison with the control group, they noted more negative images of parents or those in the position of parents, a higher frequency of loss in childhood, and traumatic psychosocial and socioeconomic experiences associated with family (Gehde E., Baltrusch H. J., 1990).

A study by M. G. Ivashkina (1998) showed that the formation of a "cancer personality" often correlates with the presence of a dominant mother. Scientists from the medical school in Hanover, Germany, concluded that the development of cancer in adulthood is caused by a deficit of a sense of security in childhood. This, in turn, is due to the degree of emotional closeness to the parents and the emotional needs in the parent-child relationship that are not satisfied, the formation of the value system of the child in the spirit of strict adherence to rigid social standards, and suppression of emotions, which leads to the potential development of the syndrome of pathological "goodness, courtesy" (Baltrusch H. J., Waltz M., 1987).

The absence of safety and love, parental coldness, and lack of attention in childhood, as causes of cancer in adulthood, was described by one of the pioneers of psycho-oncology, Claus Bahnson (1980). Dr. Morton Reiser said back in 1966 that stressful events change the body on an ongoing basis, and therefore the impact of a very early psychological trauma on psychological development may appear only after a long, latent period. Even if a stressful event has long been forgotten, it can play an important role in creating a predisposition to cancer. Dr. Douglas Brodie (2015), the founder of one of the first clinics of integrative oncology in the United States, who observed thousands of cancer patients for twenty-eight years of medical practice, writes:

> Usually, beginning in childhood, this individual has internally suppressed his/her hostility and other unacceptable emotions. More often than not, this feature of the affected personality has its origins in feelings of rejection by one or both parents. Whether these feelings or rejection are justified or not, it is the perception of rejection that matters, and this results in a lack of closeness with the "rejecting" parent or parents, followed later in life by a similar lack of closeness with spouses and others with whom close relationships would normally develop. Those at higher risk for cancer tend to develop feelings of loneliness as a result of their having been deprived of affection and acceptance earlier in life, even if this is merely their own perception. These people have a tremendous need for approval and acceptance, developing a very high sensitivity to the needs of others while suppressing their own emotional needs.

Observations of practicing physicians are also supported by studies at the genome level. The results revealed, that patients with basal cell *carcinoma*, who suffered a negative emotional attitude in their early life, and then had a serious stressful event about a year before the diagnosis, have in the tumor tissue a reduced activity of specific genes (CD25, CD3E, ICAM1, CD68), responsible for the immune reactivity (Fagundes C. P. et al., 2012b).

If, in addition to emotional coldness and neglect, children are also subjected to cruel treatment and physical abuse, then in adulthood such people are 49% more likely to develop cancer, according to researchers from the University of Toronto in Canada. They have made an adjustment for other factors affecting health, such as socioeconomic status, alcohol consumption, smoking, and lack of physical activity, but the link between maltreatment and the occurrence of cancer has remained significant. The authors of this paper believe that it is cortisol that can mediate the "violence–cancer" bond (Fuller-Thomson E., Brennenstuhl S., 2009).

American scientists from Purdue University during 1995–1996 analyzed 3,032 people between the ages of 25 and 74 to determine whether childhood adversities and their specificity affect the incidence of cancer. It has been found that the factors that increase the incidence of oncological diseases in men are physical abuse by the father, cruel treatment from both parents, and the effect of accumulating experienced misfortunes. Among women, these factors were physical abuse by the mother and cruel treatment from both parents (Morton P. M. et al., 2012). Researchers from Saudi Arabia have found that the beating and insulting of boys by their fathers greatly increases the risk of their developing cancer at the age of forty to sixty years. This risk has already occurred at a frequency of violence every six months, and peaked at monthly violence (Hyland M. E. et al., 2013).

All this corresponds to the data received and the description of the experiences of cancer patients in the process of *psychedelic therapy* by Stanislav Grof and Joan Halifax (1978). They observed a large number of people who suffered from emotional or physical deprivation in childhood or were even directly subjected to cruel physical treatment. One of the constantly emerging experiences during the therapy sessions were severely painful episodes associated with anxiety, loneliness, hunger, and cruel treatment. Sometimes dying patients perceived this abandonment in childhood as a possible cause of their disease.

But, it is not only emotional coldness or violence in the family that creates a predisposition to cancer. Stressful experiences and bereavement, such as the death of one parent or the parents' divorce, can also provoke the development of the disease in the future.

Here is an experience of my patient A. in the process of a transpersonal psychotherapy:

I was able to make contact with my grief over the loss of my father. I have understood mentally that my father abandoned me early and that the pain was too big for me to live with. I made up a story to survive, that he had to sacrifice our contact for the sake of God, and that made me feel special. I see now that that was not true, and that the grief had to be processed by me for me to move forward. I have mixed up my father with God, idealized my father, and because of this repressed my anger. I have a clearer understanding, but still don't emotionally and physically feel the grief and the feeling of being unworthy, though I know it is strong. I feel like a process has been working deep inside of me these weeks, with a lot of fear included, and I therefore automatically distract myself with other things, and resist going inward through meditation.

It's becoming clearer that this is the key to my relationships. I have more feeling-contact with my fear of rejection in relationships, and I understand that I isolate myself to calm the anxiety. I experience both deeper contact with the pain and also deeper contact with my will to be me and move forward.

A *prospective study* of cancer mortality in the UK, using more than fifty years of statistical records, found that women who said that they had experienced stress in childhood had a higher chance of dying from cancer before the age of fifty than those who had not experienced such stresses (the control group). The probability of such a death increased in accordance with the number of adversities suffered in childhood. Those who had only one negative episode before the age of sixteen had a 40% greater chance of dying from cancer by age fifty, whereas those who had two or more negative episodes in childhood had a 150% increased risk of premature death compared to the control group. For men, however, the relationship of their childhood stresses to cancer was statistically insignificant (Kelly-Irving M. et al., 2013)—perhaps because men are less likely to share emotional memories?

The same authors were exploring scientific literature to define how much the experience of acute or chronic stress factors during sensitive periods of child development affects subsequent biological and behavioral functions. They came to the conclusion that it most likely depends on the specific moments of time when the initial stresses occurred that were later supplemented by other negative events. For this reason, childhood adversity can be considered to have an important initial impact on the development of cancer in adulthood (Kelly-Irving M. et al., 2013a).

This point of view is supported by Gerald Harris (2005) of the University of Nottingham (UK): the psychological trauma experienced by a child during the critical period of his development by age seven to eight forms a kind of "time bomb." It is activated by the stressful events of later life and provokes the development of malignant neoplasia. One of the biological mechanisms of this is a disorder in the regulation of cortisol synthesis in people who suffered psychological trauma as child, and should they fall sick with breast cancer, they also exhibit larger cognitive impairment during chemotherapy (Kamen C. et al., 2017).

American researchers, after analyzing the lives of 17,337 adults, found a threefold increase in incidence of lung cancer in the people who survived childhood psychotraumatic events (Brown D. W. et al., 2010). At the University of Texas, an investigation of forty-two women with breast cancer revealed that twenty-eight of them had lost a significant close person as a child (Tacon A. M., 1998). Psychologists at the University of Southern Connecticut, as a result of a fifteen-year observation of 1,213 women, found that the death of the mother in early childhood and resulting chronic depression were associated with the development of breast cancer in later life (Jacobs J. R., Bovasso G. B., 2000). Similar results were obtained by scientists from the University of Heidelberg, Germany (Scherg H., Blohmke M., 1988), the University and Institute of Public Health of Nis, Serbia (Kocic B. et al., 2015), and Kuopio University Hospital in Finland (Eskelinen M., Ollonen P., 2010).

Hans Becker (1979) of the Psychosomatic Clinic of the University of Heidelberg, studying patients with breast tumors, showed that severe suffering in childhood due to the loss of one of the parents leads to an increased risk of developing cancer in adulthood. Arthur Schmale (1964) from the University of Rochester in New York found that many adults with a physical illness, including cancer, had lost one or both parents at an early age; the same conclusion is reached by Prof. Claus Bahnson of Eastern Pennsylvania Psychiatric Institute (1980). An epidemiological study of the University of Orebro in Sweden on a group of cancer patients for the period from 1961 to 2006 demonstrated that a childhood psychological trauma, related to parental death, leads to a significant increase in incidence of neoplasia in adulthood, especially of cancer associated with *papillomavirus*, as well as cancers of the stomach, lungs, rectum, breast, and pancreas (Kennedy B. et al., 2014).

G. Baltrusch and M. Waltz (1987) determined that the appearance of cancer in adulthood, among other things, is related to the loss of significant relationships due to the death of a loved one or parting with him or her. The reason for this, according to the observations of the psycho-oncologist Laurence LeShan (1989), is the formation of a powerful destructive belief in the child: "If I were a good boy/girl, my mom/dad would not leave me," which in turn leads to a lifelong subconscious sense of guilt and negative self-esteem. This disrupts a person's ability to cope with the stresses of life.

All the studies presented, as we see, support the diathesis–stress theory of cancer.

8.6. Psychological Causes in Pediatric Oncology

8.6.1. Psychotraumatic Childhood Events and the Personality Traits of a Child

Often the cancer "does not wait" for people to grow up, and, as we well know, it also occurs in children. Children do not always have enough protective bodily resources to convey the "incubated trauma", "time bomb" to adulthood. In all likelihood, the underlying reason for this is the less developed psychological defense mechanisms and, correspondingly, the greater intensity of stress experienced by children, as well as the appearance of several or all previously discussed factors of predisposition. This is confirmed by the observations of N. A. Uriadnitskaya (1998): children with cancer display inconsistency of character, tendency to fix on problems, self-blame, suppression of emotions, and passive-accepting behavior.

In the works of T. J. Jacobs and E. Charles (1980), as well as S. B. Lansky and colleagues (1978), a significantly higher frequency of stressful events was found in those families where children developed cancer. In an extensive study of employees of the universities of Aarhus (Denmark) and California (USA), the incidence of cancer in children under fifteen years of age, born in Sweden and Denmark between 1968 and 2007, was explored. It was found that the loss of a close relative (a situation of severe bereavement) increases the chances of developing cancer in childhood by 10% (Momen N. C. et al., 2013).

W. A. Greene and G. Miller in 1958, studying thirty-three children and adolescents with leukemia, showed that thirty-one of them had experienced one or more stressful events in life within two years prior to the manifestation of the disease, including death (or the threat of death in the course of illness) of significant relatives—the father, the grandmother, or the grandfather. Psychologists from the Russian Center for Pediatric Hematology, Oncology and Immunology found that 36% of the children with cancer had an attachment trauma occurring in early childhood, and 19.4% experienced a severe psychological trauma—the loss of a significant other (more often a mother or father) (Guseva M. A., Barchina E. T., 2015). Charles Weinstock (1977) at the Albert Einstein College of Medicine explored young patients who, during the first seven years of life, suffered from extensive emotional trauma (for example, the loss of a mother) and impaired trust in parents, while fostering the suppression of anger. He found them unable to form strong attachments in general, and often having lost a satisfying relationship during young adulthood, this resulting in hopeless depression. Cancer would then develop within six months to eight years.

However, even if the child had secure attachment (from the first year of life) before the onset of important life events, these events (such as divorce, relocation, illness or death of one parent) can transform it into an insecure one (Becker-Stoll F., 1997), which becomes a risk factor for various diseases.

Even such a seemingly happy event for the family as the birth of a second and subsequent child can in certain cases become so psychotraumatic for the first child that it will contribute to the development of the disease. As L. LeShan and M. Reznikoff (1960) found out, some adults who contracted cancer in childhood perceived the loss of a significant portion of the parental attention after the birth of a brother or sister as traumatic, especially when they were forced to devote considerable time to the younger child—to the detriment of their own interests. Subsequently, this was perceived as a "curtailed" childhood. The relationship between the birth of the "competing" sibling and cancer was also found by W. A. Greene and G. Miller (1958) of the University of Rochester School of Medicine and Dentistry. Studies of the German Cancer Center have shown that having five or more siblings vs none increases the risk of prostate and anal cancer, while eight or more siblings also add the risk of stomach cancer

(Altieri A., Hemminki K., 2007). The reason for this, as shown by Arthur Schmale (1964) in the case of adults with a physical illness, including cancer, may be that they have retained a sense of "rejection" in their life. This was due to the fact that one or both parents were excessively demanding, or these people had several brothers or sisters and therefore felt unwanted, unacceptable, and separated from their parents.

A case in point is my patient F., with cervical cancer. After the birth of her sister when F. was five years old, the attention of the parents was largely focused on the sister, also because of her poor health. F.'s life turned into "one big must" in relation to her sister.

> She received everything she wanted, and if something was not given to her, she made hysterics and still got what she wanted,—*the patient told me in tears during the session.*—I had to help her all the time, give her everything, toys, books, even my room. She grew selfish, constantly criticized me, both then and now. And our mother had since that time the habit of talking to me in an imperious tone, and even now, although she helps me when I am ill, I often feel her help as a compulsion: you have to drink this, you must eat that. And inside me everything is shrinking at her tone.

Undoubtedly, such experiences became an important factor of predisposition to the disease: they formed her habit of conceding and the so-called "subliminal ego" (we will consider this in detail in Chapter 11.1.2.4), which in her adult years determined her unsuccessful relationships with men, which became the main source of her carcinogenic stress.

The fragile psyche of a child, especially weakened by previous factors of predisposition, can even experience relatively "ordinary" life stresses as psychotraumatic. Doctor of Psychology, Medicine and Biological Physics P. A. Levine and his colleague A. Frederick (1997), who studied stress and trauma for thirty years, consider it vitally important to understand that events that may hardly be regarded by the majority as traumatic can influence children with the same force as the horrors of war.

Other traumatic events for the child that contribute to cancer, according to W. Greene and G. Miller (1958), are unwanted changes in the place of residence or school. This research is confirmed by the results of a study in Greece. In most families where children became ill with lymphoma and leukemia, serious changes were expected in the near future, such as changes to the composition of the family or living conditions. In 50% of cases cancer was diagnosed in the same month as the changes were planned. The author came to the conclusion that the experience of moving to another place of residence, which is accompanied by loss or separation with a person close to child, becomes especially emotionally traumatic for him. As it often turned out that the plans for forthcoming changes in many families were hampered or canceled in connection with the child's illness, one can understand that such children subconsciously resort in the only way available for them to prevent an unwanted event: by somatization of their unspoken suffering, to the extent of developing a serious disease like cancer (Papadatou D., 1983).

Another reason for such a negative attitude from the child to the change of residence may be the expectation of difficulties in relations in the new class, based on the observations of bullying, humiliation, beatings, and discrimination against newcomers in the current school. Given the psychosomatic personality type "C," that often forms in such children, with its desire to avoid conflicts, fear of a new collective can become a source of serious distress with a resolution found through somatization.

Of course, the oncogenic effect of such stressful events could not be manifested in a "happy" family unit. In all likelihood, by the time of stress, such children have already formed a serious attachment disorder with the corresponding physiological disorders and weakening of the body's defenses, that is, a state of diathesis. Thus, Greene and Miller (1958) revealed that at a certain period before the onset of the disease, the mothers of these children were often in a prolonged depression, which worsened their relationship with their children. As a result, some children were forced to perform the functions of taking care of their mothers that were not characteristic of their age. That is why authors called them a "small mom" or "little man," while other children remained "infants" regardless of age.

A similar conclusion while studying the psychological and family characteristics of Greek children suffering from lymphoma and leukemia and their relationships with parents, came also from the author of the cited study, Danai Papadatou (1983). In comparison with healthy children of the same age, sick children were mainly brought up in a "ruined family." Most of them at an early age experienced a loss or absence of a significant close person, most often a father, or grew up in an atmosphere of their parents' unhappy marriage. Being most often the only or the first child in the family, such children were distinguished by increased emotional sensitivity and vulnerability, but at the same time avoided showing their feelings, especially negative ones. Based on descriptions of their character by mothers, Papadatou selected two categories of children:

- "little adults": highly responsible, obedient, reliable, serious, polite, and/or "proper" children. They tend to meet the expectations of adults, follow established rules, and are excellent at learning. These children are often described as "exemplary," "ideal," "mature," never creating any problems for parents.

- "babies": children who are cosseted, "spoiled" by their very environment. They are described as egocentric, requiring inseparable attention, and often forcing other people to serve them, using their "charm." Most, if not all, of the desires of such children are fulfilled, owing to the nature of their character—they use all forms of behavior (crying, hysteria, touchiness) to get what they want.

Remarkable is the similarity, including terminology, as noted by scientists from different countries and different professional orientations. Children described by American psychiatrists Greene and Miller as "little mother" or "little man," and the Greek psycho-oncologist Danai Papadatou as "little adults," almost completely correspond to children with a hypercognitive version of CEID. Ukrainian psychiatrist Galina Pilyagina (2013) calls them "little old men": "The behavior of such children is quite predictable: extremely 'proper' and quiet obedience. Such children are easy to recognize: they are 'little professors', 'independent from the diaper age', never cause problems for parents or caregivers and often … demonstrate behavior of an adult, mature personality." "Babies," according to Greene, Miller, and Papadatou, clearly correspond to the regressive-emotional variant of CEID according to Dr. Pilyagina (2013): they are characterized by "... a constant and inadequate hyperbolization of emotions; poorly controlled, impulsive, and unpredictable emotional and behavioral response; uncontrollable affective flashes; constant fixation on the attainment of a state of pleasure; egocentrism; chaotic behavior aimed at satisfying the short-term desires."

These observations, in comparison with the personality traits of psychosomatic patients (given in Chapter 2.2), once again confirm the validity of my conclusion: the oncological type of psychosomatic personality predominantly comes from the hypercognitive version of CEID with the avoidant type of attachment disorder at its core. There are other data supporting this hypothesis: examination of advanced cancer patients sampled from the university medical centers of Hamburg and Leipzig, Germany, revealed that 64% of them were insecurely attached. Moreover, there were 48% avoidant and 16% preoccupied types. Such an insecure attachment contributed to the prediction of depression (10%) and death anxiety (14%) (Scheffold K. et al., 2018).

Anna Tacon of the University of Texas (1998) studied the child relationship with parents in patients with breast cancer from the position of the theory of attachment disorders. In comparison with non-cancer patients, a predominantly avoiding type of attachment disorders and statistically higher indices of emotional suppression (especially anger) were noted in cancer patients, while in women with an ambivalent type of attachment disorder such suppression of emotions and interrelation with cancer was not found. In her subsequent works (Tacon A., 2006), the author also concluded that the avoiding type of attachment disorder is the basis for the formation of the cancer type of personality (type "C," which we will discuss below). A similar conclusion was made by Yvane Wiart of the Descartes Paris University (2014). After examining the relationship between the type of attachment of a person and his health, she found that the risk group for oncological diseases includes, first of all, people with alexithymia, who have an avoidant type of attachment.

Psycho-oncologist Tom Laughlin (1999) notes: "Avoidance behavior in childhood ... is a background factor, something that took place during the patient's childhood, and therefore functions as a deep, underlying dynamic to the conditions existing in the patient's current life"; in other words, this is what forms the psycho-oncogenic diathesis. Researchers J. Feeney and S. Ryan (1994) and T. Kotler and co-authors (1994), who showed similar attributes of emotional repression (especially negative emotions) in both individuals with avoiding attachments and cancer patients, consider further studies in this direction to be extremely important for understanding the causes of diseases and developing therapeutic interventions.

At the same time, additional research is needed to understand the relationship with cancer of the regressive-emotional variant of CEID, which has an ambivalent type of attachment disorders at its core. Despite the fact that A. Tacon did not find such a correlation, it is known that the somatization of emotional experiences and the development of psychosomatic diseases are also characteristic for the ambivalent type of attachment disturbance (Pilyagina G. Y., Dubrovskaya E. V., 2007). D. Papadatou's study directly confirms the clear relationship of the development of cancer in children to the ambivalent type. It is possible that different types of attachment disorders have different "target organs" in somatization of the psycho-emotional conflict, with the final development of various oncological pathologies—from organ cancers to blood cancer (we will analyze the research of Dr. R. Hamer from Germany, directly confirming this hypothesis).

One question is of great interest regarding whether or not insecure attachment is an obligatory factor in the development of cancer; do people who grow up in good families and have a safe attachment suffer from cancer with the same frequency? Judging by some of the available studies, they become ill less often (although I have not yet been able to find statistical data) and cope more effectively with disease (Schmidt S. D. et al., 2012; Scheffold K. et al., 2018). An analysis of available research shows inconsistency in data regarding the type of attachment and cancer incidence (Nicholls W. et al., 2014). Apparently, in patients with secure attachment, other aspects of predisposition can be more important: epigenetic heredity, the mother's stresses during pregnancy or birth complications, and subsequent provocative events that stimulate the cancer process. We will discuss them in Part III.

8.6.2. Mechanisms of the Early Age Onset of Cancer

The data above, in my opinion, shed light on the secrets of early age oncology. We can feel bitter amazement when an infant or toddler becomes ill with cancer, or a slightly older child, of whom people say — "so beautiful and never did anything wrong." I find the causes of infant disease in a combination of factors of epigenetic heredity and the mother's stresses during pregnancy, including those continuing after childbirth. Especially dangerous for the child are constant negative emotions experienced by the mother during pregnancy, her own insecure attachment, quarrels with the child's father and, most of all, thoughts of abortion and the feeling of not wanting the child. As we learned in Chapter 6, this generates powerful stress in the fetus, including the fear of death, and such emotions induced by the mother in accordance with the laws of epigenetics disrupt his physiological harmony and the normal development of the organism. To this may be added the psychological trauma of birth: when the mother suffers stress during pregnancy, her body takes on a rigidity of musculature, a kind of "muscle armor," described by one of the founders of psychosomatic medicine Wilhelm Reich (1980). It functions as a protective mechanism, a somatic manifestation of chronically suppressed negative emotions. Such an "armor" may well cause complications in the birthing process, creating the child's basic perinatal matrices according to Stanislav Grof, as one of the elements of predisposition to cancer.

If, after the birth of the child, the psychological situation in the family does not improve, then early disorders of attachment to the mother start, which already at the age of twelve to twenty-two months can cause disturbances in the normal development of the child, regardless of the presence of organic pathology (Ward M. J. et al., 1993). Early attachment disorder can also be caused by the mother's and/or father's untreated psychological traumas, the mother's inability to communicate with her baby if she is not empathetic, or does not speak at all in interaction with the baby, or helpless and chaotic behavior on her part, and instability in caring for the infant (Brisch K., 2009).

For example, the mother can be unable to pay attention to her child's signals, as her attention is directed elsewhere. She may be self-preoccupied, overburdened, or overwhelmed by life circumstances, taking care of herself rather than her child. Her own needs for emotional regulation and soothing may distract her so much that she does not notice what her child is expressing. All this contributes to the development of an insecure, mostly avoidant, style of attachment.

Mothers of this kind may spend more time in a state of apparent positive emotion with their children, but actually they do this by suppressing and ignoring their own and the child's negative affective communications. The child does not learn then how to express and manage his true emotions, explains Professor Peter Costello of Adelphi University (2013), because

> ...when they are negative, [it] leads his mother to withdraw and become unavailable, and they thereby heighten his own attachment anxiety and insecurity. His own feelings become something to avoid, and he seeks to suppress them. The mother who avoids negative emotions therefore threefold burdens her child: with the need to deal with what is upsetting him without help, with the need to suppress

and regulate his emotions on his own, and with the need to control his anxiety about the withdrawal and unavailability of his mother.

All this brings about high stress levels in the infant, or in the words of psycho-oncologist Frederick Levenson (1985), an "overwhelming degree of irritation," when the cancer may appear as the baby's least severe reaction. The author illustrates this statement with a case of his practice:

> Peter's defense of withdrawal and self-containment was a survival mechanism from earliest infancy. His mother had not been able to relate to the boy she thought she had always wanted. When the infant Peter sensed her hostile feelings, he attempted to turn them off, with both his body and mind storing the negative stimulation. Because his mother did not like him, Peter generalized that other people did not like him either. He was afraid that they were feeling what his mother felt. His defense of withdrawal and self-containment helped kill him. At the age of ten, Peter died of acute leukemia.

In addition to disorders of psycho-emotional development, negative events in the family also contribute to the development of childhood oncological diseases. The author of the above-cited Greek study also found that in 67% of families where children were diagnosed with lymphoma or leukemia, stressful events happened during the first four years of a child's life, both temporary and permanent. Referring to the literature, Danai Papadatou (1983) assumes that between the ages of seven months and six years, the child is particularly vulnerable to psychotraumatic events associated with separation. I have also cited above the research on the ability of infants to "mirror" the stressful state of the mother's body. Whatever the mechanism of this empathic connection— based on maternal facial expressions, smell, micromovements, or energy-information exchange—it is significant that distresses occurring in the family, hidden and especially open conflicts, are reflected on the child, disrupting his psychological and then physical health.

(By the way, although today eniology, the science of energy–information interactions, is in its formative period, we can see how items of knowledge about these interactions, long known in spiritual practices and folk medicine, are gradually being confirmed. Just a few decades ago, yoga, Qi-gong, and energy therapy, whose philosophy is based on energy–information exchange, seemed to most scientists to be insignificant entertainment, while in these days numerous serious studies are devoted to their influence on health and healing (I'll talk about them in Chapter 32)).

All this suggests that in early cancer (and in general, in childhood cancer), a thorough study of family history, the process of pregnancy, birth, and the psychological characteristics of parents is always necessary. As an example, we can use the study of parents whose children with cancer received treatment in the department of oncology at Zagreb Children's Hospital. These parents as a whole had a large negative affectivity (the experience of anxiety and depression along with other negative emotions—fear, sadness, guilt). Moreover, these personality traits were not caused only by the child's illness; both in the lives of these families in general, and in the lives of the children, there were significantly more stresses before the onset of the disease than in families with healthy children. Families with sick children also had more quarrels, and children were more "obedient and well-bred" (so-called) than healthy children (Jakovljevic G. et al., 2010). Is this not a familiar picture of the hypercognitive variant of CEID and the emerging psychosomatic personality?

A survey of parents of children in treatment in the children's department of the Institute of Oncology of the Academy of Medical Sciences of Ukraine (Korol L. I., 2005) showed 53.4% of mothers' dominance in family relationships. Most mothers showed the influence of the experience gained in childhood—the dominance of their own mothers in the family, that is, the effect of transgenerational transmission. The mother and father in 47.35% of families estimated their parents' attitude to them in childhood as negative. 65.3% of fathers suffer from alcoholism or use alcohol systematically. Even without taking into account cancer in a child, in 39% of families, the parents' relations were strained and conflicting, and the onset of the disease exacerbated the relationship to that level in 75.5% of families (*probably due to the manifestation of suppressed emotions—V. M.*).

Psychologists from the Regional Children's Clinical Hospital of Kharkiv (Ukraine), studying child–parent relations in families where children had cancer, found that parents are characterized by a distortion of emotional contact with the child. This was expressed in the difficulties of communication, inadequate ability to explain their emotions in various situations, and lack of ability to stimulate the child's activity. Such parents build relationships with children in terms of domination but not partnership and equality, distance themselves or avoid contact with children, show a high level of irritability associated with their interaction and excessive strictness. There was redundant parental care, a strong restriction of any extraneous influences on children, active interference in their inner world, the imposition of the parents' own decisions, often disregarding the desires of the children, as well as attempts to control the manifestations of their aggression and sexuality. Family conflicts, reflecting the general psychological background, were observed in families of sick children more than half as often as in the control group (Piontkovskaya O. V., 2013).

In this way, chronic stress in such families, the emotional coldness of parents, neglect of the child's interests, and emotional and physical violence can increase the intensity of the systems of condensed experience, strengthen the "incubated trauma," and activate in the child all that sequence of pathogenic effects of stress and vulnerability to carcinogens that we discussed in previous chapters.

The reader may think that I speak about some particularly cold or cruel parents, rarely-met monsters. Unfortunately, I do not. In a large number of outwardly favorable families, even without parental violence, children either receive less love and attention, or/and are under strict control, limiting their natural curiosity in the exploration of the world, distorting the attachment, and suppressing the formation of their full-fledged personality. Karen Horney (1994) writes that in the life histories of many psychosomatic patients, there is a constant inhibition by parents of the development of their independence, as a result of which the balance of the relationship between child restraint and the granting of freedom has been distorted. When these children arrive at the need to separate from their parents, they fall victim to fear and depressive disorders.

Even if the physical care of the child does not cause complaint, but is formal, is subject only to external standards of behavior, and is not filled with the personal emotional involvement of the parent, the child will also have a lack of love and alienation from closeness, which hinders the development of his sense of self-sufficiency and resistance to the complexities of life. This situation even found its definition—"hidden social orphanhood". It manifests in a change in the attitude toward the child, up to the complete ousting of him from the family. Thus, modern society reproduces generations of self-enclosed, psychologically malformed, and demoralized people vulnerable to psychotraumatic situations (Filippova N. V. et al., 2015).

Even loving, well-meaning parents or caregivers can cause the dissociation of the child's personality if they do not know properly how to get in tune with him, and do not understand how to raise a child with complex needs, or again if the parents themselves have unresolved emotional problems, especially from childhood, suffer from internal or interpersonal conflicts (especially between themselves), and are in chronic psycho-emotional stress. The same happens when the child's needs do not coincide with the parenting style, and when other difficulties make it impossible to meet the child's needs—in the event of parental illness, financial problems, natural disasters, wars, etc.

All this can lead to the appearance of both psychopathological and psychosomatic personality traits, and then to the development of a variety of diseases, including cancer. A similar picture of the oncological patient's childhood is described by the pioneers of psycho-oncology and other physicians and psychologists who studied hundreds of patients—Claus Bahnson (1980), Lawrence LeShan (1989), Carl Simonton with colleagues (1978), Lydia Temoshok and Henry Dreher (1993), Bernie Siegel (1998), Michael Lerner (1996), Douglas Brodie (2015), and many other authors of scientific articles.

That is why, during the process of a child's cancer treatment, it is necessary to include family psychotherapy so that, having changed, the parents may create a new, positive atmosphere that contributes to the strengthening of the child's protective resources. Studies on the transgenerational transfer of attachment styles show that if in the process of psychotherapy the insecure attachment of the mother changes to a secure one, it permits the establishment of a secure attachment in her children, in contrast to those children whose mothers left with an insecure attachment style (Iyengar U. et al., 2014). This, undoubtedly, affects the state of the children's bodies and stress resistance.

* * *

It is important that the parents of a child with cancer, reading this book, do not start ruthlessly blaming themselves for the child's illness. This way you will not help the child. Yes, you can relate to his illness, but it's not your fault—most often you are also the victim of your parents and of your insecure attachment. The famous child psychoanalyst Françoise Dolto told the parents that everything happens because of them, but not their own fault. Life simply did not grant you the chance before this to learn how stress distorts health. You did not have the opportunity to develop other emotional reactions, or to change your character. But, it's never too late. By changing and healing yourself, you can improve the health of your child, and this book will help you to find the ways to do it.

Chapter 9

Specific Traits of The Cancer Personality

> It is often more important what person has the
> disease, than what disease a person has.
> *Sir William Osler,*
> *the father of British medicine*

Specific features of the personality formed on the basis of childhood experiences that determine the degree of their resistance to stress are also very significant factors in predisposition to diseases (Sokolova E. V. et al., 1996). According to the studies of Boris Karvasarskiy (1988, 2008), a famous Soviet and Russian psychiatrist and psychotherapist, the formation of specific symptoms in psychosomatic illnesses is determined by the following factors:

- the properties of personality and temperament;
- unconscious intra- or interpersonal conflict, dissatisfaction with some need;
- the methods of emotional processing and establishing the basic defensive mechanisms of the psyche;
- individual experience and living conditions;
- the type and strength of the current psychological trauma.

In the last chapter, we argued that attachment disorders and stresses, experienced at an early age, lead to the formation in a child, who later develops cancer, of a specific type of personality common to psychosomatic patients. The main traits of this personality are avoidance of negative emotions, alexithymia, excessive perfectionism in social etiquette, problems with self-esteem, etc.

How much do these features remain in the personality of an adult and what is their contribution to the predisposition to cancer? Are there specific personality traits of cancer patients that can be considered predisposing factors? In psychology, there are various classifications of personality types. In the context of this book, I will use the classification by the type of psychosomatic personality reaction to stress, highlighting four categories: A, B, C, and D.

9.1. The Main Types of Psychosomatic Personalities

As I mentioned before, it was Hippocrates who, in the fourth century BC, first spoke of the Four Temperaments (sanguine, choleric, melancholic, and phlegmatic). They can be considered as personality traits associated with various diseases.

American physician and psychoanalyst Helen Dunbar, one of the pioneers of psychosomatic medicine, in her book *Emotions and bodily changes* (1954) has established a connection between certain personality characteristics and the types of disease. Believing that the personality of the patient determines his emotional reactions, and this directs the development of specific somatic diseases, Dunbar identified hypertensive, coronary, allergic, and "prone to damage" types of personalities.

Cardiologists M. Friedman and R. H. Rosenman (1959) described and named the behavior of the coronary personality as "behavior of type A." Since they observed a large number of patients, they were able to find similarities in the behaviors of patients with coronary heart disease with a complication in the form of myocardial infarction.

Personality type "A" is constantly at the center of events and problems. These people are driven by a persistent desire to achieve their goals and by their willingness to compete in this effort, turning any situation into a race. About themselves, they often say that they spin "like a hamster in a wheel," being in a fevered state twenty-four hours a day, and performing several tasks at the same time. Type "A" people are basically workaholics—they love their work and completely devote themselves to it. The driving force of "A" people is the desire to be recognized; they have high ambitions and claims. Typical of them is an exaggerated self-esteem that shapes personality traits such as individualism, aggressiveness, combativeness, addiction to "clarifying relationships," dissatisfaction with their place in life (for example: with their profession or position) (Granovskaya R. M., 2007). Striving in everything to be the first or the best, they are not able to stop and relax, and often push themselves to nervous exhaustion and cardiovascular diseases, mainly angina pectoris and heart attacks.

Ambitiousness and sensitivity to loss of prestige is the most important reason for the increased morbidity in people of type "A." These persons, as a rule, are restrained, secretive, and resentful. If they cannot get recognition from the people around them, be satisfied in the process of self-affirmation, and especially if they are ignored or suppressed, then their body reacts to the corresponding chronic emotional imbalance with the development of hypertension. Infarction in such subjects usually comes after a sudden and crushing catastrophe, often associated with damage to prestige (Rotenberg V. S., Bondarenko S. M., 1989).

People of type "B" have the opposite reaction to stress. They live in a hasteless way, not hurrying, planning their day, although they're not always at odds with their schedule. They do not try to "grasp the immensity," working calmly and measuredly. They lack the desire to compete, and prestige and recognition do not have much significance. These people manage to combine work with entertainment and family responsibilities. At the weekend they do not show up at work but try to relax and do something pleasant. Personalities of type "B" can be very creative, they like to learn new ideas and concepts, reflect on the outer and inner worlds. People of this type tend to have a positive approach to life and high self-esteem, so they are able to manage emotions, successfully overcome stress, and have good health.

Personality type "D" (distress) was introduced by the professor of clinical psychology Johan Denollet from Tilburg University in The Netherlands in 1996, when problems arising from stress began to attract serious attention in medical research. This is a type of person experiencing mostly negative emotions—irritation, anxiety, gloominess, and hostility. They often feel unhappy, pessimistic, restless, and are prone to depression. However, these people are extremely reluctant to share their feelings with others because of a fear of any negative reactions, and they accumulate discontent within themselves. Within social interactions, representatives of type "D" feel insecure, therefore they have fewer personal connections with other people and feel discomfort when dealing with strangers, so they strive for closeness and security. As a result, these people lack social support and positive impressions, and experience low self-esteem and a general dissatisfaction with life (Denollet J., 2005).

If individuals of behavioral type "A" are mostly leaders inclined to dominate their interactions, people of type "D" are more dependent personalities, an antipode of type "A." Although they also have professional ambitions, their inability to correctly assess their capabilities, analyze and learn from failures, notably avoiding criticism from others, takes them to a high level of stress. Shallow life difficulties, those easily resolved by a sociable person, for people like "D" can become an insoluble problem. In the language of psychologists, individuals of type "D" have an elevated assessment on two points: negative excitability (the tendency to experience negative emotions) and social inhibition (the tendency to self-forbid the manifestation of these negative emotions in communication), so type "D" is considered to be a chronic psychological risk factor.

According to the observations of Johan Denollet, about one in five people on the Earth belong to people of type "D," i.e., 20%. However, in a study of 1,012 healthy young people of both sexes in England and Ireland, "D" type affiliation was detected in 38.5% (Williams L. et al., 2008). These people, as a rule, lead a sedentary lifestyle, are not careful regarding their health and nutrition, and are often smokers who will not even consider giving up their habit. They are less likely to turn to doctors about their health problems and to follow their recommendations. If they do not find effective ways to overcome their stresses, their physical and mental health falls into the risk zone, because the level of the stress hormone cortisol is higher in their blood and it is therefore more difficult for them to relax (Denollet J., Kupper N., 2007).

Such individuals often complain of poor health and a low quality of life, but even the presence of disease does not explain this stance. It is shown that the personality type "D" adversely affects the prognosis of the disease in cardiac patients: with ischemic heart disease, chronic heart failure, in those who have undergone myocardial infarction, and after heart transplantation. The risk of death due to an unhealthy heart in type "D" patients increased sixfold in comparison with non-type "D" patients (Sumin A. N. et al., 2012).

It has been demonstrated that type "D" is also a prognostic factor for the development of cancer (Denollet J., 1998). Among 750 patients with rectal cancer, 19% corresponded to the type of personality "D", with 15.1% of them associating the onset of their illness with lifestyle, and 11.9% with psychological distress (Mols F. et al., 2012). Type "D" was found in 22% of patients with melanoma and 19% of a mixed group of cancer patients, including uterine, rectal, lymphoma, and multiple myeloma (Mols F. et al., 2010, 2012)

For our analysis, the most interesting is the so-called personality type "C" (cancer).

9.2. The Type "C" Personality

> The precancerous personality
> is the ultimate carcinogen.
> *Dr. Frederick B. Levenson,*
> *The Causes and Prevention of Cancer*

According to historical documentation we have reviewed, in the nineteenth century doctors were already describing some typical psychological characteristics of cancer patients. Dr. Caroline Thomas of the Johns Hopkins University School of Medicine in 1946 began a long-term study that showed important results. The scientist made profiles of personalities of 1,337 medical students who studied at the same university, and year after year during the decades after graduation, observed their mental and physical health. Her original purpose was to determine the psychological factors associated with heart disease, hypertension, mental illness, and suicide. In addition, Dr. Thomas included cancer in her research as a group for comparison, since she initially thought that this disease has no psychological component. However, her observations showed that almost all cancer patients throughout life inhibited the expression of emotions, especially aggressive ones, when it came to their own needs. Using only pictures that were part of one of the psychological tests, Dr. Thomas (1974) could even predict in which part of the body the cancer would develop.

Eugene Blumberg and colleagues in 1954 described cancer patients as defensive, anxious, overly self-controlled individuals, unable to release their stresses either through motor, or verbal, or any other form of discharge. Therefore, cancer, according to these scientists, is a syndrome of "non-adaptation." In the same year, at the first symposium on the psychological aspect of cancer in California, Dr. Max Cutler reported on his studies of patients with breast cancer. Being an oncologist and indeed the director of the Cancer Institute in Chicago, he nevertheless was actively interested in the psychological causes of the appearance of tumors. He found the following main characteristics in his patients: 1) a masochistic nature, 2) suppressed sexuality, 3) suppressed motherhood, 4) inability to discharge or adequately control their anger, aggressiveness, or hostility, covered by the facade of "pleasantness," 5) an unresolved conflict of hostility with their mother, that the patients coped with by rejecting said hostility while making excessive and unrealistic sacrifices, 6) delayed treatment.

According to A. B. Cobb (1952), cancer patients refer to emotional manifestations as a danger, avoid them, and become isolated in their space because of a fear of failure and rejection. In Glasgow, from 1962 to 1969 Dr. David Kissen and colleagues studied *psychodynamic* aspects of the personality with lung cancer. They found these patients to have noticeable difficulties with emotional expression, and to be prone to depression and inhibition (Kissen D. M., 1966; Kissen D. M., Rao L. G., 1969).

Based on their own and similar research, T. Morris and S. Greer of the hospital at the Royal College of London in 1980 introduced the "C" personality type for cancer patients, believing that their main trait is emotional closeness, especially in stressful situations. Developing this concept, in 1986 Dr. Lydia Temoshok from the School of Medicine of the University of California presented a more detailed picture of the "C," type of personality, supported by the respected German experts in psychosomatics H. J. F. Baltrusch and P. Santagostino (1989). Analysis of the characteristics of several thousand oncological patients gave Dr. Temoshok grounds to call them "good" patients, because they always wanted to appear that way. The following characteristics were established as typical:

- suppression and repression of anger—the main mechanism of cancer patients' psychological defense;

- the desire to not experience and not show other negative emotions, such as fear, anxiety, or sadness;

- patience, modesty, passivity, obedience, cooperation, satisfaction with relationships at work, in the family and in society, and subordination to authorities. Without contact with their basic needs and emotions, this person is waiting for signals from other people about how to think, feel, and act;
- avoidance of any conflicts, i.e., a lack of "fighting spirit." The way to deal with stressful situations is to refuse to recognize them, that is, to pretend that nothing is happening;
- excessive interest in meeting the needs of others and insufficient satisfaction of one's own needs, frequent manifestation of self-sacrifice;
- depression, a tendency to hidden despair, apathy, frequent fatigue, difficulties in adapting;
- chronic hopelessness and helplessness, even if it is not realized. A person believes that it is in principle useless to express their own needs, since they will not be positively received by others (Temoshok L., 1986; Temoshok L., Dreher H., 1993).

Subsequently, these personality traits of cancer patients were in general repeatedly confirmed by other studies in many countries of the world. I will present only some of them.

Spanish scientists have shown that cancer patients are characterized by a higher level of neuroticism, anxiety, and some aspects of anger, and a lower level of extroversion (impulsiveness and openness of emotions). Those patients who suppress anger strongly show excessive humility and self-criticism against a background of diminished self-awareness, and in turn have an unfavorable prognosis of the development of disease (Cardenal V. et al., 2012).

Australian researchers from the University of Melbourne, studying patients with colorectal cancer, have identified a significant link between their disease and the suppression of anger and other negative emotions and the rejection of their manifestations, the desire to be a "good" or "pleasant" person and meet social norms, and to avoid conflicts and expressing resentment toward other people. At the same time, the risk of developing cancer was independent of diet, beer consumption, country of birth, marital status, religion, and history of cancer in the family (Kune G. A. et al., 1991).

Israeli psychologists came to similar conclusions about patients with rectal cancer, discovering in them: the desire to achieve peace and rest in their environment through restraint and self-regulation; the need for excellent performance of their duties and obligations; suppression of anger; rigidity in relation to themselves; combating injustice; control of others; avoidance of control by others; and the desire to please others (Figer A. et al., 2002).

A study conducted in several Russian cancer centers on patients with various types of cancer found that many patients had a predominantly childlike position in communication; difficulties in perceiving, understanding, and responding to traumatic situations, the tendency to exempt themselves of responsibility ("everything depends on external circumstances," "I do not decide anything"); dependence on external attitudes and values; propensity to long-suffering, self-sacrifice, ignoring their own needs, and difficulty in expressing feelings (Ivashkina M. G., 1998).

American scientists, who observed about a thousand women with breast cancer, concluded that a low level of emotional expression is associated with poorer survival (Reynolds P. et al., 2000). Researchers from the Netherlands showed a predominance of rationality and anti-emotionality in cancer patients associated with controlling, suppressing, or repressing of anger (Van der Ploeg H. M. et al., 1989).

C. Hurny and R. Adler (1991), analyzing the available scientific data on persons prone to cancer, identified the following common psychological characteristics:
- denial and suppression of disturbing experiences,
- reduced self-perception,
- reduced ability to discharge emotions,
- impaired ability to express anger,
- increased self-sacrifice and self-blame,
- a rigid lifestyle, subordination to others,
- belief in authority, religiosity,
- an excessive orientation to practical reality,
- shallow and vulnerable interpersonal relations,
- depressed sexuality,
- high moral standards.

A. V. Aseev (1993, 1998) of the Tver Medical Academy (Russia), studying psychological life history and using the archetypal test in 700 patients with breast cancer, identified the following as their most common features:
- difficulties in identifying one's own feelings (alexithymic radical),
- reduced ability to express aggression or resist it,
- primitiveness of ideas about means of defense against aggression,
- fixation on the obstacle, a feeling of despair in stressful situations,
- the absence of sufficiently good and adequate means of emotional discharge,
- difficulty in communicating and in forming close friendships,
- inability to understand the causes of many events, being satisfied with the knowledge of external, formal manifestations; lack of analysis of cause–effect relationships in life,
- inability to accept support from outside sources in difficult situations,
- propensity for a high level of personal and reactive anxiety,
- decreased tolerance of frustration,
- the presence of uncomfortable relationships in the family (36%), divorce (12%), widowhood (12.3%),

- the presence of non-harmonious sexual relations (46.9%), including sacrificial attitudes, to one's own detriment.

German psychologists from the universities of Heidelberg and Marburg came to a similar conclusion about the special attributes of cancer patients, as a result of a ten-year prospective observation of 1,353 people in a small Yugoslavian town. They found that individuals who developed cancer during this time, in the period preceding the illness were characterized as submissive, non-aggressive, and suppressing their needs. These people tend to adapt to non-harmonious interpersonal relationships in order to maintain a sense of security and dignity, neglecting themselves and submitting to the suppressive behavior of dominant people significant to them (Grossarth-Maticek R. et al., 1982).

Dr. Claus Bahnson of the University of Rochester (1980), on the basis of his own clinical experience, lists the following characteristics of cancer patients:

1. Childhood trauma, loss of loved ones, lack of safety and love in childhood, parental coldness and lack of attention.

2. Repetitive, intrusive, self-destructive tendencies, attitudes, and actions, often manifested on the anniversaries of specific events (for example, the death of a loved one).

3. An all-embracing, underlying pattern of hopelessness in their behaviors that leaves an imprint on the person's entire life ("everything must go wrong") in combination with a simultaneous sense of guilt due to self-criticism.

4. The formation of a double life or a double personality, where both the realistic and adaptive actions of the rational self are expressed, and the separate and independent actions of the parallel "shadowy self," which feels isolated, unloved, sick, and devastated.

For the sake of objectivity, it should be noted that not all psychologists find a link between the development of cancer and the psychological state of a person, in particular the type of personality (Nakaya N. et al., 2003), depression (Johansen C., 2010), agitation, dissatisfaction, and unhappiness (Lillberg K. et al., 2002), etc. The reason for this is probably the heterogeneity of the methods used for examining patients. Also quite a large part is played by subjectivity, and therefore the assessment by patients of their mental state and the stresses they have experienced is not always adequate (some of these stresses are simply unconsciously suppressed from the patients' memory). According to R. E. Huggan from Otago University in New Zealand (1968), it seems that we have not yet created adequate tools for measuring what cancer researchers have been trying to bring to our attention since the time of Galen. The greatest benefit, according to this author, can be brought via long-term observations of groups at risk of cancer.

Firdaus Dhabhar, with colleagues from Stanford University, arrived at a similar conclusion (2012). The heterogeneity of data in studies of the relationship between personality characteristics, stress, and the onset of cancer is attributed to the patients studied being at different stages of the disease, with differing locations and types of tumor, in different phases and states of stress intensity, as well as to methodological differences in the experiments. At the London Institute of Preventive Medicine, prominent psychologist Hans Eysenck and his staff evaluated the survey methodology which uses questionnaires to study the risk of the development of cardiac and oncological diseases in healthy people. They discovered that the degree of personal attention of the researcher influences the attitude of the subject to this procedure, the level of his openness in the tests, and, accordingly, the degree of accuracy in predicting the occurrence of diseases. The authors concluded that in research on the impact of personal factors and stress on cardiovascular disease and cancer, the survey methodology factor may be critical in the success or failure of finding interrelations (Grossarth-Maticek R. et al., 1993).

In my opinion, the most trustworthy is the work of practical physicians and psychologists who regularly observe oncological patients. C. Simonton with colleagues (1978) believe that the emotional and intellectual state plays a significant role both in the susceptibility to all diseases, including cancer, and in their elimination. In 1983, Stephen Locke and Mady Hornig-Rohan compiled an annotated bibliography of studies on the relationship between the mind and the immune system, reviewing 1,304 journal articles and about 150 books. Among these works, 49 were devoted to the psychology of cancer, and most of them recognized the importance of the psychological properties of the personality in the development of cancer. Russian psychotherapist, Sergey Kulakov (2009a), believes that among the psychosomatic mechanisms of cancer the most important are the traits of the personality, manifested in the way of life and in overcoming the stressful effects of the environment.

Australian doctor Ian Gawler (1984), who defeated his cancer and devoted himself to helping other patients, writes:

> In my experience, psychological factors are important in the causation of most cancers. There is a typical psychological profile that occurs in more than 95% of many thousands of people affected by cancer with whom I have discussed their disease. ... Deep down, there can lurk a marked lack of self-confidence with a tendency toward self-negation, almost self-destruction. Deeply bottled inside is the feeling that all is not well. True reactions, emotions especially, are often suppressed. There is a continual effort to block out basic feelings. It is like trying to push the truth from the conscious awareness, like trying to keep the lid on a constantly bubbling pressure cooker.

Psychologist Lawrence LeShan (1977), one of the classic psycho-oncologists, came to the conclusion as a result of studying patients for more than two decades that there are four basic personality characteristics associated with the development of cancer:

1. Negative experiences due to the loss of important emotional relationships,
2. Inability to express anger or resentment,

3. An unusual large volume of self-denial and distress in life,

4. Feelings of hopelessness and helplessness.

Why do these psychological characteristics lead to the development of cancer? At the beginning of her research Lydia Temoshok (1986) understood that the behavior of "C" types was the best attempt of every person to cope with psychological pain, stress, humiliation, and unsatisfied needs from early childhood. However, this behavior only had the appearance of effectiveness— later in life, this method of coping showed its detriment, in both the mental and physical aspects.

In her later book (1993), Lydia Temoshok writes about two main ways of coping with emotions: through externalization (manifestation in the outside) or internalization (keeping them inside). People who internalize emotions generally tend to exhibit bodily, not psychological, responses under stress. In accordance with the data reviewed above, we can assume that these people will demonstrate a somatic "cancerous" type of processing of an intrapersonal conflict or a traumatic situation. Indeed, Dr. Temoschok's research on patients with melanoma confirmed that patients, specifically those who could express their emotions better, had smaller skin tumors, the cells in which multiplied more slowly, and the lymphocytes of their immune systems, fighting the tumor, were detected in larger numbers, compared with those in less emotional patients. I have already cited data on the negative impact of inhibiting emotions on health, and in the following sections I will introduce the reader to important studies, confirming the conclusions of many researchers about the predominant role of avoiding negative emotions in the mechanism of cancer development.

Dr. Temoshok also believes that the types of personalities of most healthy people are somewhere in between the extremes of the classical types "A" and "C," and therefore they can be generally referred to as type "B." I would refer them as having a secure type of childhood attachment. Undoubtedly, the ability of "B" type people to express their emotions freely and cope better with stresses makes them less likely to get cancer. At the same time, it seems that there are not so very many "clean" types of personalities; rather, every person represents a certain percentage of each type, and this balance determines the individual characteristics in responding to stressful situations.

As is quite evident, there is an important similarity between the "C" and "D" types of personalities: the desire to limit the expression of negative emotions, anxiety, propensity to depression, and inability to adequately cope with stress. Since these two types of personality are the most susceptible to cancer, these properties should be perceived by psychologists as an emergency indication for preventive psychotherapeutic work, and people who discover such traits in themselves should take serious steps to change their lifestyle.

Along with the similarity, there are differences between types "C" and "D." Professor Johan Denollet, the author of the discovery of the "D" type of personality, in this regard states (1998):

- type "C" was introduced in opposition to type "A," whereas type "D" does not refer to type "A";

- type "C" reflects the totality of psychosocial variables, while type "D" is based on the interaction of two global positions (tendencies to experience negative emotions and at the same time forbid their manifestation);

- type "C" mainly focuses on the suppression of emotional self-expression, whereas type "D" is characterized by experiencing negative emotions.

The reader will probably ask: do representatives of personalities types "A" and "B" not suffer from cancer? They do, but less often than types "D" and "C," especially type "B." For example, a study of a group of 3,154 people revealed that type "A" individuals are 50% more likely to develop cancer than those of type "B," but with age, this ratio is reduced to 30% (Fox B. H. et al., 1987). The reason for the prevalence of morbidity in "A" type over "B" can be their high levels of ambition to achieve their goals. With repeated life failures, these individuals may experience frustration, followed by the development of depression as a precancerous condition. Psycho-oncologist Tom Laughlin (1999) attributes personality type "A" to exceptions among cancer patients, and indicates that their aggression and dominance are often just a mask under which they conceal the trauma of childhood. "A" is a type of defensive behavior that allows these people to suppress their childhood fear of conflict and rejection in the form of attack. As a result, they suffer from loneliness and thereby "suffocate" themselves with their own hostility, which predisposes them to developing cancer.

A talented representative of the Jungian psychotherapeutic school, Tom Laughlin created the original psychological concept behind the theory of development of a cancerous personality. He found six fundamental factors, and during a person's life, at least five of them must appear for the person to fall ill with cancer:

1. Because of living conditions as a child, or upbringing, a person develops and then retains the habit of avoiding expressing his emotions and needs in order to avoid conflict.

2. In the latter half of life, a person finds herself in conditions where she feels controlled, victimized, trapped, isolated, and helpless, this leading to a loss of hope for a change in this situation.

3. In some areas of adult life (usually in relationships with parents, children, or spouse, or at work), regardless of whether the person is aware of it or not, she is so under control and/or domination that she cannot freely express her own basic emotional or personal needs and develop the potential of her personality. This state is experienced as "suffocation."

4. Previous factors cause the formation of a "subliminal ego" in a person; that is, a person incapable of resisting those individuals or circumstances that are perceived by her as dominant and suffocating, and who therefore concedes decision-making. It is important that at a conscious level, the person still may not be aware of the true state of affairs.

5. The "subliminal ego" of a person becomes vitally dependent on the dominant personality or situation ("I cannot live without a parent / spouse / child / job ...") and this limits her life actualization. This pathological bonding to the suppressing ("suffocating") factor blocks a person's ability to get out of a relationship or situation and transforms helplessness into a precancerous state: hopelessness.

6. Conflict and mental attitudes formed by the previous five factors remain unknown to the person, since these conflicts are played out in the subconscious and the person does not realize her suffering. This forms an unconscious, subliminal depression leading to suppression of immunity and development of cancer.

Tom Laughlin (1999) also believes that the main and most important negative consequence of the formation of such a subordinate personality is the loss of the ability to manifest one's life goal, or one's vocation. As a result, the first thing lost is one's "meaning of life," and then, according to this spiritual program, life itself.

It is especially important that a person predisposed to cancer often does not even suspect the existence of those deep destructive processes that occur in his subconscious. The reason for this is that his image of life, which has arisen on the basis of personality defects acquired in childhood, does not allow him to pay himself enough attention and care, and the negative emotions that arise as result are suppressed or repressed.

As we can see, the personal characteristics of cancer patients generally correspond to the somatic type of stress and conflict processing, and, consequently, belong to psychosomatic personality. Most of the traits of the cancer patient's character and their life circumstances, as follows from the cited studies, coincide with those of psychosomatic patients in general. A more detailed analysis of individual psychological aspects, carried out in subsequent chapters, will confirm this conclusion. Similar traits have been described in a certain group of patients with neurosis, which is regarded as a precursor to psychosomatic diseases. Well-known psychotherapists Karen Horney (1992) and Claudio Naranjo (1994) have referred to such a patient as "a compliant person, oriented towards people" and an *enneatype* 9, respectively (further details in Chapter 11).

Therefore, today it is hardly advisable to talk about the existence of a specific type of oncological personality "C"; I believe that future cancer patients have a "general psychosomatic" type of personality with oncogenic potential (or, as L.

Temoshok and H. Dreher (1993) said, type "C" coping with stress). Further, for brevity, I will call it psychosomatic type "C" that may materialize its cancer potential under chronic stress, caused by traumatic processes or conflict within the psyche. We will consider these circumstances in the next part.

Conclusion

The materials presented in this part show that the stresses experienced in the pre-, intra-, and postnatal periods of development, notably in the presence of hereditary epigenetic vulnerability, determine the specific biological and psychological styles of response to subsequent stressful events, and form a specific psychosomatic personality predisposed to cancer.

In this sort of person, the main stages of ontogeny become, in the following various combinations:

- a stress-reactive epigenetic distortion inherited from the parents;
- intrauterine stress experienced because of and together with the mother;
- birth stress—the formation of the second (most likely) basic perinatal matrix;
- disorder of children's attachment to the mother, predominantly by the avoidance type;
- development of a hypercognitive variant of the child's cognitive-emotional disbalance;
- the formation of the main types of psychological defense—repression, suppression, and negation of negative information and emotions;
- a limited range of adaptive capabilities and coping with distress;
- the fixation of the internalization of psychological conflicts and their somatic processing;
- gradual increase in the activity of the psychosomatic system of condensed experience.

What is the further danger of these factors in terms of the probability of cancer developing in people with type "C" psychosomatic reactions? Undoubtedly, it depends on their number and intensity, the variety of their combination, and the effect of their accumulation. The more epigenetic changes occur, the more distorted the hypothalamic-pituitary-adrenal axis becomes, the further immunity decreases, and the more inflammation develops in the tissues, the higher is the probability of accumulation of genetic mutations and the malignant transformation of cells. The impressive discoveries of science of the last decade have clearly demonstrated the important influence of psychosocial and socioeconomic influences in early childhood on epigenome modifications that can lead to health disorders in adulthood (Borghol N. et al., 2012; Lucassen P. J. et al., 2013), including the appearance of cancer (Kelly-Irving M. et al.,

2013a). This reflects the paradigm of "lifelong accumulation," according to which genetic, epigenetic, and socioeconomic factors, multiplying as a result of prolonged exposure, strengthen one another, and worsen health (Loi M. et al., 2013).

In accordance with the diathesis-stress model, the more severe the stressful events-provocateurs (especially the psychological trauma of loss) happening in the later life of a person with a "C" psychosomatic type, the greater is the likelihood of developing chronic distress and of transformation of a predisposition to cancer into a precancerous state. We will analyze this process in detail in the following parts.

But, there is also good news from the field of epigenetics: the dangerous potential of genome modifications is not activated if the person's environmental conditions are favorable, and if stresses do not exceed her adaptive capabilities. That is, in the case of a link called "diathesis-stress," the latter component does not have destructive power over a given person. Understanding these fundamental biological laws also makes it possible to develop new strategies for psychotherapeutic intervention that will prevent or even reverse the previously established negative programs of the body's response to stress (Matthews S. G., Phillips D. I., 2010). It is especially important to do this at an early age, when children are cared for most intensively. Helping parents to improve the quality of raising children can prevent the emergence of inadequate psycho-emotional behavioral patterns in them, as well as preventing the deregulation of biological systems. This improves the children's response to stressful events and reduces the likelihood of health problems in the future (Mayes L. C. et al., 2005).

The creator of the attachment theory, John Bowlby (1984), wrote that the attachment style that emerges in childhood can change under the influence of relationships or circumstances created in later life. This is confirmed by the research mentioned previously showing that psychotherapy, which changes the mother's insecure attachment to a secure one, leads to the formation of a secure attachment in the children (Iyengar U. et al., 2014). A meta-analysis of scientific literature also shows that safe, stable, developing relationships hinder the transgenerational transmission of child abuse (Schofield T. J. et al., 2013).

Data have already appeared showing that a warm psychological climate in the family can help eliminate the adverse changes in epigenetic regulation that have occurred in early life under the influence of stresses. In particular, reduced synthesis of pro-inflammatory agents such as interleukin-6 and NF-$\varkappa$B transcription factor and the activity of the AP-1 activation factor of immunity (Chen E. E. et al., 2011). Also, studies in rats have shown that a high level of maternal care for the offspring, manifested in frequent licking and good care, is reflected in a decrease in methylation of the gene responsible for the synthesis of the of hormone cortisol receptors in the hippocampus. This leads to an increase in the receptor content and provides a calmer response to stress in the baby rats (Weaver I. C., 2007). Such behavior in the mother also prevents neuronal deficits in the offspring's hippocampus resulting from the stress experienced by the fetus during intrauterine development (Lemaire V. et al., 2006). All this helps to prevent negative health consequences that could arise in children on account of parental stresses and cruel behavior.

Even if a person has not been lucky enough to grow up in a family where parents have realized their inherited psychological defects and the danger of their transfer to children, and subsequently psychologically changed themselves, if an unhappy childhood has epigenetically imprinted on one's genes and stress-reactive systems of the body, thus forming a psychosomatic predisposition, epigenetics still permits changing of the function of genes and weakening of the predisposition to cancer even in adulthood.

An experiment at the laboratory of Ivan Pavlov in the 1950s found that ceasing to electrically stimulate nerves in mice delayed the development of the malignant process, even with a relatively long application of an electric current as a stressor—provided that the cessation of this neurotization occurs at a stage when the cancer process is still reversible (Melikhov E. F., 1956), i.e. at the stage of precancer.

As for the human, "... factors from the past have enormous significance only when the patient has once again put themselves in a situation which is a current re-creation of that childhood suffocation. The tragic legacy of such a past is that it predisposes such a person, almost 'programs' them, to become suffocated in any relationship that is emotionally important for them," writes Tom Laughlin (1999). However, he states, "How a cancer patient lived in the past would mean nothing if now they were living in a fully liberated and totally free environment, if they were free to express their emotional and other needs whenever they wished, and were also free to fulfill them in any way they felt appropriate."

The study of the possibilities for preventing the development of cancer is still divided into two approaches in science. Traditional scientists, focused on bio-medicine (or pharmaceutics), are concerned about finding new drugs that can change the direction of modification of the epigenome. More progressive (from my point of view) psychosocially oriented scientists investigate the methods of the conscious work of a person with his body and psyche, which are also able to regulate the epigenome.

A review of the effect of psychotherapy on health demonstrates that it leads to the decrease of: a previously increased response of the limbic system to stimuli; disproportions between the activity of the sympathetic and parasympathetic parts of the nervous system; distortions in learning and memory processes; elevated levels of cortisol and other stress hormones; and disorders of immune functions. These improvements are reflected in corresponding changes in gene activity (Feinstein D., Church D., 2010). Studies conducted at the Icahn School of Medicine in New York show the changes in the methylation of the NR3C1 and FKBP51 genes, which were involved in the synthesis of the glucocorticoid receptor, as a result of a successful course of psychotherapy in patients with PTSD (Yehuda R. et al., 2013). Based on this data, S. M. Stahl (2012) from the Department of Psychiatry at the University of California believes that psychotherapy today can be considered as an "epigenetic drug" that changes the synthesis of substances in the brain, a kind of therapeutic agent acting on the body in the same way as do pharmacological remedies. New achievements in neurogenetics make it possible to explore the effectiveness of psychotherapy at the molecular level objectively and in a standardized way.

In addition, it is shown that positive effects of physical exercise in humans are also mediated by epigenetic changes in gene activity (Sanchis-Gomar F. et al., 2012), as well as the effect of the Chinese physical discipline of tai-chi, which reduced the age-related decline in methylation of individual genes (Ren H. et al., 2012). Scientists from the Benson-Henry Mind-Body Institute in Massachusetts found that relaxation practices increase the expression of genes associated with energy metabolism, mitochondrial functions, telomeres, and insulin secretion, while the activity of genes associated with inflammatory and stressful reactions decreases (Bhasin M. K. et al., 2013).

Other researchers have found that as an affect of mindfulness meditation, acetylation of chromatin's histones increases, and the activity of genes responsible for inflammatory processes decreases accordingly (Kaliman P. et al., 2014). An eight-week Kriya Yoga meditation practice results in an increase in the activity of nineteen genes, including immunoglobulin genes, and a decrease in the expression of forty-nine genes, including genes encoding pro-inflammatory cytokines and genes that activate the primary response of lymphocytes to external stimuli (Black D. S. et al., 2013). A study by Indian scientists on oxidative damage of the sperm genome, cited above, found that in men practicing meditation and yoga the amount of oxidative damage to DNA gradually decreases, starting from the tenth day of classes and progressing for six months (Dada R. et al., 2015).

In scientific language, epigenetics has once again confirmed that the state of our health largely depends on us, on our minds. As the American scientist Randy Jirtle (the first to show that hereditary information is transmitted epigenetically) said, "Epigenetics is proving we have some responsibility for the integrity of our genome. Before, genes predetermined outcomes. Now everything we do, everything we eat or smoke, can affect our gene expression and that of future generations. Epigenetics introduces the concept of free will into our idea of genetics." (Watters E., 2006). Moreover, I believe that epigenetics opens the door to a completely new era of preventive medicine and psychology, shifting the emphasis from treatment to prevention of diseases—we shall talk about this in the book's conclusion.

On the basis of the data presented, we can expect that epigenetic modifications that predispose to cancer can also be transformed by changing the state of the psyche and environmental factors that affect a person after birth. Although I have not found experimental data directly confirming this possibility with regard to cancer predisposition, there are similar conclusions from other scientists (Kelly-Irving M. et al., 2013b). Professor C. A. Wendling (2016) from the university of Strasbourg, following his studies of women with breast cancer, came to the conclusion that successful psychotherapy, combining a somatic technique and a talking cure, can reverse the harmful effects of early adverse experiences through the epigenetic route. Also convincing are the results of research on cancer patients demonstrating the reality of improvement in their health and quality of life, together with the accompanying epigenetic changes, under the influence of psychotherapy, meditation, physical exercises, tai-chi movements, stress management techniques, social support, and dietary changes (see Chapter 32). If such changes are possible for sick people, they are undoubtedly achievable for those who have only a predisposition to cancer.

Therefore, if you are healthy but recognized yourself in the descriptions of type "C" or "D" personalities, if you were emotionally ignored or abused in childhood, do not panic and conclude that you are likely to develop cancer. I hope that the reader has already understood: predisposition is probabilistic in character—it manifests only when one is unable to cope with situations of acute or chronic stress and associated negative emotions. But this factor depends only on the person, and here again we return to the fact that everything determines our mind. Practice shows that everyone is able to get rid of the predisposition to disease, change their character and emotional reactions.

It is appropriate to bring Bernie Siegel's (1998) observations in this connection:

> I have seen people change the scenario once they become aware of it. ... Fatalism can be fatal. Too many people think they're doomed to reenact their parents' scripts. As a nurse told me after one of my lectures, 'I think you may have saved my life. I've been waiting to die of cancer, since my mother has it and my father had it. It never occurred to me that I didn't have to have it.'

Undoubtedly, the reader asks the question: many adults have predisposing factors; they had perinatal complications, childhood adversities, psychic traumas, and attachment disorders—many of them also have a psychosomatic personality type. Why do only some of them get cancer? The reason is that all these factors are not "narrowly specific" for cancer. Many findings confirm that exposure to adversities during childhood and adolescence may enhance one's vulnerability to biological risk, i.e. to different diseases, in adulthood (Berg M. T. et al., 2017). The same is considered to apply to character traits. For example, although alexithymia is inherent in many cancer patients, it also appears in a significant number of other psychosomatic patients, people with neuroses, as well as healthy people. Therefore, scientists prefer to believe that alexithymic behavior is a nonspecific risk factor that can be associated with other, both specific and nonspecific pathogenic factors (Brautigam W. et al., 1997). From the same point of view, we can also consider other aspects of predisposition to cancer. In addition, in the lives of those who did not get sick, although they had a predisposition, there were no provoking and initiating psycho-traumatic events or conflicts.

* * *

As is evident from the above, a deficiency of parental love and emotional care, all the way up to physical and emotional violence, on top of already existing diathesis factors, plays a crucial role in developing a predisposition to cancer. In the following chapters, I will repeatedly return to the childhood of cancer patients, since almost all the basic personality characteristics and behavioral features of an adult that contribute to the onset of the disease are laid in this period.

Analyzing the scientific data presented here on the factors of the childhood attachment disorder, it is surprising that modern "highly developed" society understands the need for professional training of doctors, psychologists, social workers, etc. in order to allow them to work with people. However, an incommensurably more important occupation—the raising of children in a family—is considered something that does not require special education. But, how can parents with a distorted psyche, and often also a distorted physiology, courtesy of their childhood, raise fully actualized children?

I would like to imagine future society to have a state-developed system of training and counseling for young people entering into marriage—to the extent of making it an obligatory element of the work of maternity hospitals. Professional psychologists could assess the level of the traumatic childhood history of young people, the stance of their adult attachment, and offer a rehabilitation program for those who have disorders. This would allow young parents not to replay on their children their own traumatic scenarios of behavior, imprinted in their subconscious in childhood. I am sure that this would become a powerful factor in reducing the incidence of all kind of diseases, including pediatric oncology, and after the maturation of this generation, a decrease in the incidence of cancer in adults.

In our schools and universities, we fill the minds of children and young people with a mass of information, a large part of which will never be needed for them, but we do not teach the fundamental questions of life: how to understand ourselves and other people, how the mind works, how to manage emotions, and especially how to take care of the body. We teach children about life sciences, but do not teach them how to live in harmony, and if we do teach these things, we often pass on our limited and inferior experience. Reform of the health care system, therefore, is impossible without the reform of the education system. Psychology and self-regulation should occupy an important place among school subjects. Very gratifying in this regard is the initiative of specialists of the Ukrainian Institute of Experimental Pathology, Oncology and Radiobiology, who developed a special educational course for schoolchildren about the role of a healthy lifestyle in the prevention of cancer, and taught it in one of Kiev's schools.

The psychology of interpersonal interaction should be an obligatory subject in universities. Child psychologists in kindergartens and schools are required to have a much higher level of training and authority; they must be able to track or detect personality defects and attachment disorders, especially the emerging psychosomatic types, and direct these children, along with their parents, to a serious rehabilitational and emotional education program. Consider how much it will reduce the morbidity of these people when they grow up!

* * *

What are the factors that arise in adulthood and aggravate the already existing predisposition to cancer, or even provoke it? In accordance with the diathesis—stress model of diseases, in order for the predisposition to work out, significant stressful events must occur in a person's life.

Part III

Factors of Provocation:
Unresolved Psychic Trauma
or Intrapersonal Conflict

We are not our wounds.
Whenever we suffer, it is because
we consider ourselves to be those who we are not.
Liz Burbo,
Five injuries that prevent you from being yourself

If any of the stressful events of life have attained a psychotraumatic power and have not been safely lived through, resolved, or, as therapists say, are not "processed," and the negative emotions associated with trauma have been suppressed or repressed into the subconscious, then the predominant state of one's organism becomes chronic distress, with the corresponding metabolic syndrome. The psyche can get into a state of anxiety, neuroticism, depression, and helplessness. Such mental trauma, especially combined with a specific intrapersonal conflict, is considered the leading cause of most psychosomatic diseases (Alexander F., 1939; Topolyanskiy V. D., Strukovskaya M. V., 1986; Aleksandrovskiy Y. A., 2005).

There is a solid base for considering that an unresolved psychological trauma can become a factor provoking oncogenic distress, because it leads to increased sensibilization[1] of the organism to the damaging effects of various carcinogens due to a progressive decrease in the effectiveness of the body's defense systems.

This is basically what the physicians and scientists of the past whom I quoted in the first chapter wrote about. Below is what the pioneers of psycho-oncology of the twentieth century say:

Carl Simonton and co-authors (1978) observed that often the onset of cancer is preceded by a severe stressful condition:

> Frequently, clusters of stress occur within a short period of time. The critical stresses we have identified are those that threaten personal identity. These may include the death of a spouse or loved one, retirement, the loss of a significant role.

Lawrence LeShan (1977) emphasizes that future cancer patients invest so much energy in some relationship or social role that it becomes the meaning of their existence. Then, for various reasons, this relationship or role disappears from their life—perhaps because of the death of a loved one, a move to a new place of residence, retirement, the beginning of their child's independent life, etc. This event reactivates the psychic trauma that had not been healed from childhood and leads to the emergence of despair.

---

[1] Sensibilization - increasing the sensitivity of the body to the influence of any environmental or internal factor.

Ian Gawler (1984) notes that practically all cancer patients he talked with admitted that, in the period before the disease, stress had become a chronic phenomenon in their life. Also,

> In about 95 percent of patients asked, this ... involves one particularly severely stressful experience precipitating a drastic drop in their well-being. The stressful event invariably occurred well before the cancer was diagnosed, but its untoward effects continued.

These observations are supported by other studies.

In Finland, psychologists at the University of Helsinki in 1981 began to monitor 10,808 women who noted in questionnaires that there had been stressful events in their lives during the previous five years (i.e., before 1981). In the period from 1982 to 1996, 180 women from this group became ill with breast cancer. Statistical analysis of their questionnaires showed a reliable correlation between significant stressful events, such as divorce or separation, the death of a spouse, or a close relative or friend, and the subsequent occurrence of disease. Factors such as body weight and its changes, smoking, alcohol consumption, and physical activity were not found significant for the onset of cancer (Lillberg K. et al., 2003).

Scientists at Purdue University in Indiana, USA, conducted a psychological examination of 826 women who came to a breast clinic for a *mammogram*. Those women who subsequently were diagnosed with a malignant tumor had more incidents involving the deaths of a husband or close relative during the previous two years, and they felt deeper loneliness, compared to healthy women or those who were found to have a fibrous cyst (Fox C. et al., 1994). In a similar study carried out in the University of Manchester in the UK, 1,596 women were psychologically examined before the mammogram. Those who experienced psychotraumatic stress (death of a loved one, loss of significant relationships, physical trauma, health problems with close relatives, and/or marital problems) some time before the examination had a significantly higher risk of developing breast cancer (Cooper C. et al., 1989).

Researchers from the University of Marburg (Germany), who examined a group of women with a tumor in the mammary gland before the biopsy, came to the same conclusion. Women whose tumor turned out to be malignant had experienced much greater stress due to the loss of a loved one than women with benign tumors (Geyer S., 1991). Swedish scientists (University of Goteborg), for twenty-four years observed 1,462 women aged 38 to 60. The analysis showed that those who experienced stress for five years at the beginning of the observation period were twice as likely to develop breast cancer as women without stress (Helgesson O. et al., 2003). In Israel, 6,284 parents whose children died in 1970–1977 due to war or accident were observed for twenty years. A significant increase in the incidence of cancer of the lymphatic system, blood, respiratory system, and skin (melanoma) was found (Levav I. et al., 2000).

In the quoted studies, it is significant that the psychological examination was carried out before the establishment of the diagnosis, which excluded the imposition on the results of the examination of the state of stress due to a fact of diagnosis.

A meta-analysis of studies on the role of psychological factors in the occurrence of breast cancer for the period from 1966 to 2002 revealed a statistically significant effect of stressful events in life, typically the death of a spouse, relative, or friend among 7,666 cases of illness (Duijts S. F. et al., 2003). A similar conclusion was reached by other scientists after a meta-analysis of 307 publications conducted from 1995 to 2012 (Lin Y. et al., 2013). Another meta-analysis of 165 cases of cancer revealed the influence of psychosocial factors causing stress on a higher incidence of the disease (Chida Y. et al., 2008).

A significant association of the occurrence of colorectal cancer with stressful events due to work, the death of a spouse, or a change of residence was noted in the analysis of 569 patients in Sweden (Courtney J. G. et al., 1993). In the same country, scientists from the Karolinska Medical Institute analyzed the incidence of cancer among 101,306 parents who had lost their children. An increase in the incidence of cancer, especially of the cervix, liver, and stomach, was found, mainly within five years of the loss (Fang F. et al., 2011). In a similar study in Denmark, among the 2,062 parents who lost a child, a slight increase in the incidence of maternal cancer in the following 7 to 18 years was found (Li J. et al., 2003).

Other researchers have shown the effect of stressful life events in the two years prior to the diagnosis of gastric and lung cancer (Lehrer S., 1980, 1981). Psychologist Bert Garssen (2004) of the Helen Dowling Institute of Psycho-oncology in Holland conducted a meta-analysis of seventy psychological studies of cancer patients for 1974–2004. He revealed the factors associated with the development of malignant tumors: the loss of loved ones, helplessness, a low level of social support, and chronic depression.

According to Russian authors, the starting period of the action of psychological trauma, such as the death or disability of close people, divorce, frequent family conflicts, change of residence, etc., varies from 1 year to 4.5 years before the diagnosis of gastric cancer and melanoma. This indicates the presence of chronic psychoemotional stress long before the clinical manifestation of the disease (Bukhtoyarov O. V., Arkhangelskiy A. E., 2008). Similar data was noted by American researchers from Yale University: the death of a spouse, divorce, bankruptcy, and being unemployed for five years before the diagnosis are prominent among precursors of the development of malignant melanoma (Havlik R. J. et al., 1992). Indian scientists found that most of the stressful events that happened in the life of cancer patients occurred one or three years before the appearance of the clinical signs of the disease (Doongaji D. R. et al., 1985).

Researchers from Turkey studying 768 patients with cancer of different locations found that 41.7% of patients underwent at least one stressful event during the year before the disease. Mainly, it was the death of a significant person, lack of livelihood, debts, quarrels, and illnesses (Tas F. et al., 2012). In the illness case history, 83% of patients studied at the St. Petersburg Oncology Research Institute (Russia) have been diagnosed with various serious mental traumas in the period from one to two years preceding the disease. In 21% of the patients, the trauma was the death of relatives, with 14% including the relatives' death from cancer (Gnezdilov A. V., 2002). At Ben-Gurion University in Negev, Israel, scientists examined 255 women with breast cancer and 367 healthy subjects as controls, studying their life experience and the psychological characteristics manifested before the diagnosis. It was found that most of the sick women had experienced negative life events at that period, had a lower level of happiness and optimism, and higher rates of anxiety and depression (Peled R. et al., 2008).

As in the situation with personality traits, some authors did not find a link between stressful life events and the onset of cancer (Bergelt C. et al., 2006; Protheroe D. et al., 1999; Schernhammer E. S. et al., 2004; Schoemaker M. J. et al., 2016, etc.). Such disagreements are explained by methodological errors of experiments, in particular in different types of psychological questionnaires, subjectivity of patients in assessing stressful events, small patient samples, and distortion in patients' memories (Olsen M. H. et al., 2012). As noted by Spanish researchers, many patients diagnosed with breast cancer said that it was very difficult for them to answer a number of questions in the questionnaire; some of the patients were crying throughout the interview, or could not even complete the questionnaire. This situation reflects their mental pain and also indicates the difficulty in expressing certain negative emotions (Cardenal V. et al., 2008). Indeed, my psychotherapeutic practice confirms the significant frequency of the suppression of memories of psychotraumatic events (especially the childhood period), from the active area of consciousness in patients to the subconscious. In this case, the details of the past can be restored mainly through hypnosis or trance techniques.

The reader already knows that the intensity of the trauma experienced depends first of all on a subjective assessment of its significance (a shock to one person can only be a nuisance for another), and on one's ability to adequately respond and cope with the stressful state. Distinguished Soviet psychiatrist Vladimir Myasishchev (1960) identified three groups of human value systems, occurring according to the degree of psychotraumatic influence of a situation. The difference is in people's priorities regarding which spheres of life were their main focus points. For the first group of people, the main value was placed on the family, so that most psychotraumatic for them were: divorce, a relative's death, a child's or parent's illness, and family conflicts. In the second group, where people were oriented toward career and job status, psychological trauma (leading to neurosis) ranged from failing examinations, to demotion and dismissal at work. In the third group, where their hobbies were of primary importance for people, a traumatic event could be, for example, the loss of their collection.

Therefore, it is not so much the specific origin of the trauma that is important as its consequences for a particular person: post-stress disorders that range from reactive states and psychoses, to neurotic and psychosomatic disorders.

M. Biondi and A. Picardi (1996) of the psychiatric clinic of the La Sapienza University of Rome, in their review note that after acute stress and loss, numerous disorders occur in one's neuroendocrine and immune systems that last for several months, making one vulnerable to physical and mental illnesses. The vulnerability to grief can be sustained for about two years after the loss, with men more at risk than women. If grief remains unresolved or psychologically complicated, then vulnerability to health disorders persists; moreover, it becomes part of the nervous system of the grieving person, as if imprinted in his neurochemical basis. This leads to the development of depression, which, as will be noted later, becomes one of the precancerous factors.

These aspects of the response to stress continue to operate even after the onset of the oncological disease. Studies of women with breast cancer, conducted at the Institute of Psychology of the Russian Academy of Sciences, showed that the greater the number of psychotraumatic situations in their life before the disease, and the greater their subjective impact, the more psychopathological changes manifested, and a higher incidence of post-traumatic stress disorder in response to such a powerful stressor as cancer. At the same time, it isn't the specificity of the past stresses that is significant, but their intensity and quantity, and especially the effect of their accumulation. The chain of accumulated stressful events before the disease, a high level of personal anxiety, and an inability to cope with stress, lead to the depletion of personal resources and the emergence of depressive state, which complicates the course of the disease (Vorona O. A., 2005).

Next, we will consider the mechanisms by which first acute and then chronic psychic trauma can provoke the formation of specific carcinogenic distress in the body.

Chapter 10

Acute Psychic Trauma as a Trigger of Chronic Stress and Its Connection with Cancer

The pain we feel when we lose something we're attached to,
or when we confront something we'd rather avoid,
is a direct result of not knowing everything
we could or should know about our own mind.
Yongey Mingyur Rinpoche,
The Joy of Living:
Unlocking the Secret and Science of Happiness

10.1. Mechanisms of Acute Psychic Trauma

In psychology, a stressful mental trauma means a person's reaction to an event that is important to him, associated with intense emotional experiences, has harmful consequences for the psyche, and leads to a deterioration in the quality of life. Psychic trauma occurs as a result of an incomplete instinctual reaction to a threatening event, when a person has not found an opportunity or a way to discharge fear, pain, and inner tension that arose at the time of the traumatic experience. By intensity, psychic trauma can be conditionally divided into shock, acute, and chronic, and they may lead to somewhat different consequences: adaptation disorders, acute stress disorder, post-traumatic stress disorder, and chronic stress.

Adaptation disorders are quite diverse and can range in manifestation from a drop in one's mood up to excessive alertness, anxiety, and a sense of inability to cope with the situation: to act correctly, and make plans in everyday life. There may also be behavioral disorders, emotional instability, a brief or prolonged depressive reaction; on a bodily level—insomnia, headache, chest pain, and palpitations. The outstanding Soviet physiologist Alexey Speranskiy as early as 1937 discovered that maladaptation is a nonspecific sign of many diseases.

Post-traumatic stress disorder is a protracted reaction to a shocking stressful event, characterized by great force and suddenness of action, usually associated with a threat to the life or well-being of a person (or his/her loved ones) arising from natural disasters, catastrophes, military actions, or criminal violence. This state also often develops after the cancer diagnosis, perceived by many as a shocking psychic trauma, and can significantly complicate the treatment (Chapter 29 will include more details about this kind of trauma).

Acute stress disorder (ASD) is the most frequent reaction to acute psychic trauma, occurring in situations of loss, grief, and/or severe conflict. Unlike shock, acute trauma is not always sudden and unexpected. Often it results from previous events in which the person participated or which he observed. An example is a serious illness and death of a loved one, the breakdown of a family with a history of previous conflicts or violence, loss of work or business, the experience of a serious offence or insult, etc. If the acute stress disorder which develops as a result of such a trauma is not resolved, it can progress into one that is chronic.

As we learned earlier, a person can react to stress predominantly in either a mental or somatic way. In accordance with this, most often in the case of the mental processing of ASD, a depressive syndrome occurs, whereas bodily disorders occur in the case of somatic processing. The latter can range from acute respiratory disease to urgent pathology, such as heart attacks, strokes, and perforated ulcers of the gastrointestinal tract (Tukaev R. D., 2012), to the extent of psychogenic death caused by heart failure (Engel G. L., 1971).

As a rule, the symptoms of ASD are short-lived. They disappear within a few hours (maximum: two or three days) without any other manifestations of mental disorders. However, owing to the above-listed personal characteristics, the intensity of anxiety, and abilities to cope with stress, ASD can lead to further complications. They range from adaptation disorders to chronic psychophysiological stress and post-traumatic stress disorder.

In the context of our research, it is necessary to understand what physiological and molecular alterations occur in the body owing to the experienced acute psychological trauma, as well as their possible connection with the onset of cancer.

The general mechanism of an acute physiological stress reaction was described in Chapter 3.1. Acute psychic trauma begins in the same way. It is accompanied by the activation of the immune system to increase the body's defense against possible simultaneous physical injuries. During the subsequent experience of a traumatic period, especially due to a severe loss, the activity of immunity decreases, and the level of cortisol in the blood increases (Irwin M. et al., 1988; Laudenslager M. L., 1988). This indicates the transition of stress to the chronic phase. For example, researchers at the University of Kentucky found that after the death of a spouse, the activity of protective immune killer cells in a widower or widow is significantly reduced (Segerstrom S. C., Miller G. E., 2004). A decrease in immune response by the sixth week after losing a wife or husband was shown by a group of scientists from Australia and the United Kingdom (Bartrop R. et al., 1977). This suppression of immune system activity in grieving spouses can continue for up to two years (Biondi M., Picardi A., 1996). At the same time, the slightest reminder of the psychic trauma that happened leads to a new surge in the activity of the stress-realizing system, thereby keeping the limbic system of the brain, responsible for emotions, in a state of chronic overstimulation (Horowitz M. J., 1997).

At the University of Ohio, scientists compared the psychological state and immunity in those widowed (on average, two years after the acute stress of loss), in people caring for spouses suffering from Alzheimer's disease (that is, in a state of chronic mild stress), and a control group (without stress). The activity of the immune response in both experimental groups was significantly lower compared to the control (Esterling B. et al., 1994).

It is also found that acute stress causes DNA damage (Gidron Y. et al., 2006) and activates the proto-oncogene encoding the regulatory protein—a nuclear factor of transcription NF-κB. This protein controls the expression of genes associated with cell division, immune response, and apoptosis, so distortion of its regulation activates inflammation and viral infections, and causes autoimmune diseases and cancer. During acute stress, the NF-κB content increases together with catecholamines and corticosteroids and can reach 341%, but within an hour its level returns to normal (Bierhaus A. et al., 2003). However, when the stress goes into the chronic phase, as for example in people caring for cancer patients, the NF-κB content remains increased continuously (Miller G. E. et al., 2008).

As a result of acute stress, the brain structure and its reparation are disordered. In particular, even a single stressful event entails a significant disruption of so-called "short-lived survival" of dividing cells and the "long-term survival" of differentiated cells in the hippocampus (Thomas R. M. et al., 2007). Acute stress that cannot be avoided leads to a decrease in cell division in the hippocampus (Malberg J. E., Duman R. S., 2003), and this disorder persists in chronic stress (Czéh B. et al., 2002). Such stress effects are mediated by its hormones—corticosteroids—and can cause various nervous disorders (McEwen B. S., 2012).[1] So, depression, which develops under chronic stress, is related to

---

[1]Fortunately, brain cell disorders are not irreversible. Perhaps not all readers know that the hypothesis of nerve cells as not able to be restored has sunk into oblivion. The phenomenon of neurogenesis, or the appearance of new nerve cells in the brain of adult

malfunctions in the hippocampal neuroplasticity (Pittenger C., Duman R. S., 2008). It is assumed that the above-mentioned nuclear transcription factor NF-$\varkappa$B, which promotes inflammatory processes in the brain (Barger S. W. et al., 2005; Ekdahl C. T. et al., 2003), can play an important role in the cellular mechanisms of neuroplasticity disorders.

Another component of the limbic system in which neurogenesis occurs is the amygdala, the functions of which include the regulation of social behavior through the creation of positive and negative emotions, especially fear and pleasure. Unlike the hippocampus, the amygdala increases in size with stress and psychic trauma, starting in childhood. In animals and humans, this leads to hyperreaction to emotional stimuli and to the development of anxiety, depression, fears, autism, and post-traumatic stress disorder (Tottenham N. et al., 2010; Shin L. M. et al., 2005).

Researchers at the Institute of Neuroscience in the University of California have established that it is the amygdala in situations of fear that signals the hippocampus to create new neurons, and in these newborn neurons, as on a blank sheet, information about the dangerous situation is imprinted. It is important that this memory retains not only the information aspect of the event, but also its emotional coloring (Kirby E. D. et al., 2012). From the hippocampus, short-term memory of the event is transmitted to the cerebral cortex for long-term storage (Feng R. et al., 2001). From the point of view of evolution, it was important that emotional memory was preserved (for example, about the behavior of predators), and this contributed to the survival of man. However, in our days, such a powerful emotional imprint becomes a source for many mental disorders.

Dr. Peter Levine and Ann Frederick (1997) note that though people rarely die from mental trauma, life can seriously deteriorate as a result of it. Consequently, many people are fixed in a state that can be described as "living dead" (which is equivalent to the oncogenic existential crisis that we will consider in chapter 15). Dr. Frederick Levenson (1985) is even more categorical: "A sudden and abrupt ending to a significant emotional entropic system is a cause of cancer."

From the presented material, we have seen how acute and, developing in its wake, chronic stress cause structural and functional disorders of neuroplasticity

---

mammals, was discovered in rats as early as 1962. By the nineteen-nineties, it was found that new neurons emerge from adult stem cells and mainly in the evolutionarily ancient parts of the brain: the hippocampal cortex and the olfactory bulbs, which play an important role in emotional behavior, the formation of short-term memory, the response to stress, and regulation of sexual functions in mammals. In 1998, this phenomenon was also confirmed in humans and became the basis for the concept of brain neuroplasticity—its ability to change following an experience (Curtis M. A. et al., 2011).

in the limbic system. This leads to distortions of mental activity, especially emerging as anxiety, depression, and post-stress disorders, which are risk factors for the development of cancer.

10.2. Early–Stage Cancer: Foe or Friend? The Theory of Dr. Hamer

However, there are other studies that have shown that acute stress can be associated with structural changes in the brain and the development of cancer in a different way. The results of these studies allowed Dr. Ryke Geerd Hamer (2000) from Germany to create what he termed Germanic New Medicine (GNM), so named because it disproves the traditional medical views on the origin of diseases, including cancer. Because of the alleged danger of the practical application of his theory, Dr. Hamer's medical license was revoked and he was persecuted in Germany and in some other European countries, where his teaching, however, found numerous supporters. Although Hamer's theory is criticized by academic science, I think it is appropriate to present here, since data have been found to confirm at least some of its assertions.

In the early 1980s, Dr. Hamer announced the discovery of several biological laws, according to which diseases are not the result of disorders or malignant processes in the body, but rather "important special biological programs of nature," evolved in order to assist the animal and human being during a period of distress. These laws claim to explain the causes of many diseases, including cancer, the course of their development, and the process of natural healing arising from them. The root cause of diseases, according to Hamer: a "conflict shock," or a situation that we could not foresee, were not prepared for, and which leads to acute distress (in other words, it is acute stress disorder or shock in conventional terminology). For example, unforeseen loss of or separation from a loved one, an unexpected outburst of anger, or severe anxiety, an unexpectedly bad diagnosis with a negative prognosis.

Hamer firstly arrived at his discoveries on the basis of his own experience; as a result of the tragic death of his son, he developed testicular cancer. Having realized the connection of his illness with the psychic trauma he had suffered, Hamer was able to cure himself. Subsequently, working in the gynecological oncology clinic of the University of Munich, he examined a large number of cases of cancer and found that, in literally all of them, the first signs of the disease appeared one to three years after the emotional trauma. As we can see, in this, Dr. Hamer is in solidarity with many psycho-oncologists.

According to his theory, a conflict shock at the time of occurrence affects a specifically predetermined area of the brain, the exact localization of which is defined by the nature of the conflict. For example, the "motor conflict" that is experienced at the time of distress as "it's impossible to escape," or "shock stupor," affects the motor cortex, responsible for controlling muscular contractions. Moreover, according to Hamer, one particular shock can affect even several areas of the brain with further dysfunction of various organs. When the cancer develops there, it can clinically look like metastases, although these are actually several different types of cancer. For instance, if someone unexpectedly loses their business, and the bank takes all their property, they can develop intestinal cancer as a result of a conflict arising from the impossibility of digesting something ("I cannot digest this situation!"), liver cancer as a consequence of the conflict arising from the threat of hunger ("I do not know how to feed myself!"), and bone cancer due to the "self-depreciation conflict" (loss of self-esteem) (Markolin C., 2007).

Another example: if a woman experiences an unforeseen parting with a loving partner, it can be experienced as a "throw-out conflict" that affects the kidneys, or as a "self-depreciating conflict" that damages the bones and leads to osteoporosis, or as a "loss of life," leading to ovarian failure. Every person experiences a typical conflict in their own way. I will not go into the numerous details of GNM described by Hamer and his students—those interested are advised to study them independently (see Hamer R. G., 2000, Markolin C., 2007). I will give only the most general and, in my opinion, significant moments that correspond to the context of this book.

From the specific zone of the brain, the conflict shock passes through the neurons to the corresponding organ associated with this zone (for more details on the "choice" of organs by cancer, wait for Chapter 12). In this organ, according to Hamer's theory, an "important special biological program" (SBP) is activated, designed to resolve this type of conflict. This is what mainstream medicine mistakenly calls a disease. The biological purpose of such a program is to improve the functions of the body involved in the conflict, to increase its capabilities, so that the individual can cope with the situation and gradually resolve the discrepancy. When, in the first phase of the SBP, more organic tissue is required to resolve the conflict, explains Hamer's disciple Dr. Caroline Markolin (2007), the cells in the appropriate organ multiply and tissue grows. This looks like a tumor. While for conflict resolution which requires less organic tissue, the appropriate organ or tissue responds to the conflict by reducing the number of cells (looks like ulceration).

This kind of physiological reaction of the organism to stress has been known to science for a long time. It is the "triad of changes" that accompanies stress: the increase in the volume of the adrenal cortex, the reduction in the size of the thymus, and the appearance of hemorrhages and even ulcers in the gastrointestinal mucosa; this was the basis for Hans Selye's concept of general adaptation syndrome. When applied to oncology, Dr. Hamer's ideas can astound many readers, since this should mean that an initial cancer that occurs in a particular organ has a positive purpose: to help a person survive stress (especially if this organ is already weakened owing to diathesis or previous stresses, as follows from the previous chapters); and after "completing its task," the early-stage cancer must degrade by itself.[1]

10.3. The Further Fate of the Initial Tumor

What determines the eventual outcome: whether the tumor will freeze, degrade, or develop? According to Hamer, this depends on whether the initial conflict has been resolved (in other words, if the patient has been able to process the situation of acute stress by their own efforts, or with the help of a psychotherapist), or has developed into chronic stress. Therefore, like many psycho-oncologists, Dr. Hamer (2000) says that it is our subjective perception of the conflict and the feelings behind the conflict that determine which part of the brain is affected by the shock, and accordingly, what physical symptoms will reflect the conflict as a result.

If the conflict (acute stressful situation) is resolved, the second phase of SBP is activated—healing at the level of the psyche, brain, and organ. Mental tension gives way to relief and relaxation; firstly, edema emerges in the brain, in the zone corresponding to the conflict, and then the growth of *glial* nervous tissue, which helps to eliminate the conflict zone. Conventional medicine considers it to be a malignant brain tumor—glioblastoma.

As modern research shows, this idea of Hamer's seems to be true. A group of Israeli-American scientists discovered that in mice, in the first few days of acute stress, the microglia (*glia*) in their brain begin to multiply and activate, increasing in size and producing inflammatory molecules. After this, during the transition of stress to the chronic phase for five weeks, the microglia begin to degenerate and die, accompanied by symptoms of depression in the animals' behavior (Kreisel T. et al, 2014).

The growth of glial tissue in general is one of the elements of normal neurogenesis, so it may indeed help the organism to adapt to a stressful situation. From another angle, both neurons and glial cells originate from a single source:

---

[1] It is interesting to note in this regard that in the developing tumor, both angiogenesis (the formation of new blood vessels) and neurogenesis (the emergence of new nerve fibers) are activated. This is shown in tumors of various origins, particularly in the mammary gland (Zhao Q. et al., 2014), the prostate (Beard C. J. et al., 2004), the pancreas (Hirai I. et al., 2002), and the rectum (Albo D. et al., 2011). Are these normal physiological processes triggered by nature solely for the purpose of destroying the host organism?

multipotent neural stem cells. Some of these cells can acquire the properties of tumor cells, therefore they are called cancer stem cells (Ignatova T. N. et al., 2002). The reasons for this transformation are unknown to scientists; however, it is assumed that this can be due to genetic mutations or damage caused by the environment (Gangemi R. et al., 2009), which is quite consistent with the phenomenon of stress. This point of view is supported by the study of Nozue and Ono from the Tokyo University of Medicine and Dentistry (1991): the injection of catecholamines into newborn mice provokes the development of gliomas. As previously noted, the sharp increase in the level of catecholamines is the underlying mechanism of acute stress.

Igor Semenov (2005), physician and neurophysiologist from the Altai State Medical University (Russia), argues that affective (i.e., caused by strong emotions) damage to the nervous system can be considered as an acute neurotrauma, which in its severity and consequences can be even more serious than a mechanical trauma. Often, it is accompanied by focal edema of some area or part of the brain:

> Under general stress, initially a small local edema of the brain, due to the addition of a general edema, can significantly increase in size ("inflate"), completely or partially affect some brain part and, increasing it in volume, press it against the dura mater. There may develop an edema in one or both hemispheres, a pseudotumor of the brain, various variants of wedging, or other complications. ... Chronic excitation of the neuronal population, as for example shown in epilepsy, is accompanied by focal gliosis and hypervascularization. At some point, this overgrown glial-vascular mass, like the neoplasm, begins to mechanically and toxically affect the substance of the brain and its membranes, disrupt the dynamics of blood and liquor, etc.

However, as the author notes, edema of the nervous tissue is not always a pathology. Moreover, sometimes this is the only, albeit temporary, salvation of a person:

> The mechanism of the protective and inhibitory effect of an edema is simple and reliable: an increase in the degree of tissue hydration automatically causes "dilution," or a decrease in the concentration of all substances contained in this area, including oxygen. This suppresses (limits the upper peak of) the activity of [nerve] cells.

This data can also be considered to be of a category similar to Germanic New Medicine.

To resolve the conflict at the level of the final organ, according to Dr. Hamer, the healing process develops in a direction opposite to the original one—since the tumors that occurred in the active phase of the conflict have already fulfilled their protective mission and are no longer needed, they are eliminated by the body with the help of fungi and tubercle bacilli. In the case of their absence or suppression by drugs, the tumors are encapsulated and do not grow further.[1] If,

---

[1] In Chapter 22 we will learn that such "frozen" or "dead" tumors are often found by pathologists at autopsies of people who have died from causes not related to cancer.

in the active phase of the conflict, there was a loss of tissue in the organs affected by the conflict, then there will be a growth of new, reimbursing, cellular tissue, which also looks like a tumor, but later this process also degrades. GNM argues that "conventional medicine mistakenly takes these actually therapeutic tumors for malignant cancerous neoplasia" (Markolin C., 2007).

Therefore, according to Hamer, with the detection of cancer in the initial stages, all that a person needs is psychotherapeutic help to resolve the conflict and to rest, as everything else will be corrected by nature; while "chemotherapy and irradiation abruptly interrupt the natural course of healing from cancer." (Markolin C., 2007). This view of GNM is supported by the above-mentioned research conducted in the middle of the last century in the laboratory of Ivan Pavlov. First, K. M. Petrova in dogs (1946) and then E. F. Melikhova in mice (1956) found that if a stressful experiment that has led to the development of a malignant tumor is interrupted, that is, researchers leave the animals alone and give them a chance to restore their natural forces, in many of them, the process of involution of a tumor initiates, i.e. a "spontaneous regression." In a sense, this situation can be considered analogous with the cases of spontaneous recovery from cancer in people due to the resolution of their intrapsychic conflict (this data will receive further focus in Chapter 22). The termination of stressful stimulation in an animal immediately completes the mental conflict of an inescapable threat. There is no longer a desperate situation. The animal does not continue this conflict by reflecting on why it happened, who was wrong, on whom and how to take revenge and how to live on. The animal simply switches to its life in the "here and now," which undoubtedly activates its immune system and anticancer protection, and is thereby get physically restored after its bout of suffering.

When patients die in the acute phase of the conflict, it actually happens, according to GNM, because of "energy exhaustion, lack of sleep, and, more often, from fear."(Marcolin C., 2007). This point of view finds support in the research of Russian scientists who described the reality and mechanisms of the psychogenic death of cancer patients (Bukhtoyarov O. V., Arkhangelsky A. E., 2008, for details see Chapter 28).

If an acute stressful conflict is not timely resolved, it enters a chronic phase (GNM calls it "a continuing conflict"). In this state, a person can even live to old age if a stress-induced tumor does not cause mechanical disturbances (an example may be a tumor in the intestine). However, as we know from the previous sections, chronic stress is often characterized by repeated psychic traumas of greater or lesser intensity. Hamer calls these situations "renewable conflicts" or "tracks" that hinder the process of natural healing, each time activating the biological mechanism of the conflict anew, albeit not with the same intensity. A similar version twenty years before Hamer was expressed by Dr. Roy R. Grinker Sr. (1966). Considering the reasons why early-stage tumors either stop in their development or progress, he wrote: "Carcinoma can often remain latent, asymptomatic, for many years ... before it is awakened by the factor of the loss of [a significant] object." According to this model, we can conclude that the non-resolution of psychosocial conflict (or psychic trauma) and subsequent chronic distress will lead to a situation where tumors and ulcers either do not reach the stage of natural arrest of growth and degradation, and will progress—or will again be activated from a latent state—until their growth brings about fatal disorders.

What are the possibilities of the practical application of Germanic New Medicine? According to Dr. Hamer, a specialist who knows the localization of cancer in the body and has detected a focus of conflict on a computer tomogram of the brain (where it can appear in the form of concentric circles) is able to pinpoint the type of conflict shock that has occurred in the patient's life. Then it can be eliminated by the methods of specialized psychotherapy, which will lead to activation of a natural healing process. The Canadian GNM website, supported by the students of Dr. Hamer (www.newmedicine.ca), contains expert opinions from the commissions of scientists from the University of Trnava (Slovakia), the University Clinic of Vienna, the Gelsenkirchen State Children's Clinic (Germany) and a number of private doctors, as well as patients, confirming the effectiveness of diagnosis based on GNM. Hamer claimed thousands of healed patients. At the same time, opponents of the GNM claim that there were a significant number of cases when patients expected natural healing in accordance with Hamer's theory and did not resort to traditional cancer therapy, resulting in premature death. (Here I have a logical question: did these people receive timely and qualified psychotherapeutic help?) Lately, Dr. Ryke Geerd Hamer settled in Norway, where he passed away in July 2017.

The future will reveal just how true are the ideas of Germanic New Medicine. There are already researchers who, regardless of Hamer, are moving in a similar direction. For example, according to the theory developed by American scientist Paul Davies, along with Australian colleague Charles Lineweaver (2011), cancer is not a random accumulation of selfish outlaw cells with bad behavior, but a highly effective programmed response to stress, honed by a long evolutionary period, and therefore it cannot be regarded as something bad that arises inside a healthy body. Cancer, in their opinion, is an active response of the body to changing the cellular, physical, and planetary environment in an unhealthy direction; this is an expression of cellular intelligence and the ability of our cells to survive in critical, threatening conditions.

Naturopath Andreas Moritz (2008), on the basis of his thirty-year practice, states that cancer is not a disease; this is the last and most desperate mechanism of survival which body has at its disposal. Cancer can only take control of the body when all other means of self-preservation have failed. In order to really heal cancer and find what it represents in a person's life, we must understand that the reason why a body allows some of its cells to reproduce in an abnormal way is to protect its interests, and not that it wants to destroy itself. Cancer is an attempt by the body to heal itself. Blocking this attempt can destroy the body, while support in its healing efforts can save it. The cells only then enter defense-mode and become malignant when they need to ensure their own survival, at least, for as long as they can. Spontaneous remission occurs when cells no longer need to protect themselves. According to Moritz's theory, cancer cells arise to collect all the toxins and waste of the metabolism, with which the body is no longer able to cope.

Dr. Hamer (2000) sums up his views in his fifth and last biological law:

> Our ignorance prevented us from recognizing that all so-called diseases have a special biological meaning. ... While we used to regard Mother Nature as fallible and had the audacity to believe that she constantly made mistakes and caused breakdowns (malignant, senseless, degenerative cancerous growth, etc.) we can now see, as the scales fall from our eyes, that it was our ignorance, arrogance and pride that were and are the only foolishness in our cosmos. We could not understand such a 'sewn up' totality, and so brought upon ourselves this senseless, soulless and brutal medicine.

> Full of wonder, we can now understand for the first time that nature is orderly (we already knew that), and every occurrence in nature is meaningful, even in the framework of the whole, and that the events we called 'diseases' are not senseless disturbances to be repaired by sorcerers' apprentices. We can see that nothing is meaningless, malignant or diseased.

* * *

Today, for a layman who has grown up on the paradigm of traditional biomedicine, it is extremely difficult to accept the possibility that, if an early-stage cancer is detected, it is possible to use only psychotherapy and alternative medicine, and not to undergo traditional surgery and/or radiotherapy and chemotherapy. However, the cases of spontaneous regression of both initial and advanced tumors, which will be noted later in this book, prove the reality of healing in this way.

For all its ambiguity in respect of both the theory and the author (particularly his offensive and ignorant political views), Germanic New Medicine is very close to the ideas that I formulate in this book. Regardless of whether we treat the initial tumor, resulting from an acute psychic trauma, as a natural adaptive physiological response of the organism (according to Hamer) or as a disorder of its functions (according to modern oncology), there are other things that are really important for the development of disease. They are a person's reaction to a stressful event, his/her ability to cope with the consequent mental overstrain, and how severe and prolonged the post-stress disorder and further chronic distress will be. It is these aspects that ultimately determine whether a malignant tumor will become life-threatening.

Dr. Ian Gawler, in his book *You Can Conquer Cancer* (1984), writes that the main thing for cancer patients is not the very problem they face, but their reaction to it. An important feature of their character is the inability to cope with a serious problem, especially if it is associated with abrupt changes in life. Failure to correctly respond to a difficult situation, to find a way out of it, and to ease the soul leads, as a result, to stress in the body's biochemistry. Gawler's conclusion is that this, in turn, weakens the immune system and thereby adds another powerful factor to other causes of cancer.

Dr. Douglas Brodie (2015) argues:

> How one reacts to stress appears to be a major factor in the development of cancer. Most cancer patients have experienced a highly stressful event, usually about 2 years prior to the onset of detectable disease. This traumatic event is often beyond the patient's control, such as the loss of a loved one, the loss of a business, job, home, or some other major disaster. The typical cancer victim has lost the ability to cope with these extreme events, because his/her coping mechanism lies in his/her ability to control the environment. When this control is lost, the patient has no other way to cope.

Bernie Siegel (1998) came to a similar conclusion: the disease does not develop in everyone who has experienced a tragic loss or stressful lifestyle change; apparently, the crucial factor is how a person copes with the problem.

Thus, we can conclude that the distress of loss, i.e. the death of a significant one, the breaking of relations, the loss of job and/or social status, financial deprivations (of business, property, or savings), like other acute psychic traumas, can indeed provoke potentially oncogenic disorders in the body. Such distress triggers a complex set of adaptive reactions that, depending on existing mental and biological resources, can proceed from an adaptive phase into a maladaptive one, with the development of chronic distress. The volume of resources at the time of a psychological trauma is determined by the activity of diathesis (the severity of the psychosomatic type of personality "C" or "D", and the amount of epigenetic changes in the organism's regulation that were previously accumulated under the influence of pre-, intra-, and postnatal factors), the intensity of previously suffered psychic traumas and conflicts in the life of the person and the degree of their resolution or treatment. In other words, as a result of acute psychic trauma the mechanisms of the already existing stress (via the diathesis-stress mechanism) are significantly activated, and the predisposition to cancer passes into a state of elevated sensitivity to carcinogens, with a high probability of escalation into a precancerous state.

How long will it be until a malignant neoplasm actually develops? As we have seen from many studies, this most often occurs in a period of from one to five years. However, everything depends on the rate of depletion of the protective biological resources of the body, the presence of physical and chemical carcinogens in the external environment, and from further changes in the psyche and the body in a state of chronic distress, as well as the absence of specialized psychotherapeutic assistance. All this leads to the formation of the so-called 'oncological dominant' against the background of depression, helplessness, hopelessness, and disillusion with how they define the meaning of life. This will determine the body's ability to cope with the emerging cancer cells. All of these aspects will be analyzed in detail in following chapters.

Chapter 11

The Chronic Oncogenic Intrapersonal Conflict and How it Can Be Formed

*All the horrors of life are not as terrible
as the ideas invented by the conscience and the mind.*
Nikolay Berdyaev,
prominent Russian philosopher

The launch of chronic stress by acute psychic trauma, followed by an oncological process, seems to be sufficiently substantiated by the data previously provided. What, then, causes disease in those cases when acute psychic trauma is not found in a person's life history? For example, researchers at the University of Rochester, examining the life histories of ninety-four women with repeated or metastatic breast cancer, found one or more traumatic events in 42% of cases, and in 28.7% found less severe stressful events that did not fall within the criteria of a psychic trauma. In both groups, the remission period was half as long as in patients without identified stress or traumatic events (Palesh O. et al., 2007). What was the source of the cancer in the remaining 29.3% of patients? What creates and maintains chronic oncogenic stress in such cases?

More than century ago, Sigmund Freud (1990) created the concept of conversion, according to which bodily symptoms reflect attempts to resolve a chronic emotional conflict. Franz Alexander (1939) argued that the manifestation of somatic disorders is caused by vegetative neuroses—a neurotic complexes suppressed into the subconscious. They are accompanied by stable changes in the autonomic nervous system and lead to persistent physiological and emotional disorders. The main factor in the development of a disease, in his opinion, is unconscious emotional conflicts, which are common to different people but at the same time in each case specific for a particular pathology.

Walter Brautigam and colleagues (1997) characterize psychosomatic illness as an initially different form of resolving of psychic conflict—a form that, from an early age, replaces another way (perhaps, verbal) of experiencing this conflict. According to the research of the emeritus Soviet physiologist, Konstantin Sudakov (2005, 2007), the director of the Normal Physiology Research Institute of the Russian Academy of Medical Sciences, unresolved conflict situations lead to emotional arousal and the formation of "stagnant negative emotion"; if these conflicts are long and continuous, they result in emotional overstrain: distress.

The Simontons (1978) note that the internal conflict caused by frustration due to serious difficulties in personal relationships, the impossibility of the realization of youthful hopes, the crisis of self-approval as a person, can play no less great a role in the formation of a precancerous psychological state than the apparent external stress. Many of Stanislav Grof's cancer patients showed a significant number of serious psychological difficulties and emotional problems that preceded the emergence and diagnosis of their disease. In several cases, the nature of these problems almost assumed a pathogenic dependence (Grof S., Halifax J., 1978).

Studying the scientific literature and observing my cancer patients, I also came to the conclusion that the second most important cause of oncogenic distress (apart from unresolved psychic trauma) is a more or less prolonged and also unresolved intrapersonal and/or interpersonal conflict. Undoubtedly, there are various combinations of trauma and conflict. For example, the psychological trauma of loss in the case of adultery by a spouse and/or divorce is often combined with the conflict of taking offence, one that is mutually reinforced. Also, turning of distress into the chronic phase and its activity causes a periodic recurrence of previous psychic trauma of lesser intensity—for example, conflicts in the family or failure at work. They form the cumulative effect of the experienced unhappiness, "cumulative trauma," in which each subsequent stress, even of a similar intensity, leads to a stronger emotional reaction in a person (Khan M. M., 1963), distorting the hypothalamic-pituitary-adrenal axis, and increasing the risk of post-traumatic complications (Contractor A. et al., 2018).

The importance of the aspect of accumulation is confirmed by the concept of condensed experience systems: earlier psychic traumas "arrange space" for later ones, as if teaching the brain to respond in a specific way. Stanislav Grof (1996) explains that even a single event can be of enormous pathogenic significance when it happens against the background of a particularly unfavorable family situation. However, the daily pathogenic interactions with a family member that last for months and years can be continuously recorded in memory, collected in a condensed form, and eventually formed into a pathological focus that is comparable to the kind that is due to substantial trauma.

The importance of the duration of the stress factor is emphasized by other authors. Rare, short-term stresses, unlike chronic ones, do not lead to overloading and reorganization of the adaptive mechanisms of the organism, and do not cause pathological conditions. However, with repeated short-term stresses, especially when they are intense, functional systems do not have enough time to adapt to the growing unfavorable conditions, therefore the consequences for the organism can be irreversible (Kitaev-Smyk L. A., 1983; Burchfield S. R., 1979). A similar point of view is shared by the founder of positive psychotherapy Nossrat Peseschkian (1991): the specificity of psychosomatic disorders is determined not so much by the intensity of the psychotraumatic impact as by its repeatability, uniformity, and duration of the experienced microtrauma.

According to the study of patients with brain tumors carried out in the Dnipropetrovsk Medical Academy (Ukraine), in most cases (76.7% of those examined) there was a gradual accumulation of stress factors or negative emotional experiences of psychotraumatic events in patients before clinical manifestations of the disease. Acute psychological traumas were noted in only 12.8% of the cases in which the disease developed within about five months of the stress events (Ogorenko V. V., 2011).

The effect of accumulation of experienced misfortunes and stressful events in the onset and course of cancer was also found by American and Russian scientists (Vorona O. A., 2005; Morton P. M. et al., 2012). Lydia Temoshok (1987) writes that the ineffective ability of individuals of type "C" to cope with stress leads to an increasing intensity of stress, which in turn enhances the personality characteristics of "C." Canadian physician Gabor Maté (2003) also notes that in most cases of breast cancer, stresses are hidden and chronic, accumulating throughout life and making a person susceptible to the disease.

An illustrative example is the history of my patient L. Born in 1940, she experienced all the severity of stresses and deprivation of war. Her father had died, and her relationship with her mother was complicated. Her marriage was not harmonious, and the relationship with her husband was tense. The elder son was run over by a truck at the age of 13 and died in the hospital in her arms. The younger son (possibly because of his brother's loss) got diabetes. A year later L. divorced her husband. To somehow distract herself from negative life experiences, she got a job at the local city council in an environmental commission. Five years of hectic work "for the benefit of nature" only aggravated her stressful condition—there was insomnia, constant body pains, and chronic fatigue syndrome. The younger son developed gangrene of the feet, with subsequent amputation, and later his kidneys began to fail. After six months of constant dialysis, the son died. Is it surprising that in a couple of years the woman who had experienced so many stresses and psychological traumas was diagnosed with breast cancer?

At the same time, as I have already noted on several occasions, it is not the stress itself that is important, but its assessment and overcoming. What most people may see as insignificant or moderate emotional disturbance, for a psychosomatic personality of "C" type, particularly with high anxiety, the periodic repetitions of any stress can accumulate and become a factor of great strength, equal in intensity to acute psychic trauma. This conclusion is confirmed by observations of those who are experiencing what is in reality minor stresses, but do not know how to control their reactions to them. They have decreased immune system activity and increased morbidity (Bauer-Wu S. M., 2002). In this way, bodily disorders gradually accumulate at all levels of the psychobiological system, resulting in a depletion of adaptive and protective resources. Finally, the body loses the ability to control emerging cancer cells.

Next, we will consider which types of chronic psychological conflicts and psychic traumas are capable of creating oncogenic distress.

11.1. The Unresolved Conflict and its Cause, an Unsatisfied Need

> When the inner situation is not made conscious,
> it appears outside of you as a fate.
> Carl Gustav Jung,
> *Collected Works, Vol. 7*

11.1.1. Sources of Intrapersonal Conflict

In the history of modern psychology, studying intrapersonal conflict is primarily connected with the name of Sigmund Freud (1990). He argued that human existence is linked to the constant overcoming of the contradiction between biological drives, desires (especially sexual), and socio-cultural norms, which is reflected first in the tension, and then in the conflict between consciousness and the unconscious.

Freud distinguished the following sources of intrapersonal conflict:

- the contradiction of motives, interests and needs ("I want to go with my friends to the cinema, but I need to prepare for the exam");

- the discrepancy of social roles ("I need to go on a business trip (the role of 'employee'), but my child is sick" (the role of "parent"));

- the opposition of social values and norms (a moral or religious attitude "do not kill" and the need to protect one's country).

Nowadays, a contradiction of self-esteem is added to this list: a conflict between an underestimated or overestimated self-assessment of one's capabilities and actual needs and achievements.

In other words, an intrapersonal conflict can arise as an opposition between "I want" (motives, need, interests), "I must" (values), and "I can" (self-esteem). To have a conflict develop, the contradictory forces affecting the individual should be equal, otherwise the person will easily choose one of the options and internal disagreement will not emerge.

Freud's student Carl Gustav Jung (1972), the creator of analytical psychology, sees the origins of an intrapersonal conflict in the irreconcilable attitude of man to his "Shadow"—the unconscious complex containing the suppressed, repressed, or estranged aspects of the conscious part of the personality. Ignoring or being unaware of the "Shadow" can cause both personality and bodily disorders, according to the above-described mechanism of distress.

The unresolved conflict, expelled to the "Shadow," as well as the emotions suppressed as a result, will color all aspects of a person's life, influencing his interaction with others. These feelings will seek to get out of the state of "incubation" and rise to the surface, waiting for the proper moment. This moment will undoubtedly come, because in the avoided emotions hidden in the "Shadow" there is a large concentration of psychic energy that requires a discharge. Like rust, it "consumes" one's adaptive reserves. The rejected contradiction returns again and again in various forms, reminding the victim (including symbolically) about itself. Ignoring and denying it, a person only strengthens his "Shadow" even more (Jung C. G., 1972). For this, as I mentioned earlier, there is a proven physiological basis: every reminder of the conflict creates a reaction in the amygdala and hippocampus of the brain, similar to the initial one. It again brings an active release of stress hormones in the body, so the initial imprint of stress gains more strength (Bloom F. E., Lazerson A., 2000). Therefore, the life of a person who suppresses the conflict can be felt as an endless struggle.

For example, when I analyzed the chronic fatigue of a patient K. and her subsequent reluctance to go to work (although she is a talented violinist who loves her profession), I discovered the reason was in her rejection by several colleagues in the orchestra. At a conscious level, the woman did not notice anything like that. However, during the trance treatment session, K. not only clearly felt her negative emotions in relation to certain properties of the character of her colleagues, but she also realized the presence of such qualities in herself. These traits were suppressed by the patient, and their discovery was a shock to her.

"That which we reject becomes the fate we live," argue American psychologists Hal Stone and Sidra Winkelman (1988), —"... From our study on many cancer patients, there is a little question in our minds that the denial of the natural instinctual heritage can be a major etiological factor among the many causes of cancer."

Carl Rogers (1995), one of the leaders of the humanistic school in psychology, considers the "self-concept"—the image of one's own self or the person's representation about the self, which arises in the process of interaction with the environment—as the main component of the personality structure. If the "self-concept" does not correspond to reality, distress arises, and an intrapersonal conflict is formed.

Domestic psychologists define intrapersonal conflict as a stance of the internal structure of the individual, expressed in the confrontation of oppositely directed motives, goals, interests, and desires which are not simultaneously satisfiable and accompanied by negative experiences and emotions (Burtovaya E. V., 2002).

Intrapersonal conflict, as a rule, continues interpersonal, social conflict—after all, almost everything that happens to us reflects our interaction with society. However, owing to personal characteristics and limiting beliefs, most often learned in childhood, internalization of the conflict takes place. One can experience it either consciously (by repressing the emotions associated), or unconsciously (with the suppression of emotions). As a result, the processing of the formed conflict can go either in a constructive (productive, optimal), or destructive (destroying human personality structures) direction (Antsupov A. Y., Shipilov A. I, 2002).

If a person has the necessary psychological stability, sufficient resources, and is able to overcome stress, then the intrapersonal conflict will be constructive. It will require minimal costs for its resolution and contribute to the development of the individual, lead to an increase in his harmony and adaptive capabilities, and will facilitate its transition to new levels of functioning. By overcoming such conflict, a person learns and moves forward in life.

Otherwise, especially with prolonged inability to resolve the conflict (which creates chronic psycho-physiological stress), and against the background of specific traits and history of the life (a factor of diathesis), frustration arises. The result is a destructive conflict that depletes the adaptive resources, creates a dissociation of the personality, leads to the development of neurotic or somatoform reactions, and grows into a life crisis, with a high probability of psychosomatic disease. "That which is suppressed from consciousness continues to operate in the body," wrote Viktor von Weizsäcker, one of the pioneers of psychosomatic medicine, as early as the 1940s. In other words, when a person cannot destroy an unacceptable situation, he destroys himself with a disease.

Such a crisis, especially associated with psycho-traumatic experiences, is characterized by: the need to resolve the global conflict, the fundamental unsolvability of the initial contradiction by means familiar to the person, and a high degree of mental tension (Vorobiev V. M., 1993). An important role in the development of the conflict into crisis is also played by the imperfection and underdevelopment of psychological defenses, used in order to reduce the intensity of negative emotions aroused because of conflict.

The situation is often complicated by a combination of several conflicts. For example, obligations to one's family make one endure a disliked job for the sake of earning money (a conflict of social roles) and do not allow one to do what one loves (a conflict of self-realization). The Simontons (1978) believe that cancer often suggests that a person has unsolved problems that have intensified or become complicated because a series of stressful situations occurred between six months and one and a half years prior to the onset of disease. Often, the origin of unresolved conflict is in one's relations with parents and/or a psychic trauma suffered in childhood. As noted in Chapter 8, this negative experience of the distant past is preserved in the "incubated" state and serves as the basis for the formation of that system of condensed experience which eventually forms a psychosomatic diathesis.

As Stanislav Grof (2000) discovered, if some *COEX* is once established, it is already predisposed to self-reproduction and can force the individual to unconsciously recreate similar types of life circumstances and, thus, adds newer and newer layers to the already existing complex of memories. This is confirmed by children's psychiatrists: the suppressed energy of an early psychological trauma can unfold in adulthood as a "compressed spring" in psychotraumatic circumstances, symbolically reminiscent of the situation and the period of childhood traumatization (Pilyagina G. Y., 2003).

Dr. Douglas Brodie (2015) notes that cancer patients are characterized by their inability to resolve the underlying emotional problems and conflicts that usually arise in childhood. Often people do not even suspect they are there. Those who survive, as a rule, are patients who are ready to explore and reveal their fundamental emotional problems and find solutions to long-standing conflicts. Dr. Brodie came to the conclusion that such an approach and character qualities are almost indispensable for recovering from cancer; if problems and conflicts are not considered and not corrected, the cancer patient, most likely, does not have a positive prognosis.

In this way, a destructive conflict, aggravated with psychosomatic diathesis, develops into a crisis. But, in order for the crisis to obtain the power of oncogenicity, it must arise as a situation of impossibility to realize the inner necessities of one's life–motives, aspirations, values, etc. Then, a person is not able either to get out of the conflict situation, or to resolve it, by finding a compromise between conflicting motives or by refusing one of them (Vasilyuk F. E., 1984).

In turn, this "impossibility" for a potential cancer patient is determined by:

a) personal self-identification—because of the unconscious ideas of what kind of person one "should be" (cognitive diathesis), one may not even assume that something in life can be changed (Simonton C. et al., 1978);

b) specific personality traits (type "C"), leading to predominance of primary psychological defenses over coping strategies (this issue is examined in Chapter 12.2);

c) an inaccessible, paralyzed, but vitally necessary need—due to a person's inability to cope with a conflict or psychotraumatic situation.

11.1.2. Unmet Needs are the Path to Disease

The basic necessities of life, or needs, were described by the famous psychologist Abraham Maslow, one of the founders of humanistic psychology. In his book *Motivation and Personality* (1954), he suggested that all human needs are inborn, and they are organized into a hierarchical system of priorities, consisting of five levels (situated by increasing complexity):

1. Physiological (biological) needs (food, water, sex, sleep, etc.)
2. The need for safety (protection, stability, order, and freedom from fear, anxiety, and failure)
3. The need for belonging (love, partner, family, friendship, personal circle, professional community)
4. The need for esteem (self-respect and respect of others, achievements, recognition, prestige and reputation, status)
5. The need for *self-actualization*—the development of potential and abilities, finding a life goal.

In subsequent works, Maslow added two more levels: the level of cognitive abilities and the level of aesthetic needs. Finally, he combined all existing needs in two classes: the needs of the deficiency (the lower ones) and the growth needs (self-actualization and self-transcendence). Despite the fact that other researchers have disputed the rigid hierarchy of the Maslow pyramid (for a number of people the aesthetic needs or the needs for self-actualization may be more significant than the lower ones in the pyramid), it is still widely used today in psychology.

Of particular importance for us is Maslow's position which states that for some characteristic to be considered as a need, it should satisfy the following conditions:

- Its absence leads to disease.
- Its presence prevents disease.
- Its recovery heals the disease.
- In certain, rather complex situations and having freedom of choice, the subject prefers satisfaction of this particular need.

- In a healthy person, it can be passive, weakly functioning, or functionally absent (undeveloped) (Goble F. G., 1980).

Though only the basic needs (physiological and safety) were noted, in my opinion, these characteristics can relate to all other needs. The experience of dissatisfaction with any of them can lead to the development of an intrapersonal conflict.

The connection between diseases and unmet needs was realized not only by this American psychologist. I am grateful to a colleague, psychotherapist Vyacheslav Gusev (2014), who in his remarkable book *Sredstvo ot Boleznej* (*Remedy for Diseases*) reminded me of the *Manual of General Human Pathology*, published under the editorship of renowned Soviet clinician, academician A. I. Strukov (1990). The authors, proceeding from the fact that "... human life is the satisfaction of material (matter-energy) and spiritual (information) needs," have precisely formulated the true causes of illness: "In any case, the disease is a disruption of the normal (optimal) way of satisfying needs. And since freedom is an opportunity to realize the reasonable personal needs, the disease is associated with the violation of these freedoms."

Further, the authors of the manual note that "... the need always acts as a deficit of something and as an active realization of human actions," and therefore "diseases can be of two kinds: diseases arising from excess and disease from lack of satisfied needs." What a pity that such wise reasoning did not stimulate the development of a psychosomatic approach to diseases! After all, the conclusion made by Dr. Gusev on the basis of these provisions is logical: the patient is a person who is not able to understand what he really needs and what in his life is worthy of rejection. In other words, a person cannot find a way to realize his needs. Therefore, what should the doctor do? "Help the patient to find the ways of realizing his needs" (Gusev V., 2014). Are these ways supposed to be the pharmaceutical suppression of the symptoms with which the body claims unrealized personality needs?

Professor Irvin Yalom (1980), one of the founders of existential psychology, argues that events that create a potential or real threat to the satisfaction of the fundamental needs of a person confront him or her with a problem that cannot be avoided, or solved in the usual way. Hence, this situation is perceived as a psychological trauma. The complications of such a conflict manifest in the form of crisis and somatization, and, therefore, have the potential of oncogenesis. Indeed, according to Laurence LeShan's observations, the depletion of life force, leading to the development of cancer, occurs due to the pressure on the patient of a problem that he must, but is not able to, resolve. As one of his patients said, "What I really wanted in life is impossible for me to ever have. What I can have, I do not really want. There never really was a way out for me" (LeShan L., 1977). It often happens that patients have so deeply suppressed their true needs that only thanks to the illness could they give their attention to these needs (Simonton C. et al., 1978).

Next, we will explore the data confirming the relationship of inner conflicts due to unrealized needs with the development of cancer.

11.1.2.1. Biological and Safety Needs

These unrealized needs were subjected to experimental research on the stress model of repeated social defeat in mice—either staying in a crowded cage or experiencing an invasion of aggressive dominant animals. Both factors evoke fear, violence, and depression in mice. Such stress disrupts the connection between the neuro-endocrine and immune systems, promotes tumor growth through the development of local inflammation (Powell N. D. et al., 2013), and leads to an increase in the weight and size of initial tumors and the number of metastases, after "inoculating" animals with cancer cells (Wu X. et al., 2015; Stefanski V., Ben-Eliyahu S., 1996). At the molecular level, this stress also demonstrates explicit epigenetic mechanisms: an increase in methylation of the promoter part of the BDNF gene, a neurotrophic brain factor, a protein that stimulates and supports the development of nerve cells (Tsankova N. M. et al., 2006), and participates in some mechanisms of tumor growth.

Researchers at the Karolinska Institute in Stockholm, together with colleagues from the Institute of Experimental Medicine in St. Petersburg (Russia), studied the health of adults who, as children and adolescents, had suffered the stress associated with the blockade of Leningrad in World War II. It turned out that the women in the study group had a 9.9-fold higher risk of breast cancer than those in the corresponding control group, while the men had a slightly higher risk of prostate cancer (Koupil I. et al., 2009).

In Germany, in 1992, British scientists studied mortality rates from cancer and other diseases among Jews who were imprisoned in the Nazi concentration camps during the Second World War. The intensity of the stress they experienced was determined by the length of their stay in the camp, by the number of relatives who died during this period, and by psychological complications. Scientists have discovered that the younger the subjects were at the time and the more intense the stress they experienced, the more often they fell ill later in life. In a group whose age then was 10–15 years, when the intensity of stress was high, the death rate reached 36.4% from cancer, 28% from heart disease, and 20.4% from other diseases. In the group aged 18 and older at that time, which had less intense stress, the mortality rate was 12.1% from cancer, 11.4% from heart disease, and 10.6% from other diseases (Grossarth-Maticek R. et al., 1994).

In a similar area of study, researchers from University of Haifa discovered that Jewish Israelis who emigrated from Europe after World War II (which means they had directly or indirectly been exposed to the Holocaust) have higher rates of all cancers, particularly breast and colorectal cancer, than those who left Europe before the war. The strongest associations between distress exposure and cancer risk were observed in the youngest birth cohort of the years 1940–1945 (Keinan-Boker L. et al., 2009).

Undoubtedly, in such dramatic life conditions people are threatened not only with loss of safety, but also with frustration of basic biological needs—for food, sleep, and rest. This also applies to animals in the described experiments. Thus, the inability to satisfy both types of these needs leads to traumatic experiences and chronic distress and contributes to the emergence of cancer.

11.1.2.2. The Need for Love and Belonging—How It Might Lead to Self-Neglect (Psychological Masochism)

The unmet need for love, as previously noted, underlies all disorders of children's attachment, and as a whole determines the formation of psycho-oncogenic diathesis. Ian Gawler (1984), reflecting on the stories of his patients' lives, emphasizes that children have a deep, inner need to love and be loved, they actually live and grow by the power of love. What they are very afraid of is to become disliked, and if this fear had a ground, they still carry it in their hearts even having grown up. Should they, as adults, find themselves in the condition of permanently hidden and restrained internal tension, any serious life crisis can engender intolerable stress.

If the need for love is not satisfied in the future, a corresponding inner conflict develops between this most important need and the impossibility of realizing it, which obtains the character of destructiveness over time. This thesis illustrates the dissertation research carried out at the Ryazan Medical University (Russia). B. Y. Volodin (2007) found that in women with breast cancer and uterine *myoma*, the leading intrapersonal conflict was the unmet need for love and affection. Both groups of patients clearly demonstrate this basic human need. However, its embodiment is hampered by the alienation of these women, their "closedness," the desire for independence, the reluctance to establish connections with other people. Patients with uterine myoma, moreover, are also hindered by fear of emotional intimacy and this, as a consequence, blocks the need for it. An unmet need for love in cancer patients is also found by other scientists (Bottomley A., Jones L., 1997; Taylor E. J., 2003; Murray S. A. et al., 2004).

The therapists of the psychological support department of the Hippocrates Health Institute in Florida, who developed the program of alternative medical care for cancer patients, have a similar opinion: the deprivation of love is the origin of physical and mental diseases. Deprivation of love can, later in life, lead to situations ranging from extreme violence to the formation of a self-image in which one feels unloved, deprived of support, or neglected (Bernay-Roman A., Hubbard-Brown J., 2011).

Dr. Claus Bahnson (1980) talks about the feelings of his cancer patient: "She said that the damaged little girl she carried within her always needed more love, care, and protection than existed in the whole world."

In order to somehow satisfy this central need, to deserve the love and approval lacking in childhood, and to receive positive emotions from interactions with others, the potential cancer patient uses rationalization and hypercompensation, ineffective primary ways to cope with the stress that has arisen because of a lack of love. This is often based on the hypercognitive variant of cognitive–emotional imbalance developed in childhood and expressed in "pathological goodness"—an excessive attempt at satisfying other peoples' needs. Probably, in this way, the need for love is compensated by the satisfaction of the need for respect and recognition. According to the observations of cancer patients by Dr. Ian Gawler (1984), though the initial childish fear of becoming unloved is often replaced and masked by other forms of fear, the essence remains the same: a person can achieve self-esteem only through the approval of other people. What is very important for such people is a certain status—whether it is the status of a rich and prosperous person, or the status of the head and breadwinner of the family.

This kind of "goodness" and "trueness" is idealized: for example, in Volodin's (2007) quoted study it is shown that overestimated moral and ethical demands for oneself, in the form of hypertrophied morality and conscience, are characteristic for both categories of sick women. As a result, caring for the needs of others is a priority for them. This phenomenon in cancer patients was also noted by C. Simonton and colleagues (1978): "It is a particularly sad course of events that many times those people who most steadfastly and responsibly attempt to live up to cultural rules develop the most serious illnesses."

This feature, which can be considered as one of the manifestations of cognitive diathesis, is also common for psychosomatic patients in general. As the psychoanalyst Jan Bastiaans (1982) writes,

> … in the anthropological sense, the psychosomatic patient not only has his ideals and conscience, but they themselves are almost an ideal and a conscience. This self-centered guideline presupposes the restriction of the self. One's own position and own actions must necessarily be emphasized. If such patients experience frustration associated with the functions of conscience or with the ideal, they have a sudden growth of anxiety, and then, under the pressure of the *Super-Ego*, improper adaptation develops in the aforementioned psychosomatic direction.

Inadequate satisfaction of needs stimulates the development of another intrapersonal conflict in the future cancer patient—between values: "I must" (be good to others), and one's own suppressed interests: "I want." This further strengthens the basic intrapersonal conflict of an unmet need for love. In addition, as observed in women with uterine body cancer, if they still try to meet their needs, the inner conflict emerges leading to a feeling of guilt, that increases their initial tendencies toward self-destruction (Volodin B. Y., 2007).

As we have seen in previous chapters, many scientists have found similar data on the conflict between the cancer personality's own needs and his or her cognitive attitudes about the greater importance of the needs of others. Summarizing their observations, we see:

- the propensity to place the interests of others as the top priority (Simonton C. et al., 1978);
- excessive interest in meeting the needs of others and insufficient satisfaction of own needs, frequent manifestation of self-sacrifice (Temoshok L., 1987; Temoshok L. et al., 1993);
- the desire to be a "good" or "pleasant" person and comply with social norms (Kune G. A. et al., 1991);
- perfectionism, self-sacrifice, adherence to religious rules, helplessness (Schmale A. H., Iker H. P., 1971);
- submission, non-aggression, suppression of one's needs, timeserving (Grossarth-Maticek R. et al., 1982);
- "pleasantness" and excessive, masochistic sacrificing (Cutler M., 1954);
- a tendency toward long-term suffering, self-sacrificing, ignoring one's own needs (Ivashkina M. G., 1998);
- the priority of caring for the needs of others (Volodin B. Y., 2007);
- not expressing one's emotions and needs in order to avoid conflicts (Laughlin T., 1999);
- exhibiting a strong tendency toward carrying other people's burdens and toward taking on extra obligations, often "worrying for others." Having a deep-seated need to make others happy, tending to be "people pleasers" (Brodie D., 2015).

These properties of character can be combined with the term "masochism." Masochism is a fixed, patterned way of self-destructive behavior, characteristic of earlier (infantile) phases of development, which emerged as a paradoxical way of adapting for a child when it is impossible to cope with the difficulties of relationships with society (Nekrut T. V., 2015). Since childhood, the future masochist has gotten used to the fact that he is not important, that he is less valuable than other people's desires, preferences, and needs, that her aspirations and needs are constantly being trampled on, postponed to "later." He feels as if standing in the last place in line, always having to remain tolerant. As a result, she develops a perfectly established mechanism for self-restriction: a detachment from her own impulses and needs. Moreover, deep down inside, such a person can even be proud of how much suffering she is able to endure, the remarkable extent to which she can tolerate, how comfortable and functional she can be, and how selflessly able she is to devote her life to serving other people, coming off at the same time as "the sweetest or quietest person."

The masochist decides that first it is necessary to devote himself completely [to others], having become so useful to them that they cannot do without him. Indispensability, being needed, service with full dedication—that's at least some guarantee that implicitly, covertly, love and care will still seep to him along with a feeling of unconditional 'goodness', if not 'holiness',—

notes the psychotherapist I. Y. Mlodik (2014).

However, expectations of retribution or positive responses from other people are often not fulfilled, because the body of such a person can begin to break down from neglect, exhausting use, and self-destructive attitudes. The anger that inevitably accumulates throughout life due to the fact that one did not live as one wanted, did not allow oneself to be really important; all this anger about one's own ineffectiveness is redirected inside, leading a person to self-destruction. Following the model of suffering in life, a person is able to "acquire" at least psychosomatic, or more severe diseases (cancer) that will bring to him maximum suffering and helplessness. Then, the sufferer involves relatives in his illness, and they have a duty to serve a masochist, giving up their own life plans. "In such an indirect way, a masochist gets what he dreamed of 'in one package': devotion, service, and the punishment of another. ... The extreme form of auto-aggression is complete self-destruction and self-punishment, and then early death" (Mlodik I. Y., 2014).

The role of masochism in the depletion of the body's physical strength, "undermining" health, "turning oneself into a void," was also discovered by T. V. Nekrut (2015). According to D. Rancour-Laferriere (1996), "any behavioral act expressed in actions, verbalization, or fantasies that, by unconscious design, are physically or psychologically injurious to oneself, self-defeating, humiliating, or unduly self-sacrificing is masochism." Karl Menninger (1956), a renowned American psychiatrist, calls masochistic sacrifice "neurotic suffering," and regards it as one of the forms of self-destructive behavior based on the unconscious desire for death. Edmund Bergler (1992), a prominent psychoanalyst of the mid-twentieth century, viewed psychic masochism as the "source of the life force of neurosis" and, in fact, as the basic human neurosis.

As I have mentioned, neurosis often precedes the development of psychosomatic diseases. Karen Horney (1992) distinguishes three types of neurotic personality types (depending on their behavior with respect to the people around them): toward people, away from people, and against them. With stable dominance in the behavior of the first type, the author speaks of the development of a specific "complaisant" or "compliant" neurotic personality, seeking love and approval at any cost. Such a subordinate type demonstrates a specific need for a partner, friend, or loving spouse, who must fulfill all the neurotic's life expectations and be responsible for everything that happens, both good and bad. This kind of person seeks to automatically adapt to the expectations of others, or to what he or she believes meets these expectations, often until the complete loss of control over his or her own feelings. One becomes "unselfish," sacrificing oneself, requiring nothing, except of one's boundless desire to be loved. One turns to become dependent, excessively attentive and valuing others, overly thankful, and benevolent.[1]

Claudio Naranjo (1994), in his classification of neurotic types of people, describes an *enneatype* 9, very similar in features to our psychosomatic type "C." This personality is characterized by "over-adaptation," "self-denial," "self-forgetfulness," "inattention to one's own needs," "susceptibility to excessive control," obedience and dependence, and adjustment of one's own behavior in order to please those on whom he or she depends. Such humility leads to rejection, renunciation of oneself and of life, "as if the individual endorsed a strategy of playing dead to stay alive (yet becoming tragically dead-in-life in the name of life)."

For this enneatype, other people's needs become his needs, and others' joys are his joy. "Living symbiotically, he lives vicariously," writes Naranjo,—"He could say, 'I am you, therefore I exist'—where the 'you' can be a loved one, a nation, a political party, a Pickwickian club, or even a football team." In the basis of this self-forgetfulness, according to the author, lies a deep subconscious thirst for love and a hidden desire to be rewarded with love, therefore this person denies those thoughts or feelings that others might not like. This individual feels great gratitude when someone notices his self-sacrifice, and therefore the search for love is mainly manifested in the desire to be recognized in his self-sacrifice and unselfish generosity. This "forgetting oneself," Naranjo (1994) believes, is the source of all pathologies.

Thus, this unrealized childhood need for love is manifested in a distorted, neurotic, helpful, masochistic, and self-destructive character, even capable of leading a person to cancer.

The known Estonian physician and healer Luume Viilma (2014) writes about cancer patients on the basis of her experience:

> ... the more positive you want to be, the more tolerant of people, that is, the more you take them into account, the more importance you attach to each of their words, the closer to the heart you take everything that happens and leave it in you, the more

---

[1] This "complaisant" or "compliant" personality, considered from the point of view of attachment theory, clearly corresponds more to the anxious-ambivalent type defined by Ainsworth and Bowlby, and the regressive-emotional variant of CEID offered by G. Y. Pilyagina. At the same time, the second main type of neurotic personality, according to Horney—distanced, manifesting behavior "away from people"—largely coincides with the avoiding type of attachment disorders and the hypercognitive version of CEID. Consequently, it can be assumed that the desire to over-satisfy the needs of others is a kind of common characteristic of cancer patients, regardless of the type of initial attachment disorder. These nuances need to be understood in order to choose the right strategy for psychotherapy.

you try to please people in life, and the more you destroy a human being in yourself. When a personality dies, the body also perishes.

For example, my patient A. with breast cancer mostly complained about her husband: "I did everything for him, I did not have time to take care of myself, and he left me alone after all this." Deep resentment of her husband literally "gnawed" at her, which led to illness. But, during the course of psychotherapy, she realized that deep down she was always afraid to offend her husband and cause his displeasure—just as in her childhood she was afraid of her mother's disapproval...

That is why in female cancer patients, often together with a masochistic personality, repressed sexuality can also be found (Cutler M., 1954; Aseev A. V., 1993, 1998; Hurny C., Adler R., 1991)—both because of the fear of not pleasing her husband, and because of the fear of pleasure (usually suppressed or barely actualized). Since the credo of a masochist is to suffer, she therefore punishes herself for the pleasure she has received, either before, in the process, or after (Mlodik I., 2014).

The extreme degree of masochism and self-sacrifice can be experienced by a sick person as a feeling like: "I feel that it would be better for others if I were dead." Such a feeling was, in a study of lung cancer patients, recognized as closely related to depression and with a worse survival rate (Buccheri G., 1998). It may reflect the vision of oneself as a physical and financial burden on family members, and a desire to quickly "rid" them of such a burden, even at the cost of one's life. Another extreme is when one in advanced stages of the disease continues to behave in the same masochistically sacrificial way. Bernie Siegel (1998) observed people on their deathbeds who continued to waste their energy recklessly. Instead of spending it on their own needs, they still try to make the whole world happy. Even when they are dying, they try to be good to everyone, while ignoring their own feelings.

Anita Moorjani (2012), a businesswoman from Hong Kong, whose amazing story of spontaneous recovery from the terminal stage of Hodgkin's lymphoma I will talk about later, considers sacrifice to be one of the reasons for her illness:

Why was I always suppressing my own creativity and intelligence to please others? I betrayed myself every time I said 'yes' when I meant 'no'! Why have I violated myself by always needing to seek approval from others just to be myself? Why haven't I followed my own beautiful heart and spoken my own truth? ... I was completely disconnected from who I was or what I wanted, because everything I did was designed to win approval—everyone's, except my own.

Very often, feeling a desperate need for the missing love, the future cancer patient seeks to find a partner for personal relationships, from whom she unconsciously expects to get love as a cure for the spiritual pain of childhood. Then a shift and projection follows of her feelings and desires from parents toward the new significant other. However, according to psycho-oncologist Tom Laughlin (1999), "... by a strange twist of fate, cancer patients find themselves back in a situation similar to their childhood. A situation where in some way they end up still being afraid to express their needs in order to avoid conflict." This phenomenon was also noted by Sigmund Freud. A "forced repetition" occurs; due to imprinting of parental behavior at an early age, this person subconsciously chooses partners similar to his parents, since, as later researchers have found, this is habitual and seems safer for the subconscious than dealing with whomever new or unknown (Hendrix H., 2007).

This situation is illustrated by the experience of my patient L. during the treatment session:

> Much of what I remembered was deeply buried and long forgotten, but now it came to the surface, clearly and painfully. It turns out that the problem of the father, and men in general, is much more important for me than I thought before. I see now that every aspect of my life was violated because of the absence of a father. My whole personality was formed around this. I had no idea that my father had such an influence on me, because my mother was very aggressive and riveted all my attention and all my disappointments to herself. I understood now the meaning of so many things that happened in my life, especially, why my ex-husband was one way, and not the other...

In fact, the masochistic properties of such a person's character often attract the personality of the opposite type: overly dominant or even sadistic, and this ultimately gives rise to the feelings of "suffocation" in the relationship in the future patient.

As a result, the conflict of the lack of love will increase and intensify, and family relations will be far from harmonious. For example, long-term prospective observation of students showed that future cancer patients noted less satisfactory interpersonal relationships and inconsistency with their expectations in these relationships (Graves P. L. et al., 1986). A study of the families of cancer patients revealed the presence of intrafamily conflicts and disturbing situations in 82% of cases (Gnezdilov A. V., 2002). In 1952, English doctor S. Peller had already found that the less satisfactory family relationships are, the earlier women will develop cancer. Chinese researchers, studying the impact of lifestyle and psychological stress on the development of early-onset breast cancer in 582 young patients, found as significant risk factors disharmonious marital situations, frequent depression, and negative emotional experiences (Li P. et al., 2016). In a psychological study of women with breast cancer carried out in Russia, 60% of patients evaluated their relationship with their spouse as unfavorable (Gritsevich T. D., Chernykh I. D., 2009).

It also often happens that one cannot get out of such family relationships because one has held on to the limiting cognitive beliefs from his childhood: "I have never been loved," "nobody needs me," "I'm not worthy of love." Therefore "I should be thankful for the available volume of love and attention." These subconscious beliefs in cancer patients are reinforced and amplified by a fear of failure, rejection, and abandonment, as a result of which they become locked in their space (Bottomley A., Jones L., 1997; Cobb B., 1952). Often, they have the feeling that it is useless in principle to express their needs, since they will not be satisfied anyway by those around them (Temoshok L., 1987, Temoshok L., Dreher H., 1993). This further intensifies the conflict of the need for love and acceptance. If, in adulthood, such a person endures the stress of a romantic break-up, a relationship failure in which a partner leaves him (especially a partner on whom the unconscious expectations of replenishment of parental love were projected), then the belief "nobody needs me," will be amplified according to the mechanism of formation the system of condensed experience (COEX, Grof S., 1996) and develops toward the life crisis and *cancer dominant*. We will talk about it in detail in Part V.

Thus, the unfulfilled need for love and belonging is undoubtedly a powerful intrapersonal conflict, which can compensatively deepen and become complicated by excessive self-sacrifice and masochistic satisfaction of the needs of other people. This conflict, as we see from the data given, contributes to the development of cancer (also because the person pays less attention to their own body and health).

11.1.2.3. The Need for Esteem and Recognition in the Form of Childlike, Dependent Behavior

The "masochistic" preference for the needs of other people serves to satisfy one more important need: for esteem and recognition, which the person subconsciously expects to receive for his efforts. However, as a result, this kind of person often becomes dependent on those whom they "serve," both because of fear of losing the source of love and recognition, and because of the desire to avoid conflicts, a tendency formed in childhood.

As a result, an internal psychological conflict of dependence–independence arises. On one hand, it manifests itself in the childish desires for dependence, and on the other, in intense aspirations to independence, giving rise to difficulties for the adult in resolving life situations. This is often observed in people with psychosomatic symptoms (Shtrahova A. V., Kulikova E. V., 2012). This phenomenon psychologists call "dependent relationships," when the childhood-born inner emptiness is filled with active external activity in favor of the important one. The person actually refuses him- or herself, believing that the life of another is more important and more valuable than their own. One of my cancer patients, faced with the need to actively work on herself, regularly independently completing various exercises during the therapeutic process, complained to me that: "I feel I have absolutely no time for myself because of all this work that I have to do for my family." An analysis of the dependency problem conducted at the University of New York has shown that dependent individuals have a tendency to somatic resolution of their problems, and accordingly to an increased risk of various diseases (Greenberg R. P., Bornstein R. F., 1988).

Unfortunately, such a situation of dependence often continues on its own, and the person does nothing to change their life, eventually losing their own individuality. "Psychosomatic pathology is [actually] a spiritually psychosomatic pathology based on a moral error or a conscious choice of non-freedom instead of freedom," comments Dr. Igor Semenov (2005). This is actively helped by the mechanism of immature psychological defense "denial"—the existence of the problem is rejected to reduce anxiety about an uncertain future. However, this leads to the development of a contradictory attitude to oneself (Rusina N. A., 2010), and to the next conflict: low self-esteem (Losiak W., 1989), which further worsens a person's ability to cope with stress (Rosen T. J. et al., 1982). The progressive decline in self-esteem can lead to self-aggression in the form of non-love for oneself and for one's own body, which, according to the psychoanalyst P. Kutter (1989), is the basis for psychosomatic diseases, creating a kind of "struggle for one's body."

The reader may ask: "Can this kind of dependence exist among public figures who get cancer? Observing the bright lives of many well-known businessmen, politicians, and artists, how can we talk about such conflicts?" The problem is that at the external level we see only one side of their personality, the most developed subpersonality, effective in their narrow industry. In other life situations, another, insufficiently developed subpersonality may be involved. Tom Laughlin (1999) notes, for example, that the disease of the head of a large and successful corporation can be connected to the fact that, at home, he turns into a dependent child, subordinated to his wife.

In such cases, a fundamental intrapersonal conflict inevitably grows between the need for freedom, respect and recognition, and the desire to maintain relationships—even if they create dependency. Although such relationships, as in childhood, suppress and restrict a person, very often this conflict, as well as its associated negative emotions (especially anger), is forced into the "shadows." As a result, there is a gradual weakening of the person's adaptive resources with the corresponding physiological consequences of chronic stress. However, despite the raging volcano in the subconscious, the satisfaction of the other people's needs remains a priority, because it creates the illusion on an external level that this person is needed, as well as the feeling of recognition of his efforts.

Dr. Bernie Siegel (1998) stresses the great importance of awareness and recognition by cancer patients of this conflict's existence. Usually for them, it means to discover the way they treat the needs of other people, perceiving them as the only ones that are of any importance, and thus hiding their own needs from themselves. Dr. Siegel gives an example of what happens when a patient denies the seriousness of this conflict:

I saw this most clearly and tragically in the case of Norma, an ECaP *("Exceptional Cancer Patient"*—*V. M.)* member with an abusive husband. Her disease started to disappear as she became more "self-caring." Then her husband developed heart disease and was hospitalized. Norma was faced with a choice. Rather than force her husband to choose between growing with her or fostering his illness, she chose to return to her old self. He resumed his abuse and got well, while she went home to die...

Another example is given by Carl Simonton. When one of his patients began to work on herself to stop ignoring her needs, this caused her husband to worry. "I just want my sweet wife back," he told her. However, this patient was able to make another choice: "If she comes back to life, I'll die," answered the woman (Simonton O. C., Henson R. M., 1992).

Unfortunately, many cancer patients are too dependent and are by definition not autonomous, and therefore unconsciously, at any cost, try to avoid responsibility for their own destiny, do not take on personal commitments to the actualization of their life plans, and feel the impossibility of influencing what happens to them (Rusina N., 2010). This behavior is based on the mechanism of a primary psychological defense called "regression" (a return to early, immature, childish forms of behavior). This type of defense, as I already reported, is typical for many psychosomatic patients in general, and cancer patients in particular (Korotneva E. V., Varshavskiy A. V., 2007; Shmakova T. et al., 2009), and reflects in the special psychological trait known as infantilism.

The infantilism[1] of one's personality (from Latin *infantilis*—belonging to infants or children) is a peculiar deviation of mental and personal development and behavioral activity, manifested in a propensity to childish (inappropriate to the actual age) ways of behavior, views, and assessment of the surrounding reality, as well as one's place and roles in it. This level of personal immaturity is reflected in the insufficiently formed emotional–volitional sphere of the individual, in comparison with his given age. At the same time, personal or psychological infantilism does not at all imply the presence of mental problems—it can be combined with normal, delayed, or advanced intellectual development (Kondratiev M. Y., Ilyin V. A., 2007), i.e. hypercognitive variant of CEID.

For a dependent person, the specificity of the fear of being abandoned by a person with whom there is a close relationship is based on a feeling of helplessness, a lack of independence, and an inability to make everyday decisions. At the same time, such fear is an infantile reaction to a potential separation/parting. Like a child, the dependent person is worried and concerned about being alone, lonely, and is unable to cope with life's difficulties. Because of this, there is a formation of behavior that demonstrates a close connection and dependence on a significant person—

---

[1]It is necessary not to associate the psychological term "infantilism of personality" with the common understanding of infantilism as a synonym for debility.

shifting the most important decisions to him, subordinating one's own interests to the needs of relatives or friends, submitting to their desires, and refusing to make any of his own demands to those around ...—writes V. D. Mendelevich (2003).

Often the dependent person "realizes" himself in psychosomatic diseases. According to M. V. Bogdanova (2005), people with long-term illnesses, who can be considered from the standpoint of a psychosomatic paradigm, often demonstrate destructive, infantile, and sometimes self-destructive tendencies in their behavior.

Similar information was received by German and English scientists, studying the features of the behavior of cancer patients. They found a constant tendency in patients to regard a highly valued object (be it another person, profession, or job position) as an important condition for their own well-being and happiness. This type of person lacks autonomy, is not able to distance himself from the object, and becomes dependent on it. If this object disappeared from their life or was absent for a long time, there was distress experienced as an emotionally traumatic event. At the same time, individuals of this type rarely succeed in achieving the desired proximity to an emotionally important object, and remain distanced or isolated from it. Such a failure leads to even greater distress (Grossarth-Maticek R. et al., 1988).

A study conducted by psycho-oncologists in Krasnodar (Russia) also established the similarity of personal characteristics of cancer patients to those of children. This is manifested through the use of the "child's vision of the world," and the inability to cope with emerging problems and difficulties through the prism of adulthood. Patients with such a "childish attitude" tend to associate their successes, achievements, and joys not with their personality, but with external circumstances: good fortune, or the help of others. At the same time, they see their health and illness as the result of an accident, and in accordance with this they expect that the recovery will come from the actions of other people, especially doctors. Therefore, patients with infantile positions do not make their own efforts to recover and do not consider themselves responsible for it, which is not normal for an adult (Egikyan M. A., 2014).

According to other authors, the infantilism of cancer patients is expressed: in the predominance of the reality-attached, habitual (concrete) image of the world and themselves; in the difficulty of understanding the proposed concepts; in the prevalence of the external locus of control (attributing responsibility for the events of one's life to external factors of the environment, fate, or surrounding people); and in the difficulties in perception, awareness, and reaction to psycho-traumatic situations (Ivashkina M. G., 1998; Sirota N. A. et al., 2014). According to N. I. Nepomnyashchaya (1998), the specific infantilism of people prone to oncological diseases is manifested in "a decrease in the emotional and to some extent rational perception and reaction to events and situations that constitute an active and serious threat to 'the comfort of the psyche'."

Similar are the observations of the psycho-oncologist N. N. Tarnovskaya (2014) of the Mari State University (Russia): cancer patients often demonstrate a desire to "go with the flow," to withdraw from participation in their own lives, and to absolve themselves of responsibility for any outcome of the situation. L. T. Baranskaya and M. A. Polyanskiy (2001), exploring men diagnosed with cancer of the stomach and rectum in the Ural Oncology Medical Scientific and Practical Center (Russia), discovered infantility (immaturity of personality traits) as one of the stable characteristics of their personal structure. This was expressed in egocentrism (egoism), resentment, capriciousness, reactions of childish capitulation to difficulties, and an inability to create mature interpersonal relationships.

The reasons for such infantilism lie in distorted child–parent relations. Both constant punishment (especially the repression of the initiative) and excessive care (extra encouragement, the desire to protect from any effort, etc.) block the child's exploratory behavior—its innate desire to explore the world independently, by trial and error. Exploratory activity teaches the child, while experimenting and making mistakes, to find the right decision in conditions of uncertainty, and plays an important role in adaptation to stress and health preservation (Arshavskiy V. V., Rotenberg V. S., 1984). Owing to parental dominance, this important human trait remains undeveloped, leading to dependence on others (on whom the image of the "powerful and dangerous" parent is projected), and to capitulation in the face of a difficult situation or conflict. In other words, this is a pathological adaptation: the natural adaptive forms of a child's behavior in the process of chronic frustration of its vital needs are pathologically transformed, in order for the individual to stop feeling psychological pain (Pilyagina G. Y., 2003, 2013). One of the consequences, as we saw in the previous section, is the development of masochistic personality traits.

Because of the impossibility of a normal development in accordance with the age dynamic and unattainability of the desired interpersonal relations, this kind of behavior takes on a biased, self-destructive character. The point of application of self-destruction, owing to the distortion of somatic regulation, often becomes the body (Pilyagina G. Y., 2003). Moreover, as we saw in Chapter 8, as a result of psychic trauma and/or attachment disorders, the dissociation of the child's personality emerges, when time for him seems to stop, and becomes fixed at the period of negative experiences. Then, some part of the personality—as a rule, the emotional part—is blocked in its development. This promotes the formation of the aforementioned hypercognitive variant of cognitive–emotional imbalance, when the cognitive functions of a person accelerate progressively while the emotional ones regress, creating and fixing models of infantile behavior (Pilyagina G. Y., 2003). In turn, it leads to a decrease in emotional intelligence and the development of alexithymia.

Vladimir Mendelevich (2003) notes that many researchers who studied mental infantilism explain its origin from the point of view of somatic developmental defects, including endocrinological disorders. Taking into account the distortion of the structure and function of the brain, especially the hypothalamic–pituitary–adrenal axis in children with attachment disorders, discussed in Chapter 8.4, such an assumption seems quite justified.

It is the infantile way of reacting, according to the concept of de- and re-somatization of Max Schur (1955), that forms the basis of psychosomatic disorders. Infants, because of their underdeveloped mental and somatic structures, react to external influences as a single whole, discharging tensions in both a bodily and an emotional way. In the process of normal child development, desomatization occurs, which the author understands as a separation of affect and somatic reactions. That is, the child learns to display aggressive tension not through vegetative, bodily processes, but in more conscious, cognitive ways: speech, control of emotions, and inner experiences. However, under the pathological development associated with psychological traumatization and the inadequate development of personality, there is a reverse process: resomatization, or a return from cognitive forms of processing emotions to a somatic response. According to Walter Brautigam and his colleagues (1997), in the process of psychosomatic regression, the "I" returns to a primitive protective level with aggressive and autodestructive tendencies in the form of somatization.

N. I. Nepomnyashchaya (1998) sees a similar manifestation of infantilization in the biological mechanisms of cancer development. According to her hypothesis, after a deep psychological infantilization, in response to a stressful situation, somatic infantilization can often occur: a return to the mechanisms of the child's cell growth, which turns into cancerous cell growth. In this connection, the data of Italian researcher Pier Maria Biava (2009), which note the marked similarity of cancer cells to embryonic cells, is of interest. Both types of cells have similar modes of metabolism, factors of intercellular interaction, and both synthesize similar proteins and enzymes (in particular, alpha-fetoprotein and placental alkaline phosphatase). "One is under the impression," the author writes, "that the cancer cell returns back to a state of subordination to embryonic purposes, and thus restores the activity of embryonic genes—those which have long been deactivated."

As an example, I quote a letter from my patient K., age 35, who has suffered from herpes breakouts since childhood and has already had several treatment sessions with me:

> On Wednesday, I had to solve one very important question for myself. I was sure of what I wanted and what I needed, but was afraid to make a decision and act according to it. During these hours of uncertainty, I began to feel familiar symptoms of herpes on the body, as I had in the past. Despite the unpleasant sensations, I tried to assess what is happening to me. Finally, I remembered that I felt the same way in my childhood when I was forced to do something. But best of all, I understood what

happened five years ago, when I was also sick. At that time, I was also unable to fight and say what I need and what I want. I agreed with my partner's decision, although I did not like it at all. But now, this Wednesday, I finally decided on what I need, and all the symptoms disappeared! I also realized that now I can make decisions in the same way in the future, and no longer feel like a victim. In the days that follow, I feel very good and have no complaints.

Considering the danger of infantilization, S. G. Pleshchits and others (2012) note that for the human being living in a [subjectively] simple and easy world, any slightest violation of the here-and-now satisfaction is a critical situation that places all of existence into question. For such a person, any very simple dissatisfaction instantly develops into a psychological catastrophe. Hence, inside, for every infantile being, every stress is a crisis. The more power the infantile installation has in the psyche of a given person, the more it determines his life perception, the more likely that any situational failure or unpleasantness will be felt as a global life crisis.

According to the research of M. Y. Kondratiev and V. A. Ilyin (2007), regression and personal infantilism can reach a pathological character not only in the socio-psychological field. They can threaten the health and life of a person through his unconscious "escape into illness," that is, the activation of somatization mechanisms or mental disorders, most often of a depressive nature, down to suicidal attempts. B. D. Karvasarskiy (2008) believes that the infantile personality structure and a neurotic life position are the main characteristics of the personality of the psychosomatic patient, since the somatic expression of emotional experiences is an infantile form of expression.

This also applies to cancer patients. Emotional immaturity, an unconstructive style of worrying—which reduces the level of anxiety, but retains a pronounced emotional tension—as well as restriction of emotions, according to psycho-oncologist N. A. Rusina (2012), becomes the basis of inefficient strategies for their behavior. In all likelihood, it is infantilism and regression, and exploratory behavior that has been suppressed since childhood, which lay the foundations for the increased inclination of cancer patients to experience helplessness and hopelessness. This is also, as we shall see later, characteristic of the precancerous state. This attitude also aggravates the course of the disease, because these patients do not believe in their ability to cope with difficulties and live with the habit of relying on someone who is stronger, more meaningful, and can do everything for them—doctors, healers, etc. It's like a child waiting for help from his elders, who does little for itself. In this regard, the psycho-oncologist V. V. Yatskevich (2007) writes: "The choice [of the cancer patient] is only, without changing inside, to try to find the 'wondrous healer', shifting all responsibility for the result to his shoulders."

The desire to remain a "good child" in order to deserve the recognition of parents affects the entire subsequent life of a potential patient, forming a deep conflict between this need to be good for others and the need to build one's own destiny. This conflict continues in the relationships of the person in the family and at work, leading to dependence on others and the emergence of the desire to relieve oneself of responsibility. It also creates a lack of self-respect and self-confidence, and maintains an inadequate image of the self and a feeling of ineffective existence in society. As a result, as noted by Dr. Douglas Brodie (2015), cancer patients have a huge need for approval and acceptance.

Hence, the dissatisfaction of the need for esteem, coupled with the subsequent inner conflict (as follows from the material examined), can also be considered as a provoking cancer factor.

11.1.2.4. The Need for Self-Realization and Pathological Subordination

Pathological accommodation, dependence, and psychological infantilism lead to a loss of ability to develop one's personality and make one's life. As Elida Evans noted in 1926, cancer patients refer to a psychological type that tends to limit them to one single object or role—a person, job, or home—rather than developing their own personality. This often leads to the formation, prior to the disease, of the state of subordination that Tom Laughlin (1999) calls the "subliminal ego": when the authority to make decisions in the most important spheres of life is transferred to the other person, and the refusal to make one's own decisions suppresses the natural and correct development of the individual.

Laughlin explains how the subliminal ego is formed in the individual:

... instead of growing up and becoming emotionally independent and self-sufficient, a [future] cancer patient remains infantilely dependent upon the parent, still spending his or her life trying to please the parent, still looking to the parent for approval, love, and emotional support. This symbiotic emotional connection to the parent sucks the life blood out of the dependent child and prevents such dependent patients from developing their own ego, their own personality that remains dormant in their unconscious. Most repressed of all is their need to grow up and become a self-sufficient adult.

In later life, many cancer patients fall into the same dependence on their spouses as, in their childhood, on parents, and this tendency sometimes even occurring as a lifelong addiction. This creates a state of chronic "suffocation" that leads to subconscious depression (Laughlin T., 1999).

German researcher Ronald Grossarth-Maticek and his colleagues (1982), during a ten-year observation of more than a thousand people, also determined that being a passive receiver of repression from others is one of the most important traits in the personality of cancer patients. It occurs when for a long time a person experiences repeated social pressure, which limits or blocks the alternative directions of action that are subjectively important to him or her. In other words, it does not provide a way out of the situation. At the same time such social pressure is often not fully realized by the person.

An illustration is the study of patients with gynecological cancer, conducted in the oncology dispensary of the city of Kursk (Russia). It revealed the predominance of their obediently shy, compromising style of communication and passivity in comparison with a group of healthy women and gynecological patients of a general profile. This allowed the authors to talk about the decrease in the activity of patients in social interaction and the appearance of passive subordination in communication (Vasilenko T. D., 2011). In a similar study of patients with cervical, uterine, and ovarian carcinomas, conducted by R. Mastrovito and colleagues (1979) in Sloan Kettering Memorial Cancer Center, less aggressiveness, greater emotional control, and a habit of compromise were found, compared to patients with non-oncological diseases in the reproductive system.

In the previously cited study of the characteristics of men with cancer of the stomach and rectum, their personality revealed passivity, rigidity in social norms, dependence on the other, lack of self-value, complete submission, and a constant tendency to be suppressed, which the authors also, like M. Cutler, called the masochistic trend (Baranskaya L. T., Polyanskiy M. A., 2001).

The masochistic behavior of psychosomatic patients can be generally likened to one of the basic reactions to a stressful situation, namely, "freezing" (total passivity). If the patient is able to express his feelings, then the aggression, that is, the "fight" reaction, rather than the anxiety or feelings associated with flight or passivity, will be brought to the forefront. This characterizes the more active and unstable psychosomatic patients (Bastiaans J., 1982) and, undoubtedly, improves the prognosis of treatment.

Antonio Meneghetti (1977), from the point of view of pathology, considers the tumor a form of latent rebellion, an uprising against historical passivity. A person afflicted with cancer always agrees with everything on a social level. For this, he or she avenges him/herself on a mental level.

NLP expert Robert Dilts (2006) talks about a similar situation in his mother's life before the occurrence of cancer. Some part of her identity was built around the role of a mother, so for many years she gave herself to others. Since she refused to do things for herself and competently took care of others, some part of her personality did not have the opportunity to develop for a long time. As her children grew up, she had more and more time for herself. But, she followed the old habit and started to nurse other people's children to somehow fill up her time, i.e., to care for others again. This situation Dilts considers as a conflict between the part of his mother's personality that knew what to do in order to be a mother, and the part that wanted to do something for herself: to travel, visit interesting places, and have hobbies. However, her belief system said that it's selfish to be self-centered, and that her mission is different: to take care of other people. As result, she gave constant permission for other people to manage her life and did not ever let herself do what she wanted.

In my opinion, as a result of this "conformism," the potential patient gets the most fundamental and chronic conflict of the unmet need for self-actualization, when the capabilities and talents of a person cannot be realized, his uniqueness is not manifested and, in the words of psycho-oncologist Laurence LeShan (1977), "the song of life is not sung." According to his observations, it is precisely this unsatisfied need that underlies such people's perception of life as unhappy.

The need for self-actualization, according to Abraham Maslow, is based on the active desire of a person to develop individual abilities, to achieve the realization of personal goals and interests, and thereby to form and develop oneself as a person. Self-actualization is the continuous realization of potential opportunities, abilities, and talents, the accomplishment of one's mission or vocation, destiny, etc. Maslow (with B. G. Maslow, 1993; 1999) reflects that it brings a more complete cognition and, therefore, acceptance of one's own original nature, as a relentless pursuit of unity, integration, or internal synergy of the person. It is self-actualization, according to the scientist, which leads to the development of such a personality, which frees one from the problems arising from a deficiency in growth, and from the neurotic (or infantile, or imaginary, or "unnecessary," or "false") problems of life (Maslow A. H., 1959).

Self-actualization is not just finding the best profession or job, but something broader, meaningful. It is the realization of what brings passion and meaning into our lives.

Aristotle, in the fourth century BC, developing his system of teleological causation, spoke of the doctrine of internal conditionality. According to it, "the proper end and aim of every object and every being is to come to fruition and to realize its own being. Thus, the acorn is realized in the oak, and the infant in a fully actualized adult" (Yalom I., 1980).

The well-known Russian philosopher and religious thinker of the IXth century Vladimir Soloviev (1990) asserted that the personality is not a self-sufficient and perfect being, it exists in a state of permanent self-transformation, self-development, and transition to a new quality: "The person, and, therefore, every human, is the opportunity for the realization of unlimited reality, or a special form of infinite content." Contemporary Spanish philosopher and sociologist Jose Ortega y Gasset (1972), Nobel laureate in literature, speaks of a human as a being whose existence, first of all, consists of what is not yet present—that is, in a pure design, a program of one's own being, and also in the desire of this being to realize itself.

Dr. Alfred Barrios (2012), an American psycho-oncologist, also attaches great importance to the self-actualization of patients, because a self-actualized person is almost always much happier, less depressed, full of life, and has a strong will to live. This, according to Barrios, is of great importance for a strong immune system or a natural protective system.

Carl Rogers (1995a) believed that the aspiration to self-actualization is one of the general formative characteristics of the universe at all of its levels, not only in living systems:

On an even larger scale, I believe we are tuning in to a potent creative tendency which has formed our universe, from the smallest snowflake to the largest galaxy, from the lowly amoeba to the most sensitive and gifted of people. And perhaps we are touching the cutting edge of our ability to transcend ourselves, to create new and more spiritual directions in human evolution.

According to the theory of self-determination of E. L. Deci and R. M. Ryan (1985); Ryan R. M., (1995), a person has an innate tendency to develop his abilities, in the form of internal motivation and freedom of choice in activity and behavior. Factors that destroy this innate propensity or associated self-image will not only stop the internal motivation, but also negatively affect the overall well-being of the person. Abraham Maslow (1999) considered this discrepancy between a person's desire for self-actualization and a real result is the most important reason behind intrapersonal conflict.

In family relationships, such a conflict for a potential cancer patient, having a "subliminal ego," consists in a situation of choosing between his or her authenticity and the loneliness associated with it on one hand, and, on the other, denying him/herself to follow the interests of their significant other, "in exchange" for the emotions that were not received in childhood. Moreover, there often arises a pathological attachment to the repressing ("suffocating") partner (Laughlin T., 1999). As Lawrence LeShan (1989) wrote about one of his patients, "she could not sell her soul … for love, nor could she live without the water of love. Seeing only these two possible alternatives, she was filled with a deep despair about ever having a life worth living."

Such conflicts between self-repression and the desire for freedom, reflecting the need for self-realization, don't arise only in marital relations.

Born from disorders of children's attachment, the conflict between the parent and child, according to Tom Laughlin (1999), is often still the main driver for the future cancer patient, although usually neither side fully understands this. It is about young and even adult people who, despite their age, remain emotionally or financially dependent on the parent(s). This dominance is especially characteristic of "*narcissistic*" parents. For them, the child is the source of satisfying their ambitions of being the educator and patron; it is the performer of unfulfilled dreams, desires, and fantasies. A parent who "knows what's best" for a child (perceiving it as a continuation of himself), by this behavior unconsciously cripples the child and develops in it a subliminal ego. As a result, the child, even in later years, remains completely dependent on the parents (the same infantilism).

This parental behavior blocks the subsequent growth of the personality of the future patient, their freedom to choose a partner and profession. After a treatment session, one of my female patients said:

I had a very bright and realistic vision of my father. He always tried to intervene and limit all my relationships with the boys when I was a student. I remembered a very revealing case. One time, when I was at home for the holidays, I received a letter from a fellow student. My father saw the name of the sender and pronounced the phrase, which I again clearly heard in a trance: 'You will not have any relationship with this person, he is a Jew'—without even asking me what kind of relationship we have. I was so shocked that I felt as if I was being strangled. And I've never met this student again, not knowing why.

But, what is even worse is that parents of this type do not allow their children to develop talents and will-power, limit their self-actualization, and program them to fall into submission and dependence in emotionally meaningful relationships in the future. This emotional dependence of future cancer patients, as noted by R. Grossarth-Maticek and H. J. Eysenck (1991), forms the absence of autonomy, preventing such people from making independent decisions when it comes to their own best interests. "Failing such autonomy, the patient's needs, having high emotional importance for him, are blocked and remain unsatisfied, with the result that symptoms like depression, hopelessness, anxiety, excitement, and self-aggression appear. Individuals of this type enter into social relationships which arouse conflict, and develop behaviors which are detrimental to health," the authors concluded.

Paradoxically, in the mind of a child, and then of an adult, the notion of what defines a "good" parent is often retained, i.e. the perception of a parent as one who "sacrificed" his life for the child's sake, and who "never complained, asked for nothing in return, and was always near." Resistance and anger caused by suppression coming from the parents remain completely pushed into the subconscious (Laughlin T., 1999).

Tom Laughlin gives a vivid clinical example of this suppression of self-actualization:

Jerry, a pleasant young man of twenty, successfully graduated from college, showing great interest in the telecommunications industry and demonstrating a clear talent in this field. However, his father did not even want to hear about it, insisting that Jerry should join him in the family business. As a "bribe," the father gave Jerry and his friend a three-month tour of Europe after graduating college, after which he had to start working with his father. But, at the end of the trip a strong headache led Jerry to the hospital, where, as a result of an examination, a brain tumor was detected. He successfully underwent the necessary treatment and about a year after that started working in his father's firm.

Jerry came to see Laughlin after he had a relapse of the disease. At first he called his parents "incredible, excellent," because they have done so much for him. However, during the exploration of his subconscious, a depressing picture of the constant, "suffocating" domination of his parents throughout his life was revealed, especially noting the lack of freedom to play as a child, and the fear of objecting (*I would say that this is a typical story of the formation of a personality type "C"—*

V. M.). Moreover, when Jerry started working at his father's company after the first treatment, he put the son in a position where he was subordinate to a less-qualified employee and had worse working conditions, which made the young man feel humiliated all the time.

As a result of psychotherapy, Jerry first realized the entirety of the amount of anger, resistance, rejection, and depression that concentrated in his subconscious and led to illness. He made a firm decision to live his own way... However, the father, who, of course, did not like this therapy, used all his power to stop the sessions and find other doctors. This brought Jerry to his death.

Laughlin (1999) calls such relations the worst form of tyranny—"a tyranny of love"—and insists that psychotherapy must be applied to both the cancer patient and his "tyrant" (be it a parent, spouse, or boss). As a result, the "tormentor" must realize his suffocating behavior and change it. Otherwise, a return of the patient to the previous life situation will lead to an imminent relapse.

For my patient N. with a brain tumor, viewing the performances of favorite singers on the Internet was one of the few pleasures available to her because of the illness. However, the doctors believed that she should not look at the monitor because of the flickering of the screen, leading to excessive activation of brain neurons. Her family tried to follow these regulations, limiting the patient's access to the computer. At one of our treatment sessions during this period, in a state of trance, the woman realized:

> My sense of grief over the ban on watching videos on YouTube was exactly the same as when I was a child. For the first 17 years of my life, my mother told me every day that I'm lazy, selfish, and should not be doing what I was doing, regardless of what it was. I wanted to sing, but I wasn't allowed. So, these prohibitions really took a toll, and I always had a feeling that all my personal affairs are useless, that I'm not allowed to have fun or be happy. This is how she negated my self-expression! ... Trying to force me to be obedient now, they will only achieve making me want to die.

The oncogenic conflict between children and parents also illustrates the research of patients with breast cancer, conducted in the middle of the last century by Dr. Max Cutler (1954). He found that almost all of the women surveyed had an unresolved conflict and, as a result, pathological relationships with their mothers. This was usually reflected in the experience of a sense of extreme commitment, leading them to a high degree of self-sacrifice for the sake of their mother. However, this sacrifice was based on a feeling of hostility, almost always unconscious, but clearly visible to researchers. Such behavior was interpreted by them as a reactive formation—a kind of psychological defense, consisting in substitution in one's mind and behavior of feelings and motives, creating tension or conflict, for the opposite.

Very few women could express their anger toward the mother—most of them suppressed it, compensating with excessive "pleasantness" and masochistic self-sacrifice. At the heart of such a deep psychological conflict, according to the psychoanalytic interpretation (mainly used in the middle of the last century), is suppressed competition with the mother in the field of sexuality and pregnancy (Cutler M., 1954). In this connection, I can also mention the study of H. Wrye (1979). Relationships with parents were studied in a group of sixteen patients with breast cancer, and in a corresponding control group. The results showed that cancer patients perceived their mothers as incapable of fulfilling their maternal role, while their relationship with their father was stressful or inadequate. According to Frederick Levenson (1985), throughout life, the precancerous individual resists truly close contact with the irritating mother. This attitude becomes generalized to the world in general as well as to significant others: a spouse, siblings, children, and friends.

All this once again confirms my opinion: in any child's oncology, first of all, psychotherapy of relations in the family is necessary.

The third basic variant of dependence and repression, according to Tom Laughlin (1999), arises in the future cancer patient in connection with a profession that does not suit them. Sometimes, it is that the job or profession did not please the person from the very beginning, but he was involved in it to satisfy the parent or the spouse, to finance the family. Continuing to deal with the unloved occupation from day to day, a man suppresses the innate talents, creating a conflict of self-actualization. The result of this we saw above in the example of Jerry.

A similar story of a man who in his youth dreamed of becoming a violinist is told by Bernie Siegel (1989). At the insistence of the parents, this young man was forced to become a lawyer, for only then could they be proud of their son. In adulthood, he too developed a brain tumor, and, according to the doctors' forecasts, had about a year to live. "'At that point, he said, I'll play my violin for the year'. A year later he had a job as a violinist in a concert orchestra and no brain tumor. I know many stories like his," Siegel writes.

These stories about brain cancer are confirmed by the data of the National Cancer Registry of Ukraine for 2013–2014: morbidity and mortality from tumors of this localization in children and adolescents aged five to nineteen years are in second place after lymphomas and leukemia (Byuleten…, 2015). In the US, according to government statistics, the level of child mortality from brain cancer came out on top (Curtin S. C. et al., 2016). That is the price children pay for getting "upbringing" and education, for coping with the stress of the constantly increasing volume of information that they study, and competition starting from one's school desk.

I also believe that it is the suppression of self-actualization that explains most of the cases of employee "burnout." The real reason for this phenomenon may be that a person is not in his or her place, or cannot express their true abilities. The suppression of this internal conflict in the subconscious and keeping it out of awareness, as we already know, absorbs a lot of psychological energy, which then is not enough for effective working activity, thus leading to said "burnout."

There is also another source of pathogenic overstrain: a person falls into dependence on the boss who represses him in the same way as a parent did during childhood. According to studies conducted at the University of Indiana, relations with one's superiors are as important for one's well-being as the relationship with a spouse, and the disruption of these relations can lead to depression and other psychiatric problems (Gilbreath B., Benson, P. G., 2004). Another study concluded that being under the leadership of a boss who is not respected, considered dishonest and incompetent, and is not trusted, leads to chronic stress. This manifests in disorders of the cardiovascular system and chronically increased arterial pressure, with a risk of stroke (Wager N. et al., 2003). This situation can also lead to a predisposition to cancer. For example, Rintala P. E. et al., (2002) reported that women in Finland who were diagnosed with breast cancer were experiencing a substantial overload of duties and responsibilities at home and at work.

The top manager may also find him/herself repressed by his job or position, which is no longer interesting and has become a burden. However, he or she cannot leave the job because he or she considers him/herself "irreplaceable," or the company's success depends too much on him or her. Psycho-oncologist Susan Silberstein talks about the case of Warren, the hospital president. He experienced strong anger and even fury over the changes in healthcare, because he had a lot of work to organize interaction between the industry, his administration, and medical staff. The result of his emotions was cancer of the colon with metastases to the lungs. When Susan asked him: "Who are you and what are you doing when you feel totally alive?"—the patient spoke about twenty acres of land with gardens that he owned in Wisconsin. He loved it, though he could only visit this place about once a year. Susan suggested Warren to quit his job and move to Wisconsin. He did so, and as a result he completely recovered and now lives a totally different and happier life (Chatfield C., 2015).

In the same group of patients are women who, under the influence of social stereotypes, consider their main goal to be a household and motherhood, but unconsciously are in need of active work in society, in the realization of their talents and interests. The opposite is equally true about other women engaged in business—they experience subconscious suffering from the lack of family or the need to pretend to be an "iron lady" (Laughlin T., 1999).

Dr. Paul Rosch, president of the American Institute of Stress, writing about the latest data from government, reported a mysterious increase in the incidence of breast cancer in middle-aged women. He believes this can be associated with the stress of "civilization." It was also found that women who are career-oriented, especially without children, have a higher incidence of fatal ovarian cancer. Single working women have a fourteenfold greater risk of developing ovarian cancer than the corresponding groups of housewives. The job itself can be a stress factor, particularly because of overt or covert sexual harassment. As to married women, many of them

> ...have to juggle work responsibilities with being a wife, supermom, single parent, or providing custodial duties for an aging parent or relative. In addition, they find that despite equal or superior training, experience and ability, they are paid less than their male counterparts, and usually reach a dead end when they try to reach the upper rungs of the corporate ladder,

noted Dr. Rosch (2014). Thus, work can be a source of numerous psychological conflicts.

Although external factors cause limitations or repression of the individual's potential, the type of personality, limiting beliefs, stereotypes of thinking, the inability to "give up the principles," and the fixed images of oneself and the world are a prerequisite for manifesting these factors as action. Generated, as a rule, due to childhood and social programming, they lead to an intrapersonal conflict between the individual's needs and social values. A striking example of this was the increase in the incidence of cancer among state employees, military, and security personnel who were dismissed after the collapse of the Soviet Union: their beliefs and worldviews were too rigid to adapt to the new reality and to find new means of self-actualization (Danilin A. G., 2011).

This is confirmed by A. Meneghetti (2011), who found that inside an individual suffering from a tumor in an explicit or as yet latent form, there is a psychic bifurcation, a reluctance to adapt more to the current historical situation, rejecting that affective game and relationship in which the subject existed previously. As shown by the study of women with rectal cancer, their main psychological problems are the repression of spontaneity of mental reactions, restraint of active self-realization, control over aggressiveness, and hyper-social orientation of interests (Averyanova S. V., 2012).

At the same time, Tom Laughlin (1999) argues that it is not so important who or what exactly represses (in his terms: "suffocates") the personality of the cancer patient, but what is repressed, i.e. the spiritual, creative beginning in man, one's development potential, the need to find the meaning of life, one's destiny, and one's talent:

> What makes this extremely dangerous for a cancer patient is that the talent or skill that is being denied development is absolutely essential for the life of the suffocate. ... if the suffocatee is to become the complete person he or she was meant to be according to their individual blueprint in their DNA.

As a patient of Stephen Levine (1989) once said: "I know what my cancer is made of. It is made of paintings I didn't paint, the sculptures I didn't sculpt, the lovers I didn't love. My cancer is beautiful. It is simply misdirected creative force, energy turned inward and impacted in a cramped space instead of flowing outward into the world." Anita Moorjani (2012) writes similarly: "I understood that the cancer was not a punishment or anything like that. It was just my own energy, manifested as cancer because my fears weren't allowing me to express as the magnificent force I was meant to be."

The Taiwanese psycho-oncologist, Dr. Tien-Sheng Hsu (2010), also believes that cancer is the result of a blocked and distorted life energy, which we rarely pay attention to. This creative energy, when distorted, leads to a genetic mutation and initiates the growth of cancer cells. A similar idea was expressed by Dr. Roy Grinker from Chicago back in 1966: he suggested that people who cannot personally grow and develop feel shame and anxiety in connection with this. This unrealized creativity can be limited to activity in an isolated group of cells or an organ, thus leading to growth of the tumor; whereas the psychological development of the individual, which evolves self-pride, productivity, and creativity, is the counteraction to the disease. Also, according to Dr. Galyna Pilyagina (2002), the person who sublimates the repressed need for self-realization may realize oneself in the disease.

Still, the conflict of self-realization can arise not only because of repressing and "suffocating" factors, but also because of the low level of one's spirituality, the lack of understanding of the meaning of life as a whole. Viktor Frankl (1984) believed that the most important reason for an intrapersonal conflict is the so-called *noogenic* neurosis: a disorder of the internal structure, a special "spiritual core" of the personality, caused by the lack of a person's sense of life. This leads to a state of existential vacuum: the absence of meaning and value in human existence, which are of paramount importance for the individual.

11.2. The False Personality and Existential Vacuum as the Basis of the Conflict of Self-Realization

> There are two great days in a person's life —
> the day we are born and the day we discover why.
> William Barclay,
> *Scottish theologian*

The meaning of life is the most important component of human spirituality, creating the potential for one's formation, determining goals, and promoting a harmonious existence. The desire to find the meaning of one's existence is the main motivational force of personality development.

Viktor Frankl considered the lack of having a meaning of life to be the main, widespread stress of our days. After passing through personal experience of survival in a concentration camp during World War II, Frankl became convinced of the possibility of finding meaning in all, even the most terrible, manifestations of life. The desire to search for and realize a person's sense of life is something he considered an innate aspiration, motivation, and the main engine of personal development inherent in all people. According to Frankl, the "existential crisis" (loss of meaning of life) was observed in more than 50 percent of his patients in a Viennese hospital. He therefore developed what he called logotherapy—an existential analysis (a kind of psychotherapy) aimed at recreating the uniqueness and originality of human life in an indissoluble connection with the world and other people (Frankl V., 1984; Yalom I., 1980).

It seems that during the half a century that has passed since Frankl's research, people's awareness of their need for a meaning of life has not yet increased. For example, according to a study conducted in 2008 by the US Centers for Disease Control and Prevention, four out of ten US residents either do not have a clear idea of their life goals or are completely neutral to the concept (Kobau R. et al., 2010). As the well-known psychologist and one of the founders of body-oriented therapy Moshe Feldenkrais (2009) put it, modern society is satisfied with the minimal development of the individual. The fundamental development of one's abilities ceases in early adolescence, because society requires that the young generation become useful members of society as soon as possible, so the development continues only in extremely rare cases. Only an unusual person, believes Feldenkrais, will continue to improve himself and realize potential abilities—despite the fact that the basic biological tendency of any organism is the development of its capabilities to the greatest extent.

It is interesting that Hans Selye (1975), the creator of the stress theory, also linked stress to the lack of meaning in life, emphasizing that lack of motivation—expressed in the form of a thirst for accomplishment, which brings satisfaction and does not harm anyone—is the greatest spiritual tragedy that destroys all life's foundations.

Another prominent representative of existential psychotherapy, Irvin Yalom (1980), professor of psychiatry at Stanford University, considers the absence of the meaning of life to be an existential disease, in which a person does not search for meaning in high affairs and noble motives, but plunges deeply into the experience of purposelessness and apathy. A similar position, quoting Yalom, is shared by other well-known authors:

Carl Jung (1966) believed that senselessness impedes the fullness of life and therefore is the equivalent of the disease, playing a critical role in the origin of neurosis. Therefore, neurosis should be understood as the suffering of a soul that does not find its meaning. About a third of Jung's patients were suffering not from some clinically definable neurosis, but from the meaninglessness and purposelessness of their own life.

Salvatore Maddi (1967) describes an "existential neurosis," whose cognitive component is "senselessness," or a chronic inability to absorb the truth, importance, usefulness, or interest in anything a person participates. Benjamin Wolman (1975) defines existential neurosis in a similar way: as inability to find meaning in life, leading to the feeling that there is nothing to live for, nothing to fight for, nothing to hope for—the feeling that no matter how hard one works, there is nothing inspiring to work for.

11.2.1. How Childhood Adversities Form a False Personality

The noogenic conflict and its consequence, existential neurosis, in my opinion, is the fruit of the formation of this type of personality which can be called "false," where type "C" can be considered as one of its varieties. It is based on the same psychological infantilism and pathological accommodation that we have discussed above. According to the research of Alfred Adler (1932), the meaning of life is a personal construct made at an early age, which has already formed on the unconscious level by the age of four to five. The meaning of life becomes an integrative basis for the personality of the child, because it connects in a single pattern (the style of life) its behavior, mental processes, and personality traits.

Gunter Ammon (1972) writes that when a child feels that the parents express their love only under certain conditions (for example, if he meets their expectations), that he is important not by default but because of "proper behavior," when he feels that he should be different from how he is in reality, then the true feelings and desires of the child, due to fear of rejection, are suppressed, the search behavior is blocked, and the development of the potential of his true personality becomes limited or even impossible. If, on this basis, the child also blocks the expression of natural aggression against the suppression of his personality, this can lead to his experiencing the absence of needs, interests, and tasks, the appearance of a feeling of inner emptiness and boredom, and difficulties in self-regulation and self-actualization, claims Ammon.

Forcing the child to excessive obedience will further exacerbate such a psychic state, in which the child loses the understanding of his or her own abilities, their life goals go into the background, and so the trait of over-satisfying other people's needs is formed. As a result, according to the opinion of the child psychiatrist and psychoanalyst Donald Winnicott (1994), instead of the correct personality structure, or "true Self," a false compensatory ego, or "false Self," develops, stimulating maturation and intellectualization far too early. Such a state, although it protects the child from an unfavorable situation, at the same time prompts the rejection of the surrounding hostile world, giving rise to the feeling that everything is in vain, devoid of meaning, and invalid.

According to Winnicott, excessive intellectualization (*we have already been introduced to this in Chapter 8 in the form of a hypercognitive version of CEID—V. M.*)

leads to a confrontation between consciousness and psychosomatic unity, which adversely affects health.

In society, a person who has grown up from an extra-obedient child, who suppresses his aggressive emotions, is very much in demand and encouraged; as Edward Hanna (1990) writes, a false personality is not recognized because it is socially desirable and is perceived as a sign of success, particularly if the individual has grown accustomed to caring for others from a very early age.

An original Russian philosopher and spiritual teacher of the early twentieth century, George Gurdjieff, argued that a false personality composes most of what we consider to be our personality, and consists of a collection of unconscious elements and actions borrowed from other people who limit our true identity: pride, affection, conceit, vanity, fantasy, etc. (Ouspensky P., 1969). Developed according to the behavior adopted in childhood with the aim of accommodation to the environment, the false personality combines a multitude of different beliefs and principles that are shared only because the social group to which the person belongs shares and considers them correct.

Gurdjieff believed that a false personality does not allow one to see the true meaning of life, because if we look closely at our inner world, thoughts, and actions, we will see that we are almost in the same state as during sleep. One does not see the real world, it is hidden by the wall of one's own imagination. What one calls "clear consciousness" is a dream, which is much more dangerous than the dreams one has when asleep (Ouspensky P., 1969). In my opinion, this "dream" is dangerous because it leads to an existential vacuum.

In order to satisfy the hidden mental pain caused by this vacuum, the false personality swells more and more as life goes on, covering the true personality with a hopeless curtain of fancies and delusions. It compensates for life's frustrations by striving for power and enrichment, forcing a person to see the meaning of life in an infinite pursuit of prosperity and career growth, and/or desire for pleasure, pouring out into an endless change of sexual partners, buying lots of unnecessary things, addiction to food, alcohol or drugs. This meaning of life can be called false or involutionary—inhibiting human development or even reversing it, to the extent of degradation.

This situation is well described by Russian psychiatrist Y. R. Vagin (2003):

The whole problem of the personality ontogenesis lies in the fact that after reaching biological maturity, the inner, nuclear potential of the individual begins inevitably and irreversibly, like The Magic Skin, to lessen, shrink, dwindle, and wrinkle. The living soul begins to gradually die; and the only way not to slow down, but to hide this terrible irreversible process from oneself and others is to erect the decor, strengthening the facade of the personality. Money, property, power, connections, titles and ranks, national pride and patriotism, faith and morals are all the eternal methods of illusory inflation of one's own personality, not only in the eyes of others, but also in one's own. In those cases when we see a person deeply, intimately interested in and concerned with the above issues, we see a dying person.

... the paradox of human existence arises, which Ananiev[1] once drew attention to, saying that in many cases forms of human existence cease to exist even when a human lives as an individual; their dying comes earlier than physical decrepitude from old age.

A similar opinion was expressed by George Gurdjieff: a false personality gradually consumes almost the entirety of a person's life energy, his inner light gradually fades away, and life becomes a mechanical, automated set of habits that generate depression and emptiness (Ouspensky P., 1969). This conclusion is confirmed by modern studies showing that people who zealously strive for external aspects of well-being: money, fame, and attractiveness, but neglect internal and personal growth, communication, and belonging to the group, demonstrate a lesser vitality (Kasser T., Ryan R. M., 1993, 1996), understood as subjectively experienced life energy, which serves as an important personal resource for maintaining health and psychological well-being. In turn, the general decrease in the sense of vitality (*vigor vitalis*) is one of the most significant structural components of a neurotic condition (including a disorder of general sensitivity, asthenia, and anxiety) and is capable of developing into depression (Anufriev A. K., 1985). This is one of the symptoms of chronic stress.

In this way the lack of meaning and purpose of life is growing, which is characteristic of modern society, oriented toward consumption and the material aspects of life. In many respects, it is the basis for the development of various psychological conflicts, followed by mental and bodily diseases. And of course a parent, governed by a false personality, is unlikely to be able to form a secure attachment in their own child and assist in developing in that child the knowledge of the true meaning of life. Most likely, the imprint of the false identity of the parent (or both parents) will lay the foundation for the false personality and involuntary direction of life for the child as well. Indeed, if the parents themselves did not make sense in life, then how could they help create it in their child? As Irvin Yalom (1980) writes, "If a child is unfortunate enough to have parents so caught up in their own neurotic struggle that they can neither provide security nor encourage autonomous growth, then severe conflict ensues." Such spiritual and moral disharmony in the family becomes one of the factors predisposing a person to cancer in later life (Sidorov P. I, Sovershaeva E. P., 2015).

11.2.2. A False Personality Experiences False Happiness?

Although understanding the meaning of life for many people remains difficult, the goal of life everyone probably sees is being happy. However, a

---

[1] Boris Ananiev (1907–1972) well-known Russian and Soviet psychologist, academician, one of the originators of the Saint Petersburg scientific psychology school.

person, led by a false personality and a vague sense of life, in his effort to achieve happiness often achieves the opposite result. Thus, in studies conducted at the University of Denver, it was found that people fixated on achieving happiness are 50% less likely to experience positive emotions, 35% less satisfied with their lives, and 75% more likely to fall into deep depression (Mauss I. B. et al., 2011). This was also noted by Viktor Frankl (1984): the constant pursuit of happiness hinders its emergence.

The reason for this, in my opinion, is the erroneous understanding of the essence of happiness: if it is understood only as material well-being, then unceasing intense activity in this direction, the pursuit of "a bird in the bush" creates a state of chronic stress, asthenia, neurosis, and then comes somatization and the occurrence of chronic diseases. That is, the result is the opposite of what is expected.

Karl Gustav Jung (1989) noted in this connection:

I have frequently seen people become neurotic when they content themselves with inadequate or wrong answers to the questions of life. They seek position, marriage, reputation, outward success or money, and remain unhappy and neurotic even when they have attained what they were seeking. Such people are usually confined within too narrow a spiritual horizon. Their life has insufficient content and insufficient meaning. If they are enabled to develop into more spacious personalities, the neurosis generally disappears. For that reason the idea of development was always of the highest importance to me.

In general, Buddha said on this topic two and a half thousand years ago: although people believe that they are looking for true happiness, they are not particularly successful in this, because they are misguided and do not know where to look for it (Traleg Kyabgon, 2001). Buddhists believe that there are two kinds of happiness: temporary and permanent. Temporary happiness affects the mind like a pill, easing emotional pain for a limited time, while constant happiness comes when the underlying causes of suffering —the ignorance of one's true nature—are eliminated (Yongey Mingyur R., Swanson E., 2008).

Similar ideas are developed by Tom Laughlin (1999), who argues that one of the important causes of predisposition to cancer arises when we keep trying to pretend to be something we are not, or to claim that we have qualities or traits that we do not actually have. Doing this for the purpose of living in accordance with someone's expectations, we force our conscious personality to constantly experience a state of intolerable conflict with what we consider to be the truth in the depths of ourselves. In some way we "sense" that we have a false "person" who tries to cover us up, disguises our flaws, weaknesses, and defects, and forces us to pretend that we do not have these weaknesses and shortcomings. The tension that arises from the activities of a false personality and those qualities that exist in our personal negative shadow leads to various manifestations of anxiety, misfortunes, and neurotic behavior, even to the extent of physical illness.

Moreover, a person who is preoccupied with a one-pointed pursuit for some material purposes, does not know that he has other, hidden talents or opportunities that seek to be actualized and realized in his life. Thus, he so much infringes his true nature that it causes a state of subconscious "suffocation." "Suffocation of this newly emerging talent or ability is the single most important psychological cause of cancer," Laughlin stresses.

Anita Moorjani (2012), after her spontaneous healing from lymphoma, realized:

> I believe that my cancer was related to my self-identity, and it feels as though it was my body's way of telling me that my soul was grieving for the loss of its own worths—of its identity. If I'd known the truth of who I actually am, I wouldn't have gotten cancer! ... I understood that true joy and happiness could only be found by loving myself, going inward, by following my heart, and doing what brought me joy.

Many cancer patients of Stanislav Grof, during psychedelic therapy, realized that they had a "mechanistic" existence, constantly experiencing a deep sense of discontent with themselves and their situation. Therefore, most of their thinking was aimed at "chewing over" the past and its moral assessment, regrets about earlier decisions, and dreams of what could be, or what they should have done better. This incessant cogitative cycle only perpetuated their dissatisfaction with life, because they misunderstood the nature of their needs. Such people concentrated on external substitutes: money, position, fame, or sexual achievements, which, however, never brought them the expected satisfaction upon completion. That is why they often felt a sense of meaninglessness of being (Grof S., Halifax J., 1978).

Here's how one of the patients of psycho-oncologist Laurence LeShan (1989) spoke about himself: "My life is good and it's pleasant. I have everything I thought I'd have when I grew up. But I look around and say, 'Is this all there is?' I look at my life and I ask 'Why?' I enjoy myself mostly, but it all seems rather empty. There's no purpose, no reason." Reid Henson, one of the "exceptional patients" of the psycho-oncologist Dr. Carl Simonton, had a very similar experience. Henson writes: "I eventually received all the material things I thought I wanted. However, once I had them, I realized they were of very little real value in enhancing my happiness in life. My experience with cancer brought this into sharp focus" (Simonton O. C., Henson R. M., 1992).

N. A. Rusina (2012), studying the life history and the personality of cancer patients, found that socially they were successful, actualized in life and work. At the same time, there is a discrepancy between the declared and deep-seated meanings of the personality. There is a contradiction between their high self-esteem, bordering with conformance and dependence on social norms, together with the internal conflictual structure of the individual, from one side, and their awareness of their life's meaning's inconsistency and dissatisfaction with the past, from another.

Danish psycho-oncologist Søren Ventegodt, with co-workers (2003) describes the experiences of their patient:

> Some day you realize that this is not how you want to live. Enough of lies and politeness and pretension. Air! You need fresh air, renewal, new inspiration. The way you live brings you slow death and this is not how life was meant to be.

The reason for this paradox is explained by scientists from the University of Florida. They studied the attitude of about 400 Americans aged from eighteen to seventy-eight years regarding having a sense of purpose or meaning, happiness, and other factors. Researchers have established that the meaning of life and happiness are not always interconnected: happiness without meaning is characteristic of a very shallow, self-centered, or even egoistic life where things are going well, needs and desires are easily met, and difficulties are avoided. The meaning arises when we take care of the people around us. Therefore, according to the authors of the study, happy people are those who are used to "taking," while those who live in search of meaning are used to "giving" (Baumeister R. F. et al., 2013).

Aristotle also wrote about this, classifying happiness as hedonistic (focuses on well-being in terms of achieving pleasure and avoiding pain) and eudemonic (focuses on sense and self-realization, and defines well-being in terms of achieving full potential in his activity). The philosopher considered hedonistic happiness vulgar, forcing a person to follow slavish desires, and the eudemonic to be its true form, manifested in the expression of virtues—that is, doing what is worth doing (Ryan R. M., Deci E. L., 2001).

Janusz Reikovskiy (1979) notes that when personal interests and needs dominate, and achieving personal goals becomes the main source of vital activity, then favorable conditions for psychosomatic illnesses are created. In his opinion, in such a person with an internally contradictory structure, with limited abilities for self-realization and for solving problems associated with it, the dominant egocentric attitudes can be a source of frequent and very strong emotional reactions that are difficult to control. In turn, it can become a stable source of disturbances in the emotional and vegetative functioning of a person. Also, self-centeredness, narrowed-down interests, limited and distorted hierarchy of values, goals, and needs, leading to inadequate claims that constitute the life purpose of a psychosomatic patient, were among those discovered in N. A. Rusina's research (2011).

Karen Horney (1992) argues that the "compliant" neurotic personality, externally "unselfish," sacrificing itself, demanding nothing, super-attentive, super-thankful and generous (*almost a portrait of the "proper," "good" cancer personality that most psycho-oncologists paint—V. M.*) is actually self-centered—it hides from itself the fact that deep down it is indifferent to others. These observations are confirmed by the studies of V. D. Mendelevich (2003): "The whole structure of the dependent personality is permeated with egocentrism: fixing attention to oneself, one's interests, feelings, etc. After all, the basic need of a dependent person is hedonistic (getting pleasure, joy, and/or satisfaction), hence it cannot be non-egocentric." Despite the fact that the behavior of the dependent person has an external resemblance to altruism—in their subordinating their interests to the needs of relatives or friends, compliance with those others' desires and refusing to present any demands to others—these actions are imbued with egocentrism and selfishness. The propensity of the dependent person to absolve himself of responsibility for his or her own life is just a good excuse when problems arise.

According to the observations of I. Y. Mlodik (2014), masochistic people are convinced that the readiness to serve others, endless patience, and self-deprivation make them altruistic; however,

> … in the Shadow of their psyche there is so much self-satisfaction from their own 'goodness', so much conviction in their own right and kindness! Their great pride can be discerned by a desire to take upon themselves all the suffering of the world and the expectation of a great reward for this, and also on the intransigence and intolerance which they relate with to those who do not want to suffer and endure.

Such egocentric attitudes are often the result of personality infantilism. The well-known Soviet philosopher Merab Mamardashvili (1990) considered infantilism as the concentration of the whole world in relation to oneself: a person assumes that everything in the world is happening either to make him happy or to upset him. However, an adult view of life that calls for the courage of the soul is a recognition that things are happening on their own in the world and have no intentions toward us, while those intentions that we see in this things are what we attribute to them. The behavior that occurs in such an egocentric infantile individual is to strive for ever greater pleasures, thus including itself in the "infinity of running," in the search for an environment in which "I would have more and more cakes."

It is interesting to note that a similar view of infantilism arose in Buddhism. Here, these kind of people are called "child-beings," characterized by unfreedom, unconscious attachment to life because of personal egoistic desires (passions), motivated by only "desire for oneself": narcissism and lust. They are completely immersed in the naive sensory experiencing of the world as it seems to be and are conditioned by eight "worldly interests": pleasant—unpleasant, finding—loss, praise—blasphemy, glory—dishonor. This leads, according to Buddhism, to suffering as a result of unfulfilled desires (Kozhevnikova M., 2006).

Such observations are confirmed by a study of the understanding of happiness in psychosomatic patients conducted at the Far Eastern Federal University (Russia). It showed that the "features of true happiness" of a psychosomatic patient are to live in such a way that "everything turns out well," "everything must be achieved immediately," and for that, life should be "without obstacles." Such an idealistic perception of happiness explains its actual rather low level in comparison with the control group of healthy people, therefore psychosomatic patients always "find" a reason to be unhappy. As a result, they have lower self-acceptance, autonomy, and personal growth, a poorer ability to manage the environment, to have a positive attitude, and to achieve a life goal (Vinichuk N. V., 2012).

The fact that the egocentrism of psychosomatic (including cancer) patients arises on the basis of psychological infantilism directly points to the origin of these personal distortions from disorders of child attachment. In my opinion, this egocentrism is a compensatory reaction of the individual to under-received love and care in childhood. As a result, in the later life such a person strives with all his or her might to find the pleasure and joy that he or she lacked in childhood, and above all, to do it in the simplest way: through the achievement of material wealth and the search for a partner. However, as we have seen before, this behavior often takes on distorted, shifted, excessive forms, ultimately affecting health.

For example, according to a study by psychology professor David McClelland of the University of Harvard (1980), in people who are motivated by a desire for power, the level of immunoglobulin A (immunity index) in saliva is lower than that of people who care for others. According to McClelland, this means that one of the ways to avoid stress and illness associated with a strong desire for power, is a mental growth, in terms of the transformation of this into a desire for power for the benefit of others. Maturity, love, and unselfishness reduce sympathetic nervous system activation with its potentially pathogenic effects on health.

An attentive reader can find a seeming contradiction here: in the previous section, I argued that an intense desire to meet the needs of others can create an oncogenic conflict, and now I'm writing that one of the important aspects of the meaning of life is to "give" and care for other people. However, these situations have a cardinal difference: the satisfaction of others' needs by the potential cancer patient is based on forcefully ignoring their own needs and "masochistic" sacrifice, which is based on egocentrism (Temoshok L., 1987, Temoshok L., Dreher H., 1993; Cutler M., 1954; Ivashkina M. G., 1998; Baranskaya L. T., Polyanskiy M. A., 2001; Danilin A. G., 2011) and is the product of a false personality.

For example, German expert in the field of psychosomatic diseases, Dr. Ruediger Dahlke, in his book *Krankheit als Sprache der Seele* (*Illness as the Language of the Soul*) (1997) writes about cancer patients as willingly taking on a lot of duties when there is an absence of the inner meaning of life, in order to give it an external meaning. The altruism of psychosomatic patients serves their self-defense or self-affirmation, claims psychoanalyst Jan Bastiaans (1982). Psycho-oncologist Alexander Danilin (2011) notes that the purpose and meaning of human life can be found only outside it, therefore cancer appears when a person denies the need to care for people, things, or ideas, convinced that they are all structured incorrectly, or are "guilty," from his point of view.

On the contrary, the desire to help people as an integral part of the meaning of life comes from a true personality, which, as a rule, is generally satisfied with its basic and social needs. In other words, the likely cancer patient cares for others from a lack of vitality, primarily because of a deficit of love; in order to get it in his life, he forces himself to do this, thereby creating an intrapersonal conflict. In contrast, a harmonious, spiritual person realizes the sense of life by taking care of others from the excess of vitality, sharing with others the fullness of his love.

One of the "exceptional patients" of Dr. Siegel (1998) came to the same understanding. Summarizing the changes in life that contributed to her healing, among other things she pointed to the transition from the provision of services in the name of recognition and gratitude to true service to other people. But, for this to happen, the patient must first restore his own harmony. The modern Buddhist teacher Chogyal Namkhai Norbu (2003) writes that "the only source of any kind of benefit for others is awareness of our own condition. When we know how to help ourselves and how to work with our situation, we can really benefit others, and our feeling of compassion will arise spontaneously."

It was this revelation that Anita Moorjani (2012) got while being in a state close to death in the oncological clinic:

> In order to truly care for someone unconditionally, I have to feel that way toward myself. I can't give away what I don't have. ... Only when we love ourselves unconditionally, accepting ourselves as the magnificent creatures we are with great respect and compassion, can we ever hope to offer the same to anyone else. Cherishing the self comes first, and caring for others is the inevitable outcome.

Similar ideas are developed by another Buddhist teacher, Lama Zopa Rinpoche (2001). He believes that the best way to enjoy life is to voluntarily devote ourselves to serving others, not because someone forced us to do this, but because of the freedom that is granted us with love, compassion, and wisdom. Then our life will suddenly become joyful and filled with deep meaning; it becomes a life that is worth living.

This was very clearly realized by Reid Henson, who also came close to death with cancer: "It became quite obvious to me that the really important things in our life are the unselfish things we do in a loving way for other people. Even the smallest act, done not selfishly and with love, has a profound effect on the Universe ... Intent is the key issue" (Simonton O. C., Henson R. M., 1992).

Thus, the true personality, as opposed to the false one, can be defined as one which confidently realizes its potential and its comprehension of the meaning of life, its talents and destiny, and builds on this basis its values, beliefs, and faith, an understanding of "what I am," "who I am," and "what I will and will not do." A true personality is critical of the "common" opinion: it is spiritual, but not always religious. It is open to new ideas, flexible, and can therefore change from within, on the basis of new knowledge and experience, is constantly evolving. It is easy to assume that such a person, as a rule, had a secure attachment to his parents, or went through a profound transformation of consciousness in the course of life. This person is resistant to stress, accepts and forgives himself and others, is able to constructively process a sense of guilt, and can constructively resolve conflicts. As a result, a true person has good health, a high quality of life, and deep satisfaction with it, in other words—this person is harmonious. The meaning of his existence is creativity and evolution in all spheres of life for the benefit of both himself and the surrounding world.

Therefore, in what follows, by "true meaning of life" I understand the evolutionary, spiritual meaning that appears when we discover our Essence.

A study in point has showed that people who have a meaning of life in the form of a clearly defined goal, assess their satisfaction with life higher even when they are unwell, compared to those who do not have a clearly defined life goal (Mauss I. B. et al., 2011). As Viktor Frankl (1984) wrote, "If there is a meaning in life at all, then there must be a meaning in suffering."

Danish doctor, psycho-oncologist, researcher of holistic and integrative medicine Søren Ventegodt, with colleagues (2003, 2004a) developed the theory of "life mission", according to which every person has his or her purpose in life, and if it is found and realized, it takes the form of a great talent. Living in accordance with one's life purpose, expressing one's fundamental talent, is real happiness. To achieve it, in the process of personal development, natural conditions must exist in which a person recognizes himself and undertakes everything necessary to fulfill his most important goals. Otherwise, the quality of life declines, which, if considered at a deep level, is the real cause of most diseases, particularly cancer, cardiovascular disease, allergies, etc. However, these diseases can be prevented through a targeted improvement in the quality of life.

11.3. Self-Transcendence as the Ultimate Meaning of Life

> What lies behind us and what lies ahead of us
> are tiny matters compared to what lies within us.
> Henry S. Haskins,
> *Meditations in Wall Street*

Studying the spiritual and philosophical heritage of mankind, one cannot ignore one of the most important provisions that is present in practically all the teachings and schools: the true personality is considered the expression of our Essence—our true nature. In religious traditions, it is called the "spirit" of a human being, i.e. that which connects one with the spiritual dimension of life, which exceeds the mundane interests of the person and even their self-actualization. Essence, unlike personality, is present in us from birth, laying the potential for higher, spiritual traits and opportunities. Most of them can never manifest themselves if appropriate circumstances do not arise in the world where the person lives, or will not be created by him in his life, since the development of the Essence is suppressed by a false person (Tart C., 1987).

Buddhism, the ancient philosophical and psychological doctrine, which was turned by overzealous followers into a religion, considers the underlying goodness and perfection of the human being as "the essence of the Buddha," the true nature of man, possessing wisdom, compassion, and power. In ordinary people, this state is hidden behind the conceptual ideas of their ego (often based on a false personality), its selfish or self-exaggerating manifestations, and is marred by ignorance, fear, affection, and disgust. It is the ignorance of this true nature that Buddhism sees as the cause (origin) of all human suffering. However, through spiritual practice, "the essence of the Buddha" is manifested as a state of full realization or enlightenment, when all layers of obscurations are removed, and from where complete and final liberation from all suffering and their causes comes (Ray R. A, 2002).

The eminent Ukrainian philosopher of the eighteenth century, Grigory Skovoroda (1973), speaking in fact about the Essence, explains that the "inner person" is the nature of every personality, and that in each of us initially there is a "new person"; everybody is able to discover it inside and re-create it from the "old me." The search for this "inner human" is a personal act, which, if successful (if a person "acquires" for himself his true self), becomes his destiny. The path of the search of the true self is the personal spiritual history of that person, while the content of this story is the realization of the person's choice of what defines himself: "I lost the old, but found a new. Farewell, my shadow! Hello, cherished truth!" proclaimed Skovoroda.

It is no coincidence that the happiness and satisfaction that make a deeper and more fundamental "I" possible are different from the happiness and satisfaction that the everyday "I" wants, writes the American physician and spiritual seeker Harry Benjamin (1989), a follower of George Gurdjieff. A human seeks happiness on the wrong path and with improper means and, therefore, inevitably suffers defeat, regardless of his talent and abilities. Until one gives oneself the opportunity to act as the basic and deep "I," one's life will always be heavy and full of disappointments. The growth of personality and Essence is not interconnected, notes Benjamin; on the contrary, the more a personality is distorted toward a false one, the fewer opportunities exist for the development of the Essence.

But, it is the Essence of a person that creates the true, self-transcendental meaning of his or her life. By self-transcendence, I understand a stage of one's development that leads to comprehension of one's spiritual nature, the meaning of life, the creative power of the universe, the unity of the universe, and, ultimately, "going beyond oneself," desiring to contribute to the evolution of the universe. By realizing our uniqueness and expressing it, we literally contribute to the development of the world, asserts Pierre Teilhard de Chardin (2008) in his bestseller *The Phenomenon of Man*. Self-transcendence is the way in which a person realizes his spiritual potential. This path can be philosophical, religious, esoteric, or empirical—in the end, it is not that important; the content does not change in any form. Whatever we call the creative energy of the universe—God, Nature, Allah, Tao, the Absolute, emptiness, or just our true nature—words will remain words until we experience the manifestation of this energy in ourselves, through personal experience.

If self-actualization is related to development of personality, then self-transcendence is the direction of the development of the Essence. It is connected with the deep thirst of a human being to surpass him/herself, to rush to something or someone outside his or her personality which is "higher". Moreover, according to Viktor Frankl (2016), self-actualization is unattainable if it becomes an end in itself; it can only be an accompanying effect of self-transcendence.

This view is supported by a study of the relationship between the types of emotions reflecting meanings of life, depression and hope, conducted by psychologists at the University of Texas Medical School. They found that although both kinds of meaning of life give rise to hope in a person, it is the spiritual, existential meaning of life, but not the trivial personal, that serves as a buffer between the stresses of life and depression (Mascaro N., Rosen D. H., 2006). The spiritual meaning of life also contributes to better coping with stress, less anxiety, better physical and mental health, and generally higher psychosocial well-being (Mickley J. et al., 1995; Watson P. et al., 1994).

According to anthropological notions, a person in his development toward freedom always encounters borders, both of reality and of his own internal possibilities. To pass these boundaries, a sufficient degree of openness is necessary, which is only possible when these boundaries are known to a person, when he or she can accept them, and is no longer afraid to violate them. From these positions, psychosomatic patients can be seen as stunted in their development toward full creativity and dedication (Bastiaans J., 1982). The Essence can remain in an infant state throughout life, even if the person has gained fame in some field to which he or she has dedicated him/herself (Benjamin H., 1989).

The aspect of spirituality is also illustrated by the work of P. Reker and G. Wong (1988) of the Psychology Department of the University of Trent, Canada, where they distinguish four levels of depth of the meaning of life. The first, most superficial level, reflects those meanings that are inherent in hedonic values and the needs of personal comfort. At the next level, the meanings of life embrace the values of self-actualization: personal growth, self-development, and self-realization. At the third level, life's meaning is centered on serving group, social, and human interests. The fourth and deepest level is constructed by transcendental meanings of life, directed to the ultimate human values: cosmic, divine, etc. The authors believe that the greater the importance of transcendental values for the person, the more he will feel the meaningfulness of life.

Nikolai Berdyaev (1996), a prominent Russian philosopher, described the desire for ultimate values:

> I, a unique individual in the world, must participate in the realization of the world's universal hopes, to absolute perfection. I can never give up the thirst for my final strength, final freedom, ultimate knowledge, and beauty, otherwise the world will perish.

The coryphaeus of modern psychology, Carl Jung (1989), who had a deeply religious worldview, saw his personal goal of life in the completion of the divine work of creation:

> Man is indispensable for the completion of creation; that, in fact, he himself is the second creator of the world, who alone has given to the world its objective existence without which, unheard, unseen, silently eating, giving birth, dying, heads nodding through hundreds of millions of years, it would have gone on in the profoundest night of non-being down to its unknown end.

Claudio Naranjo (1994), speaking of the psychological enneatype 9 (in many respects corresponding to the psychosomatic "C" type of personality), considers its leading passion to be spiritual laziness (accidie). By this, he understands the loss of inner awareness, deafness in relation to one's spirit, and loss of a sense of being, up to a state of spiritual coarsening—forgetting God. Alfred Adler (1932) argues that if the meaning of life has a self-transcendent (spiritual) orientation, then it favors good adaptation, health, and high productivity in solving basic life problems, whereas the egocentric or soulless orientation of the meaning of life, on the contrary, leads to disadaptation, crises, neurotic breakdowns, and inability to overcome life difficulties.

This is confirmed by studies of psychosomatic patients with a pronounced alexithymic radical, conducted by G. N. Pilipenko and colleagues (2009). These people are characterized by stiffness of the inner emotional life, ill-will, addressing only themselves, fixation on somatic health and bodily sensations, poor inner peace and lack of closeness to others, self-limiting tendencies, conformism, conservatism, and moralism. Self-restraint and lack of capacity for self-expression, a significant predominance of personality traits aimed at realizing the social role, but not personal perfection and somatic well-being, are manifested. The internal sensations of these individuals are described as boredom, emptiness, fatigue, tension, and excitement, resulting in the closure of unreacted emotions at the somatic level.

Well-known crises of "middle age" and "what is the meaning of life," in fact, arise when a person begins to acutely feel an existential vacuum, manifested as a noogenic neurosis. A. H. Maslow and B. G. Maslow (1993) generally believe that most neuroses are a failure of personal growth due to spiritual disorders: doubts about the purposes and meaning of life, regret or anger over lost love, loss of courage or hope, despair in the face of the future, a feeling that life was lived in vain, or that there is no chance of joy and love, etc. All this is considered by Maslow as a fall from the height of complete humanity, from the full embodiment of human nature; this is the loss of human capabilities—those that could have been and those that could have been retained.

According to the research of Grodno University psychologists (Belarus), a meaning of life with low significance of self-transcendental values against the background of a predominance of egocentric values becomes the most crisis-prone, and therefore the most harmful for development, adaptation, health, subjective well-being, and a person's productive life. Spiritless meaning, as a particular kind of non-optimal meaning of life, is conditioned by mundane, distorted, or even perverted spiritual values, and leads to a spiritual crisis. However, if a person consciously accepts self-transcendent values as sources of the meaning of life, the intensity of experiencing a meaningful crisis will decrease (Karpinskiy K. V., 2011).

In the body, the noogenic conflict, like any long-acting intrapsychic conflict, creates a state of chronic stress, metabolic syndrome, and depletion of the resources of the psyche and organism (Davis C. G. et al., 1998; Haustova E. A., 2008; Ventegodt S. et al., 2005a); in other words, by analogy with psychosomatic—existential-somatic disease.

11.4. The Meaning of Life, Spirituality, Health, and Cancer

> Disease is a reminder of the purpose of life.
> Dr. Gottard Booth,
> *expert in psychosomatics*

Scientists are increasingly confirming that the presence of meaning and purpose of life is necessary for good health. This increases a general human resistance to adversity, reduces distress, aggressiveness, negative emotional responses, anxiety, depression, and a tendency to abuse alcohol or drugs, gives rise to the feeling of being happy and promotes the flowering of life (Frankl V., 1984; Bronk K. C. et al., 2009; Brassai L. et al., 2011; Mascaro N., Rosen D. H., 2005; Wong P. T., 1998; Zika S., Chamberlain K., 1992). For example, cardiologists, having analyzed the survey data of 137,000 people, reliably established that a high level of meaningfulness of life reduces the risk of mortality from cardiovascular diseases by 23%, including a decrease in the risk of heart attack and stroke by 19% (Cohen R. et al., 2015). Similar conclusions were drawn by other researchers: people who live their purpose enjoy greater health, life satisfaction, and overall well-being (Kashdan T. B., McKnight P. E., 2009).

Such observations led to the understanding that the meaning of life is an integral part of a healthy lifestyle, based on a combination of physical and mental health, proper nutrition, optimal exercise, and avoidance of bad habits. This style of life was called wellness. The basis of wellness is the integration of mind, body, and spirit into the fulfillment of a person's life mission (Dunn H. L., 1961; Myers J. E. et al., 2000), so the wellness acts as the unifying force of life, the ability of a person to cope with challenges creatively, and form an emotionally open relationship, to be inspired by hope (Egbert E., 1980).

"More and more people seem to be realizing that true spirituality is based on personal experience and is an extremely important and vital dimension of life," write S. and C. Grof (1989):

> We might be paying a great price for having rejected and discarded a force that nourishes, empowers, and gives meaning to human life. On the individual level, the result seems to be an impoverished, unhappy, and unfulfilling way of life, as well as an increased number of emotional and psychosomatic problems. On the other hand, deep, positive, and liberating transpersonal experiences, such as the return of blessed intrauterine memories, or feelings of oneness with nature, with other people, or with the Divine, have a remarkable healing effect. They often give us a greater sense of well-being, an updated point of view on current problems, and a greater sense of purpose and meaning in life.

Since the optimal meaning of life is inseparable from spirituality, the results of studies showing that people with a expressed sense of spiritual well-being are better able to cope with their bodily and psychic problems, seem very reasonable (Graham S. et al., 2001; Specht J. A. et al., 2005). According to a review of several hundred studies conducted by Harold Koenig (2012), such people are less prone to coronary heart disease, hypertension, cerebral vascular disease, and depression, and they have more effective immune and endocrine systems.

In accordance with the spiritual and genetic health paradigm of V. D. Troshin (2011), a human being is considered to be a "spiritually genetic, biological, integrative, multi-level, self-regulating, open system. All levels of this system (spiritual, neuro-psychological, and somatic) are in a dynamic relationship, formed during onto- filo-, and cosmogenesis as a result of the improvement of the structural and functional, regulatory, and adaptive mechanisms of man in the conditions of constant influences of stressors and environmental factors." From this point of view, it is not surprising that psychosomatic patients have a low level of meaningfulness of life, their sense of life has an abstract character and is in principle unrealizable, and motivation for its realization is insufficient (Shevelenkova T. D., Fesenko P. P., 2005).

It is natural that the absence of the meaning of life, especially in the transcendent sense, is closely related to the incidence of cancer.

Psycho-oncologist Alexander Danilin (2011) considers one of the main features of the cancer personality to be its self-focus because of the lack of clear goals of existence. N. A. Rusina (2010), studying the effectiveness of life or satisfaction with self-realization among cancer patients, found extremely low parameters of this indicator, which shows the dissatisfaction of the life they lived.

"In fact, commercial civilization entered the era of mass death of the population from diseases which develop for socio-psychological and cultural-psychological reasons. Among them, illnesses that express anthropoptosis[1] constitute the main category," writes psychotherapist S. P. Semenov (2007). In his opinion, one of the main factors triggering the mechanism of malignant neoplasm is psychosocial deprivation: in this state, a person is psychologically devoid of a natural connection with the social organism and cannot fulfill his purpose. This purpose is not confined to the birth of children and their upbringing:

> ... it assumes a constant and constructive interaction with those close to him and with society, during which a person, realizing his individuality, acts for the benefit of others and is satisfied with his efforts. If the organism loses its purpose, its vegetative regulation turns out to be very unsettled: the generative process gives way to the leadership of death, which emerges in the form of a disastrous disease.

P. I. Sidorov and E. P. Sovershaeva (2015), developing a synergetic biopsychosocial–spiritual concept of oncological diseases, noted in cancer patients the infertility of the animagenesis process: the ontogenetic spiritual and moral development of the individual. Disharmony begins in childhood owing to the spiritual and moral deficits of the family; in the course of life, a deformation of the development of moral feelings occurs, contributing to oncogenic diathesis; a precancerous condition is characterized by a distortion of the personality's moral structure; and by the time the clinical picture of the disease unfolds, the spiritual and moral position of the patient is being destroyed.

S. A. Kulakov (2009a) developed a similar biopsychosocial–spiritual concept in oncology. In his studies, disturbances were found relating to *noogenesis*: the dynamics of a personality's spiritual development, as well as an existential vacuum or frustration in the spiritual sphere of cancer patients. At the same time, the prognosis of the disease depends largely on how far the patient is from the transcendental level of his spiritual development.

According to N. V. Finagentova (2010), cancer patients have a lower level of social and personal awareness, especially in the sphere of somatics, social activity, creativity, and values-based (spiritual) comprehension of reality. An American

---

[1]Anthropoptosis—human self-destruction, by analogy with apoptosis—the process of programmed cell death.

physician and author, Professor Rachel Naomi Remen (2008), founder of the Institute for the Study of Health and Illness, writes that after thirty years of work as a therapist with cancer patients and listening to their stories, she believes that such a significant disease as cancer almost always has a spiritual dimension. Physical improvements in this illness are accompanied by "movements of the spirit" in patients.

Australian psychologists have found that women with ovarian cancer who have an insufficient level of spirituality and who fall into religious struggle in search of meaning, see the world as an unreliable and malicious place, and therefore they can not effectively cope with stress, and display great anxiety and depressiveness (Boscaglia N. et al., 2005). On the other hand, American scientists have demonstrated that patients with the same diagnosis, sharing the eudemonic approach to happiness, have a lower content of norepinephrine in the tumor tissue, which may indicate that it is less aggressive, owing to the higher psychological and physiological resistance of such patients (Davis L. Z. et al., 2015). According to the research performed in Italy, patients with intestinal cancer, exhibiting a lower level of spirituality, and who have a high risk of depression and self-criticism, neglect themselves in both physical and emotional planning, which prevents their adaptation to therapy (Vespa A. et al., 2011).

Carl Jung also noted the connection of the appearance of cancer with problems of spiritual development. This development he called individuation: the self-realization of man in a holistic, unique individual, who does not follow the collective psychology (Jung C., 1972). This is a lifelong process of mental growth and maturation, turning into a full human being, attaining comprehension of the full "I," that is, of the Essence. Jung (2015) shares observations from his practice:

> I have in fact seen cases where carcinoma broke out ... when a person comes to a halt at some essential point in his individuation or cannot get over an obstacle. Unfortunately, nobody can do it for him, and it cannot be forced. An inner process of growth must begin, and if this spontaneous creative activity is not performed by nature itself, the outcome can only be fatal.

Psycho-oncologist Tom Laughlin, Jung's follower, believes that in such cases, what did not get the opportunity to be included in the conscious personality is repressed (in his terminology "suffocated"), and as a result remains dormant—this is the Supreme Person, the spiritual principle in man, the embodiment of the Supreme Mind of the universe. Its role is to create a completely unique human being in each of us, different from all the others that have ever existed, a human being with its own meaning and purpose in life. In its attempts to awaken, to be heard, this repressed Supreme Spiritual Person sends us signals first in the form of ailments, various physical symptoms, addictions, emotional, and behavioral disorders. If these signals to a change in lifestyle are not recognized, are ignored for a long time, then the Supreme Person will lead the body to a heart attack or cancer, as the last attempt to induce a person to fundamentally reassess his or her life (Laughlin T., 1999).

Carl Simonton, observing his patients, also saw cancer as the way that the body, through shock, induces a person to change in life. Therefore he concluded: "cancer is the message to stop doing the things that bring you pain, and start doing the things that bring you joy—things that are more in line with who you are and what you want your life to become" (Simonton O., Henson R., 1992).

Indeed, Dr. Johannes Schilder and colleagues (2004), who studied spontaneous cancer regression, believe that this happens because the crisis caused by the illness can call forth those parts of the personality that were suppressed earlier in life. These parts, once recruited with all their drives, resources, and skill sets, may bring into being virtually a different personality, which shows up in unusual behaviors and activities.

Jan Bastiaans (1982), considering psychosomatic patients as halted in their development on the path to full creativity and dedication, believes that their treatment should focus on eliminating such inhibition, and on releasing a person from an individual and personal "prison of fixation."

The reason for this stunting of human development, as we have seen above, is the obscuring impact of a false personality. According to Donald Winnicott (1994), in the extreme cases of the false "I" development in childhood, the true "I" hides so well that spontaneity in general ceases to be inherent in the child. However, only the true "I" can be creative and felt as real, whereas the existence of a false "I" gives rise to a feeling of unreality and emptiness.

Bernie Siegel (1989) considers that "cancer, being a kind of growth gone wild, lives something of the life that is unlived by those with repressed, constricted personalities. It is almost as if the absence of growth and excitement externally leads to its internal expression. All that energy that is kept inside seems to fuel the cancer, for it has no place else to go."

Lawrence LeShan (1989) concurs with this approach. He repeatedly observed: if a person is not in his place, life will not be his joy. And even if his life situation is externally successful, his soul gradually loses hope that this joy and meaning will ever appear. The reaction of the body to the absence of hope is cancer. Throughout many years of his practice, LeShan found this pattern of loss of hope in the range of 70% to 80% of all his cancer patients, and only about 10% in his non-cancer patients. Again, he views the disease as the last warning, prompting a person to remember his true destiny, to recognize his needs. If this happens, the body begins to find strength to fight cancer, mobilizing its protective mechanisms as much as possible.

Perhaps this is why cancer arises in those famous artists and politicians who have seemingly fully realized their talents, gone through a difficult path of self-actualization, and reached a position inaccessible for many in society. Of course, without a thorough personal examination of such patients, it is impossible to draw conclusions about the degree of distortion of their true personality. However, it is quite feasible that at a certain stage of life, because of unresolved psychological problems and chronic stress, their Essence stalled in its development, which resulted in the formation of an existential/spiritual crisis, often even unconscious. Such observations are not uncommon in the practice of psycho-oncologists (Ventegodt S. et al., 2005a; LeShan L., 1989), and in the concluding chapter we will take as an example the life of the famous Hollywood actress Audrey Hepburn. Another quite plausible explanation is the forced adherence by public individuals to a "positive mask of goodness," goodwill, and pleasantness. This, as we discussed earlier, is inherent in many potential cancer patients. Often this mask contradicts their real nature and leads to intrapersonal conflict and suppression of negative emotions, which we will discuss in the following chapter.

Chapter 12

Emotional Mechanisms of Unresolved Conflict and Psychic Trauma: Anxiety, Fear, Anger, and Aggression

> When desire and fear clash,
> the mind and body become a battleground.
> Joseph Murphy,
> *The Power of your Subconscious Mind*

As we already know from Chapter 3, in most cases stress arises as a reaction to a threatening situation, hence it is inextricably linked to the experience of fear. In the animal world, fear always has a clear, natural origin and a fixed period of duration, culminating with a threat; but in a human being's case, where stress is primarily psychosocial, fear can have stages of development, on each of which the individual can "get stuck" for a prolonged time. They are: worry, unrest, anxiety, fear itself, and horror. Each of these stages is reflected in the corresponding intensity of physiological distress. We also know that the human body can respond equally to the situation of both real and imagined threats.

Sigmund Freud (1920) considered the issue of fear a key point in which the most diverse and most important issues converge, and a secret, whose solution should shed a bright light on our entire psychic life. According to Irvin Yalom (1980), fear and anxiety, which are indispensable companions of a psychological trauma, have a destructive effect on the psyche.

In fact, it is through anxiety and fear that unmet needs are felt as an intrapersonal conflict. This is a fear for one's life and health when the biological needs are unsatisfied; fear of insecurity speaks for itself; fear of not being loved, not being needed, not having a family; fear of being irrelevant and unclaimed; the fear of living a life that is meaningless, and a fear of not "finding oneself."

One's problem is that the source of fear often remains unconscious, as unresolved intrapersonal conflicts are suppressed into the "Shadow." In this case, emotional stress is perceived as an apparently unmotivated, unconscious anxiety. Because of its uncertainty, anxiety is subjectively felt as painful and difficult to bear, resulting in a "neurosis of anxiety." Anxiety can lead to frustration, which is considered as a primary link in the development of mental stress (Sokolova E. D. et al., 1996). It is suggested that anxiety can be the main factor determining whether the conflict will move into the neurotic or psychosomatic course. If neurotic processing does not occur (because of the neuropsychological immaturity of higher mental functions that form alexithymia), the neurosis of anxiety becomes a psychosomatic disorder (Sidorova O. A., 2001; Velikanova L. P., 2006). Therefore, it is natural that anxiety becomes the leading pathogenetic factor in psychosomatic pathology (Kosenkov N. I., 1997). Most often even with such a bodily complication, anxiety is not perceived and not regulated at a conscious level (Atamanov A. A., Buikov V. A., 2000) and, as a rule, leads to depression (Kovalev Y. V., 2004). This may contribute to the formation of oncogenic potential.

In the process of this somatization, anxiety acquires bodily concretion and makes it possible for one to separate from unpleasant events. Disorder of physical health becomes an "indulgence" of life's difficulties, so the anxiety created by them is reduced, and the chance appears to find a socially acceptable way out of the stressful situation, avoiding psychic insolvency in the face of society's demands (Berezin F. B. et al., 1998). Thus, anxiety is attributed by the patient to somatic, not to psychosocial factors. Franz Alexander (1939) explained that psychosomatic disease, as a rule, is the physiological expression of permanently acting over-intensive protection of the emotion of fear.

But even if the conflict is conscious, but there is no solution to it (for example, the fear of parting with a repressive husband because of children or economic dependence), then anxiety (in the context of the example—this woman's for the future) can also reach beyond to an intolerable level, often leading to hysterical or asthenic neuroses. Fixed with time, anxiety becomes a stable formation and progresses into a personality trait, which is an important component of chronic distress, and manifests a lack of functional reserves in a person to overcome life problems. An increased personal anxiety trait, according to the observations of V. D. Mendelevich (2001), is closely related to intrapersonal conflicts, neuroticism, and depression, as well as psychosomatic pathology. Other authors have identified a high level of anxiety and a pathological inability to reduce it in conventional ways as a risk factor for post-traumatic stress disorder (Shelby R. A. et al., 2008)

Psycho-oncologists found that anxiety was particularly high in women who were subsequently diagnosed with breast cancer (Ando N. et al., 2009). An association was also found between anxiety and activation of synthesis in cells of HSP70 protein involved in the mechanism of uterine cancer development (Pereira D. B. et al., 2010). Psychiatrists, led by Dr. Arnstein Mykletun from the University of Bergen, examined over sixty thousand people during the largest medical examination of the population in Norway. They found a statistically significant association between the high degree of anxiety detected in a part of those surveyed ten years ago and the subsequent development of precancerous conditions (Haug T. T. et al., 2004).

Another study in the UK involved statistical data on mortality in a group of 163,363 people. An association between anxiety, depression, and cancer (most notably for carcinoma of the colon or rectum, prostate, pancreas, and esophagus, and leukaemia) has been demonstrated (Batty G. D. et al., 2017). It is important to understand that the cited research speaks not about the state of anxiety resulting from heavy illness, but mostly about the anxiety trait that was present before the diagnosis.

Obviously, it becomes even stronger in these people after diagnosis. In particular, women with rectal cancer demonstrated a neurotic personality profile with a "free-floating anxiety" that has not been formed into any clinical pathopsychic manifestation (Averyanova S. V., 2012). Studying the immune system of women with ovarian cancer, American scientists have found that anxiety and depression are associated with significant violations of adaptive immunity in the blood and in the tumor microenvironment (Lutgendorf S. K. et al., 2008). In another research, it has been defined that anxiety is one of the leading psychological characteristics in 48% of patients with tumors of different localizations (Stark D. et al., 2002). High level of anxiety was also found as significant prognostic factors for the worst survival rates in patients with cancers of different locations. The researchers concluded that the development of cancer in humans can be a consequence of the physiological effects of prolonged intrapersonal stress, unresolved owing to a lack of external assistance or inefficient adaptation (Blumberg E. et al., 1954).

The anxiety trait, as the basis of fear, is often formed in future cancer patients in childhood, when the child does not dare to show his or her feelings and desires, out of fear of being rejected or punished. Jan Gawler (1984) tells that in the typical childhood history of a cancer patient, we can find a fear, causing severe stress—sometimes the fear of physical punishment, but much more often the fear of not being loved, if the child does not do what the parents expect from him or her. Thus, experiencing suffering due to distortions of attachment, physical or emotional violence, dissatisfaction with appropriate age needs (and above all in the need for love of parents), the child ceases to feel safe, feels uncertainty, becomes highly sensitive, and perceives a constant threat to his or her self-esteem. This is how the increased anxiety develops (Hjelle L. A., Ziegler D. J., 1992), which, according to Karen Horney (1994), is the basic feeling underlying all neuroses.

For example, patient S. addressed me with complaints about anxiety, difficulties, and sometimes even panic in situations when her new partner asked her to do something and later asked about the results. During therapy, the woman recollected: she experienced this state in her childhood when her strict father demanded her report card, and if the results dissatisfied him, the daughter was punished.

Often, a child has an inner conflict between fear of a dominant, overwhelming parent and fear of rejection. In this situation, which M. Main and E. Hesse (1992) called "fear without solution," the child is forced to maintain contact with the parent or caregiver, despite the experienced fear. So, a tendency to avoid conflicts and suppress negative emotions develops, which, in fact, reflects the fear of the consequences of the conflict or manifestation of one's own emotions. It is noted that the state of fear leads to an underdevelopment of children's ability to express themselves through speech under stress. That is why they are more silent in the conflict situation—because they do not find the right words to resolve it. Therefore, such individuals sometimes feel helpless and are inclined to psychosomatic illnesses (Bastiaans J., 1982). Probably, this is one of the mechanisms behind the formation of alexithymia.

Molecular studies show that the conditioning of fear is associated with the emergence of a variety of short-term and long-term epigenetic changes. In particular, the level of methylation of the genes encoding the REL and PP1 proteins is changing and the synthesis of enzymes of DNA methyltransferases is increasing, which is associated with fixing memory traces to frightening events (Miller C. A., Sweatt J. D., 2007). In the future of such people, this can become the basis for the formation of a system of a condensed psychotraumatic experience that maintains a state of chronic stress.

Describing the mechanism of forming the state of "suffocation" in cancer patients, Tom Laughlin notes that the severity of the parents causes the child to feel an underlying fear, even horror, and quickly teaches him or her not to cross a certain line of what is permissible. The parent may not even raise his voice, but the child clearly understands what is expected of him, what is not allowed and what he should never express. Therefore, the child never crosses this border because of a fear of consequences. "There is no tyranny more powerful than the tyranny of love, especially the love of a child for a parent, whose tyrannical control can express itself in hundreds of different ways," writes Laughlin (1999).

For example, if a child does not live up to his or her parents' expectations, then he or she has a chance of hearing a reproach from the parent: "You do not love me." So, a disguised installation goes into the child's subconscious, programming him or her that to behave "correctly," that is, in accordance with the expectations of the parents, means to love them, whereas behaving "incorrectly" means not loving them. As a consequence, the child learns that the only possible way to prove one's love for one's parents is by full submission, and by the refusal of one's own manifestations.

The connection of the experience of fear in childhood with the development of cancer is found even in animal experiments. In rats prone to developing malignant neoplasms, an individual degree of fear was determined at an early age when they were studied in a new environment devoid of visible threats. When the rodents reached adulthood, it turned out that 80% of the "cowardly" individuals got cancer, while only 38% did of those who "courageously" studied the new environment (Cavigelli S. A. et al., 2006).

As the patient W. who had a disease of the hematopoietic system told me, when he was a child, his mother constantly criticized him. He had a fixed feeling that he was not good enough "because of the shit that my mother poured into me," in his words. As result, as a big, adult man, when even a small problem arose he used to became very anxious and upset. During the therapeutic session, in a trance, his subconscious showed him the image of accumulated maternal humiliation and his fear of her as black frogspawn, which seeded his brain. This spawn, during the session, he returned to his mother, "the owner." Unique in this case was the strange apparition of his elderly mother, which arose around the time of our session: the next day she called her son and told her that, in her eyes, she saw small floating black spheres, never seen before and similar to ... frogs' eggs! This vision lasted all day, and so the woman even decided to visit the ophthalmologist, who, of course, did not find anything. This is the strength of the connection between mother and child, which persists forever[1]...

As a rule, up until adolescence, anxiety in children takes the form of sustainable personal formation, ever consolidated and strengthened through a "closed psychological circle." The accumulation and deepening of negative emotional experience in this circle generates negative assessments of the future

---

[1] This is not the sole case of an "invisible transpersonal connection" in my practice. For example, the back problems of an elderly woman appeared to be associated with negative emotions that were "stuck" in her for thirty years after her divorce. A week after the session the patient told me that her son, who had not mentioned his father for almost a decade, had suddenly started asking her about him and what had happened between them. In another case, a mother was desperately worried about her daughter, who lived in a mental care house and was extremely negative toward her, completely refusing to communicate. After several therapy sessions, where we worked with the negative emotions of the mother herself and her traumas, the woman wrote me in great surprise that her daughter called her for the first time in a year on her own initiative and they talked normally. From that moment on, their relationship began to improve.

and a negative image of oneself that in turn contributes to the increase and preservation of anxiety (Prikhozhan A. M., 1998).

As a result, an adult who is a frightened and lonely child at heart will always unconsciously be in search of someone or something that will give him a feeling of parental warmth. Dissatisfaction with childhood needs for love, security, recognition, etc. is projected and transferred in adulthood to partners, work, and making money. For some of these people the desired and significant parental figure becomes God and the church, for others—the idea (saving the world, nationalism, hobbies, cults, fan clubs, etc.), while the group sharing this idea turns into a surrogate family. Finding what seems to be suitable and calming down this deep fear, a person, as we already know, can become pathologically dependent on this object and even elevate it to an overvalued idea: the dominant purpose of life (we'll get into it further on). Still, individuals who cannot reach the necessary autonomy and remain in an object-dependent relationship, usually experience a great anxiety about being abandoned by the affected object or person, thus feeling unhappiness (Grossarth-Maticek R., Eysenck H., 1991).

If, however, the found subject or object is lost or ruined, or when it turns out that this goal or even the life of a person as a whole does not correspond to his expectations, then intrapsychic conflicts arise, followed by disappointment (frustration), to the extent of an existential neurosis. Such states are often not consciously realized, but create a negative emotional background, which causes even greater anxiety and chronic stress.

In my opinion, suppressed or repressed anger acts as the leading and the main psychoemotional mechanism of oncogenic distress (this will be proved further), while suppressed or repressed anxiety and fear constitute the second most important reason. This second mechanism, apparently, prevails in patients with a regressive-emotional type of CEID, which is based on an anxious–ambivalent disorder of child attachment.

Anita Moorjani (2012), in the course of her healing spiritual experience, investigated the question of why she fell ill with cancer:

> I can sum up the answer in one word: fear. What was I afraid of? Just about everything, including failing, being disliked, letting people down, and not being good enough. … My life was driven by fear … Slowly, I found myself terrified of both dying and living. It was almost as if I were being caged by my fears.

To avoid the psychalgia—psychic pain associated with this inner tension—subliminal conflicts that are suppressed into the subconscious often give rise to aggressive reactions or motives, in other words, to anger: someone must be to blame for what's wrong with me! And if a person finds or "assigns" an object of anxiety, then he develops a new fear, which, in contrast to anxiety, is specified (Sadock B. J., Sadock V. A., 2007). This "personification" of anxiety is aimed at reducing its severity, that is, it serves as a method of psychological defense.

However, now there is a new problem: aggression, fueled by fear and felt like anger and hatred, can come into conflict with the moral principles of the subject and his childish cognitive beliefs—"to manifest negative emotions is impermissible and/or dangerous." This further blocks the ability of the individual to express his emotions and needs. Thus, one of the main intrapersonal conflicts arises; between the emotional nature of person and the rejection of this nature (Kholmogorova A. B., Garanyan N. G., 1999), which, as we saw above, is the most important characteristic of cancer patients.

Nossrat Peseschkian (1991), the founder of positive psychotherapy, considers the dichotomy of "fear–aggression" as a central conflict, as the key point of occurrence of a psychosomatic symptom. In human behavior, this conflict is reflected in the dichotomy of courtesy vs straightforwardness, where courtesy means the ability to be attentive, obedient, saying "Yes" at the cost of intuitive self-refusal (emotional reaction to fear), and straightforwardness means the ability to openly express needs, stand up for oneself, and assert oneself, with the accompanying risk of aggression.

Because of the special importance of this topic, we need to analyze in detail the mechanisms of the formation of aggression, the ways of its manifestation both in the inner world of man and in his relations with the surrounding world (through feelings of guilt and resentment), and to determine the ways in which aggression realizes the oncogenic potential in cases of its suppression or repression.

12.1. How Repressed Aggression is Transformed into Stress

The feeling of aggression is necessary for any living creature to survive and react to a stressful situation, including for the choice of "fight or flight." The child, in order to carry out his search activity, according to the founder of dynamic psychiatry, Gunther Ammon (1972), needs constructive aggression, understood as the child's initial openness to the environment, curiosity, and the desire for discovering contact. Such aggression, according to the scientist, is a central humane function located in the unconscious nucleus of a growing person. It leads to the formation of a healthy, creatively oriented personality, contributing to the building of personal boundaries.

However, under the influence of a destructive atmosphere or events in the family, constructive aggression turns into its destructive antipode, playing an important role in the illnesses of the personality. Even in mouse experiments, it has been shown that chronic psychosocial stress in younglings (in a cage with aggressive adult males) leads to the formation of aggressiveness and restlessness, which persist in adulthood (Kovalenko I. L. et al., 2014). In humans, such destructive aggression can be directed both outside, to the extent of antisocial, criminal behavior, and inside a person, leading to mental and psychosomatic disorders, self-harm, suicide, or a tendency toward accidents (Ammon G., 1972). This reflects the externalization or internalization of the corresponding internal conflict, which depends, in all likelihood, on the type of cognitive-emotional deficiency or imbalance determined by the type of attachment disorder to parent or caregiver.

Aggression to such close people who do not meet the needs of the child serves as "fuel" for the appearance of anger, but the child avoids an open manifestation of this feeling. After all, in his early experience, he knew that it could alienate the much-needed adults from him, cause their counter-aggression and lead to punishment or rejection. The powerful primary psychological defense comes into play: suppression and repression of aggressive emotions—at the same time the search behavior stops, active interaction with external objects is limited. This leads to the child's lack of development of the ability to actively shape and change the delineation of his or her "I" from his parents, and the function of consideration is not achieved (Ammon G., 1972).

It is noteworthy that aggression toward parents can arise at a very early age. That was the revelation my client S., 38 years old, with a precancerous state of the digestive system (chronic inflammation of the large intestine) experienced in the therapeutic session:

> I remembered myself at the age of about four years, filled with extreme anger. I was trembling all over, like a strained bowstring. I was nothing but embodied anger, and the reason for this was that my body, my feelings, and my thoughts were not taken into account; no one respected me, and everyone either only used me for their own purposes or completely ignored me. I cannot remember that I have ever felt such pure anger, but I was able to remember a specific situation, at about the same age, when I accidentally broke a window. I was also angry then, and precisely because I was not taken into account. The anger that I choked in myself has done much harm to my body and it frightens me ... Now, I know where my abdominal problems originated.

It is possible that it is in this way that this state of splitting and dissociation of the child's personality arises, through which the future cancer patients will reach the degree of psychological infantilism and dependence considered in the previous chapter. Very close to the clinical picture of such infantilism is the concept of "deficient aggression," that develops, according to G. Ammon (1972), as one of the consequences of blocking constructive aggression. Undeveloped abilities for an external expression of feelings, manifested in passivity, in this case are combined with an intense internal experience of aggression. These are manifested in the inhibition of active behavior in general, the absence of needs, interests, and tasks; the tendency to concede in competitive and conflict situations; the loss of the desire for personal autonomy; and the unwillingness to get out of "symbiosis" with the mother. Often there is a sense of inner emptiness and boredom, difficulties in self-regulation and self-actualization, and a sense of guilt. The creative potential of a person is reduced, asthenic and depressive states are formed, together with obsessive-compulsive disorders and autoaggressive phenomena (Antonyan Y., 1997). We see that such a picture largely corresponds to the psychosomatic type of personality "C" and explains the sources of development of the existential vacuum.

Lawrence LeShan (1977) notes that for a cancer patient, it is more likely not a general inability to manifest aggression, but an inability to be aggressive in protecting one's own needs, desires, and feelings. At the same time, they can show strength and aggression in protecting the rights of other people or meaningful ideas. This can be one of the mechanisms of the behavior formation associated with the preferences for other people's interests over their own.

According to the model of basic (initial) fault of Michael Balint (1970), the self-perception of a psychosomatic patient depends on the need for a constant presence of another person that protects and supports him or her, giving a sense of wholeness. But, because of this, it becomes difficult for such a patient to openly express his aggression because of fear of provoking a conflict and parting with a supportive object, which is so necessary for him. Such aggression simultaneously means autoaggression, as it infringes on the integrity of the patient's world, so she is forced to suppress her negative emotions and, as a consequence, manifest her psychic problems at the body level.

Günter Ammon (1972) believes that psychosomatic illness can also be understood as a disrupted ability to say "no," because in this case constructive aggression becomes destructive, directed against one's own body. In turn, Carl Simonton, with colleagues, (1978) notes that the inability of a potential cancer patient to say "no" to the conflict situation leads to the fact that cancer "speaks" for him or her.

This is confirmed by more modern studies of psychosomatic patients who were found to have elevated levels of anxious-depressive feelings and aggressiveness, correlating with each other (Ragozinskaya V. G., 2010). Another reason for the aggression of these patients is the loss of a significant object, when the inability to process the emotions of loss leads first to frustration and violation of self-esteem, and then to anger, irritation, and self-hatred. This scale can even reach hostility with respect to the lost object (Shtrakhova A. V., Kulikova E. V., 2012). Increased hostility, depression, anger, and latent forms of aggression play a special role in the formation of the metabolic syndrome, which serves as the pathophysiological basis for many psychosomatic diseases (Miller T. Q. et al., 1996; Goldbacher E. M., Matthews K. A., 2007), including oncological: for example, suppressed aggression increases the likelihood of developing prostate cancer (White V. M. et al., 2007).

The propensity of cancer patients to express their aggression through somatization is apparently laid down in childhood. This type of child finds the opportunity to satisfy his needs mainly by manifesting a psychosomatic disturbance, demonstrating helplessness and passivity, and thus making the mother and/or relatives give him the attention he or she did not receive before. If such a disorder is not "expressive" enough, it is possible to develop psychosomatic diseases as a way of replacing parental love with the attention of the medical staff, received by the young patient during numerous diagnostic and therapeutic activities. In this way the psychosomatically reacting child actually says "no" to him, as the dependence on caregivers, created by the psychosomatic symptom, contradicts his own vital needs to find him, and develop his identity and creativity, which requires constructive–aggressive behavior (Ammon G., 1972; Kohut H., 2000).

Subsequently, such a disadaptive skill contributes to the unconscious choice of the disease as a "secondary benefit," allowing the patient to escape from the solution of complex or conflicting life situations. Thus, in psychosomatic patients with pronounced alexithymia, researchers discovered, along with self-aggression, certain unconscious causes, because of which patients are "interested" in their own illness; therefore, they psychologically participate in the creation of the ailment (Pilipenko G. N. et al., 2009).

Because of limited abilities to cope with stress, both destructive and deficient aggression will increase throughout a person's life, weakening the possibilities of his or her adaptive systems. In the desire to "break out of the Shadow," but being prohibited from addressing the true source of the conflict, aggression and its consequences in the form of anger, as I mentioned before, can be directed either to the outside world, or, by the projection mechanism, to the future patient. In this way, a deep fear, lying in the source of aggression, is personified in him/herself.

In case of preferential internalization of aggression (addressing to one's own "I"), dissatisfaction will develop in the forms of self-dislike and self-rejection, low self-esteem and self-image, and permanent feelings of guilt. If aggression is externalized (directed at the objects of the outside world—parents, spouse, superiors, and/or the state), a person's deepest feelings most often become resentment, condemnation, and unforgiveness. There are, of course, mixed forms in different ratios. Lynn Payne (1991) believes that the main barriers to the acquisition of integrity are the inability to accept oneself, the inability to forgive others, and the inability to accept forgiveness.

According to the observations of J. M. and C. K. Teutsch (1975), hatred, resentment, and guilt lie at the base of most forms of cancer. This opinion is shared by therapist Debbie Shapiro (1990), who considers cancer to be the manifestation of a long-standing internal conflict, feelings of guilt, resentment, confusion, or tension. In the mental status of cancer patients, psycho-oncologist S. A. Kulakov (2009a) found, among various emotional deviations, destructive reactions to their ruminations, such as guilt, resentment, and vindictiveness, which lead to violations of significant relationships. Bernie Siegel (1998) notes that the more a person feels rejected and unloved, the more fear and irritation he or she accumulates, which then turn into resentment or hatred.

The practice of psycho-oncology shows that working with repressed offence and guilt is a primary therapist's task leading to the disclosure of destructive intrapsychic conflicts in cancer patients.

12.1.1. Autoaggression: Guilt, Self-Criticism, Self-Dislike

> Echoes of our own reproaches for our behavior
> constantly sound in our head.
> We are embarrassed to put up with it,
> probably because we are convinced
> that only punishment will help us change ourselves.
> Dr. Mario Alonso Puig,
> *Reinvent yourself: Your second chance*

Autoaggression can be viewed as a pathological form of human existence, arising from one's psychological, biological, and social maladjustment. It has both internal forms: a negative attitude toward oneself, manifested in self-destructive thoughts, attitudes, ideas, and emotions (rejection, self-criticism, guilt, self-dislike); and external forms: self-destructive behavior (abuse of intoxicants, risky behavior, ignoring symptoms disease, self-harm, and suicide) (Yuryeva L. N., 2006; Pilyagina G. Y., 1999).

The Simontons (1978), considering the psychological features of cancer patients, draw our attention to the fact that in the relationship between parents and children, there is almost always an unresolved feeling of guilt or resentment. The experience of guilt is born and remains with the child when his suppressed aggression of protest, due to violence or lack of attention from the parents, breaks out in some form into his consciousness or behavior. Hostility of this kind comes into conflict with the conviction about the "goodness" of the parents, i.e. with social attitudes, and is reinforced as a result of disapproval or punishment by parents or caregivers. Forcing a child to excessive "repentance" leads to the consolidation of the tendency to self-criticism and self-punishment as a way of obtaining parental approval.

Erich Fromm (1990), a prominent German psychologist and philosopher, one of the founders of neo-Freudianism, believed that at the age of five or six years the child develops an all-pervasive, constantly active source of guilt as a consequence of the conflict between his natural inclinations and their moral assessment by parents. In families with inflated demands and high levels of criticism, the child eventually becomes unable to meet the expectations of the parents. Having idealized the image of the parents, such a child feels guilty for not being a "worthy" son or daughter. He or she strives with all their might to match that fictitious self-image, which, in his or her opinion, corresponds to the vision of the parents, to the detriment of the development of the child's own personality.

The presence of such a mechanism in the occurrence of cancer in adolescents is confirmed by Russian psycho-oncologists. Before the onset of the disease, teens often experienced depression, which they described as helplessness in the face of a load of expectations and demands from their parents. These parents, as a rule, showed perfectionism, were strict with themselves and others, and had high anxiety. The children felt guilty about their inadequacy to meet the requirements of the parents (to be ideal students, assistants, etc.) and their inability to resolve problems in the family (Fisun E., 2010). N. A. Uriadnitskaya (1998), studying the peculiarities of the children's psyche before diagnosing cancer, found in them a maladaptive emotional coping mechanism in the form of self-blame.

Neurophysiologists at the School of Medicine, University of Washington, found that children who experienced an excessive sense of guilt and self-blame during the preschool period retained an insula (in the cerebral hemisphere) of smaller size than those of their "normal" peers. This phenomenon is closely related to the depression often experienced by such children (Belden A. C. et al., 2015). Given that the functions of the insula include the regulation of emotions, perception, cognition, and self-awareness, it may well be that its "underdevelopment" causes the phenomenon of cognitive-emotional deficiency or imbalance, dissociation, and infantilization, when the emotional part of the child's personality is blocked in its development.

Alexander Lowen (2006), a celebrated American psychotherapist and creator of the "Bioenergetic Analysis" method, explains the origin of the guilt in a child as her assumption that she is not worthy of love until she deserves it via good deeds and refrains from "bad" feelings. But, the fact that child feels anger toward those who hurt her, or hate those who betrayed her love, does not make her bad. Such reactions are biologically natural, therefore, they should be treated as morally acceptable. Unfortunately, children who depend on parents and other adults can be easily persuaded that in fact everything is different. When a child feels that his parents do not like him, he thinks that there has been some mistake, because in his mind there is no thought that the mother and father who gave him life could treat him like that. If he begins to have doubt in them, it is not difficult for parents to convince him that it is "bad" when he feels anger or hatred toward them. If "good behavior" guarantees parental love, the child will do everything in his power to be "good," together with the suppression of "bad" feelings. Thus a sense of guilt programs her behavior for the rest of her life, forbidding her negative feelings toward those who should be loved.

Also, guilt, as established by Lawrence LeShan (1977), often arises in the childhood of cancer patients following the experience of emotional pain, as a result of which they later began to step away from emotional intimacy as a potential source of such pain. These children, because of a lack of understanding of the nature of what is happening, perceive the resulting feeling of loneliness as their rejection, which gives rise to their experience of guilt and self-blame.

12.1.1.1. The Nonconstructive Sense of Guilt of Cancer Patients

Such a guilt, according to E. V. Belinskaya (2015), should be classified as "nonconstructive," producing disharmony and ill health. It arises as a result of the fusion of beliefs and rules uncritically introjected in childhood from authoritative people, and stuck with a dead weight of false conscience and useless complexes that trigger automatic behavior in response to unreacted emotions. Experiencing such guilt, one is usually afraid of being rejected and lonely because of violating the "norms," which prevents one from being a person having one's own positions and values, depletes support within one.

"Nonconstructive" guilt is radically different from the "constructive" form, which protect a person's true values, helping them to realize mistakes and correct them, and change their behavior. This kind of genuine, beneficial guilt is experienced only when this feeling arises from a conscious effort to identify the driving forces of one's behavior, to understand the origin of one's beliefs—if they are one's own or external—and to develop one's own individual ethical principles instead of foreign moral clichés. Only a free and integral person, who knows his or her boundaries and makes life decisions responsibly and independently, becomes able to experience guilt constructively (Belinskaya E. V., 2015).

It is obvious that a constructive experience of guilt contributes to the constructive resolution of conflicts, to learning and increasing the adaptive abilities, whereas non-constructive guilt leads to a conflict transition to the destructive phase, to maladaptation and the development of chronic stress.

Apparently, people who developed a reliable and secure attachment in childhood, or who have passed through a deep personal and spiritual transformation as adults, can be constructively aware of guilt. In most other cases, unconstructive guilt contributes to the emergence of the alexithymic mechanism of suppression and repression of negative emotions and the formation of deficient aggression. Then the need for "redemption of one's guilt" brings one over time to excessive satisfying of other people's interests, avoidance of conflicts, formation of a "subliminal ego," and the preservation of children's forms of behavior. As Karen Horney (1994) notes, a person prone to a frequent experience of guilt can invariably and indiscriminately do something for others: lend them money, provide work, carry out their assignments, and at the same time he or she is completely incapable of doing something for him/herself.

The research of I. A. Belik (2006) shows that people with an inadequate experience of guilt are incapable of analyzing their specific behavior; they are characterized by a negative emotional-value attitude toward themselves, a low level of meaningfulness of life, emotional instability, and a tendency toward indirect aggression, irritability, and hostility.

According to the research of Novosibirsk's (Russia) psychologists, alexithymic psychosomatic patients possess high natural aggressiveness and intolerance of other people's mistakes, conflictedness, rigidity, severity, and callousness. However, this is combined with high normative behavior, suppression of aggressive impulses, self-restriction, incompetence, anxiety, suspicion, resentment, increased latent vulnerability, and an unbearable attitude to change. Often, these properties accompany a pronounced sense of guilt, which goes back to deep childhood. The listed personality traits contribute to the suppression of aggression and to the direction of the aggression vector on oneself, as well as to scrupulously concealed hostility. Researchers believe that autoaggressiveness is one of the main properties of the alexithymic individual (Pilipenko G. N. et al., 2009).

Self-directed aggression, arising in childhood under the influence of a fixed unconscious sense of guilt, leads to self-destructive inclinations, because of which a child, and then an adult, can cause misfortunes or harm without fully realizing that it is he who forces himself to suffer. In its extreme manifestation, this sense of guilt can lead to the transition of internal forms of autoaggression to external ones in the form of self-injury, self-destruction through disease, and even suicide. Karl Menninger (1956), developing the theory of diseases as a manifestation of self-aggression, cites numerous clinical examples that show how an intolerable feeling of guilt, fear of punishment, and an unavoidable desire for it go hand in hand, manifested in bodily ailments.

In addition, autoaggression is accompanied by "shifting" the responsibility for solving the psychotraumatic situation to the outer world (external locus of control) with the development of the corresponding hypertrophied and distorted subordinate behavior as a function of pathological adaptation. At the same time, such forms of autoaggression as self-punishment, self-sacrifice, and negative balance of life are mainly characteristic of the hypercognitive variant of CEID (Pilyagina G. Y., 2000, 2013). We have already noted previously that such personality and behavioral traits are also characteristic of cancer patients.

This is illustrated by studies of patients with breast tumors who were shown to have aggressive tendencies against the background of emotional rigidity (Moskvitina S. A., 2012), difficulties in identifying their own feelings (alexithymic radical), and a reduced ability to express aggression or resist it, a primitive idea of how to protect against aggression (Aseev A., 1998). When a woman with uterine cancer tries to satisfy her own interests, it creates in her yet another source of guilt for such supposedly "selfish" behavior and, as a result, cultivates hypertrophied moral and ethical requirements of herself. In this way, this initial tendency to self-destruction increases. Autodestructive propensities in such women are among their most important characteristics, which are supported by their inherently passive way of coping with the difficulties of life, including with the disease that has emerged (Volodin B. Y., 2007).

Similar observations were made by R. Grossarth-Maticek and H. J. Eysenck (1991). When dependent cancer patients try to achieve autonomy, they often experience social pressure from the person on whom they are dependent, followed by intense feelings of anxiety and guilt. Erroneously, patients interpret the autonomy as egotism or separation from others, risking the loss of social contacts.

Concurring with these results is the study of women with breast tumors, which I mentioned earlier (where patients show masochistic self-sacrifice in relation to their mothers). Dr. Max Cutler (1954) revealed in them a distinct sense of guilt (*probably for unconsciously felt aggression toward the mother—V. M.*), which they were realizing a year before the appearance of the tumor. This sense of guilt could be the reason for their starting their treatment late, as a reflection of self-punishment for their hostility.

Karen Horney (1992), analyzing the subordinate type of a neurotic personality, discovered many diverse and deeply repressed aggressive drives. However, since any form of aggressive behavior is excluded from recognition by these personalities, any desire to take revenge or to win is so deeply repressed that the neurotic person often marvels at her own ability to tolerate and to hide the feeling of resentment for a long time. Particularly important is or her tendency to automatically take the guilt on herself. Almost independently of her feelings, whether he really feels guilty or not, such a person will try to place blame, critically evaluate him and not others, and feel guilty.

Rada Granovskaya (1988) draws attention to the fact that internal conflict (especially prolonged, leading to a neurosis) can create not only a sense of guilt, but often a conviction that the psychotraumatic situation has arisen because of one's omission. Another source of guilt is long-term suffering for one's misdeeds, when the emphasis from what was done is transferred to one's personality, with the development of "toxic" shame.

A good example is the case history of my patient I., whose son was an alcoholic. She had long been divorced and lived with her son, repeatedly kicking him out of the house and taking him back; eventually he died in the hospital. Here's what she said:

> In my youth, I often had to leave home to finish my education, and I left my son with my ex-husband. I know that it was very hard for my son, and I never felt calm. And when I was at home, I was quite busy and could not give him enough attention. After he died, I often remembered how I was doing my own things, and he had to wait for hours. These memories tear me apart. My poor boy! The sense of guilt that I have been experiencing since almost killed me! If there is one thing that I can take with me to the other world as an experience of

this life, it's an understanding of how important it is to take care of our children, and never be selfish—regardless of the situation in which you live!

Also, the feeling of guilt appears when the person preoccupied with those aspects of his or her personality that he or she does not like and therefore denies in him/herself, suppresses in the "Shadow"—especially a feeling of anger. Therefore, unconstructive guilt, in fact, is a manifestation of autoaggressive behavior, formed in conditions of maladaptation and chronic stress. On the other hand, this behavior can be considered as a specific defensive-adaptive reaction, depending on one's individual accommodative capabilities. Such a defense manifests the development of pathological somatization during an insoluble psychological conflict (Pilyagina G. Y., 1999), to an extreme degree of which can be attributed cancer.

In particular, N. A. Rusina (2012) determined internal conflict and self-accusation in cancer patients with different tumor localizations as a mechanism for protecting the "I" from negative unconsciously repressed emotions. At the same time, the predominance of overcontrol and emotional lability, passive attitude to conflicts, avoidance of problem-solving, and restriction of emotions are often accompanied by "escape to the disease," thereby manifesting autoaggressive mechanisms that are realized in the malignant somatic process. V. V. Solozhenkin (2003) came to the similar conclusion that psychosomatic pathology is a problem of autoaggression: "A person transfers aggression from the world to himself, to his internal organs … One 'fights his body' instead of struggling with the outside world."

S. Grof and J. Halifax (1978) frequently witnessed striking cases when cancer patients constantly felt an acute sense of guilt, self-hatred, and the desire for self-punishment, over the years or decades before the manifestation of the illness. Often during sessions of psychedelic therapy, these patients saw a direct relationship between such trends in themselves and the onset of a malignant tumor. Some of these people had a tendency to interpret the already existing disease as punishment. Lawrence LeShan (1977) notes that many cancer patients do not like and do not trust themselves. They do not respect their own achievements and often use self-descriptions such as "dumb," "lazy," "mediocre," "destructive," etc., despite the fact that other people treat them much more positively than they do themselves.

Reid Henson, after he learned about his diagnosis, remembered sitting in his apartment a few years before the onset of illness, thinking about his son's problems. Browsing a handy magazine, he saw in it an article about leukemia, and thought that he deserved something like that for destroying his son's life. "Was it just a terrible coincidence, or was there real connection between that deep feeling of self-blame and my current diagnosis?" reflected Henson. He decided that the disease was the result of his violation of Divine laws (the way he understood them at that time) and therefore he must be punished, while medicine should not help him, because otherwise it would be a violation of "Divine Justice" (Simonton O., Henson R., 1992).

Dr. Johann Heinroth, who was the first to use the term psychosomatic as early as in 1818, considered cancer to be a result of feelings of anger and shame. C. L. Bacon and his co-workers (1952) studied the psychological characteristics of a group of women, in which forty were diagnosed with breast cancer during the year after examination. They found that half of these patients had a heightened sense of guilt, acute or chronic depression, disseminated anxiety, self-criticism, and self-condemnation even before the diagnosis. In the studies of other scientists, a sense of guilt was found in 93% of sixty patients with cancers of different locations. The source of this feeling was the experience of a lack of relationships and the repression of the ability to communicate, a sense of inferiority, inadequacy, dependence, rejection, and in some cases a delay in seeking medical help (Abrams R. D., Finesinger J. E., 1953).

Expressed feelings of guilt were revealed to be a form of autoaggressiveness in cancer patients in the Research Institute of Therapy of the Siberian Branch of the Russian Academy of Medical Sciences (Chukhrova M. G. et al., 2010). According to the data of psychologists from Ekaterinburg, men with a diagnosis of cancer of the stomach and rectum, noting a history of depression, have self-destructiveness and autoaggression suppressed under normal conditions. These reactions were interpreted by the authors of the study as an adaptation to the unconscious sense of guilt (Baranskaya L. T., Polyansky M. A., 2001). One of my patients, experiencing a sense of guilt because of her daughter's death, said: "It's impossible to live with such guilt," thus setting the program of death to her subconscious ...

Similarly, one of Bernie Siegel's patients (1989) shared that the guilt she felt was so great that she did not know how to live on without going through some heavy redemption. She felt like such a terrible person that she could not continue living without experiencing some kind of suffering. And because of her belief that she could not be forgiven, she could not overcome the guilt until she fell ill with cancer.

A high level of self-accusation, which includes feelings of guilt and a decrease in self-value, was revealed by Moscow scientists in patients with ovarian cancer, and, to a lesser extent, in patients with breast cancer (Sirota N. A. et al., 2014). A psychological study of women with ovarian, cervical, and uterine cancer was conducted in the Lugansk Regional Oncology Dispensary (Ukraine). It was found that the patients are characterized by high and above average levels of anxiety (83.3% of those surveyed), indirect aggression (55.9%), and suspiciousness (50.5%). On the scale of feeling guilt, 78.5% of women in all scored very high (21.5%), high (19%), and above average (38%) levels (Vereina L. V, Prohorova L. V., 2012).

"Guilt always seeks punishment, and punishment creates pain," says Louise Hay (1984). A typical example of this is seen in the excerpt from a letter of introspection sent to me by a patient with breast cancer, A.:

> ... somewhere inside I feel as if I have done something wrong, and therefore deserve all this pain. And I feel very guilty that I have not recovered yet, especially after my beautiful family has put so much effort and time helping me to be healed (and so have you!). Besides, I tortured myself with the thought that if my pain is 70% psychological, and if it does not decrease, then it's 70% my fault. And it makes me feel very disappointed and angry with myself.

12.1.1.2. A Sense of Guilt Destroys Self-Esteem and Self-Acceptance

As studies confirm, a prolonged experience of guilt has a consequence of self-criticism and self-condemnation, both of which develop stress (Berry J. W. et al., 2001), impair the image of the self, have a negative impact on the functioning of the individual, blocking the development of abilities, satisfaction of desires, and maintenance of self-evaluation. As a result, such an aggression directed against oneself contributes to the emergence of depression (Bleichmar H., 1996). Claus Bahnson (1980) writes that the "shadowy me" of a cancer patient that feels isolated, unloved, sick, and devastated, leads to a mindset of hopelessness, the expectation that everything must necessarily go wrong, self-criticism and a simultaneous sense of guilt because of it.

Anxiety, emotional tension, and lack of self-esteem were revealed in cancer patients by Polish researchers (Losiak W., 1989). Ukrainian psychologists found in a mixed group of cancer patients low self-esteem, dissatisfaction with themselves and their own behavior, a tendency to assess themselves as not strong enough, dependence on circumstances, and not enough active behavior (Gurskaya T. B., Ivanova O. B., 2013). Low self-esteem, guilt, constant anxiety, a tendency to self-punishment, and redemption are characteristic of a group of anxious-hypochondriac, psychasthenic oncological patients, according to Russian scientists (Gnezdilov A. V., 1996). Similar data—showing decreased self-esteem and *intropunitive* reactions—were obtained during the examination of patients with intestinal tumors (Melchenko N. I., Deineka N. V., 2011).

The sense of guilt, as my practice shows, can be felt even for the fact that you are a woman – if the father passionately wanted a boy and has shown this to the daughter. This leads to the subconscious rejection by the girl of her feminine nature, the desire to be like the boys, and in adulthood can lead to having a lesbian orientation or, in its extreme manifestation, to cancer of the female reproductive system, as the body's response to the abandonment of its nature.

A habitual sense of guilt can contribute to the conviction of the patients in their guilt about the appearance of cancer. This leads to self-blame, a bad mood, and a decrease in the quality of life. Self-blame also associated with a lack of self-compassion, passive and avoidant coping behavior, obedience to what is perceived to be fate, and repressed anger. These characteristics significantly worsen the prognosis of treatment (Bennett K. K. et al., 2005; Friedman L. C. et al., 2007; Cardenal V. et al., 2012; Przezdziecki A. et al., 2013). According to N. V. Finagentova (2010), emotions and concepts that indicate self-accusation and depression ("remorse," "fault," "sadness"), are combined with a less favorable course of the oncological disease, while the ability to express negative emotions of anger is characteristic of a favorable trend.

Anita Moorjani (2012) in the book about her victory over cancer shares:

> Just look at my life path! Why, or, why, have I always been so harsh with myself? Why was I always beating up myself? Why was I always forsaken myself? Why did I never stand for myself and show the world the beauty of my own soul? ... I finally understood that it was me I hadn't forgiven, not other people. I was the one who was judging me, whom I'd forsaken, and whom I did not love enough. It had nothing to do with anyone else.

A conscious or repressed experience of guilt, shame, self-criticism, and self-condemnation, and the consequent low self-esteem, lead to the loss of proper pride, the destruction of the image of oneself, the loss of one's identity and eventually dislike of oneself. Meanwhile, a positive image of oneself, in other words "the power of the I," is an important condition for the success of the resolution of an internal conflict, since with a weak "I" the ability of the individual to adapt to the situation will also be weak. This can lead to the onset of symptoms of serious diseases (Brautigam W. et al., 1997). Destruction of the image of self and self-dislike, in turn, underlie the existential crisis and the loss of the meaning of life, which, as we discussed earlier, is one of the most important mechanisms of oncogenic sensibilization. The data of N. A. Rusina (2012) show in cancer patients of different profiles a general negative emotional attitude to themselves and self-depreciation, which are manifested as a combination of self-blame and high internal conflict because of the difficulty of localizing the true source of their problems.

One of my patients, who had several tumors in the brain, said after the treatment session:

> Throughout my life, I believed in a very big lie: that for some kind of sins, which I didn't even know, did not understand, and probably did not even commit, I was punished with unbearable suffering for many years. So, to this day, when I suffer, I believe that I am being punished for something ... but I do not know what I did wrong. Besides, I could never believe that I deserved a life without suffering. The effect of my acceptance of such a great lie is the emergence of this iron helmet on my head (*a metaphorical image of cancer, seen by this patient during the trance immersion—V. M.*). Even the divine power can not penetrate there, because I guarded it with my belief that was installed in me. The reason why my iron helmet still exists (this is completely unreasonable, I know, but nonetheless) is a deeply rooted feeling that I was left by God in the face of an unpleasant fate, because I caused somehow His displeasure.

O. D. Rozhkova (2015), studying women with breast cancer, noted among other things their floating or low self-esteem, lack of personal boundaries in the family, and low life competence. There is often a sense of guilt—both for oneself and for the behavior of other family members. The experience of hidden dissatisfaction with oneself is often combined with the desire to prove one's value to the parents or family in order to earn their love. For this, and also for the purpose of normalizing their emotional state, such women need constant external approval, and the means of getting it becomes a concentration of efforts on the lives of other people, particularly family members. Against the background of a vague understanding of their own desires and goals, these women develop a sense of self-denial, a refusal to pay attention to their own needs, and a merger of their goals and someone else's desires. As another one of my patients realized, "I could never allow myself to feel good if someone next to me was not well ..." A similar observation in a group of women diagnosed with lymphoma and leukemia was published by W. A. Greene (1966). These patients were ashamed of themselves, because they did not fit their idea of their "ideal self" and of the image that they think their significant other would like. All this made them feel that they could not be loved.

It is obvious that such character properties do not arise because of the disease, but are formed long before its manifestation. Since self-denial, as we have already discussed, creates a conflict in the future patient with his or her deep need of self-actualization, the next round of subconscious self-condemnation and guilt arises; this happens because a person has subordinated his or her life to the interests of another or others, even if it is done to receive love and attention (LeShan L., 1977).

Thus, we see once again, this time from the standpoint of guilt and self-criticism, the development of the pathological adaptation, psychological infantilism, masochism, and the "subliminal ego" that all form the psychosomatic personality type "C." To eliminate or reduce the psychological discomfort caused by autoaggressive experiences, the subconscious of such a person uses defensive mechanisms of denial and hypercompensation, leading to excessive satisfaction of the needs of other people and overstating moral and ethical requirements to oneself (Volodin B. Y., 2007). This gives rise to the illusion of the well-being of the future patient, as reported by Jan Gawler (1984): though it may seem that such a person knows his own worth and is self-confident, in fact he always tries to disguise the lack of self-esteem. Sometimes doubts, a desire for self-punishment, and even an urge for self-destruction arise in his soul. He is tormented by a suppressed feeling that not everything in his life is as good as he would like to see it. Lydia Temoshok (1987), describing the propensity of type "C" persons not to express their emotions and needs, says that they thereby conceal these feelings under the guise of normality and self-sufficiency.

This was also observed in cancer patients by Rudiger Dahlke (1997): a pleasant or noble self-restraint that the surrounding world observes in them can in fact be a suppression of life impulses, and ultimately will poison their life. Just as a cell in a body subjected to the strongest continuous irritation makes every effort to fulfill its function, so patients try to match the role of the daughter, son, mother, father, employee, etc., regardless of their own needs and to everyone's satisfaction. Their own development is pushed to the background. The resulting mood of such a "lifeless life" becomes a state of depression.

Such a state of the soul of a future patient who, owing to an unresolved conflict and an inability to cope with it, experiences an autoaggression in the form of feelings of guilt and self-condemnation (especially accompanied by obsessive, negative thoughts about the past), according to some authors becomes the leading factor in the formation of chronic distress (Berry J. W. et al., 2001; Barber L. et al., 2005; Worthington E. L., 2013). The reason for this is, as we already know, that the essence of autoaggression is negative emotions of anger and dissatisfaction with oneself, which destructively affect the body. In addition, a person with low self-esteem under the influence of a threat develops a higher level of fear or anxiety than a person with high self-esteem; the former believes that he lacks the ability to confront the threat. Therefore, she shows less activity in taking preventive measures (although she tries to avoid difficulties), because she is sure that she is not able to cope with the threat. There may also be a fatal belief that the person himself can do nothing to prevent the negative consequences of the problems experienced (Rosen T. J. et al., 1982).

The state of physiological distress in experiencing guilt and low self-esteem is confirmed experimentally. It is reflected in the growth of the content of cortisol, the decrease in the activity of immune killer cells and the amount of immunoglobulin A (Strauman T. J. et al., 1993; Liu S. Y. et al., 2014; Lowe G. et al., 1999), and a more intense inflammatory reaction (O'Donnell K. J. et al., 2008). It has also been shown that stress caused by self-criticism, as a form of self-aggression, leads to DNA damage (Irie M. et al., 2001). In Chapter 19 we will see that all these phenomena are characteristic of the conditions in the body in which tumor growth occurs.

12.1.1.3. The Healing Power of Self-Forgiveness

The discussed data speak about the significant importance of psychological help to cancer patients in changing their attitudes toward themselves, acquiring a positive image of "I," and eliminating self-aggression in the form of non-constructive guilt. According to M. E. Litvak (2004), the removal of the feelings of guilt is one of the main tasks of modern psychotherapy. Jan Bastiaans (1982) writes that sometimes the psychosomatic symptoms in psychosomatic patients disappear even when they get rid of the childish feelings of guilt toward the parents, which largely influenced the formation of their personality. The most important step in this direction is the patient's achievement of self-forgiveness, which contributes to the growth of self-esteem, increased coping abilities with stress and better management of emotions (Lyutova M., 2012), whereas the inability to forgive oneself is closely related to increased anxiety, depression, and neuroticism (Maltby J. et al., 2001).

The inability to forgive oneself significantly worsens both mental and physical health, according to the dissertation research of C. M. Avery (2008) of the University of Hartford. C. Simonton and co-authors (1978) note that the worst factor of all cancer patients is their inability to forgive themselves. Bernie Siegel (1989) holds the same opinion: "This is what our [cancer] patients need too— not our forgiveness but their own. If they forgive themselves, they won't need to seek diseases of mind and body."

It is no wonder that researchers from the University of East Tennessee found that forgiving yourself is the most important factor in health (Svalina S. S., Webb J. R., 2012). Self-forgiveness leads to a reduction in anxiety, anger, and depression, and helps to free one from psychic trauma, suicidal behavior, and alcohol dependence, as well as increasing positive emotions and satisfaction with life (Thompson L. Y. et al., 2005; Hirsch J. K. et al., 2012; Davis D. E. et al., 2015). Dr. Luule Viilma (2014) advises in this connection:

> Forgive yourself for failing to free up your problem earlier. Forgive so that you can feel that your soul has become easier and your head cleared. You will be convinced that not only your well-being has changed, but also your relationships with people. Forgiveness of yourself is the most important element of the process of forgiveness. He who has forgiven himself is able to forgive others.

The latter empirical conclusion is also supported by statistical data from the above-cited study by C. M. Avery (2008).

According to the classical study of J. H. Hall and F. D. Fincham (2005), self-forgiveness has the following characteristics:

- It is based on the recognition and acceptance of responsibility for a real misdemeanor or crime, which could be directed either against others or against oneself;
- Can be applied to shortcomings of character, and not just to specific actions;
- Causes love of and respect for oneself, despite one's own misconduct;
- Reduces or eliminates hatred or contempt for oneself;
- Includes recognition of one's own intrinsic value and its independence from one's misconduct;
- Contains a transition from self-estrangement to self-acceptance;
- Leads to a decrease in manifestations of "retribution on oneself," that are replaced by more benevolent behavior toward oneself;
- This process involves a conscious effort, undertaken with due intent;

- Unlike interpersonal forgiveness, which psychologically does not necessarily entail reconciliation with the offender, self-forgiveness necessarily includes reconciliation with oneself.

Thus, forgiveness of oneself can be considered as one of the effective methods of coping with stress (Worthington E. L., 2013), caused by an internal conflict in the form of feelings of guilt. Therefore, scientists recommend teaching the staff who are caring for patients with chronic and fatal diseases methods of achieving self-forgiveness (Gonyea J. G. et al., 2008).

Louise Hay (1984) admits that people who suffer from cancer are very self-critical. But, she was convinced from her own experience that an acquired ability to love and accept herself helped her cure her cancer.

In the study of patients with breast tumors, it was found that forgiving oneself favors coping with the situation of the disease and improves the quality of the patient's life (Romero C. et al., 2006). As a result of the group course for positive changes carried out by psychologists at Vanderbilt University in Tennessee, self-esteem increased in women with breast cancer, and they began to experience a personal transformation and improved quality of life (Carpenter J. S. et al., 1999). The psychospiritual program for cancer patients, "Restore: The Journey Toward Self-Forgiveness," developed in the department of psychology of the Luther College in Decorah, Iowa, leads to a significant increase in self-forgiveness, acceptance, self-improvement, a decrease in pessimism, and an increase in self-development (Toussaint L. et al., 2014). Closely associated with self-forgiveness is the experience of compassion for oneself, including benevolence, self-understanding, and the absence of self-condemnation. Patients with breast cancer who have more compassion for themselves are less distressed due to the crippling operation and the changed image of their body (Przezdziecki A. et al., 2013).

"Learning to forgive yourself is necessary to be able to heal the wounds of the soul," advises Dr. Mario Alonso Puig (2012) in the book *Reinventarse: Tu segunda oportunidad* (*Reinvent yourself: Your second chance*). In professional terms, self-forgiveness is necessary for liberation from an intrapsychic conflict, resulting in self-aggression and feelings of guilt and self-criticism, and the suppressed or repressed negative emotions associated with them.

Reid Henson, whom I mentioned earlier, as a result of the self-exploration process, came to the conclusion that his illness was caused not by his son's problems with drugs, but by his own reaction to these problems, his inability to cope with them, and his false beliefs. He decided to treat this past as a student's mistakes in the path of knowledge, who at every moment of his life acts in the best possible way, proceeding from the information and understandings available at that time. This approach opened the opportunity for him to change his attitudes toward himself and free himself from feelings of guilt—together with his illness (Simonton O., Henson R., 1992).

Another important aspect of the problem of guilt is obtaining forgiveness for the real harm and suffering caused to other people. Repentance and confession have long been known to people as a means of healing from the pangs of conscience and guilt associated with misconduct. Psychologists from the same Luther College conducted another study in which 1,500 elderly people first underwent initial psychological testing, and three years later 1,024 available people from this group were retested. An analysis of the data showed that in those participants who reported having received forgiveness from other people, the cancer morbidity during the three years between the two interviews was 50% less. The authors of the study associate the revealed effect of forgiveness with the reduction of stress, negative emotions, and favorable influence on the nervous, endocrine, and immune systems (Toussaint L. et al., 2010).

* * *

In the context of this topic of guilt, given the tendency of cancer patients to blame themselves for the occurrence of the disease ("I deserve it") (Bennett K. K. et al., 2005; Abrams R. D., Finesinger J. E., 1953), I strongly urge the reader who is a patient against gaining a distorted perception from this book. A superficial interpretation of the materials can lead to the conclusion that one is guilty in respect of the disease. Many of the studies analyzed here show that, in the future patient, a special personality structure and its limited way of coping with stresses and conflicts, predisposing to a decrease in the protective anti-malignant forces of the body, are laid down in childhood. This is not the fault of the patients or even of their parents, but of our society, which does not make proper efforts for psychological literacy or to provide comprehensive assistance to families with psychological problems. Improving the health of the nation cannot be achieved by progress via medical technologies only. The true basis of health is the study in school of how to be healthy, the psychology of emotions and relationships, and the number of hours that ought to be spent teaching these subjects!

12.1.2. Exo-Aggression (to the Outside World): Resentment and Unforgiveness

> Hatred and unforgiveness is like a cancer.
> It constantly eats away at you until it annihilates you.
> R. K. Hopkins,
> *Terrorists of the mind*

Resentment is the usual emotional reaction of a person to psycho-traumatic events of interpersonal conflict (insult, deception, betrayal, injustice, violence, etc.), leading to a state of frustration and aggression toward the offender. Resentment is resolved when a person feels satisfaction and relief in solving a conflict peacefully (having received an apology from or genuinely forgiving the offender) or by violent means (physical vengeance, prosecution). If the person does not find a resolution of the conflict, then feelings of frustration, anxiety and anger grow, often leading to melancholy and depression. Thus, initially the external conflict turns into an intrapersonal conflict (between the need to solve the problem and inability to do it), which is based on unforgiveness.

Like guilt, the feeling of resentment can arise and become fixed at an early age owing to disorders of attachment and experiencing violence. But the child, as a rule, is not able to adequately express his or her negative emotions toward his parents. As a consequence, the aggression of resentment is forced into the subconscious and manifests itself either in antisocial actions or in chronic psychophysical overstrain, from the effort to suppress this aggression and frustration (Pilyagina G. Y., 2003). So, in the child's "Shadow," there emerges an intrapersonal conflict between the experienced negative emotions and social attitudes and fear of rejection, which forbid children to manifest these emotions toward the parents.

Here is a vivid example of how the repressed emotions of resentment "work out." A teenage daughter of a client who has divorced a despotic, "suffocating" husband, was required by court order to meet with her father once a week. At these meetings the man still tried to "raise" his daughter, insisting on things she "has" to do and those she should not. The girl always tried to avoid the meetings, saying that she hated her father, and the mother had to work hard to persuade her to go. One evening after such a meeting, the girl had a strong burning pain in her nipples, which could be soothed only by applying ice. The next morning, a headache and strong vomiting began. Home remedies did not help, and the girl was eventually taken by ambulance to the hospital, where only intravenous injections managed to improve her condition.

The examination revealed only low blood pressure and high negative indicators of liver function tests. How could I not be reminded of the ancient Chinese treatise "The Yellow Emperor's Classic of Medicine," written around the fourth century BC, where it is claimed that anger affects the liver? (Vinogrodskiy B., 2014). Two days later, as the girl's condition improved significantly, she was discharged home. From the point of view of psychosomatic medicine, it was a typical somatization of affect, that is, the expression of repressed emotions through the body.

Scientists have established that it is the period around the age of ten that is critical for children who have experienced deep offence— their mental imbalance leaves a mark on their later life and can lead to avoidance strategies using alcohol and drugs (Muller R. T. et al., 2008). If such conflict happens within a family, it is often supplemented, as we saw in the previous chapter, by a sense of guilt when related emotions break out to the level of awareness. My psychotherapeutic practice shows that many patients have a feeling of profound resentment toward one or both parents, even if the relations are normalized at adulthood and the person forgets his childhood experiences (though it is more correct to say that they are suppressed into the subconscious).

For example, during a treatment session, the patient T. with cervical cancer first realized how much resentment accumulated in her childhood toward the emotionally cold father. During her trance, she saw herself as a little girl, playing alone on the floor, and her father, who always reads the newspaper on the couch. For the first time in her life she was able to approach him, pull the newspaper out of his hands and say, "Daddy, play with me." This act, albeit in the imagination, led to a significant release of the stacked and repressed anger, and allowed her to start communicating with her father, relations with whom had previously been purely formal.

Louise Hay (1984) from her experience came to the conclusion that cancer is a disease caused by a deep accumulated resentment, which literally "begins to eat the body." The adversity experienced in childhood undermines one's faith in life and can never be forgotten, so a person lives with a feeling of great self-pity and experiences endless disappointments. The resulting hopeless state of mind leads easily to blaming others for one's problems.

The last aspect—the accusation of others regarding one's own problems, resulting from resentment—as we have been discussing above, is closely related to the prevalence of the external locus of control, often observed in cancer patients (Ivashkina M., 1998) and has roots in entrenched infantile forms of response to life's difficulties. According to O. D. Rozhkova (2015), since many cancer patients do not have contact with themselves and do not realize their own feelings, most often at the beginning of therapy they act either in the position of "victim" or "complainer."

Also the mechanism of the appearance of the resentment depends on one's view of the world, something acquired during childhood. If through the demonstration of taking offense the child has learned to manipulate his parents in order to fulfill his desires, then in adulthood it will be natural for such a person to magnify expectations from other people, claiming that they are obliged to take care of him and express interest in his life. The inconsistency of these unjustified hopes with a real-life situation becomes the reason for the inclination to resentment. The same picture is also observed in masochistic personalities: as they largely live by the expectations of gratitude or responses to their selflessness from other people, the resentments are their eternal companion (Mlodik I. Y., 2014).

On the other hand, as we already know, if a person is accustomed in childhood to avoiding conflicts and direct collision, he or she may develop a negative self-image, including self-accusations and self-criticism. Then a protective projection mechanism often arises in the psyche, when the emotions of anger toward oneself are transferred to other people, and their behavior is perceived as offensive or unkind. This helps to avoid the awareness of these emotions in one's own psyche. Therefore, aggression toward others often grows out of aggression toward oneself, and resentment of others is accompanied by a feeling of guilt.

All the above also contributes to the development of hostility as a personality trait: a "negative cognitive scheme" of perception of other people, which forms the basis for anger, hatred, and violence (Beck A., 1999). Otto Kernberg (1999), one of the leading modern psychoanalysts, stresses that the tragedy of patients who experienced the effects of chronic aggression in early childhood is that they tend to constantly react to others with hatred. In turn, hostility, anger, and hatred create a high predisposition for a person to perceive the words and deeds of others as offenses and insults. Suppression of these aggressive emotions, as we have seen, creates a state of chronic stress.

Bernie Siegel (1998) assures us that anger is a normal emotion if it is expressed when it is felt. If one does not express it, it can develop into resentment or hatred, either one of which is able to bring about very destructive consequences. A similar observation was made by the physician and healer Luule Viilma (2014):

> Cancer is the result of the accumulation of the energy of ill-willed malice. ... The one in whom this malice resides is the one who falls ill with cancer, because he does not understand who is the real thief of his freedom. As a person enslaves himself with his thoughts, his anger against the restraint of his freedom imperceptibly turns into anger against himself, and the person then develops cancer.

From the point of view of classical psychology, the experience of "ill-willed malice" is close to the concept of rumination: obsessive negative thoughts, heavy memories, and an angry "mental chewing gum" in search of "who is to blame and what to do," all the way up to the construction of plans for revenge. Rumination, when experiencing an offense, escalates the state of physiological stress in the body through an increase in the allostatic load and cortisol levels, and chronic hyperactivity of the sympathetic nervous system (Thoresen C. E. et al., 2000; McCullough M. E. et al., 2007). To the same increase in cortisol and, accordingly, higher level of stress leads a constant emotional recall of past problems and psychic traumas, such as natural disasters, accidents, and sexual violence (Aardal-Eriksson E. et al., 2001; Delahanty D. et al., 2003; Elzinga B. M. et al., 2003). The indulgence of the rumination leads the person away from the possibility of resolving the resentment through forgiveness and eventually creates a high probability of depression (Barber L. et al., 2005; Ahadi B., Ariapooran S., 2009).

Therefore, scientists today consider the state of resentment and unforgiveness as one of the types of chronic stress (Orlov Y. M., 2005; Worthington E. L. et al., 2007), closely related to the suppression of anger (Berry J. W., Worthington E. L., 2001). This conclusion is based on the fact that, in a state of unforgiveness, the body is in the same physiological state as during stress: the brain and sympathetic nervous system demonstrates a similar specific activity, the electromyogram reflects increased tension in the facial musculature, arterial pressure and heart rhythm raises, biochemical blood indices (of plasma proteins, cholesterol, fatty acids, triglycerides) change in the same direction, decreases the activity of the immune system, the level of cortisol and epinephrine rises, and the ratio of pro-inflammatory cytokines changes (Pietrini P. et al., 2000; Witvliet C. W. et al., 2001; Seybold K. S. et al., 2001; Berry J., Worthington E. L., 2001; Worthington E. L. Jr. et al., 2005).

Unforgiveness brings general stress beyond the initial stress of conflict, as it increases the reactivity of the cardiovascular system during recalling and conversations about the incident and the psychic pain associated with it, and reduces the ability of the cardiovascular system to recover even when people try to focus on other topics (Worthington E. L. Jr. et al., 2007). It is not surprising that resentment is closely related to psychosomatic diseases, and one of the main characteristics of a psychosomatic personality is the feeling of "touchiness," that is, the propensity to take offence. As a result, it excessively raises the sense of dignity and self-centeredness, narrows the range of interests, and distorts the values, goals, and needs of a person (Rusina N., 2011).

More and more scientific data indicate that the state of prolonged resentment and unforgiveness has adverse health consequences (Harris A., Thoresen C., 2005; Seawell A. et al., 2014; Fincham, F., 2015). For example, according to A. Friedman's (1970) research, if a person experiences resentment with an above average intensity and perceives other people's attitude toward himself as unfair, but at the same time does not wish to or cannot openly express his emotions, his inner state becomes uncomfortable and unhealthy, and leads to depression.

Thus, we can consider the state of prolonged resentment-unforgiveness and the accompanying negative emotions as factors of chronic distress, creating an oncological sensibilization. This conclusion is confirmed by the observations of C. Simonton and co-authors (1978) that cancer patients often carry resentment in their soul, as well as other painful experiences that connect them with the past, and feel unable to find a way out: "People who carry such resentment continually re-create a painful event or events in their heads. This may even go on long after the offending person dies."

Russian psycho-oncologist Alexander Danilin (2011) claims that for cancer patients the experience of resentment is more global than just offense against friends, bosses, or parents. These resentments can merge into something much larger—an offense against destiny or God. It can be said about such a person that he or she "is resentful toward the whole world." This opinion is supported by the research of M. G. Ivashkina (2010) on patients with cancer of different localizations, for which characteristic features are defined by resentment and difficulties in forgiveness.

Anxiety, irritability, and excessive sensitivity to offenses, along with other personality disorders, are found in women who have had breast cancer (Moskvitina S. A., 2012). In this connection, the observation of Dr. Rudiger Dahlke (1997) is appropriate: "No matter how upset and angry a woman is at the offense or trauma inflicted on her, she does not get rid of these emotions, but rather is inclined to keep them in her breast, where they reincarnate and can lead to cancer." Sixty-five percent of patients with a mixed oncological pathology examined in dispensaries in the Ukrainian city of Odessa, and the region of the same name, admitted their vulnerability and sensitivity (Gurskaya T. B., Ivanova O. B., 2013).

Dr. Michael Barry (2010) participated in an extensive medical, theological, and sociological survey of patients in several Cancer Treatment Centers of America. He found that 61% of these patients had psychological problems associated with unforgiveness, and in half of these patients such problems were quite serious. In his book "The Forgiveness Project," Dr. Barry says that unforgiveness is like a spiritual carcinogen for the soul, "unforgiveness is equivalent to emotional suffocation, often resulting in a feeling that our lives are not worth living."

A study of seventy-five cancer patients conducted by clinical psychologists in St. Petersburg (Russia) showed the following: against a background of high anxiety, emotionally unfavorable reactions to stress and illness, difficulties in communication and in establishing close relationships, low self-confidence, inability to protect one's own interests, and dependence of self-esteem on other's assessments, there are also conflict areas related to resentment, disappointment, and inability to forgive others and oneself (Finagentova N. V., 2010). According to G. A. Tkachenko (2008), typical traits of women suffering from breast cancer are anxiety, emotional lability, insecurity, depression, and sensitivity to offenses and all kinds of injustice.

Colin Tipping (2000), the author of the bestselling book *Radical Forgiveness* and the psychological method of the same name, who cofounded the Georgia Cancer Help Program, discovered as a result of his practical work that almost all cancer patients, besides their life-long tendency of suppressing and repressing the emotions, are markedly unable to forgive. "I now believe," he says in the book, "that a lack of forgiveness contributes to, and may even be a principal cause of, most cancers."

In the above-cited study of women with ovarian, cervical, or uterine cancer performed in the city of Lugansk, it was also found that in addition to aggression, anxiety, and suspiciousness, on the "resentment" scale, 9.5% of patients show it as very high, 33.3% as high, and 33.3% at above average levels—76.1% of the overall group examined (Vereina L. V., Prokhorova L. V., 2012).

To protect themselves from potential "offenders," some of the future patients learn to express their aggression. According to data of Karl Goodkin with colleagues (1986) from the medical school of the University of Stanford, women with cervical cancer are distinguished by hostility, earthiness, social rudeness, projection of their feelings on others, as well as accusatory and punitive attitudes toward people. However, Tom Laughlin (1999) notes that the outwardly aggressive, controlling, and dominant personality that we observe in a certain number of the cancer patients is nothing more than a hypercompensation designed to hide a deep-seated inferiority complex called the "rejection complex."

Russian psycho-oncologist A. V. Gnezdilov (1996) found a prolonged sense of aggression in a number of oncological patients, expressed in their inability to forgive, in their animosity, and in their desire to get revenge. These feelings, in the patients' words, constantly "grind and destroy" them, becoming the basis of the psychological orientation that is "against life." The well-known Ukrainian psychotherapist and homeopath Valery Sinelnikov (2012) expresses the same solidarity with his colleagues. He says that

cancer is a long-lasting, hidden resentment, one of anger and malice, with a desire for revenge, which "eats" the body away. It is a deep, subconscious, spiritual wond that does not heal. This is a strong and far-reaching internal conflict with oneself and with the surrounding world.

Such unforgiveness can lead to the fact that patients, during terminal stages of cancer, experience significant emotional pain due to unresolved conflicts or psychic traumas of the past (Hansen M. J., 2002).

L. J. Phillips and J. W. Osborne (1989), who conducted group psychotherapy for cancer patients, noted that in order to free themselves from conflicts related to unforgiveness, patients had to fight with their own guilt, accusations, and vindictiveness, and re-learn how to have proper relationships with people. In the process of body-oriented therapy as the method of rehabilitating her cancer patients, I. V. Biryukova (2005) found unhealthy relations from an early age, emotionally unprocessed losses, suppressed anger, and covert resentment.

All the data presented indicate how important it is for a sick person to find a solution to the psychological conflict that engenders resentment and hatred, and to achieve a state of forgiveness and reconciliation in order to eliminate chronic stress. Actually, this is not a discovery—all religions and many philosophical schools have been telling us this from time immemorial. For example, "Forgive, and you will be forgiven" is one of the paramount ideas of Christianity (Luke 6.37) which largely determined the development of this religion.

Many stories of "miraculous" healing of cancer patients are associated with getting rid of resentments and forgiving offenders. Louise Hay (1984) admits in her life story, that the most difficult thing for her was to stop blaming others. Though there were solid reasons for this in her childhood, owing to people abusing her mentally, physically, and sexually, she nevertheless understood the need to get rid of these emotions: "I have found that forgiving and releasing resentment will dissolve even cancer. While this may sound simplistic, I have seen and experienced it working."

Brandon Bays (2012) (the story of her spontaneous healing will be addressed later) experienced a similar revelation in the process of deep trance immersion into her subconscious: "From the depths of the silence, I heard the words (or rather somehow experienced them)—'You need to forgive your parents.' It hit me like a stone. I knew it was the truth." Brandon was able to reach an authentic forgiveness that came from the very depths of her soul: "Tears streamed down my cheeks. Peace washed through my body, the peace of completion. A simple knowing arose from within, a knowing that THE STORY WAS OVER!"

In recent decades, the importance of forgiveness has also been recognized by academic science, now conducting serious research on the positive impact of forgiveness on health and well-being (Lawler-Row K. A. et al., 2008; Worthington E. L. et al., 2007). There are special psychological programs that help cancer patients get rid of old resentments and achieve forgiveness, which significantly improves their sense of self and quality of life (Phillips L. J., Osborne J. W., 1989; Hansen M. J., 2002).

The psychological and healing aspects of forgiveness will be described in more detail in my next book, which I devote to the practical application of the ideas developed here. At the same time, forgiveness is only the first step on the path of liberation from the suffering associated with a false personality. A Buddhist parable says:

- Teacher, how can I learn to forgive?

- What's the use in getting rid of the symptoms? Learn not to take offense!

But, in order to not to take offense, to get rid of the destructive influence of resentment and other negative emotions on the body, not only is psychotherapy necessary, but along with it a radical restructuring of one's consciousness, self-transcendence, and spiritual growth, as we shall see in the following chapters.

12.2. Negative Emotions and Their Avoidance: a Key Link

> People do not try to understand the need,
> but try to get rid of emotions.
> ... To get rid of a negative emotion,
> without understanding what it is about,
> is like throwing out the banana along with the peel!
> Dr. Vyacheslav Gusev,
> *Remedy for Diseases*

As previously noted, an unresolved psychic trauma or intrapersonal conflict, reflecting one's unmet need(s), manifests in negative emotions— initially anxiety and fear, and their aggressive or self-aggressive development—in the form of anger, guilt, and/or resentment. Despite these feelings being experienced by virtually all people, why do negative feelings contribute to cancer in some of them? In general, the answer is already known: these kinds of people forbid themselves to experience or to express negative emotions, suppressing or repressing them. This behavior, in turn, is determined by the type and activity of psychological defenses acquired by a person in childhood and is dependent on how secure or insecure was one's attachment to parents or caregivers. According to A. N. Schore (2001) of the School of Medicine at the University of California, strong unresolved emotions combined with a lack of ability to regulate them arise from the adverse events of childhood. If, as a result, primitive unproductive defenses such as suppression, denial, regression, etc. are fixed, then this largely determines the formation of the personality in the direction of psychosomatic types "D" or "C." It is the avoidance of emotions, according to scientists, that can lead to the development of distress that, influencing the endocrine and immune systems, can contribute to development of cancer (Greer S. et al., 1990; Nakaya N. et al., 2005).

12.2.1. Defensive Mechanisms of the Psyche

In general, psychological defense is an adaptive mental process directed against negative emotional overload. Psychological defense serves to save personal integrality and to have a more appropriate interaction with the outside world—this is how they begin to form in the unfavorable conditions of childhood. But as we grow older, the defensive strategy of avoiding negative emotions becomes habitual, rigid, maladaptive; the chronic conflict that creates these emotions is not resolved but also avoided, as well as unrealized drives, desires, and needs tied to it. Such defense, temporarily allowing a person to perceive his actual misfortune in an illusory "positive" way, becomes less effective as the negative experience of its use increases, together with a critical attitude of others and failures in the process of socialization.

In order to cope with anxiety, fear, and anger produced by internal conflict, a person needs a mechanism that serves either to contain these emotions or to express/satisfy conflicting needs in another, indirect way. Repression and suppression of negative emotions are, in fact, mechanisms for protecting the human psyche from the threat of stressors. This makes it possible to reduce the significance of the negative event and its psychotraumatic impact, change attitudes toward it, reduce internal discomfort and anxiety, and maintain a positive image of oneself. According to L. R. Grebennikov (1994), suppression as a mechanism of psychological defense hides the emotion of fear, which is unacceptable for positive self-perception.

However, the transfer of unresolved conflicts from the consciousness area to the "Shadow" is ineffective: as a result, the person does not get out of chronic distress. Existing in a state of "incubation," a conflict, or psychic trauma, generates negative emotions and ripens like an abscess, sooner or later leading to exceeding the threshold of stress tolerance and destroying the barrier of mental adaptation, while at the biological level producing a depletion of the protective organism's resources (in particular, the failure of anticancer resistance systems).

The barrier of mental adaptation is one of the main mechanisms of the general adaptation syndrome, which serves one's adaptation to the action of adverse factors in the external environment. It is unique in every person, formed as a result of the interaction of social and biological factors, and provides a person with the opportunity to choose an adequate and purposeful response to traumatic situations (Aleksandrovskiy Y. A., 1976). The barrier of mental adaptation has dynamics, its magnitude is constantly decreasing and again increases in response to stressful influences in the external environment. These changes can reach different degrees of intensity (Molichuk I. G., 2007):

- First level. A person experiences moderate periodic stressful impacts, whose influences are not absolutely negative. Under these moderate loads, the limits of mental adaptation expand. Such effects, in my opinion, create a physiological stage of alarm in the body, as described by Hans Selye (1975).

- Second level. With acute and especially prolonged stress, the barrier of mental adaptation approaches its critical value and is overstrained. Pre-neurotic conditions arise: anxiety, agitation, increased sensitivity to standard irritants, insomnia, manifestations of inhibition, or fussiness in behavior. These distortions are temporary, and the socially appropriate personality remains. This state corresponds to the second stage of the physiological stress reaction—the stage of resistance.

- Third level. In the chronic course of stress, the reserve capabilities of the psyche are exhausted, and the barrier of a person's mental adaptation is destroyed. Psychic activity no longer adapts to the environment, so the boundaries of adequate and purposeful human behavior are narrowing. Neurotic disorders develop. At the physiological level, this can lead to the last stage of general adaptation syndrome: the stage of exhaustion, when the protective processes of the body are inhibited and pathological changes appear.

Consequently, the most important task of psychosomatic medicine in general and psycho-oncology in particular is to determine the state of the barrier of a patient's mental adaptation and his ineffective primary defenses in order to develop the right strategy of psychotherapeutic assistance.

We already know about the existence of two types of primary defense against negative feelings: their repression (conscious) and suppression (unconscious). In Chapter 3.2 we were convinced that avoidance of emotions can be very dangerous for health in general. We also learned that this mental trait is an important sign in cancer patients. It's time to sort out the following: does the avoidance of negative emotions have a primary or secondary role? Can they act on the body so destructively that this eventually leads to cancer, or is it just a character trait that accompanies ill health?

12.2.2. Negative Emotions and Cancer

Dr. Bradley Nelson (2014), a respected American specialist in alternative medicine, shares his experience:

> While there are a variety of things that are thought to cause cancer, I firmly believe that trapped emotions are a contributing factor to the disease process, as I believe they are to many, if not most other, diseases. Every cancer patient I treated was found to have trapped emotions embedded in the malignant tissues. ... trapped emotions are, in my opinion, an underlying cause of cancer. It is vital that these trapped emotions be removed. Even though they may have already contributed to the cancer, once removed, they cannot cause any further damage in the years to come.

A significant amount of research supports this view. In 1982, T. Cox and C. Mackay of the University of Nottingham (UK), exploring the studies conducted at the time, came to the conclusion that the main psychosocial factor in cancer is the person's inability to express emotions, especially anger. The same conclusion was reached by English researchers S. Greer and M. Watson (as a result, in 1985 they developed a psychobiological model for the onset and development of cancer), as well as by German and Italian specialists in the field of psychosomatics (Baltrusch H. J., Santagostino P., 1989).

Dr. Lydia Temoshok (1985), studying patients with melanoma, found that those who could openly express their sadness and anger during the interview (which was recorded on video) had a better protective function of immunity compared to those who could not show their emotions; in addition, the people in the "non-emotional" group had a higher degree of cellular division, and, respectively, their tumors grew faster. A higher level of stress in patients experienced as anxiety, unhappiness, and/or *dysphoric* emotions (including envy and hatred toward healthy people, and outbursts of anger with a tendency to blame others for their illness), also corresponded to a more active growth of malignant melanoma. Suppressed anger and depressiveness in men with prostate cancer also reflected in a decrease in the activity of protective immune cells, while optimism and the expression of feelings improved immunity (Penedo F. J. et al., 2006). Researchers at the Royal School of Medicine and Dentistry in London, examining the immunity of patients with breast tumors (both malignant and benign), found that the level of immunoglobulin A (an indicator of chronic inflammation) was elevated in women who suppressed their anger (Pettingale K. et al., 1977).

In Beijing, a large-scale study was conducted on the relationship between psychosocial factors and the development of lung cancer. From 1990 to 1993, scientists examined about 750,000 people, among whom were detected 309 cases of cancer in the preclinical stage. Three statistically significant factors in them were established: emotional outbursts and overall problems with emotional regulation; poor working conditions, including relations with colleagues (*which implies a constant emotional tension—V. M.*); and a prolonged state of depression (Fan R. L. et al., 1997). In a US veterans' hospital, while a group of about three thousand people were observed for 55.6 months on average, seventy-five people with cancer of different locations were identified. A comparison of their psychological characteristics with those who did not develop cancer revealed in the former a much stronger feature of suppressing emotions (Dattore P. J. et al., 1980).

Another study, conducted over a period of seventeen years in the United States, found that women restraining their anger at men had an increased mortality from various diseases, including cancer. At the same time, men are at an increased risk of cancer when they suppress their aggression toward an authority figure (Harburg E. et al., 2003). The ability to express emotions of anger, anxiety, and depression, according to studies in Netherlands conducted by M. A. Tuinman (2008), is significantly lower in men with testicular cancer. Holding back emotions is defined by Russian scientists as the basis of ineffective behavior strategies in the study of patients with tumors of various localizations. It was manifested in their emotional immaturity, unconstructive style of emotional expression, lack of resources for coping with stress, and conflicting self-attitude (Rusina N., 2012).

The most important information about the role of emotions is provided by prospective studies in which the psychological characteristics of people are determined before the diagnosis is established. This sort of study was conducted in the USA on 729 people from 1996 to 2008. It showed that people deceased during this time from lung, pancreas, and rectum cancer, and leukemia had a higher level of emotional suppression at the time of the initial survey in 1996. The authors concluded that this character trait increases the risk of death from cancer by 70% (Chapman B. P. et al., 2013).

In Yugoslavia in 1965, 1,353 people were psychologically surveyed, with such personal characteristics defined as avoidance of manifestations of feelings and needs; also psychological stress in the form of continuing depression, anger, irritation, hopelessness; rationalized repression of emotions, and other features. Subsequent follow-up of these people over a period of ten years revealed a consistent relationship of emotional imbalance with the occurrence of cancer and other diseases, that could be predicted on the basis of questionnaires with 95% accuracy (Grossarth-Maticek R., 1980).

Owing to their greater innate emotionality, women usually more clearly manifest the connection between avoiding emotions and cancer. I have already mentioned the research of the oncologist Max Cutler (1954), who discovered an inability in patients with breast tumors to discharge or adequately control their anger, aggressiveness, or hostility. At the University of Freiburg, a preliminary psychological examination was conducted of fifty-six women who came to the hospital for a biopsy of the breast in order to diagnose the nature of the tumor. In thirty-eight cases, the tumor turned out to be benign, and in eighteen it was malignant—in the latter group, the inhibition of emotion was significantly higher (Wirsching M. et al., 1985). Parallel results were obtained in similarly organized studies in Italy (Todarello O. et al., 1989) and Japan (Iwamitsu Y. et al., 2005).

Scientists from the University of Manchester (UK) found that women who are closed off in their world, suppressing emotions and preferring to "turn away" from problems, have a much higher risk of developing breast cancer than women living an intensive and stressful life, but are nevertheless capable of openly expressing their feelings (Cooper C. L., Faragher E. B., 1993). Closed women, after learning about their diagnosis, develop a state of high anxiety, confusion, and depression, in comparison with emotionally open women (Edelman S., Kidman A. D., 1997), which undoubtedly complicates the process of their treatment.

It is obvious from the data presented in the previous chapters, that the most important of the suppressed or repressed emotions is anger—this is characteristic of people with various cancers and in particular of breast cancer (Cutler M., 1954; Cox T., Mackay C., 1982; Temoshok L., 1987; Temoshok L., Dreher H., 1993; Baltrusch H. et al., 1991; Cardenal V. et al., 2012; Van der Ploeg H. M. et al., 1989; Kune G. A. et al., 1991; Thomas S. P. et al., 2000; Brodie D., 2015). Another example: in the center for cancer research at King's College Hospital in London, a study was held of the psychological characteristics of 160 women with breast tumors. The main difference found between 69 patients with a malignant tumor and 91 patients with a benign tumor was excessive suppression of anger by the first group. In the same group, in women past the age of forty, there was also a significant suppression of other emotions (Greer S., Morris T., 1975).

On the other hand, scientists have found that patients with breast cancer who are able to freely express their anger, depression, guilt, and fear live substantially longer than those who show little of such emotions (Derogatis L. R. et al., 1979). The authors of one of the studies cited above, H. Van Der Ploeg with colleagues from the University of Leiden in the Netherlands, state (1989):

> The non-expression of emotions [in cancer], suppression or control appears to be a core concept. Our results suggest that the control of anger may be an essential part of it. And that it is the control or suppression of anger rather than the absence of anger which is important.

It is significant that the same conclusion was reached by scientists who studied the features of the emotional regulation of healthy students with an avoiding attachment style: emotional distress does not affect physical health by itself but it does so in the case of the simultaneous presence of a high degree of emotional control, expressed in the suppression of negative emotions (Kotler T. et al., 1994).

These conclusions were also confirmed by another study conducted at the University of Naples, where the emotional characteristics of cancer patients and patients with hepatitis (inflammatory liver disease) were compared. The basic level of anger (anger as a character trait), the predisposition to expression of anger, and the frequency of its experience (as a temporary state) were statistically higher in patients with hepatitis than in cancer patients (again, matching the ancient Chinese treatise on the effect of anger on the liver!). However, the ability to express and display their anger is also statistically higher in patients with hepatitis than in cancer patients, who controlled the expression of their anger significantly more tightly (Cotrufo P., Galiani R., 2014). Patients with hepatitis are able to show their anger outwardly, and this, in my opinion, saves them from the progression of the inflammatory pathology of the liver toward malignant transformation.

Summarizing this topic, I would like to cite the long-term practical observations of the Dr. Douglas Brodie, who considers hidden, long-suppressed toxic emotions, such as anger, indignation, and/or hostility, as the main characteristics of cancer patients. As a rule, individuals predisposed to cancer internalize such emotions (*that is, make them part of their character—V. M.*) and express them outside with great difficulty (Brodie D., 2015). However, this does not mean that these emotions are weakened by suppression or repression. On the contrary, as Lawrence LeShan (1977) discovered, having studied more than 500 oncological patients, their "clogged" emotional energy was stronger than in people in the control group, and not only due to "accumulation," but also because it was stronger initially.

In addition to inefficient coping with the emotion of anger, the second cause of oncogenic distress, as I have already mentioned, is the suppressed or repressed emotions of anxiety and fear (Ando N. et al., 2009; Lutgendorf S. K. et al., 2008; Averyanova S. V., 2012; Haug T. T. et al., 2004; Pereira D. B. et al., 2010). However, this factor in psycho-oncology is studied in less detail. In general, the above-mentioned disorders of children's attachment as factors of predisposition to cancer make it possible to link suppression and repression of anger with a hypercognitive variant of CEID (with the avoiding-attachment type in the base), and suppression and repression of anxiety and fear with a regressive-emotional version of CEID (with anxious-ambivalent attachment in the base). Understanding the differences in the type of attachment of cancer patients is extremely important for practical psycho-oncologists, since it allows us to choose the right strategy of psychotherapy, directed, in addition to eliminating the consequences of childhood psychic traumas, toward developing the awareness and expression of appropriate emotions and coping with stressful situations.

It should be noted that in this area of psychological research some authors have not found a relationship between the suppression of emotions and the development of cancer, in particular breast cancer (Bleiker E. M. et al., 1997; Ragland D. R. et al., 1992; Scherg H. et al., 1981). Reasons for such disagreements, mainly related to differences in the methodology of surveys, have already been discussed in Chapter 9 and at the beginning of the current part. In addition, the propensity of the individual to suppress emotions and to avoid their manifestations leads to the fact that even in psychological studies, such as anonymous questionnaires, people follow this trend, which complicate an objective evaluation of the results (Garssen B., 2007).

As Lydia Temoshok (1987) writes, individuals with "C" type behavior never say directly in self-filled questionnaires that their interaction with other people is ambiguous (contradictory) or features avoiding. This reflects the effect of the factor that the scientist called "denial." Even if according to the interview the level of stress in a patient does not differ from that in healthy people, but in parallel a more pronounced suppression of emotions is determined, this may indicate a de facto high level of distress, which is also suppressed. This tendency to avoid emotions can affect both the ability of a cancer patient to seek help under the occurrence of somatic symptoms and, in general, the quality of his or her life (Koller M. et al., 1999).

We have every reason to believe that suppressed and repressed negative emotions become an important mechanism for the formation of chronic distress, oncogenic sensibilization, and the subsequent development of cancer. The reason lies in the fact that modern people in the process of education learn to control only external manifestations of emotions, but not their bodily, vegetative component. Meanwhile, L. P. Velikanova and Y. S. Shevchenko (2005) emphasize that emotional states are subject to fixed cause-effect relationships and occur within the framework of strict neuro-dynamic relationships. As a result of the suppression of emotions, there is a persistent increase in the strain of the internal organs involved, followed by the formation of somatic (psychosomatic) pathology. This clearly indicates the social, civilizational nature of diseases that arise more often when human behavior is at odds with the natural emotional-vegetative context of responding to sources of stress.

Therefore, it is once again evident that it is not the stress itself that is important, but how a person reacts to it. Even if the level of stress in the life of an individual is high, but the emotions associated with it are recognized and expressed correctly, not suppressed or repressed, then the likelihood of cancer is significantly less.

The well-known American healer Tom Kenyon (2013) says:

> Cancer occurs when cells begin multiplying out of control. Unchecked, they can eventually kill off healthy cells and eventually even kill their host. Emotional cancers operate in a very similar way. An unrecognized emotional pattern begins proliferating. ... I believe that toxic emotions do, in fact, transform into disease.

12.2.3. Other Types of Ineffective Psychological Defenses

Cancer patients often use other types of primary psychological defense, for example rationalization. In this case, the person realizes and uses only that part of the perceived information which makes his behavior appear well-controlled and does not contradict the objective situation. At the same time, the information unacceptable to consciousness is removed or transformed and can then be realized in a modified form. This often happens in situations of frustration, when rationalization blocks the actual need, but allows one to retain self-esteem, find an acceptable reason for getting out of an unpleasant situation, allowing to "save face," but does not change anything within one. Under such conditions, withdrawal into the disease will release a person from the responsibility of solving problems, and rationalization is used to justify his insolvency by using the illness (Nabiullina R. R., Tukhtarova I. V., 2003).

In this way, another ineffective defensive mechanism is added to rationalization: somatization, which I have already described above. Progressing, the psycho-emotional stress transforms first into psycho-vegetative imbalance, then into somatoform disorders, and, eventually, into psychosomatic diseases. A similar mechanism has been shown to be inherent in patients with tumors of different locations: a combination of the predominance of overcontrol and emotional lability, a passive attitude toward conflicts, and escape from solving problems is often accompanied by "withdrawal to illness" (Rusina N. A., 2012). For example, with the emergence of "deadlock" family situations due to the inability to resolve deep conflicts, the threat of family disintegration can lead to carcinogenic somatization, which automatically pushes former problems into the background, and allows the family status to be maintained (Bahnson C. B., 1969).

In another study, the rates of rationalization as a way of avoiding emotions were significantly higher in patients with malignant than in those with benign tumors (Wirsching M. et al., 1985). When psychologically examining women before the diagnosis of breast pathology, it was established that those who appeared to have a malignant tumor manifested significantly higher levels of rationalization, emotional closeness, and emotional control than women without oncological pathology. These character traits remained practically unchanged after a second examination in a year and a half after treatment (Bleiker E. M. et al., 1995), which, in my opinion, creates the risk of recurrence of the disease.

The psychological study of 157 men with cancer of different locations (except skin) revealed a higher level of rationalization and emotional defense than was found in men without cancer (Swan G. E. et al., 1991). In the above-cited study conducted in the 1970s in Yugoslavia, British scientists found that a high level of rationality and anti-emotionality increases the risk of cancer by forty (!) times (Grossarth-Maticek R. et al., 1985). Psychologists of the Yaroslavl State Medical

Academy (Russia) defined intellectualization (a kind of rationalization) as the main method of psychological defense in patients with tumors of different localization—in the intestine, reproductive organs, mammary gland, larynx, and throat (Rusina N. A., 2012). In the same country, high rates of rationalization and emotional suppression were also found in the study of defense types in oncohematological patients (Korotneva E. V., Varshavskiy A. V., 2007; Shmakova T. V. et al., 2009).

Denial (negation) is another type of psychological defense, seen by some scholars as a specific form of suppression of emotions. It is expressed in the desire to reject and not to accept information that is incompatible with the existing positive ideas one holds about oneself. Changing in this way one's perception of the world around, one reduces anxiety by simply ignoring the disturbing factors. This type of defense can do a disservice in the beginning period of the disease: a person avoids recognizing the importance of disturbing bodily symptoms from the position "nothing terrible, it will pass by itself." And even when the disease has already developed and been diagnosed, such erroneous protection can induce a person to deny its seriousness.

S. Greer and colleagues (1979) describe the mechanism of denial in patients with breast cancer as a "clearly active rejection of any evidence of their diagnosis": despite the operation for removing the mammary gland, some women retain the position that "it was not serious, they just removed my breast as a precautionary measure." This "defense" predicts an increased risk of recurrence and death between ten and fifteen years after surgery (Pettingale K., 1984; Pettingale K. et al., 1985).

Researchers from the Faculty of Psychology of St. Petersburg University (Russia) identified a significant correlation between the psychological characteristics of "avoidance and denial" and the bodily state of patients with chronic leukemia (Stepanchuk E. et al., 2013). Polish scientists revealed a marked denial and suppression of emotions in cancer patients, along with restlessness, emotional stress, and low self-esteem (Losiak W., 1989).

Psychologists of another Russian city, Irkutsk, studying cancer patients, found that the most highly expressed type of defense was denial—35%, 24%—suppression of emotions, and 18%—rationalization and substitution. The latter type is used to relieve inner tension by transferring and redirecting the anger and aggression to a weaker "available" subject or object, or to oneself (Kukina M., 2009). Avoidance strategy is often used by women with ovarian cancer and to a lesser extent those with breast cancer, probably on account of their fears and negative expectations regarding the illness. In particular, a number of patients who knew about the diagnosis did not want to listen to the information about their actual condition, recognizing that they deliberately avoid talking about their illness whenever possible (Sirota N. A. et al., 2014).

Denial and suppression are also prevalent in the psychological defense of thyroid cancer patients (Dubskiy S. V. et al., 2008) and those with blood cancer, along with such types of defense as a replacement of emotions with distracting thoughts or actions, and projection—attributing to others their own unacceptable desires as rational basis for their rejection and condemnation, against self-acceptance in a positive way. Also, there are hypercompensation (prevention of the expression of unpleasant or unacceptable thoughts, feelings, or actions by an exaggerated development of opposing aspirations) and regression (return to earlier, immature, simple, and accessible reactions manifested through helplessness, dependence, and childish behavior to reduce anxiety and escape from the actual situation). Regression underlies the previously discussed infantilism (Korotneva E. V., Varshavskiy A. V. (2007); Shmakova T. V. et al., 2009).

Resignation is another passive and ineffective type of psychological defense of cancer patients, which probably also results from childish behavior. A person stops actively fighting for his life, believing that he cannot change anything in this situation (Cardenal V. et al., 2012). Resignation is fraught with the transition to the most dangerous psychological state for cancer patients—helplessness and hopelessness, which, as we shall understand later, is the actual capitulation before possible death.

We are not born with ready-made psychological defense mechanisms that might parallel biological ones such as the immune system or the DNA repair system. In the process of growing up and raising, under social influences, defensive mechanisms arise, change, and reconstruct. The inefficient psychological defense, first of all, leads to disorders of childhood attachment. In fact, the latter can be considered as a form of protecting the child from the suffering experienced, as a pathological adaptation to the traumatic conditions of life. Studies conducted at Duke University in Durham, NC (USA) have shown that psychological and physical abuse of children, leading to their emotional incompetence, develops into chronic restriction of emotions in adulthood, that manifests, among other things, in an avoidance reaction to stress. However, this avoidance is not an effective strategy, since in adults who restrain emotions the overall level of distress is much higher and is accompanied by symptoms of depression and anxiety (Krause E. D. et al., 2003). This is how one of the most important factors of predisposition to cancer arises.

If cancer has already developed, the dominant ineffective psychological defense hinders the healing process. According to Dr. Bruno Klopfer (1957), a patient spends so much vital energy to protect his insecure ego (*I would refer this definition to a false personality—V. M.*) that the body simply does not have sufficient energy to fight the disease.

Let us summarize the material of this chapter. Most of the types of psychological defense considered here are concentrated around two main ones:

suppression or repression of negative emotions, with the avoiding type of attachment disorder as the basis. It is in this attachment type, according to the data presented, that the tendency to omit and suppress a negative experience is mostly inherent, which contributes to the development of alexithymia, the hypercognitive variant of CEID and rationalization as its basis. As a result, this kind of person has decreased emotional intelligence and adaptive potential, and his or her ability to resolve life's problems effectively and successfully is lost, while the incidence of mental and psychosomatic diseases increases.

The main conflict of the alexithymic personality, according to G. N. Pilipenko and colleagues (2009), is to constrain strong hostile impulses arising from the subconscious because of fear of manifesting them externally in the form of hostility or aggressive actions. This conflict leads to emotional rigidity and an inability to express feelings of anger, generates self-restraint, static anxiety, and difficulties in communicating even with people close to the individual. As a result, the inner conflict is projected onto the somatic sphere.

German psychoanalyst Peter Kutter (2008) argues that psychosomatic disorder is the result of unsatisfactory functioning of psychological defenses. As Anna Freud (1937) noted, continuing the work of her father, in the process of personal development, the protective mechanisms that serve to prevent danger can turn into that very danger. This is what we see in a psychosomatic personality, emerging as a type "C": the basis of its behavior is a defective and dangerous defense system—meeting the needs of others excessively against a background of lack of satisfaction of one's own deep needs, with corresponding suppression of the associated negative emotions and inability to adequately cope with stress (Kneier A. W., Temoshok L., 1984).

One of its greatest dangers is the late request for medical care from people with a high level of alexithymia, as shown by Max Cutler (1954) in the example of patients with breast cancer. The authors of a contemporary study who confirmed this tendency believe that women who do not differentiate their emotions and do not know how to express and process them, as a result either do not feel their body and do not attach significance to the changes happening in it, or their suppression of frustration and anxiety is so strong that it leads to an excessively high level of stress. Inability to cope with it does not allow such women to recognize the problem and to start dealing with it (Kuper E. R., Korneva T. V., 2013).

These people simply do not know how to handle their emotions: they were brought up this way, and this behavior is built into their psyche because of childhood adversities. They need hard work to turn an erroneous defense mechanism into an effective system of coping with stress, or, as psychologists say, into a coping strategy, which is understood as acquired forms of behavior in the process of one's adaptation to a stressful situation. A primary psychological defense is a passive and largely unconscious mechanism, while coping strategies are active and conscious, although they can be both effective and ineffective. This is a defense of a higher level, and therefore we can regulate it. Examples of coping strategies are confrontation, acceptance of responsibility, search for social support, systematic solution of the problem, self-control, positive reassessment, and distancing.

Richard Lazarus (1966), one of the leading researchers of the stress problem, sees coping as a central issue of the stress problem, as an important stabilizing factor that can help a person to sustain psychosocial adaptation during the period of stress. Unfortunately, cancer patients are characterized by a limited repertoire of coping-with-stress behavior. This hampers their psychological adaptation to the situation of the disease that threatens life (Finagentova N. V., 2010).

Lydia Temoshok (1993), like other scientists, argues that the problem is not the stress of life but how we cope with the stressful circumstances; this is what determines the state of our health. Behavior of the "C" type is an erroneous variant of coping which many people use to appease others, to deny their own true feelings and to meet social standards. Temoshok's studies of patients with melanoma brought her to convincing evidence that our physical health is threatened if we chronically suppress our needs and feelings in order to adapt to other people. She found confirmation that this coping style weakens the immune defenses and leaves one more vulnerable to cancer.

As we shall see later, effective coping is also an important aspect of successful therapy and rehabilitation of cancer patients, and significantly affects their survival and the likelihood of recurrence of the disease.

12.3. Do Emotions Determine the "Choice" by the Cancer of the Target Organ?

Since the primary psychological defense is ineffective in coping with negative emotions, ultimately the psychophysiological strain created by the latter must find some exit channel, a zone of "discharge" in the body. Gradually, this place becomes a "weak spot," where the pathological changes (usually inflammatory) first appear, and then the tumor can develop. What determines the specific localization of this process?

The most developed theory of tumor localization (although not proven by conventional medicine), was suggested by Dr. R. G. Hamer (2000), according to which every type of psychological conflict is associated with a specific organ involved in this conflict. In the aspect of linking emotional stress to specific organs, Dr. Hamer is not a pioneer; as we saw in the previous chapter, it was already observed and recorded by ancient Chinese healers. Soviet doctors also observed the connection between the predominance of certain emotions and the predisposition to diseases of specific organs. Professor M. I. Astvatsaturov wrote in 1935 that the heart more often suffers from fear, the liver from anger and fury, and stomach from apathy and a depressed state. The reason for this is that stress through emotional, nervous, and hormonal mechanisms activates many organs and systems that execute "fight-or-flight" reactions. When there is a chronic overload in these organs, they show clinical signs of a distress process. Such "final destinations" for stress are most often the cardiovascular system, the gastrointestinal tract, the skin, and the respiratory and reproductive system, as well as other organs.

Strictly speaking, it was these facts that formed the basis of Walter Cannon's (1916) concept of adaptive reactions, developed back at the beginning of the twentieth century and serving as the basis for Hans Selye's theory of stress. With the long-term emotional readiness of a person to meet danger and the absence of actions associated with it, the functional activity of the relevant organs is constantly increasing, leading to an imbalance. For instance, increase in arterial pressure changes precapillary arteries and ends with hypertension; constant anxiety leads to overstrain and rigidity of skeletal muscles; the chronically excessive release of gastric juice contributes to the development of the ulcerative process, and the chronically suppressed "outburst of anger," as we see here, can lead to cancer.

Although, with the help of the mind and the associated cerebral cortex, a person can suppress external, arbitrary-behavioral manifestations of emotions, he or she is unable to regulate the peripheral components of the body's functional system that correspond to these emotions. Because of this, as modern research confirms, there is a persistent increase in the tone of the internal organs involved, leading to psychosomatic pathology. In this way, negative experiences find their somatic "end" (Garbuzov V. I., 1999). This "end," as a rule, is the most important for the vital activity organ (from the point of view of a given person and his specific situation), which, consequently, becomes the most vulnerable. Also, the place where emotional overstrain is ultimately reflected depends on the characteristics of a particular emotion, the specific nature of the person's nervous constitution, and the history of his life (Malkina-Pykh I., 2013).

According to psychoanalysis, somatic manifestations reflect that which is unacceptable in the opinion of the ego, and therefore express suppressed or repressed desires and emotions. The following position was further developed by practitioners of psychosomatics: an attack of bronchial asthma may show a blocked crying or an appeal for maternal care; digestive disorders—the inability to "digest life's circumstances," and peptic ulcer disease—self-blame due to a person's feelings of guilt and self-punishment, a kind of "digestion of oneself" (Sandomirskiy M. E., 2005).

This opinion is shared by the authors of some popular systems of healing and alternative medicine, such as Louise Hay in the USA (1984), Rudiger Dahlke in Germany (1997), and Valery Sinelnikov in Ukraine (2012). Based on their experience, they came to the conclusion that depending on the "grade" of the emotion experienced, diseases of a certain type can emerge. For example, when a person looks to the future with anxiety, he begins to develop short-sightedness, or diseases of the legs, which literally carry him through life—they also get sick because a person does not realize that he is "walking on the wrong road" or does not want to move on. Problems with the spine may arise when we take on an excessive responsibility or some big business, to which we refer as "I do not want to, but I have to." The heart gives up when there is a lack of emotional warmth and joy in life.

Alfred Adler (1907), a well-known Austrian psychologist and psychiatrist, creator of the system of individual psychology, investigated the mechanisms by which neurosis affects certain target organs. He put forward the theory that the subjectively experienced "inferiority" of the personality, formed in childhood due to the experience of helplessness and insecurity that underlying the neuroses, is reflected in the "inferiority" of the organ, making it excessively vulnerable to the development of psychosomatic disorders.

Drs Claus and Marjorie Bahnson (1964), considering the problem of tumor localization, believe that emotions can lead to changes in the functions of organs and systems depending on the symbolic meaning that the given organ or system carries (consciously or unconsciously) in the formation and discharge of specific emotional potentials. For example, anger can activate certain actions associated with it, involving the relevant body parts and organ systems in such a way that they become symbolically more excited than others, even in conditions where explicit physical action is not required or impossible.

A similar symbolism in the connection of mental factors with the localization of somatic disorders was seen by G. L. Engel and A. H. Schmale (1967). Giving as an example skin diseases (in particular eczema), the authors consider it as a violation of one's interaction with other people, which originates from maternal contact issues in the first year of life. A prominent Soviet physiologist and academician, K. M. Bykov (1960), a student of Ivan Pavlov, with his co-worker I. T. Kurtsin studied the effects of the cerebral cortex on internal organs. They also came to the conclusion that a disease arises in the consciousness as a disorder of one's relationship with the world, and according to the law of similarity has its symbolic expression in the body in the form of biochemical, functional, and organic changes. The founder of ontopsychology Antonio Meneghetti (2011), analyzing the causes of a tumor in one organ or another, specifies: "Here we are in the field of the patient's free associations, i.e. what the patient is thinking. That organ is chosen because of its symbolical proximity—according to the patient's idea —to the real thing in itself' (*i.e. related to the ongoing conflict—V. M.*).

Let us recall in this connection the information discussed in Chapter 3.1 on how our mind, when creating images (while symbols is what triggers the process of constructing images), activates physiological responses. It is quite plausible the following sequence of events in the type "C" personality: under an unresolved psychic trauma or conflict, anything that symbolically reminds a person of this problem will trigger a physiological reaction of excitation, fear, or anger that the associated psychological defense will habitually repress or suppress, often without even emerging to the level of awareness. This is what can nourish and maintain an active state of chronic stress in general and over-excitement in a specific organ in particular. And the higher the subjective significance of an unresolved conflict, the more intense it is emotionally, the higher the likelihood of somatic disorders in this organ.

Stanislav Grof and Joan Halifax (1978) often noted that the area primarily affected by cancer was the object of increased attention by the patient for many years before the development of the tumor. Sometimes, this organ manifested a variety of psychosomatic symptoms beginning in childhood or even early infancy. Researchers identified the existence of important psychotraumatic circumstances associated with such areas of the body in a significant number of patients. Some of them explained that the place where the malignant tumor developed was always the weakest and most vulnerable area in the body that specifically reacted to various emotional stress in their lives. For example, it was often found that in women the onset of cancer in the reproductive system was preceded by acute psychic traumas and conflicts on sexual grounds.

A significant psychological pathology that involved areas of the mouth, the process of eating, and digestion, in several cases preceded the onset of stomach cancer. Authors observed an ulcer of the stomach as an intermediate phase between gastritis, which arose on a neurotic base, and the appearance of carcinoma; chronic gastrointestinal disorders that preceded the onset of pancreatic cancer, and serious and prolonged anal disorders as harbingers of malignant transformation in the colon.

In my practice, there was a case of treatment of a patient with an almost "lost" voice. The otorhinolaryngologist did not reveal any disorders. In the process of therapy, we found that by way of speaking in a whisper she forced members of their family (consisting of men only) to listen to what she said, which she could not achieve from them earlier. In the next session, she remembered that in her childhood she had to scream to get her father's attention and make him hear her needs. The loss of her voice has finally turned out to be a problem of low self-esteem and self-confidence.

Surgeon and psycho-oncologist Bernie Siegel (1998) believes that parts of the body that have a special significance in one's conflicts and psychic traumas become the most likely areas of disease occurrence. Siegel cites Franz Alexander, who noted more than forty years ago that "just as certain pathological microorganisms have a specific affinity for certain organs, so do certain emotional conflicts possess specificities and accordingly tend to afflict certain internal organs."

12.4. Variants of Development of Intrapersonal Conflict: the Psyche or the Body? Schizophrenia or Cancer?

We have already discussed the existence of the two main types of psychoemotional problem processing—the mental one, when the conflict is being externalized, and the somatic one, when it is internalized, and we have come to the conclusion that such a difference depends on disorders in children's attachment. In the process of pathological adaptation to the traumatic environment, the child finds the only way to reduce the psychophysical tension and maintain the homeostatic balance—to suppress the negative emotions in order to stop feeling psychological pain. This is achieved by unconscious transformation of this pain into a shifted activity — either external, with disorders of external forms of behavior, or internal, with disorders of the somatic state (Pilyagina G. Y., 2003). Such a shift depends on which direction the cognitive-emotional imbalance or deficit is moving to, which in turn is determined by the avoiding or ambivalent type of attachment disorder. It is this shift in responding to negative emotions that determines in an adult whether a psychological conflict or trauma will finally manifest in somatic or mental illness.

A. Meneghetti (1977) considers that an impossibility of rational conflict resolution causes either a psychotic reaction (rage, hysteria, etc.), or a neurotic one (functional or organic neurosis). Moreover, in his opinion, the origin of the tumor can be defined as a somatic, outward-expressed, version of the most severe forms of schizophrenia. In this case, schizophrenia does not directly affect the brain or mental area, but manifests at a somatic level.

A similar position is shared by one of the pioneers of psycho-oncology, Claus Bahnson. In 1969, he presented a theory of psycho-physiological complementarity, according to which the direction of a psychoemotional conflict resolution depends on the type of psychological defense used. Such types of defenses as suppression and denial underlie the unfolding of somato-pathological process—from conversion hysteria and hypochondriac conditions through psychosomatic readiness to organic diseases, with cancer as an extreme degree of imbalance. Another option, psychopathology, arises from the use of such types of defenses as displacement and projection, beginning with anxiety hysteria and anxiety neurosis, through phobias and obsessive-compulsive neurosis to eventually *psychosis*—a deep disorder of the psyche. The stronger the conflict, the stronger becomes the controlling defense, and the more serious is the developing pathology; what is more, its somatic variant often limits or even excludes the psychopathic and vice versa.

The fact that the two poles of the conflict's processing often counteract the development of the pathology associated with its opposite has attracted scientists by its mystery for a long time. As early as 1893(a), Dr. H. Snow pointed out that insane people and lunatics are extremely rarely susceptible to any form of cancer. In the hospital of St. Elizabeth in Washington, D.C. for ten years of observations from 1930, among 9,503 psychiatric patients, only 227 cases of cancer of different localization were diagnosed, i.e. 2.4% (Peller S., Stephenson C. S., 1941), which is significantly lower than the average statistical level. D. Rice (1979) published data indicating that he was unable to detect the occurrence of bronchogenic carcinoma in patients with chronic schizophrenia, despite their abuse of tobacco.

Dr. A. Hoffer, who treated schizophrenia in 4,000 patients for more than half a century of practice (since 1952), noted only 5% of cancer cases (Hoffer A., Foster H. D., 2000). A meta-analysis of five studies examining the relationship between prostate cancer and schizophrenia showed a significantly lower incidence of this cancer in psychiatric patients (Torrey E. F., 2006). Similar results were obtained in Israel, where the level of oncological illness was studied among patients with schizophrenia in groups of different ethnic origins (local, European-American, and Asian-African) (Grinshpoon A. et al., 2005). L. Y. Guseva (1969), investigating the death rate of schizophrenic patients over a fifteen-year period, reported that neoplasms in them were found almost half as often as in the average person. There are also observations that if cancer patients develop severe paranoid symptoms, the progression of cancer is inhibited or even that remission occurs; authors speculate this may be due to the fact that their aggression toward themselves is turned outward in a paranoid state (Ehrentheil O. F., 1956; Miller T. R., 1977).

An analysis of 3,214 deaths conducted by the Texas Department of Mental Health revealed only 4% of cancer deaths in psychiatric patients (including the mentally retarded), in contrast to 18% of cancer deaths in patients without psychiatric pathology, regardless of age, sex, race, and method of treatment (in hospitals or outpatient departments). It is interesting that a study of the mental state of people from this group on the basis of their IQ indices revealed that the closer their level of mental development was to the norm, the more often cancer was found (Achterberg J. et al., 1978). Similar data was obtained in 1935 by Soviet scientists L. A. Prozorov and S. A. Tapelson: malignant neoplasms were revealed only in one of 268 patients with congenital or early acquired dementia (oligophrenia), in seven of the 1,123 patients with schizophrenia (0.6 %) and in none of the 403 patients with epilepsy; whereas for manic-depressive psychosis a positive relationship with cancer was found (cited by Krasnushkin E. K., 1960).

As we can see, the less a person's mind is "overloaded" with psychological traumas and conflicts (which is obvious in mental retardation), the less likely is the probability of cancer. Paradoxically, the reverse is also true: when the mind is "overloaded" with psychological suffering, but it is "channeled" through the mind, not the body, then a mental illness arises, as a way to resolve suffering. The above data once again confirm my basic thesis: the source of cancer is not in the problems of the body, but in the misconfiguration of the mind, its inability to cope with distress, as a result of which the boundless possibilities of the mind are directed toward disharmony and pathology.

Scientists have proposed several mechanisms trying to find an explanation for the phenomenon of the negative correlation of cancer and mental pathology. A. Hoffer (1994, 1998) refers to the increased content in the urine of patients with schizophrenia of the product of oxidative decomposition of epinephrine: adrenochrome, similar in structure to hallucinogens. Developing the hypothesis that schizophrenia a kind of mental defense against psychoemotional stress, the author suggests that an increase of epinephrine in the blood during the stress leads to a corresponding increase in the level of adrenochrome. On the one hand, it protects the heart from the danger of fibrillation under the influence of epinephrine, but on the other hand it damages the brain, with consequent hallucinations. In addition, A. Hoffer believes, because of its affinity with free radicals, adrenochrome can serve as a factor that destroys the spontaneously arising cancer cells in the body, which explains the phenomenon discussed. This hypothesis, taking into account the data on the participation of oxidative stress in the mechanisms of tumor development, given in Chapter 19.4, is currently unconvincing.

Another mechanism was discovered by scientists from Australia: the ability of fibroblast cells of the skin in schizophrenic patients to undergo apoptosis (programmed cell death) was significantly higher than in the control group (Catts V. S. et al., 2006). On the one hand, if this mechanism is inherent in all the cells, it can explain the loss of *neuropil* in the prefrontal cerebral cortex of patients with schizophrenia (Selemon L. D. et al., 1995) and can be a source of disorders of their cognitive abilities. On the other hand, as we will see below, the decline of the cells' ability for apoptosis is one of the most important reasons for their uncontrolled reproduction in cancer.

In the Department of Psychiatry Research of the Hillside Hospital, NY (USA), a study of the relationship between schizophrenia and oncological diseases was carried out by analyzing the variations of the MET proto-oncogene, that is active in cells of both cancer and schizophrenic patients. Scientists have found that certain changes in the sequence of nucleotides of the MET gene significantly increase the risk of developing schizophrenia and affect the mental abilities of a person, while other changes increase the risk of cancer. According to Dr. Kathryn Burdick (2010), who led the study, these results give many reason to believe that with the inheritance of a predisposition to schizophrenia and other mental disorders, a person receives a kind of "protection" from cancer.

Still, whatever the molecular mechanisms are in the phenomenon of cancer frequency reduction at schizophrenia, for us the greater interest is in the fact that both types of pathology have a similar origin. This raises the question of new approaches to their treatment. It turns out that at the base of schizophrenia there are practically the same predisposing factors as in cancer: increased reactivity to stress and similar epigenetic processes, i.e. effects on the activity of genes of adverse psychosocial factors of the external environment (Svrakic D. M. et al., 2013; Read J. et al., 2009; Labrie V. et al., 2012). In the early stages of this disease, emotional changes such as depression, guilt, and fear can appear, and then it is possible to develop defense mechanisms in the form of regression and infantilization. Some other psychological aspects are similar: Sigmund Freud (1920) saw in schizophrenia manifestations of deep intrapsychic conflict. Other authors noted the role of parental restrictions in the "double prohibition" form, leading to the loss of a child's willpower and the development of learned helplessness (Bateson G., 1960). In schizophrenic patients, we can also find alexithymia (Maggini C., Raballo A., 2004), obedience, self-accusation, and aggressiveness (Isaeva E. R., 2009).

Therefore, we again return to a common psychosomatic approach to all diseases. A. P. Kotsyubinskiy and associates (2013), comparing the psychopathological and psychosomatic forms of diathesis, found similarities in their period of appearance, in their forms of manifestations, and in the deep affinity of their semiotics (characteristics). On this basis the authors came to the conclusion that the division of pathologies based on bodily or psychic manifestations is quite conditional.

The most important of the predisposing pathogenic psychosocial factors is undoubtedly the disorder of childhood attachments, which determines the corresponding type of personality. This means there must be data confirming the relationship of these disorders with the formation of not only a cancer-prone type of personality, but also a schizotypic[1] one.

Indeed, Israeli psychiatrists have found that schizophrenic patients are characterized by a preoccupied (anxious-ambivalent) disorder of attachment (Ponizovsky A. M. et al., 2013). It is this type, as we've previously noted, that leads to the formation of an emotionally regressive version of CEID, which is different from the hypercognitive one prevailing in cancer patients. N. Tiliopoulos and K. Goodall (2009) of the University of Sydney have established

---

[1] The schizotypal personality disorder, also called "slowly progressing schizophrenia," is established when symptoms for the diagnosis of typical schizophrenia are weak and insufficient.

that the schizotypic personality type, which is prone to psychotic and affective manifestations, is associated with attachment disorders of the anxious and fearful-avoidant type. Similar data was obtained by Swedish scientists in their study of psychotic patients (Strand J. et al., 2015). Australian researchers in the cited work concluded that the connection between the disorder of attachment and schizotypy suggests the existence of fundamental and perhaps biological relationships between them that deserve the closer attention of scientists. These relationships can provide valuable information about the formation and development of schizotypal traits that result in schizotypal personality disorder, and, finally, schizophrenia (Tiliopoulos N., Goodall K., 2009).

On the other hand, N. D. Linde (2000) shows the presence in schizophrenic patients of the restriction or repression of strong emotions, which they are unable to resist if these emotions are actualized in their body and mind. Equal observations were made by E. R. Isaeva (2009) and by E. Antokhin with colleagues (2008). This type of psychological defense, as we already know, is characteristic mainly of the avoiding type of attachment disorders. Given that presently schizophrenic pathology is understood as a set of heterogeneous mental disorders, their origin may come from different types of attachment disorders—yet, the same can be true for various types of oncological pathology.

At the same time, some authors in psychological studies do not find a decrease in the incidence of oncological diseases in schizophrenia and have even found the opposite trend (Shchepin V., Masyakin A., 2014; McGinty E. E. et al., 2012; Tran E. et al., 2009). Such discrepancies, in addition to the above-mentioned methodological differences, can be explained by the existence of two variants in the course of schizophrenia, according to the patient's type of mental manifestations. The first one is regressive, and includes catatonic[1] and hebephrenic forms, where somatic symptoms of atrophy, hypoplasia, and fibrosis are common but malignant phenomena are rarely observed. Another one is supercompensatory, and includes the paranoid form; on a somatic level it is manifested in hypertrophy, hyperplasia, and malignant growth (Lewis N. D. C., 1936). It is possible that these differences were not taken into account in the contradictory studies cited above. A. E. Scheflen (1951) and W. A. White (1929) also submitted statistical data that cancer is much less common in catatonic and hebephrenic forms of schizophrenia than in the paranoid form.

---

[1] Leading symptoms in the catatonic form of schizophrenia are motor disorders with a formally clear consciousness (manifested as inhibition (stupor) or excitation); in the hebephrenic form, disorders of the emotional-volitional sphere (pronounced inadequacy, inappropriate foolishness, flattening of emotions) are present; in the paranoid form, delirium and hallucinations (mostly auditory, known as "voices").

The most intriguing data is that indicating the possibility of transition of the mental variant of the reaction to an internal conflict into a physical one and vice versa (in this case, secondary psychoses that arise as a complication of somatic diseases or are due to the use of psychoactive substances are not taken into account (Keshavan M. S., Kaneko Y., 2013)).

For example, after surgery for colitis, when the psychological defense loses its object of somatization owing to the resection of the colon, one's disorder progresses to a psychotic symptom formation (O'Connor J. F., Stern L. O., 1967). On the contrary, according to the observations of psychiatric hospitals, if psychotic patients develop somatic diseases, such as pneumonia, their psychotic symptoms may temporarily soften or even almost disappear (Obukhov Y. L., 1997).

According to the clinical observations of psychoanalysts, psychosomatic diseases can also be seen as a result of a person's desire to behave "non-hysterically." If decompensation of a psychosomatic patient progresses toward the mental disease, then his current bodily syndromes often shift toward hysteria. Therefore, during the treatment of such patients it is sometimes possible, following removal of the psychosomatic defense, to observe their hysterical symptoms become more evident, and vice versa (Bastiaans J., 1982).

Boris Luban-Plozza and colleagues (2013) also often noted in the psychosomatic clinic the exchange of neurotic symptoms and bodily disorders: "Neurotic symptoms clearly recede with the formation of bodily disease and often return after recovery from it." E. Y. Zubova (2012) describes the disappearance of psychotic symptoms after the onset of tuberculosis and during periods of its progression. Otto Kernberg (1993), observing many psychotic patients, discovered that after a decline in the exacerbation of the psychotic state, they experience psychosomatic disorders such as neurodermatitis, psoriasis, and stomach ulcers.

Studying similar cases, French psychiatrist Henry Baruk (1964) developed the concept of psychosomatic balancing: the inverse proportionality between mental and somatic manifestations of pathology. Showing the variety of such balancing forms, Baruk has elevated them to the rank of "universal law prevailing in the relationship between mental and physical diseases." A well-known Soviet psychiatrist, Prof. E. K. Krasnushkin (1960), after analyzing a large quantity of data on psychosomatic balancing (including that between schizophrenia and some inflammatory diseases), came to the conclusion that further study of this phenomenon "opens up great prospects and promises great opportunities in the treatment of mental illness." According to other psychiatrists, psychosomatic balancing was observed in almost a third of disease cases in adult patients (Sorokina T. T., Evsegneev R. A., 1986).

Proceeding from the above, can cancer and schizophrenia be considered as two "rigid" poles of psychosomatic balance, as Claus Bahnson (1969) suggests?

If we accept the positive answer for the hypothesis, then the next question arises: is it possible to "shift" this balance in the opposite direction for therapeutic purposes? Is it possible to create a kind of "controlled psychosis" for inhibiting a malignant growth of cells?

The data considered again lead us to a conclusion about the primary nature of disorders of childhood attachment and associated intrapersonal conflict/trauma as the basis of all types of pathology. It is these disorders that determine the type of personality and its psychological defenses, which will primarily cause a manifestation of either a "feeling-free mind," with somatization of the conflict right up to the development of cancer, or "mind-free feelings," with the increase of psychopathic changes up to schizophrenia.

Conclusion

Undoubtedly, the variants of the distresses described in this part do not cover the whole range of human psychic conflicts; we have analyzed just the main and most common problems. It can be concluded that the key links of chronic distress and subsequent oncogenic sensibilization are:

- an unresolved psychic trauma, and/or
- a deep intrapersonal conflict between the most important human needs, especially the needs for love, self-actualization, and self-transcendence, and an inability to meet these needs.

In turn, these psychological factors are only able to reach the power of oncogenic provocation in the presence of epigenetic predisposition and/or perinatal disorders, distortions of childhood attachment, and psychosomatic personality types—mainly "C" or "D."

Apparently, the vast majority of our distresses can be reduced to the experiences of loss. But, in the case of acute psychic trauma, the distress associated with it is felt as grief—because of the loss of a real object; while in the case of an intrapersonal conflict, it is felt as an anxiety or fear of a potential loss. This fear arises when the object connected to fear is available, but can be lost. Or it is a fear of never getting back what is lost, when the need for it is not satisfied. Finally, it is the fear of never having an object of need (particularly if it was not possessed before), that can lead to a loss of hope for a better life. Such an object of loss is usually similar in all listed cases: a close person, love, relationships, property, finances, respect for oneself, status, job, etc. Grief and fear, as well as the feelings of guilt and resentment associated with them, must therefore be the primary, most important objects of the therapist's attention.

In light of the foregoing, we can assume that inability to resolve the trauma(s) and/or conflict(s), against the background of ineffective coping with the stress experienced as grief or fear, often aggravated by feelings of guilt and/or resentment, becomes a powerful source of of inwardly or outwardly directed aggression, anger and hatred. Being unable to process or release these negative emotions, the person suppresses or represses them, with subsequent deepening of his chronic physiological distress (Anokhin P., 1980; Vasilyuk F. E., 1984; Temoshok L., 1987; Simonton C. et al., 1978). This leads to the destruction of the barrier of mental adaptation and the transition of the conflict to the destructive stage, suppressing the protective anticancer mechanisms of the body and deepening the state of oncogenic sensibilization.

It appears that acute, strong, psychotraumatic stress leads to a more rapid development of chronic distress, reflected in post-traumatic, psychological, and somatic disorders. In a chronic conflict, in contrast, there is a gradual accumulation of distortions at all levels of the psychobiological system, which eventually reaches the stage of depletion of adaptive and protective resources.

In this state, future cancer patients may feel as if they are caught in trap which cannot be avoided. According to Bernie Siegel (1998) "a drawn-out, living death happens when feelings are unspoken, conflicts remain unresolved, and life goes on only for the sake of others." The contradiction between the desire to change the course of life and the possibility of doing it independently is growing (Rusina N., 2010). Therefore, a person suffers a state of "suffocation," leading to the next phase of the cancer process: precancerous, marked by feelings of helplessness, hopelessness, and depression that aggravate oncogenic distress.

$$* * *$$

Despite their undoubted contribution to onset of cancer, unresolved psychic trauma and/or conflict, like the psychosomatic "C" personality type, are not specific only to cancer. During the analysis of the problem, we repeatedly observed that many psychological characteristics and life circumstances of cancer patients, including those that existed before the disease, are typical for psychosomatic patients suffering from other types of pathology.

Returning to the data of Chapter 2, we can see that in the life history of both types of patients there are disorders of childhood attachment and/or psychic traumas. Both types tend to avoid stressful situations and retain the desire not to fall into conflict situations (Abitov I. R., Mendelevich V. D., 2008).

Excessive control over negative emotions, especially repression of anger, hostility, and anxiety, is noted in such psychosomatic diseases as bronchial asthma (Malatesta C. Z. et al., 1987), rheumatoid arthritis (Crawford J. S., 1981), migraine (Passchier J. et al., 1988), and cardiovascular disease (Siegman A. W. et al., 1998). Repressed aggression and a strong need for love and support are often found not only in oncology, but also in patients with bronchial asthma (Mayer A. E., Weitermeyer W. U., 1967; Bastiaans J., Groen J., 1954). Masochistic-depressive manifestations with a pronounced need for self-sacrifice and an excessive desire to help others, together with super-moral behavior, are also observed in rheumatoid arthritis patients (Braütigam W. et al., 1997).

As a result of the loss of the "key figure" that played a significant role in the life of the individual, other types of somatic and mental illness often occur (Engel G. L., Schmale J., 1967; Adamson J. D., Schmale A. H. Jr., 1965; Braütigam W. et al., 1997). Some authors even believe that the subjectively processed loss of significant objects becomes a leading factor in the development of psychosomatic disorders (Freyberger H., 1977). According to studies on more than 189,000 Danish people, the experience of the death of a parent before the age of 18 increases mortality from various pathologies by 50% (Li J. et al., 2014), and also increases the risk of psychosis and suicide (Beadle B., 2014; Barraclough B. et al., 1974). Equally important in the emergence of various diseases are individually significant interpersonal or intrapersonal conflicts (Shevchenko Y., Velikanova L., 2014).

The following question naturally arises: will the psychological changes in personality that occur at the next biological stage of development of cancer—precancerous—perhaps be narrowly specific for oncological pathology? We will sort this out in the next part.

Part IV

The Precancerous State

As I have already mentioned, biomedicine understands the precancerous state to be defined by mainly chronic inflammatory and dystrophic diseases, as well as benign neoplasms predisposed to malignant transformation. In the latter cases, atypical changes in cells and their focal growths without signs of penetration into the underlying tissues (for example, dysplasia and atypical epithelial growths) are observed. Examples of precancerous diseases include atrophic gastritis; gastric ulcer; ulcerative colitis; chronic hepatitis and cirrhosis; cervical erosion; polyps of the stomach, colon, and female genital organs; cystic diseases of the mammary glands; long-term trophic skin ulcers; diffuse and nodular goiter in the thyroid gland; and others. Many of them are presently considered as having a psychosomatic origin.

It is important to understand that not every precancerous condition or disease necessarily becomes cancer. Such diseases can exist for a sufficiently long time without any malignant transformation of the cells. The leading name in Soviet oncology, Nikolay Petrov (1958), argued that precancerous changes are reversible changes, and under appropriate conditions can develop in the opposite direction, concluding with recovery. In other cases, they turn into cancer, which, as a rule, is associated with the ongoing action of a carcinogenic factor. Without rejecting the importance of external carcinogens (we'll talk about them in more detail in Chapter 20), I'm sure that the main "ongoing carcinogenic factor" is chronic distress. That is why an exclusively surgical–pharmacological approach eliminates only the symptoms, and not the root cause of precancer. For instance, after the removal of polyps, new polyps often appear in patients, and after cauterization of cervical erosion, after a while there may be new formations—in the mammary or thyroid gland.

In accordance with the concept of this book, for the radical cure of precancer it is necessary to resolve psychotraumatic experiences and eliminate chronic distress. Epigenetic regulation plays an important role in precancerous changes in tissues—in particular, changes in gene methylation have been detected in leukoplakia (mucosal lesions) of the oral cavity and esophagus (López M. et al., 2003; Roth M. et al., 2007), chronic gastritis (Sugano K., 2008), and mastopathy (Berman H. et al., 2005). This explains how precancerous changes can develop in the opposite direction.

It is known that psychological factors—for example, anxiety and depression—accompany such precancerous conditions as peptic ulcers of the stomach and duodenum, gastritis, gastroesophageal reflux disease, chronic hepatitis and cirrhosis of the liver, and proliferative mastopathy (Baranovskiy A. Y., 2011; Alekseeva A. S., 2010; Grishechkina I. A., 2011; Lapochkina N. P., 2007). According to the observations of M. I. Davydov (2005), under a state of psychoemotional stress, the risk of a transition of the non-proliferative form of nodal mastopathy into the proliferative form (at which cell multiplication is activated, so it considered to be a precancer) increases 3.3 times.

In this part, I will demonstrate that, from the point of view of psycho-oncology, the precancerous state of the organism develops when chronic distress, arisen due to an unresolved psychic trauma or intrapersonal conflict, reaches a critical disadaptive stage. On a personality level, this may manifest as a state of anxiety, helplessness, hopelessness, and depression.

Chapter 13

Helplessness and Hopelessness

If a man lacks enthusiasm,
either his body or mind is in a deceased condition.
B. R. Ambedkar,
Writings And Speeches

13.1. When All Attempts are in Vain ...

Gerald Caplan (1963), describing the stages of the development of a psychological crisis, notes that its last stage occurs if all attempts of a person to cope with the problem prove futile. It is characterized by increased anxiety and depression, feelings of helplessness and hopelessness, and, as a result, the disorganization of the personality. Such a state can be a consequence of a traumatic event: if a psychic trauma that occurs when a person collides with a sudden threatening event surpasses his ability to control the situation or respond to it in any effective way, then an extremely strong sense of helplessness arises (Yalom I., 1980).

The famous German researcher George Engel (1968) developed the psychosomatic concept of "giving up" and "given up". According to Engel, after the real or imaginary loss of an object important to the patient and as a result of a consequent psychological abandonment of the future, accompanied by a loss of faith and hope, the mechanisms of affect somatization are activated and the development of the disease is precipitated.

A similar condition, according to the observations of psycho-oncologists, often occurs in future cancer patients who are unable to resolve a long-term psychic trauma or conflict. Most of the Simontons' (1978) cancer patients admitted that even before the onset of the disease they felt helpless, unable to solve or change life situations, and had given up. They perceived themselves as "victims"; everything that happened seemed to them to be occurring without their participation and merely confirmed that they could not expect anything good from life. As a result, these people refuse to solve their problems, lose their flexibility, and are immersed in helplessness and hopelessness. The reason for this sense of being trapped, according to the Simontons, is that such people are limited by their accustomed ways of responding to stressful situations and are effectively unable to change them.

S. Locke and M. Hornig-Rohan (1983) noted that the dominant and defining psychological properties of a cancer-predisposed personality are depression, helplessness, and hopelessness; they also pointed out in those with this personality a loss of significant connections both in childhood and shortly before the onset of the disease. Dr. Yoichi Chida and colleagues (2008) from the London University College psychobiology group analyzed 165 studies carried out by other researchers. They concluded that the deaths of close people, job loss, divorce, and other stress factors, especially when accompanied by a sense of helplessness, are clearly related to both the development of cancer in previously healthy people and the survival rate in those who have it.

Experts from the independent Western Consortium for Public Health, USA, having studied about 2,500 people, found that those who had been found to experience hopelessness had 3.5 times more chance of dying from cancer or heart disease in the next six years (Everson S. A. et al., 1996).[1] Associatees of the University of Rochester examined a group of sixty-eight women before the biopsy for the diagnosis of cervical cancer. Based on the received psychological data, they were able to predict, with an accuracy of 73%, which of these women would be diagnosed with cancer. The main factor appeared to be hopelessness (Schmale A. H., Iker H. P., 1964).

Lawrence LeShan (1977, 1989), who worked with more than five hundred cancer patients, came to the same conclusion: serious, disabling psychological exhaustion and depression due to unresolved life problems form a sense of despair even before the appearance of clinical signs of cancer. After diagnosis, a state of helplessness and hopelessness is diagnosed in 95% of patients.

Similar results—the presence of depression, hopelessness, and despair before the onset of the disease—were obtained by W. A. Greene (1966) in a study of people who subsequently received diagnoses of leukemia and lymphoma. An analysis of scientific literature performed by B. Garssen (2004) over thirty years revealed helplessness and repression of emotions as the most important psychological factors associated with cancer. At the University Clinic of Trondheim in Norway, psychologists studied 253 cancer patients and found that their physical condition, age, and economic situation are closely related to the

---

[1] Another interesting conclusion of this study: people with a high degree of hopelessness have a threefold increase in the risk of dying from violence or trauma! This data supports the view that there are no "accidental" problems in our life—everything that happens is determined by the state of our mind and subconscious.

feelings of hopelessness experienced by most of the patients (Ringdal G. I., 1995).

Israeli scientists examined 113 patients who were at different stages of cancer: immediately after diagnosis, after a course of chemotherapy, and after a relapse of illness. They found that the hopelessness experienced by patients does not depend on the stage of the disease, but is closely related to the onset of depression. At the same time, patients who received significant social support had less expressed hopelessness (Gil S., Gilbar O., 2001). Russian authors, as a result of many years of research, found that before the actual diagnosis of cancer, the majority of patients were in a state of helplessness, despair, and hopelessness, often not consciously realized (Bukhtoyarov O. V., Arkhangelskiy A. E., 2008).

Let us sum this up. A person who cannot cope with stress eventually ceases to see a possible exit from the prevailing psychotraumatic situation. This state of things is experienced by him as a crisis, with the loss of hope that his deep-seated problem can ever be resolved. This state of the psyche is called learned, or acquired, helplessness. As we are going to see, even in experimental conditions such helplessness can lead to cancer.

13.2. Learned Helplessness

In the late 1960s, the American psycho-physiologist Martin Seligman conducted experiments on dogs. The task was to have these dogs form a conditioned reflex of fear in response to high-pitched sound, following the scheme of Pavlov's classical experiments. After a loud sound, dogs received weak but sensitive electric shocks, first in closed and then in open boxes. It was expected that in the open boxes animals would react to sound as they would in closed ones—they would try to find a way out of the box. However, the dogs did not do this: instead of simply jumping out of the box, they lay down on the floor and whined, making no attempt to avoid the electric current. This is how animals that had been subjected to unremitting punishment for a long time (which clearly developed into a state of chronic distress), learned the futility of their efforts: they developed learned helplessness, which became the main modality of their behavior in the future, regardless of the surrounding conditions (Maier S. F., Seligman M. E., 1976).

Since then, numerous studies have discovered the existence of this phenomenon in humans. For example, Donald Hiroto (1974) conducted a similar experiment on the effect of an unpleasant loud sound on three groups of volunteers. Two experimental groups, unlike the control one, were "pretreated" with a preliminary task. In the first group, by applying persistence, subjects could pick up the right combination of keys on the control panel and interrupt the sound. In the second group, subjects could not find the right combination because the panel was switched off, but this was not announced. Then the experiment continued in another room, where the participants in all the groups had to put their hand in a specially equipped box that produced an unpleasant sound. If a subject touched a specific place in the box, the sound ceased.

It was found that people in the first group who had the possibility of turning off the unpleasant sound at the beginning of the experiment could also find a way to stop it in the second test. So could the people from the control group who did not participate in the first series. But most of those who experienced helplessness in the first part of the experiment brought this learned experience into a new situation: they even did not try to turn off the sound–just sat near the console and waited for the test to end.

Martin Seligman and coworkers also showed in a compelling experiment that learned helplessness becomes a serious factor in the occurrence of cancer. Of the three experimental groups of rats, one group received a mild electric shock, which the animals could learn to stop. The second group received the same shock, but could not avoid it, and the third, the control group, was not exposed to electricity. After that, the experimenters injected the animals with cancer cells. This procedure, as a rule, is followed by the development of cancer in about 50% of rats. Within a month, indeed, this happened with the control group. But, in the experimental rats, the results were strikingly different: in the group where animals learned to stop the effect of the current, in other words, they were winners in a stressful situation, only 30% of the rats developed cancer, whereas in the group where learned helplessness was formed, 73% of the rats fell ill! The organism of those animals who could not find a way out of the situation was significantly less able to fight the tumor—because, as the authors believe, that stress weakened their immune system (Visintainer M. A. et al., 1982).

This assumption was confirmed by similar experiments conducted by M. L. Laudenslager and his colleagues (1983), where it was found that after a period of exposure to an unavoidable electric shock, rats developed a marked suppression of the immune response, whereas in the control group, who learned to avoid electric shock, immunity did not suffer. Moreover, the acquired ability of rats in the control group to avoid a stress stimulus led to an even higher reactivity of the immune system.

Martin Seligman, who, in 1976, received the American Psychological Association Award for his outstanding achievements, defines helplessness as a condition that arises in situations where a person feels that external events do not depend on him, and he can do nothing to prevent or modify them. Seligman (1975) believes that learned helplessness is established by the age of eight and reflects one's belief in the effectiveness of one's actions. The scientist discovered three sources of this sense of helplessness:

1) The direct experience of unfavorable events with a lack of control over them—for example, abusive parents or caregivers, divorcing parents, family

scandals, the death of a loved one (human or an animal), the loss of a job, and/or a serious illness (*here we see a clear similarity with the history of many cancer patients—V. M.*). The negative imprint acquired in one such difficult situation is later transferred to other situations in which a real possibility of control exists.

2) Observing the helplessness of other people—in reality or in the mass media;

3) Lack of independence in childhood, as is the case with excessive parental care and their willingness to do everything themselves instead of letting the child do things.

The latter situation blocks the natural search activity of the child—his or her ability to actively act and study the environment (Arshavskiy V. V., Rotenberg V. S., 1984). As we have seen, the despotism of parents, their over-control, the rigid imposition of rules for nutrition, clothing, sleep patterns, games, choice of friends, and subsequently the profession, leads to the repression of the free will of the child (teenager) and his or her creative potential. This becomes, together with emotional and physical violence, the cause of the development of states of dependence, subordination, and infantilism. Then, helplessness becomes a logical addition to this complex. According to Gunther Ammon (1972), a child tolerated and superficially praised and loved by the mother only as a passively dependent being will direct his constructive aggression destructively against himself and expend all his life energy in order to stay in a passive and helpless condition. It is not surprising that the passivity in the face of stressful stimulation from the outside constitutes the essential personality feature of the cancer-prone individual (Grossarth-Maticek R., Eysenck H. J., 1991).

Another reason for the development of helplessness is suggested by D. A. Ciring (2009). According to his observations, mothers of helpless children (in comparison with mothers of independent children) are more active in hyper-protection, they devote too much time, effort, and attention to their children, up to the point that raising a child can become the most important thing in their life. Such mothers usually dominate, make excessive claims on and prohibitions for the child, while fathers are characterized by ambivalent behavior: on the one hand, they do not establish clear boundaries and requirements for the child, and on the other, they are prone to excessive rigidity and punishment in education.

Both parents often project their own undesirable qualities on the child, believing them to be incorrigible; since the child cannot change what is happening he or she develops one of the main prerequisites for the formation of his or her helplessness. In addition, the fathers of such children prefer the following childish qualities in the child: spontaneity, naivety, and playfulness, and encourage their children to preserve these traits. Such fathers are afraid of seeing their children grow up, and, as a result, children do not have sufficient experience of overcoming difficulties, taking on responsibility, and having an active influence on the situation (Ciring D. A., 2009). Hence, it can be seen that helplessness often results from psychological infantilism.

Also, the roots of child helplessness can grow even from the period of delivery, from the passage of the child through the second perinatal matrix: Stanislav Grof (1996) believes that for the infant, this high-stress situation forms a stereotype of having "no way out." Reactivation of similar feelings in adulthood, especially in the case of psychological frustrations (a sense of abandonment, emotional rejection or isolation, threatening events, and situations of suppression in a closed family) leads to a "characteristic spiritual experience of 'no exit', or 'hell'." Martin Seligman and colleagues in the course of their research concluded that childhood helplessness is a lifelong behavior and becomes a risk factor for the development of depression, social failure, and physical illnesses (Burns M. O., Seligman M. E., 1989).

Modern studies of brain neuroplasticity confirmed the role of childhood adversity in the development of learned helplessness, showing that it is accompanied by the inhibition of neurogenesis (the appearance of new nerve cells) in the hippocampus (Ho Y. C., Wang S., 2010) and disorders of the structure of the synapses of nerve cells (the endings of cells connecting neurons to each other) in the same area (Hajszan T. et al., 2009). Similar mechanisms, as we saw above, also work during chronic stress. I have mentioned that the hippocampus is closely related to the prefrontal cortex of the brain, forming a system for managing our emotional and cognitive responses. It was found that learned helplessness is mediated by a change in activity in the middle part of the prefrontal cortex (Forgeard M. J. et al., 2011), the same part of the brain that is damaged during chronic stress (Cook S. C., Wellman C. L., 2004). This area of the cortex, together with the hippocampus, also suffers as a result of the experienced stress in childhood, contributing to the development of chronic depression in adulthood (Frodl T. et al., 2010).

Another physiological mechanism underlying learned helplessness is the increase in the content of IL-1β cytokine-interleukin. Its content increases during stress under the influence of cortisol, and provokes an increase in the inflammatory response, which, among other things, stimulates the development and metastasis of a malignant tumor (Nakane T. et al., 1990). Researchers at Ben-Gurion University in Israel found that it is this cytokine that contributes to the formation of helplessness under the influence of unavoidable shock, as blocking its action with a specific pharmacological drug significantly reduces the development of helplessness (Argaman M. et al., 2005).

A shock that cannot be avoided is the extreme degree of non-avoidable fear, or "fear without solution." As we have already seen, it arises in the child as a result of the conflict between attachment to parents and avoidance of them. Such a shock is close to the third stage of stress: freezing, when neither flight nor struggle is possible. In fact, it is close to an experience of despair, sometimes equivalent to a sense of imminent death.

Dr. Claus Bahnson (1980) of the Institute of Psychiatry in Pennsylvania, who studied the psychology of cancer patients from the 1960s, indicates that the prolonged state of loneliness and helplessness stems from a lack of protection and love in childhood. The personality traits formed as a result manifested in suppression, repression, and rejection of emotions, rigidity (difficulties in changing the program of actions under conditions that objectively require its adjustment). Bahnson believes that the combination of stress with loss and depression creates a vulnerability to the development of cancer.

Brandon Bays (2012), whose story I will tell in Chapter 33.2, in the process of self-healing from cancer was able to re-experience the immense defenselessness and helplessness that she felt as a child but did not allow herself to express. Somehow, she learned at that early age that she cannot show her true feelings or even acknowledge them in herself.

Thus, we are once again witnesses to the confirmation that the emotional distortions of the psyche arising in childhood play an important role in creating a precancerous state of the body. As noted by Claus Bahnson (1980), the all-encompassing complex of hopelessness underlying the behavior of a cancer patient leaves an imprint on his entire life. Lydia Temoshok (1987) came to the conclusion that chronic hopelessness and helplessness, even if they are not acknowledged, constitute one of the fundamental characteristics of a "C"-type personality.

Lawrence LeShan (1977) in many of his patients observed the depth of hopelessness and despair as traits of their personality to such an extent that even a diagnosis of cancer did not bring about changes in their daily lives. Cancer was not considered by them as something new in their life, but only as the last, final confirmation of the basic hopelessness that had long been a part of their existence. Tom Laughlin (1999) adds that when the feeling of helplessness about changing the situation becomes permanent and a person starts to believe that he can do absolutely nothing to get out of such an intolerable situation, then his sense of helplessness turns into hopelessness. "It is the specific feeling of being hopeless that is the key element that turns this unconscious depression into a life-threatening condition, leading to the possibility of shutting down the immune system," writes the psycho-oncologist.

In my practice, I metaphorically call the states of hopelessness, helplessness, and despair observed in patients with both a precancerous condition and a cancer diagnosis as three "demons" who get into a person, and must be "expelled" in order to start on the return to health.

Chapter 14

Depression—Manifested or Hidden

Depression is like a woman in black.
If she turns up, don't shoo her away.
Invite her in, offer her a seat, treat her like a guest
and listen to what she wants to say.
Carl Gustav Jung

The most important consequence of learned helplessness is depression (Abramson L. Y. et al., 1989)—a mental disorder in which people usually lose their ability to experience joy, and feel longing, anxiety, and irritability. Similarly, in animals subjected to unavoidable shocking stress in accordance with the above-described model of experiments, after the appearance of learned helplessness, a state of depression develops (Henn F. A., Vollmayr B., 2005).

Martin Seligman (1975) even believe that learned helplessness should be regarded as an analog of depression, when a person reduces efforts to maintain his sustainable position in the environment. Since previous attempts of the individual to control what was happening were unsuccessful, he expects a negative result in emerging situations. Over time, this breeds hopelessness and helplessness, and leads to passivity and inhibition of activity. From this point of view, depression means a crash of the pre-existing psychological defense strategy in a difficult life situation.

A person experiencing depression, as a rule, has distorted perception: negative judgments about him/herself, others, and what is happening; his or her self-esteem is reduced, pessimism and indecision emerges, as does discontent with oneself. There can be a sense of meaninglessness of life and loss of interest in it. At the physical level, there is often motor retardation, sleep and appetite disorders, weakness, decreased sexual desire, metabolic syndrome, and various ailments. Recently, depression has become one of the leading causes of health disorders and disability in the Western world (Lopez A. D., Mathers C. D., 2006), which generally corresponds to the growth of stressful conditions in modern society. On the other hand, stress and depression are often diagnosed in people with chronic physical illnesses (Kiecolt-Glaser J. K. et al., 2003). As shown later, we'll go over how depression also becomes a precancerous factor.

Depression is viewed as a consequence of inadequate behavioral, psychological, social, and biological coping resources in a person experiencing distress in life on the basis of his personal assessment of the level of such distress (Bedi R. P., 1999). Depression which develops owing to stressful life events and the emotions caused by them, is called reactive, because it arises as a reaction to some external event. In other cases, when an obvious cause of this disease cannot be detected, the depression is called endogenous—"generated within [the body]" (although, in my opinion, there is still a deeply suppressed intrapersonal conflict that is undetected).

Acute stress associated with the loss of a loved one is one of the main causes of the development of depression during the year following the event (Finlay-Jones R., Brown G. W., 1981). This disorder also results from chronic stress caused by unresolved conflicts, in particular the conflict of guilt (Shave D. W., 1974), and the conflict of social rejection. The latter activates brain regions involved in the processing of negative emotions and leads to the prevalence of a negative self-image with corresponding experiences of shame and humiliation (Slavich G. M. et al., 2010). Among the sources of the feelings behind social rejection are the lack of education and low social status that provoke constant negative emotions, which the sufferer represses in order not to expose them. Such emotional repression is a direct predecessor of depression (Langner C. A. et al., 2012). These depressive consequences are often brought about by conflictual relationships between males and females, which is also considered as a form of chronic stress (Kiecolt-Glaser J. K., Newton T. L., 2001). Professor Kenneth Pelletier (2002) of the University of Arizona has come to the conclusion that negative emotions such as fear, despair, and depression have a significant effect on the brain and can significantly alter the biochemistry of the body.

It can be assumed, therefore, that one of the sources of depression is unexpressed aggression. A. Friedman (1970) confirms that patients' inability to openly, spontaneously, and at the appropriate moment express hostility to people toward whom they feel it becomes an element of predisposition to depression. The analysis of numerous studies presented in a review of L. A. Feldman and H. Gotlib (1993) shows that depressive patients, in comparison with healthy people, are characterized by a stronger feeling of anger, but also, at the same time, by a pronounced desire to repress this anger.

In order to reject his hidden aggressive and destructive tendencies, the depressed patient often aspires to "do good," demonstrating this by his closeness to other people, by his activity and impeccable way of life. Reproaching himself for his aggression, the patient exposes himself to self-punishment in the form of isolation from the object of attachment, which leads to depression. As a consequence, W. Brautigam and colleagues (1997) believe, this broken symbiotic dependence on the external object is shifted to dependence on the internal object—one of the organs of the patient's body, which leads to the disruption of its functions, i.e. somatization of repressed feelings. Hence here we are met again with the familiar mechanism of preferring the needs of other people as a way to suppress one's aggressive emotions and avoiding conflicts.

This opinion is supported by other authors, showing that aggression, if it does not find a way out from patients with depression, can turn into autoaggression in the form of self-accusations, self-abasement, and self-destructive tendencies (Biaggio M. K., Godwin W. H., 1987; Kholmogorova A. B., Garanyan N. G., 1999). Such negative ideas can reach a degree of delusion of guilt and can lead to suicidal actions (Brautigam W. et al., 1997). On the other hand, high rates of hostility and anger are informative signs, making it possible to reliably predict the increased risk of developing depression. These people are inclined to an influx of thoughts with negative content, blaming themselves and others for unpleasant events, but at the same time seeking social support (Ingram R. et al., 2007).

It is obvious that a person with a low level of spirituality, living in an existential vacuum, is, in difficult situations, more inclined to experience helplessness and depression, since he lacks the necessary internal support. A lack of meaning and purpose in life is the most important factor of a low level of spirituality, leading to depression (Briggs M. K., Shoffner M. F., 2006; Westgate C., 1996). Research by A. V. Nemtsev (2012) shows that where there is initially insufficient development of spiritual meaning, depressive disorder manifests this deficiency, preventing a person from being freed from the "vicious circle" of the disease. In turn, the resulting depression blocks the realization of the spiritual meanings in the person's life, and does not allow elimination of the disease; but at the same time, it can also induce the suffering person to seek spirituality, to find meaning in life.

14.1. The Roots of Depression—in Childhood

We already know that important character traits of future cancer patients such as psychological infantilism, dependence, repressed aggression, avoidance of conflicts, and helplessness are laid in childhood. It will be logical to assume that the depression that arises as a result of these feelings is also associated with the beginning of one's life.

Indeed, scientists have established that the prerequisites for the onset of depression in adults are created during pregnancy, childbirth, and childhood. In a psychiatric research center at the University of Maryland (USA) it was found that psychological stress in pregnant women leads to a disruption in the formation of synaptic connections of brain neurons in the fetus, and this contributes to the formation in the child's later and adult life of psychiatric abnormalities such as depressive disorders, anxiety, learned helplessness, and schizophrenia (Markham J. A., Koenig J. I, 2011).

According to Stanislav Grof (1996), the source of the depressed state in an adult person is birth process complications, that, similarly to helplessness, correspond to the second basic perinatal matrix and lead to a "hidden depression without tears." This is confirmed by experience of this matrix by patients in the transpersonal sessions, followed by a deep depression. A person is obsessed with a variety of unpleasant feelings: anxiety, guilt, inferiority, and shame dominate his thoughts about the past. His current life seems unbearable to him, and he is overwhelmed with insoluble problems, devoid of any meaning and joy, while the future seems completely hopeless.

The depressive reaction, believes Gunter Ammon, appears as a result of the repression by the mother or caregivers of the process of the child's active exploration of surrounding objects or his creative behavior. Therefore, in the future, such a depressed patient will suffer from a lack of love and attention from the "supreme love object," whoever this is. There is a kind of "hunger" for the object: when a person is alone, he suffers from unbearable loneliness and abandonment that drive him to a nonstop, often life-long search for an object from whom he continuously demands the love and attention that his mother did not give him (Ammon G., 1972). It is not surprising therefore that the interests of such a "supreme love object" will be assessed by the depressed person as more important than his own, as we see in many cancer patients.

E. Bibring (1953) points out that depression is a reactivation of the state of helplessness experienced in childhood due to a frequent or prolonged deprivation of vital needs—for care, nutrition, and love. Such deprivations in early childhood form a predisposition to depression in a later period of life. Its depth is determined by such factors as resistance to disappointments, the frequency and severity of the feelings of helplessness in childhood, and the readiness with which the state of helplessness can be resumed in adulthood. As a result of this tendency to experience helplessness, a depressed patient feels the need for firm support, in particular from a doctor who will decide everything for him, take control of his stay in the hospital, and ease his condition and life itself (Brautigam W. et al., 1997).

Childhood psychic trauma can also become a risk factor for the development of depression in adulthood, especially in response to additional stress. In particular, T. Harris and colleagues (1986), in most of the women they surveyed, found that the loss of a mother before the age of eleven, or parental divorce was associated with the subsequent depression. In this way, the fact of loss became a factor of vulnerability to the development of depression, that occurred only in the presence of a subsequent provocative event, such as poverty or other life stresses. Once again, here we see the work of the diathesis-stress mechanism.

Physical or sexual abuse experienced in childhood, according to psychiatrists from the medical school of the University of Massachusetts, is a risk factor for depression at any age (Brown P., Finkelhor D., 1986). This is accompanied by changes in a number of the child's brain structures, such as the hippocampus and prefrontal cortex (Frodl T. et al., 2010), and by disruption in the integration of neural connections between the emotional, neuroendocrine, and autonomic nervous systems in reactions to stress agents (Heim C. et al., 2008). There is also dysfunction of the hypothalamic-pituitary-adrenal system, leading to excessive release of the stress hormone cortisol in response to stimuli in adulthood (Mello A. A. et al., 2003; Carvalho F. et al., 2012). Depressive disorders are also the first among mental diseases in the number of their somatic manifestations (Brautigam W. et al., 1997).

Recent studies have found that the stresses which arose at an early age are associated with adult depression through epigenetic changes (Heim C. et al., 2008). In particular, in experiments with mice, the unpredictable and long-term separation of pups from the mother causes depressed reactions in the growing rodents and changes behavioral responses to stressful environmental influences. Most of these behavioral disorders subsequently appear in the offspring of males exposed in childhood to the separation from the mother, despite the fact that this progeny was raised normally. This hereditary effect may be associated with a detected change in DNA methylation of several genes in mice subjected to stress. Moreover, comparable changes in DNA methylation were also present in the brains of their progeny and associated with the expression of a modified gene (Franklin T. B. et al., 2010).

Inflammation, as we will shortly learn, is one of important biological mechanisms of depression. Above, we already met the research data that childhood adversities contributes to occurring of pro-inflammatory phenotype that, in turn, promote the development of depression in adulthood (Miller G. E. et al., 2011; Cohen-Woods S. et al., 2017).

Depression is often combined with signs of asthenia: increased fatigue and irritability, reduced efficiency, reversible decline in intellectual functions, emotional weakness in the form of tearfulness, capriciousness, etc. This indicates the depletion of the central nervous system, corresponding to the destruction of the third level of the barrier of psychic adaptation and the approach of the last stage of the general adaptation syndrome: the stage of exhaustion. Therefore, we can consider depression as a precancerous condition.

14.2. Depression and Cancer

It would be a logical conclusion to assume that depression is associated with a higher risk of developing cancer. This was indeed noticed, as I mentioned above, as early as in the first century AD by Galen (Kühn K. G., 1821–1833) and in 1701 by M. Deshaies-Gendron. Dr. James Paget in his book *Surgical Pathology* (1870) stressed:

> The cases are so frequent in which deep anxiety, deferred hope and disappointment are quickly followed by growth and increase of cancer, that we can hardly doubt that mental depression is a weighty additive to the other influences favoring the development of the cancerous constitution.

Dr. Bernie Siegel (1998) describes the presence of depression in future cancer patients as an analog to the fact that the person stops resisting, or in other words, surrenders, when faced with a difficult life situation. This often occurs when an individual feels that his or her current conditions and future perspectives are unbearable. Such a depressed person behaves as if they were "rebelling" against life, by beginning to do less and less, losing interest in people, work, hobbies, etc.

These observations have been confirmed by the monitoring of larger groups of people. Upon observing 2,018 employees of the Western Electric Company (USA) for 20 years, it was revealed that there was a relationship between depression and mortality from cancer (Persky V. W. et al., 1987). In another epidemiological study, where 4,825 elderly people participated, it was concluded that those who suffered from depression for four years had an 88% higher risk of dying from cancer (Penninx B. W. et al., 1998). For twenty-four years researchers from Johns Hopkins Bloomberg School of Public Health in Baltimore observed 3,177 cancer-free patients who were diagnosed with depression. It was revealed that these individuals were at a higher risk for cancer in general and had a statistically higher increase in the risk for breast cancer (Gross A. L. et al., 2010).

Iranian scientists conducted psychological testing on 3,000 women who came to the breast cancer center to be examined. The test was carried out prior to conducting the medical diagnosis. Among 243 of those who were diagnosed with cancer, it was confirmed that 16% had depression and 22% suffered from a sense of helplessness (Montazeri A. et al., 2004). In a similar study at the Cancer Center at the University of Pennsylvania, only 9% of those diagnosed with breast cancer were found to be suffering from depression (Coyne J. C. et al., 2004). However, a meta-analysis of thirteen eligible studies showed a significant increase in breast cancer risk, appearing ten years or more after being depressed (Oerlemans M. E. et al., 2007).

A life study conducted on patients with pancreatic cancer showed that about 50% of them suffered from depression prior to being diagnosed with cancer (Green A. I., Austin C. P., 1993). In addition, being depressed for a prolonged amount of time was found to be a significant factor in the development of lung cancer, among 309 patients diagnosed in the preclinical stage (Fan R. et al., 1997).

A large-scale psychological study conducted on a group of 2,500 people in Sweden in 1947 allowed Olle Hagnell of the University of Lund (1966) to detect forty-two people who developed cancer during the ten years of the observation. In comparison with the control group, these patients showed increased "pleasantness," socialization, and depressiveness even a decade before the onset of cancer. Another large-scale study made use of data from the Taiwan National Health Insurance Research Database and was able to identify 778 patients who were hospitalized with depression from 1998 to 2003. Results of five-year follow-up observations suggested that depression is very closely associated with an increased risk of cancer (Chen Y. H., Lin H. C., 2011).

Scientists from the Harvard Medical School and the MD Anderson Cancer Center explored the data of 183,903 women from two prospective US cohorts with about 700 ovarian cancer cases. Persistent depression, revealed two to four years prior to the diagnosis of cancer, was associated with an approximately 30% increase in the risk of ovarian cancer (Huang T. et al., 2015). A meta-analysis of twenty-five studies, which was conducted in the Jilin University of China, looked at 89,716 incident cases of cancer, and concluded that depression significantly increases the overall risk of cancer and particularly the risk of liver and lung cancer (Jia Y. et al., 2017).

D. Spence (1979) used computer technology to count words related to depression and hopelessness in the speech of patients who came to the clinic for a cervical biopsy. The analysis of the results revealed a credible coincidence of computer diagnostics with the biopsy results: patients with a high level of depression and hopelessness were confirmed to have malignant processes. University of Texas staff, having examined 24,696 patients with breast cancer, found that 7.5% of them had been diagnosed with depression prior to the onset of cancer. These patients died much faster than those who did not develop depression after the oncological diagnosis was made (Goodwin J. S. et al., 2004).

The data presented indicates that many future cancer patients experience depression even before the disease gets diagnosed. A team of researchers from Novosibirsk (Russia) came to a similar conclusion, examining patients who were recently diagnosed with breast, stomach, colon, rectum, and lung cancer. The depressive state revealed in them was not a reaction to the fact of the disease, since it develops over a period of time, and this was taken into account in the questionnaire used by the scientists. According to the authors, depression in cancer is not a concomitant disease, but a condition that has common pathogenetic mechanisms with the underlying oncological disease (Chukhrova M. G. et al., 2010). The predominantly depressed type of personality is defined as a risk factor for developing cancer by other Russian scientists, who conducted a study on men with stomach and rectal cancer (Baranskaya L. T., Polyanskiy M.

A., 2001). Lydia Temoshok (1987) comments that when a person with a type "C" personality has depression, it is not strongly associated with any negative past experience but is the result of an accumulated severity of unexpressed feelings and needs, which are not adequately satisfied.

Undoubtedly, many cancer patients who did not even show signs of depression before the diagnosis was made, often develop this mental disorder as a reaction to the psychic trauma of the diagnosis, which in turn worsens the prognosis of the disease. This aspect is discussed in more detail in Chapter 27.

Much as in the above-discussed studies on the psychological state of people prone to cancer, other scientists have not found a link between depression and the development of cancer (Hahn R. C., Petitti D. B., 1988; Kaplan G. A., Reynolds P., 1988; Zonderman A. B. et al., 1989; and others). This difference in results is explained by the diverse understandings of depression, the unequal criteria for its definition and the different methodological approaches in the evaluation of depression, as well as the differences in the surveyed populations of people (Massie M. J., 2004). The authors of the above-mentioned study, which observed 4,825 elderly people, direct their colleagues' attention to the fact that a one-time examination of the subject is not sufficient when the objective is to determine the relationship between depression and cancer: in their research, accurate results were only obtained after three deferred examinations over the course of six years, whereas data from one survey did not confirm such a result (Penninx B. et al., 1998).

14.3. Is the Explanation a Hidden Form of Depression?

However, there is another important factor: depression in people during the precancerous state and in those with cancer diagnoses often does not have clinically significant characteristics. This was first spotted by Dr. Ephraim Cutter in his book, published back in 1887: mental depression during cancer is an element that is often overlooked. Psycho-oncologist Tom Laughlin (1999) asserted that depression found in cancer patients is not the standard form of depression that psychologists are used to dealing with in clients without cancer. This depression develops unnoticeably, and is often concealed by those that have a high likelihood of developing cancer. When commenting on one of the studies in which researchers from the US National Institute of Aging did not find a higher incidence of cancer in depressed patients, Laughlin points out that they indeed could not detect it because they were basing their observations on classical clinical depression symptoms rather than the subthreshold ones.

Bernie Siegel (1998) agrees with this opinion. He noted that there is a specific form of depression that is closely associated with malignant neoplasms. While the average patient suffering from depression (one that doesn't have cancer) tends to react in some way to a life situation that is unbearable for them, often by reducing their normal activity, many individuals who have yet to be diagnosed with cancer continue to lead their seemingly normal way of life, demonstrating external signs of happiness. However, these people feel that life has lost its meaning and live in a state of "calm despair." Despite treating others gently and with respect, these people are hiding feelings of rage and frustration. They rarely get diagnosed with clinical depression because on the surface they manage to function as before.

Similar perspective developed Lawrence LeShan (1977). Despite the fact that future cancer patients continue with their daily activities, which may reflect their desire to "look good and pleasant," their form of depression is much more hopeless and devastating than that of ordinary depressed patients. LeShan calls this depression "despair," which is rooted in a deep sense of loneliness. It develops either because of the inability to create full-fledged and satisfying relationships with other people (because deep down these people do not consider themselves to be worthy of such relationships and are confident that they will eventually be rejected), or because of their suppressing their true desires and talents for the sake of preserving the relationship. According to R. Grossarth-Maticek and H. J. Eysenck (1991), the form of depression suffered by cancer patients is subclinical and can be defined as the "depression of hopelessness."

In all likelihood, this hidden depression can be associated with the so-called "masked depression" known in psychiatry, also referred to as "larval," "somatized," "alexithymic," or "depressive (thymopathic) equivalent" (López Ibor J. J., 1972; Kielholz P., 1973). It has been established that this type of depression is often related to chronic stress (Tarnavskiy Y. B., 1990). In this case, the classical symptoms of clinical depression, such as a decreased emotional background, avoiding contact with the outside world, apathy, etc., may be insignificant or even completely absent, therefore it is also referred to as asymptomatic depression or dolor occultus—"hidden pain." Patients usually are not aware their depressive state, which, as a rule, is associated with the alexithymic radical. The explanation for this is that if it is difficult for an individual to understand their feelings in general, then they will not feel their depression either. Such individuals may, as a substitute, have various neurotic or somatic symptoms and are inclined to believe they have any of a range of complex and difficult to diagnose somatic diseases.

For example, L. A. Bieliauskas and colleagues (1979) in one of the above-cited studies, analyzed the data on the incidence of cancer in employees of the Western Electric Company, and found that the depression preceding the disease was not actually detected based on the results of a psychological survey, but by using the employees' somatic manifestations, vegetative disorders in particular.

G. N. Pilipenko and associates (2009) examined psychosomatic patients with strong alexithymia manifestations and were able to reveal that their inherent anxious-depressive state reflects a hidden personality complex. These people's depression is introjective (*as if "learned"*—*V. M.*) and tends to not be associated with a specific situation; instead the situation was used by them to explain their oppressed state. These patients were not aware of their depressive states, but instead the depression was diagnosed in the process of questioning the patients and by behavioral signs. The authors concluded that a hidden, unconscious anxious-depressive personality disorder is a definite sign of the alexithymic personality.

Unmanifested, or subthreshold depression, that so-called normal people (i.e. those who do not get treated by psychiatrists and psychotherapists) do not notice, can be present in a quarter of the population, according to research conducted on seemingly mentally healthy residents of Moscow (Padun M. A., 2007). Other data shows that the frequency of such latent forms of depression exceeds the number of those with visible depression by 10–20 times (Gindikin V. Y., 2000). Medical statistics indicate that this issue is increasingly observed by both general practitioners and narrowly specialized professionals: between 1/3 to 2/3 of all patients suffer from masked depression (Smulevich A., 2007).

Therefore, it is very likely that this form of depression is even more common among future cancer patients. In their study of the relationship between depression and cancer, Italian scientists noted that an insignificant number of major depressive disorders and a high level of minor depressive disorders diagnosed in cancer patients are associated with subthreshold forms of depression, and that is why these issues are at risk of not being diagnosed or treated, especially in elderly patients (Spoletini I. et al., 2008). Other scientists also draw attention to the fact that although anxiety and depressive disorders form the basis of the mental problems of cancer patients, they rarely get diagnosed (Berard R. M., 2001; Chochinov H. M., 2001).

Some psychologists believe that the bodily symptoms manifested in depressed patients are a defense against an intense emotion (a so-called affect) that they cannot consciously manifest because of personal restrictions. This results in a suppressed depression. For a person in distress, it is easier to express depression through somatic symptoms because, according to sociocultural norms, bodily problems tend to be met with more empathy and result in more serious concerns than mental disorders. Due to this, the phenomenon of the so-called "secondary benefit of the symptom" arises (Kholmogorova A. B., Garanyan N. G., 2008).

Hidden depression, similarly to anxiety ("hidden fear") acts as a link between psychogenic and somatogenic disorders; that is why they are often grouped together as anxious-depressive disorders. Therefore, such depression also represents psychosomatic balancing, where at one pole there is the classical depression, and at the other its somatic equivalents (manifestations) can be found. Weaker forms of depression result in more serious somatic disorders, and vice versa—explicitly expressed somatic symptoms, which at first can only imitate a somatic disease, get replaced by depression. This suggests that there are common mechanisms at the base of "purely" depressive and somatic manifestations (Desyatnikov V. F., Sorokina T. T., 1981).

Walter Brautigam and his colleagues (1997) report that there even is a tendency to consider all of the complexity and significance of psychosomatic connections, and accordingly all psychosomatic complaints (or at least the majority of them) as a manifestation of larval depression. The somatic symptoms that prevail in depressive patients at clinics actually express their emotions of fear and depression that cannot be reflected in the psychic sphere, and as a result recede into the background and often go unnoticed. This leads to countless unnecessary and costly somatic examinations. A well-known Spanish psychiatrist, J. J. López Ibor (1972), was firmly convinced that psychosomatic disorders in many cases can be referred to as equivalents of depression. According to W. Rief (2005), depression, anxiety, and somatic disorders are so closely related to one another that a number of researchers today attribute them to a single disorder.

The following potential "masks" of latent depression should attract the attention of physicians and psychologists and can be used as reasons for further diagnosis of the possible presence of a state of helplessness and the psychosomatic type "C" personality as a precancerous condition:

- oppressed moral state, *anhedonia*, anxiety, panic attacks, obsessions, *hypochondria*, *neurasthenia*, or contrariwise, hysterical reaction: resentment, tearfulness, tendency to dramatize situations, impulsiveness, conflictedness, outbreaks of aggression, the desire to draw attention to one's ailments;

- vascular dystonia, dizziness, weakness, sweating, hot flashes, cold limbs, lack of air, pulse and blood pressure lability, arrhythmia, tachycardia, dyspeptic disorders (dry mouth, nausea, vomiting, flatulence, constipation or diarrhea), various tics, muscle twitching;

- diversified pains of unknown origin, localized in the head, heart, abdomen, joints, or spine (psychalgia),

- biological rhythms and sleep disorders (insomnia or drowsiness, nightmares), sexual disorders (Tiganov A. S. et al., 1986; Tarnavskiy Y. B., 1990; Burlachuk L. F. et al., 1999).

According to V. Y. Gindikin, signs that indirectly speak about the presence of latent depression may be depleted facial expressions, a facial expression of grief, lowering of the corners of the mouth, triangular distortion of the upper eyelid above the inner third of the eye ("O. Veraguth's fold"), monotonous and low-modulated speech, quiet voice. A focused survey makes it possible to reveal emotional changes: a slightly sulky mood, a lack of vital activity, sadness, alexithymia, a tendency to consider oneself to somehow be defective, nervousness; sometimes the patient agrees that he is down in the dumps. The patient's well-being may change during the day—for example, they may feel worse in the morning (slackness, inhibition, fatigue) or in the evening (which is more typical); one can often observe restlessness, anxious sleep, and asthenia. Such a patient assesses the present and the future pessimistically, shows some anxiety, tearfulness, and, most importantly, a feeling of hopelessness with suicidal thoughts and even attempts. If the patient is an artist, then motives of sadness, sorrow, and despair dominate their work (Gindikin V. Y., 2000). The last observation serves as a rationale for applying projective methods in the diagnostic process, by getting the patient to draw spontaneous images (including on sand), and by using metaphorical cards (with different images that evoke associations from the subconscious).

In my opinion, the type of depression that most corresponds to precancerous depression is a kind of "masked" depression, named "depression of exhaustion" by Paul Kielholz (1973). As a general rule, it arises as a reaction to prolonged emotional stress and therefore can be considered to be a gradually developing form of decompensation of the emotional sphere of one's personality, equal to the destruction of the third barrier of psychic adaptation. According to Kielholz, what causes this depression are unresolved conflicts at work or financial problems (mainly for men), or failures in personal or family life, loneliness or an excessive workload—at work and at home (more for women). Initially, this form of depression manifests itself mostly as neurasthenic and asthenic disorders (irritability, fatigue, sleep disturbances, etc.). Later they are joined by a variety of somatic and vegetative disorders. When this state is aggravated by a state of chronic stress, the next stage develops, which is clinical depression.

Tom Laughlin (1999) believes that subthreshold depression is of great significance. This depression is unique not only because it is the result of "suffocating" factors, the conditioned ego and lifelong dependence that exist in the future cancer patient's relationship. These factors are present in every marriage, love affair, and set of parents' relationship with their kids to an extent. But:

> The key factor that changes these other factors into a dangerous situation is that the agony and suffering caused by this unconscious depression is unknown to the patient, as well as to the patient's doctor... The pain, agony, fear, resentment, anger and rage work their deadly poison on the body by festering unnoticed day after day, year after year in this invisible part of the patient's personality. It is precisely because this depression is unknown and unrecognized that it may lead to a possible cancer,

emphasizes Laughlin.

Thus the inability to recognize one's own depressive state (as well as the suppressed emotions of anger), which is probably due to alexithymia, shifts the psychosomatic balance toward a bodily disorder, with its extreme manifestation in the form of cancer. As V. F. Desyatnikov and T. T. Sorokin (1981) argue, when there is no awareness of depression, "... that is, the main channel for transmitting information about disbalance in the affective sphere of the psyche does not work properly, ... [the body has] to sound the alarm, by using pains and unpleasant bodily sensations to inform 'the upper levels of the management' (in the cerebral cortex) of formidable problems." Over time, as the chronic stress approaches the stage of exhaustion, somatoform symptoms turn into a somatic pathology—metaphorically speaking, a depressive "mask" sprouts in the body, antedating the similar behaviour of a tumor.

But even if a person is aware of their depression but attempts to not show it, rather to suppress it, then it has the same potentiating effect on the development of cancer as the suppression of negative emotions in general does—this conclusion can be made on the basis of a study conducted by Dutch scientists who discovered that excessively controlling depressive feelings is a risk factor for cancer (Tijhuis M. A. et al., 2000).

14.4. Similarities Between Biological Mechanisms of Chronic Stress and Depression

Initially, scientists only associated mechanisms of depression with disorders of the turnover of catecholamines, such as norepinephrine, dopamine, and serotonin. In Chapter 19, I will discuss their significant role in the mechanisms of cancer. However, recently a sufficient number of studies have been conducted that indicate that in the development of depression, the imbalance of catecholamines is mediated by inflammation processes, which, as we already know, also occur during chronic stress and helplessness. It is also one of the main factors in the precancerous state. Generally, this is not surprising, since depression and helplessness are products of the stressful state of mind, so the mechanisms of their development should be similar. For example, researchers from Emory University in Atlanta discovered that stress-induced depression is accompanied by the activation of inflammation processes in the body and this factor promotes tumor growth (Cowles M. K., 2009). This inflammatory depression theory resulted in a revolution in psychology, psychiatry, and neuroscience.

We also already know that stress hormones suppress the defensive functions of the immune system and induce inflammation by means of biologically active mediators—cytokines. Depression also decreases one's immunity (Kiecolt-Glaser J. K., Glaser R., 2002; Bufalino C. et al., 2013). Therefore, it appears to be logical that a reduced number of protective immune killer cells and a more active vascular growth in the tumor was found in patients with liver cancer who had the concomitant depression. This was reflected on the shortened survival time of such patients (Steel J. L. et al., 2007).

A meta-analysis of twenty-four scientific studies conducted at the University of Toronto revealed an increase in the concentration of IL-6 and TNF-α cytokines in people with depression (Dowlati Y. et al., 2010). Experimental administration of cytokines IL-1β, TNF-α, IL-10 to animals also results in a kind of "disturbed behavior," which is similar to depressive symptoms (Dantzer R. et al., 2008). Treating humans with cytokine IFN-a results in similar symptoms (as a side effect), which influences the content of other interleukins and reduces the neurotransmitter serotonin content (Valentine A. D., Meyers C. A., 2005). Consequently, cytokines can be considered as biological "stressors" that, like psychological stressors, can have time-dependent activation effects: their reintroduction in the experiment leads to significantly greater neurochemical changes, that is, the phenomenon of sensitization arises (Anisman H. et al., 2002).

The relationship between depression and inflammation is bilateral: inflammation provokes depression, and depression increases inflammation (Miller A. H. et al., 2009). The same mechanism is observed with stress—if a person is already in a state of stress, that has triggered the inflammation process, then depression that arises as a result further increases the inflammation (Fagundes C. P. et al., 2013). On the other hand, if stress and depression lead to inflammation, then treatment aimed at their reduction should reduce inflammation. Indeed, the use of antidepressants leads to a reduction in inflammatory phenomena in patients with serious depression (O'Brien S. M. et al., 2006); The same effect can be achieved by practicing meditation, which eliminates emotional distress (Pace T. W. et al., 2009).

Depression is accompanied by other physiological and biochemical changes, which are characteristics of chronic stress and contribute to the development of cancer. Depressed people have:

- an increased daily average release of norepinephrine in the urine (Hughes J. W. et al., 2004);

- cortisol hypersecretion, adrenal hypertrophy and excessive cortisol reaction to the adrenocorticotropic hormone (Gold P. W. et al., 1988);

- increased level of inflammation and oxidative stress which results in the shortening of chromosome telomeres in leukocytes corresponding to the duration of the disease and accelerated aging (Wolkowitz O. M. et al., 2011);

- worsened restoration of damaged DNA in lymphocytes (Kiecolt-Glaser J. K. et al., 1985);

- insulin resistance with a corresponding increase in the insulin and glucose levels in blood (Winokur A. et al., 1988; Chen Y. C. et al., 2007);

- other disorders common to both stress and depression (see Reiche E. M. et al., 2005).

Conclusion

In this part we have confirmed that the consequences of unresolved psychic trauma or intrapersonal conflicts are expressed in the form of helplessness, hopelessness, and depression (especially the subthreshold type), which are often accompanied by somatic disorders, ranging from somatoform manifestations to precancerous diseases. This marks the transition of chronic distress to the stage of depletion of physiological resources, with the destruction of the third barrier of psychic adaptation.

However, this condition also does not necessarily result in an oncological disease. As we know, precancerous conditions are reversible. In addition, as discussed above, helplessness and depression (whether it is clinically manifested or not) are present in other psychosomatic diseases and psychopathologies that do not result in the development of cancer. Psychosomatic patients, as well as those suffering from neurotic disorders, are particularly prone to feeling a sense of confusion and helplessness in difficult situations (Abitov I. R., Mendelevich V. D., 2008).

According to G. L. Engel and A. H. Schmale (1967), the feeling of helplessness and hopelessness is observed before the onset of various somatic diseases. The authors associate psychological rejection of the future, loss of faith and optimism with the weakening of immune defenses. The patient's life situation at the time of the onset of the disease is of great importance in the view of the authors and they pay attention especially to actual loss of attachment object or the threat of losing such an object. Typical affective states emerging during this period include grief, sadness, a feeling of irreparable loss, despair, helplessness, hopelessness, and depression. In addition, learned helplessness contributes to the development of a post-traumatic stress disorder, schizophrenia, and acute psychiatric illnesses (Forgeard M. J. et al., 2011; Adamson J. D., Schmale A. H., 1965).

Psychosomatic patients often have a seemingly innate, constitutional tendency to develop depression. Together with "operational thinking" (rigid patterns of thoughts, speech, and actions), this often causes them to narrow their circle of interests and leads to an overall loss of interest in life, creating a subconscious belief in their own triviality and insolvency as individuals (Marty P., de M'uzan M., 1963; Sandomirskiy M. E., 2005).

A. V. Shtrakhova and E. V. Kulikova (2012) demonstrated that in psychosomatic patients who were not able to overcome the suffering of a loss of a significant object, frustrated aggression turns into depression, which can be manifested in the form of depressive fear (mainly the fear of rejection), a depressive feeling of helplessness (the so-called "asthenic discouragement" or "asthenic decline of the spirit"), and/or hopelessness ("apathic-gloomy obedience"). Depressive and anxious reactions, the most typical and common psychic reactions to stress, in turn contribute to the development of various pathological somatic conditions (Velikanova L. P., Shevchenko Y. S., 2005).

It was also noted that when depression occurs in patients with mental disorders, it does not increase the incidence of malignant diseases (Evans N. J. et al., 1974; Niemi T., Jaaskelainen J., 1978), which may be due to the psychosomatic balancing discussed above.

Therefore, although helplessness and depression significantly contribute to the formation of a precancerous state, they are not solely responsible for triggering an oncological disease.

Moreover, as can be seen from the materials presented in the previous parts, so far it is difficult to single out psychological characteristics that would be unique to cancer. Lydia Temoshok and Henry Dreher (1993) also noted that the behavior of individuals with type "C" personalities, which she described, is associated not only with cancer, but also with numerous other diseases caused by immunity disorders. Dr. B. R. Cassileth (1995) adds that an individual's psychological properties and the life circumstances specific to cancer patients can often be observed in other chronic diseases: these include passivity, serious personal loss, stress, depression, anxiety, guilt, and the suppression of emotions. These characteristics can also be found in patients with diabetes, arthritis, and dermatological diseases. Roy Grinker (1966) points out that breast cancer patients' characteristics such as masochism, suppression of sexuality, lack of maternal feelings, and the inability to express hostility toward their own mothers can be also found in patients with multiple sclerosis. Life circumstances such as an authoritarian father, competing siblings, early responsibility for family members, and frequent loss of loved ones are present in the life stories of not only cancer patients but those with thyrotoxicosis as well.

It is possible that only a full combination of all of the previously discussed aspects—the four psychosomatic predisposition factors, unresolved conflict or psychic trauma (provocation factor), and helplessness, hopelessness, and depression (precancerous state) work together to create a depletion of protective resources, which is enough to launch the onset of cancer. British scientists led by Hans Eysenck also express a similar opinion: depression, based on helplessness and multiplied by additional stress is equal to cancer (Grossarth-Maticek R. et al., 1994).

Dr. Claus Bahnson (1981) came to the following conclusion after many years of research:

> It is not loss and depression alone that usher in clinical onset of cancer, but the combination of depleting life events with a particular ego-defensive and coping style. Because both ego-defensive style and a special sensitivity to object loss are determined by early life experiences, it follows that long-term conditions of stress and adaptation, rooted far back in the life history, are every bit as important in

predisposing a person to cancer as are short-term recent stresses that can be delineated without reference to a particular life history.

The combination of the four factors examined above can be enough to result in a malignant transformation in animals. However, in my opinion, there is at least one other factor crucial to initiating the disease in humans. Whether the oncogenic potential gets implemented at the time of the precancerous state or not depends on whether or not it is followed by the next phase: the spiritual crisis of the loss of the will to live. This matter will be further discussed in the next part.

Part V

Initialization:
Losing One's Will to Live
and Unconscious Suicide

> If a person has a deep desire to die
> and mobilizes considerable potential of the power of intention for this feat,
> no other force will be capable of keeping him on Earth, unfortunately.
> The person will die, for such is the Power of Intention.
>
> K. V. Yatskevich,
> *Cancer is not a sentence*

Helplessness, hopelessness, despair, and subconscious depression against the background of a type "C" psychosomatic personality have yet another, extremely dangerous consequence for an individual, which is loss of interest and will to live.

It is this giving up on the life that plays a role in interfering with the immune system and can, through changes in the hormonal balance, lead to an increase in the production of abnormal cells. Physically, it creates a climate that is right for the development of cancer,

argue C. Simonton and colleagues (1978). This situation represents a fundamental crisis of human life, which, as we previously mentioned, is related to a sense of impossibility of satisfying one's most important needs or the loss of the sense of purpose behind these needs. The individual becomes convinced (this certainty is most often unconscious) that all of their attempts to change their life are useless, and that life itself is hopeless and no longer attractive.

Psycho-oncologist Lawrence LeShan (1977) conducted a "blind" analysis (which means that he was not aware of the diagnoses of the people who filled in the questionnaires) of the results of Worthington's personal history test in which twenty-eight somatically ill patients took part, including fifteen cancer patients and thirteen patients with different diseases. By focusing on three main criteria— the loss of the meaning of life, the inability to express anger and indignation, and the death of a parent during one's childhood, the scientist was able to correctly determine the presence of cancer in fourteen out of the fifteen cancer patients. Such people, LeShan writes, continue to execute their daily responsibility, but no longer have a "taste" for life. It is as if they have nothing to keep living for: "They were simply waiting to die. For that seemed to them the only way out. They were ready for death. In one very real sense, they had already died ... inside—empty of feeling and devoid of self." The Simontons (1978) confirm that it may seem that the person lives a perfectly normal life on the outside, but for him or her existence has already lost any other meaning, except for the fulfillment of everyday duties. Serious illness or death then presents a way out of this situation, a solution for the problem, or its postponement.

So why is it that people who are predisposed to psychosomatic and especially oncological diseases experience a severe mental trauma or conflict so strong that it results not just in depression but in a loss of interest in life and the subsequent development of deadly disease? I will try to answer this question by taking the most frequently encountered oncogenic situation as an example: the loss of an important object to which one is strongly attached, such as the death of or separation from a person loved by the future patient.

Chapter 15

An Object of Paramount Importance as the Dominant Purpose of Life

We already know that the following characteristics can be observed in the majority of potential cancer patients: childish behavior (psychological infantilism), subordination, dependence, the desire to excessively satisfy other people's needs, avoidance of conflicts, and suppression (or repression) of emotions. These character traits, as was shown above, are developed during one's childhood on the basis of unmet need for love and disorders of attachment to parents or caregivers. In this case, the spouse/partner (or other attachment object) found later in life becomes the embodiment of the future patient's hope of receiving that love, which is often the individual's only or main need, and they devote their entire life to satisfying it. Then, if the object is lost or if there is a risk of not being able to satisfy the need for love, the individual treats such an experience as a crisis (Pleshchits S. G., 2012).

Karen Horney (1994) notes that for those with a subordinate type of personality, love often seems to be the only meaningful goal to go after, the value for which they should live. For such an individual, love can turn into a phantom, and the pursuit of it turns into a single aspiration, which is motivated by the feeling that they themselves are weak, helpless, and alone in the hostile and threatening world. But if the individual manages to succeed in finding someone who loves him/her more than anyone else, there is no longer any danger, since this someone will protect them.

And when such an object of paramount importance ("the all-powerful love object," according to Gunter Ammon, 1972) appears in the life of an individual, this object becomes the so-called dominant object in his consciousness, a temporarily dominating reflex, which ensures the satisfaction of the basic, i.e., dominant, needs. All other needs became secondary, and the reflex activities corresponding to them get suppressed. "Having at last found an outlet for their emotions," argues Lawrence LeShan (1977), "they (*the future cancer patients—V.*

M.) tended to put all their eggs into one basket. All meaning, all creativity, all happiness was seen as being bound up in this particular situation or relationship."

The doctrine of the dominant was developed by a remarkable Soviet scientist of the early twentieth century, Alexey Ukhtomskiy. "While the dominant is bright and alive in the individual's soul, it keeps the entire field of psychic life under its power," Ukhtomskiy (2002) wrote. "Everything is reminiscent of it and of the images and realities associated with it." Throughout their life, a person may have different current dominants that affect the functional state of their body, but some of them play the leading role. According to Ukhtomskiy (2002), the cortex associates a specific group of stimuli with the given biologically important dominant, allocates a certain image for it, a definite "completed auditory or visual face," which now becomes an exclusive excitative agent of the given dominant and is perceived as "some self-contained separateness from all other reality."

In the absence of other priorities (and especially spiritual ones), in the state of an existential vacuum, the dominant of the highly important subject or object takes on the functions of the dominant of the life goal (DLG) which is the main dominant of the individual that defines their mental state and life in general, to which all the current dominants are subordinated. The DLG concept, in the development of Ukhtomskiy's ideas, was elaborated by psycho-oncologist and immunologist Oleg Bukhtoyarov and his colleague, psychiatrist Dmitry Samarin (2010) from the Institute of Clinical Immunology of the Russian Academy of Medical Sciences:

> The dominant purpose of life is an immaterial construction, with a material expression. It is formed in the mental sphere and is manifested by means of the maximal integration of mental and physical processes, the subordination of the current person's subdomains, the maximal *sanogenic* and adaptive capabilities of the organism, which allows it most successfully withstand the constant pressure of environmental factors when achieving a vital goal. It is the DLG that ensures the coherence of the asynchronous operation of the organs and systems, the mental and somatic processes, determines the vector of seemingly chaotic, numerous reflexes of the organism, its current subdominants (biological, psychic, social, etc.) and the trajectory of everyday human behavior.

At the physiological level, the dominant corresponds to the center of excitation in the central nervous system, which includes various nerve centers that attract excitation waves from various sources in the body and are the basis for acts of attention and objective thinking (Ukhtomskiy A., 2002).

One of the main subdominants is the health subdominant, which, in situations of severe and traumatic stress and psychic trauma, can be lost together along with the DLG. In such situations, the person will find themselves in a transitional, non-dominant state, without any existence goals and at the mercy of everyday subdomains. In fact, this turns into a chronic exhausting psycho-emotional stress, with the corresponding mental and physical manifestations. An individual can remain in the non-dominant state from a mere few minutes to several years (Bukhtoyarov O. V., Samarin D. M., 2010), and this persistent state can obviously be referred to as an existential vacuum. One experiences a psychological crisis, a sense of an internal impasse that blocks the usual course of life. "Rachel cries for her children and cannot be consoled; does not want to be consoled, because they are not there! For Rachel, children are exceptional realities that cannot be substituted for anything!"—Ukhtomskiy (2002) gives as an example.

It is in this way that dependent relationships manifest their dangerous potential when, at their end, they leave a psychosomatic type "C" person in a state of total loneliness, particularly when he or she has not yet developed sufficient skills to cope with difficulties independently. All the life that the individual based around the lost relationship is destroyed when the relationship comes to an end. S. A. Kulakov (2009) notes that psychosomatic patients with a dependent personality disorder are particularly sensitive to loss of love and help. According to the theory of object relations created by the well-known psychoanalyst Heinz Kohut (2000), the founder of self-psychology, when individuals with the dependent self-structure which they carry with them from childhood lose objects of attachment, very strong feelings of helplessness, hopelessness, and longing tend to follow. This leads to the disruption of internal homeostasis, increases the body's vulnerability and the risk of diseases. Such a non-dominant state is very similar to the precancerous state discussed above, which is characterized by helplessness, hopelessness, and depression. But the main danger in it is the probability of losing one's meaning of life.

Walter Brautigam and colleagues (1997) consider the loss (real or imagined) of a "key figure" or object as a common provocative situation that occurs at the beginning of a disease or when it worsens. It was discovered that the reason for this is that the psychosomatic patient fully identifies with the object of attachment, is childishly dependent on it, and it is as if their overall existence is made possible thanks to the presence of this "key figure," that is, another person. Therefore, there is an increased sensitivity to separation, which can result in depression.

Here are some other examples of the non-dominant state. Bernie Siegel (1998) quotes an excerpt from a letter from a woman who developed cancer after her children left home: "I had an empty place in me, and cancer grew to fill it." Let us return to the case of Robert Dilts's (2006) mother. Here we learn that she also began to develop cancer when the youngest of her five sons moved out. After being a mother for more than thirty years, she suddenly found herself in a new situation, where she no longer needed the part of her character that was so accustomed to playing the role of the mother.

Upon analysis of the same matter, why the idea of loss has such catastrophic consequences for potential cancer patients, C. B. and M. B. Bahnson (1964) connect the reason with the retraumatization caused by a childhood experience.

After repeatedly losing significant relationships, a person begins to lose the hope of developing similar relationships again in the future. Psychodynamically, the reactivation of hopelessness leads to an intense regression reaction and switching of the emotional response to "inside of oneself," which can be evolutionarily reflected in an attempt to survive in a traumatic situation through "self-reproduction," that expresses through malignant cell growth. Therefore, the authors have developed the theory of "compensatory growth," according to which the rapid growth of undifferentiated (cancerous) tissue can be referred to as the organism's regressive attempt to replace the recent loss.

Jan Gawler (1984) believes that the fear which gave rise to a stressful reaction in a cancer patient originates from a fear of being unloved, rejected, insulted in his feelings. If the circumstances of one's life change against this background, and a person loses the means to keep fear under control and begins to experience despair, this will result in a terrible consequence: the loss of the will to live. According to observations made by O. D. Rozhkova (2015), cancer patients usually choose non-constructive life strategies, relying on an external object or task (be it a person, job, home, family). However, they fail to develop their own personality and life competence. When such an external means of support disappears (which may occur for various reasons), the risk of developing a depressive state and deteriorating health becomes very high.

In such cases, when a person is shaken by the death of a loved one or an irretrievable loss of someone or something that has a vital meaning for them, an intense experience of loss can take pathogenic forms and is viewed by psychologists as a state of "complicated grief." This state is characterized by an excessive duration and intensity, and leads to significant deterioration in health, working, and social functioning; that is, it results in chronic distress, which we discussed in Chapter 3. It has been revealed that for people experiencing grief in such a complicated manner, immunity is suppressed more than in people who are grieving in the "ordinary" manner (O'Connor M. F. et al., 2014). Such individuals have an increased risk of cardiovascular and oncological diseases, hypertension, suicide, alcohol and drug addictions (Szanto K. et al., 2006).

Individuals with childhood attachment disorders in general (Neimeyer R. A. et al., 2002; Prigerson H. G. et al., 1997) and anxious-ambivalent types in particular (Vanderwerker L. C. et al., 2006; Fagundes C. P., et al., 2012), are especially predisposed to developing complicated grief. For the type of people with avoiding attachment type, on the other hand, somatization is the more pronounced form of manifesting mourning (Wayment H. A., Vierthaler J., 2002), which corresponds to the data previously discussed.

If an individual cannot effectively cope with the grief of loss, find a new dominant purpose in life, and restore the subdominant of health, then, according to O. V. Bukhtoyarov and D. M. Samarin (2010), they fall under the influence of the dominant of the disease or even the dominant of self-destruction.

Chapter 16

The Dominant of Self-Destruction

The dominant of self-destruction is the pathological functional state of the body, which is characterized by the emergence of a dominant state of an aspiration for death instead of the DLG. We call it the death dominant, which includes, along with numerous pathological supporting subdomains, maximal disintegration of brain systems and psychosomatic processes, the disruption of sanogenetic and adaptive processes, which in turn lead to the death of the body,

— explain O. V. Bukhtoyarov and D. M. Samarin (2010).

In his book *The Will to Live*, American psychiatrist Arnold Hutschnecker (1983), former personal psychotherapist of President Richard Nixon, states that a person dies because they subconsciously want to die, although consciously capable of convincing themselves and others that they have everything that they require. Albert Camus (1990) was convinced that there only exists one serious philosophical question and that is whether one should continue to live when the meaninglessness of one's life is fully comprehended. He saw many people die because life was no longer worth living for them.

Sometimes the dominant of self-destruction starts to develop during childhood, when intolerable psychological pain causes a child to think, "it would be better for me to die." While initially being in a state of "incubation," this growing dominant is activated at full power in the psychotraumatic experiences that occur at a later age, that retraumatize the individual's childhood experiences. To illustrate this, I quote a story of a patient of mine.

Marina, a pretty and energetic ballet teacher of forty-eight years of age, came to see me because six months ago it seemed to her that her life had "suddenly collapsed." She quit her favorite job, because she could no longer stand her "inadequate boss," and then within two weeks her partner, with whom she had lived well for seven years, left. A couple of months later her health gave in—her old back and liver problems returned, she developed the initial stage of diabetes, and her thyroid function decreased. Marina felt depressed and helpless. She assumed that her health problems were the result of stressful events, but she could not understand why all of this happened to her at once, and how to live on. Separation from her partner caused Marina to suffer greatly. All her attempts to "assemble herself" and to "return to her normal life" were unsuccessful.

Following an examination, I found that the woman's psychosomatic system was in a critical condition. There was a high level of chronic stress and anxiety, low self-acceptance, aggression toward herself, a weak will to live, and a subconscious desire for death as a way out of her problems. I defined this condition as a precancerous one. Oddly enough, Marina was not too shocked by this news. It seemed as if she was ready for life to present her with even more unpleasant surprises. Fortunately, we had time to avoid panicking and to calmly find the sources of her problems and to develop a strategy for de-escalating the developed oncogenic distress.

The most important and urgent task was to eliminate something that I call the "death imprint" in her subconscious, which is a trace of a clear desire to die. This was what first initiated the formation of a self-destruction dominant. I was able to determine that this dominant began forming at the age of twelve to thirteen and the reason for this was Marina's relationship with her father.

During the course of further communication with Marina, an unhappy childhood story, overshadowed by fear of her strict and authoritarian father, unfolded. This kind of "upbringing" resulted in her attempt to throw herself out of her bedroom window at the age of thirteen. Her quiet and timid mother was not capable of becoming her support and protection. It was thanks to great luck that Marina's personality was not so "suffocated" as to fully obey her father, and after graduation Marina left home and entered ballet school, against her father's wishes. However, the sufferings experienced during childhood largely influenced her later life.

During the trance psychotherapy process, she realized that she had to fight and overcome life's difficulties throughout her life, just as she did during her childhood. This struggle did not make her stronger, but instead, created a state of chronic stress and disbelief in herself. The desire for death as a way to solve her problems was always present in her subconscious. When the level of the unconscious distress and the anxiety which reflected it outwardly, reached a maximum, and the resources of adaptation to external stimuli reduced to a minimum, she became unable to maintain constructive relationships. This is, in my opinion, what caused her relationships at job and at home to break down. As H. Stone and S. Winkelman (1988) write, "Disowning the 'chaos' within each of us causes disruption in our surroundings because these disowned energies operate subconsciously." For Marina's consciousness, this situation came as a surprise—a new psychic trauma, which led to the dominant of self-destruction being activated and critical disorders of her body functions emerged. During the age regression, Marina saw herself at the age of thirteen near the window, and we had to undertake the major task of removing the "death imprint" from her subconscious.

That is how after the loss of significant relationships, in a situation of hopelessness and despair, on top of chronic distress and a "non-dominant emptiness," a powerful pathological dominant of self-destruction can arise in the form of a psychosomatic disease, which O. V. Bukhtoyarov and A. E. Arkhangelskiy (2008) pertinently suggest calling the oncological dominant, in the case of its cancer variant. This oncodominant firmly takes the place of the purpose of life dominant and creates deep deformations of the psychosomatic system, while amplified and supported by the subdominants of anxiety, fear, insomnia, pain, etc.

The idea of an oncodominant is harmoniously derived from the theory proposed by Alexey Ukhtomskiy (2002):

> My doctrine of dominants in the central nervous [system] activity brings them to the higher levels of the nervous system and this coincides with the doctrine of 'mental complexes'... Here, the dominants are linked and individualized precisely through an emotive tone, to which the ideological content of one's life is predetermined to a certain extent, as well as the general range of one's activity under the given unilateral excitation. Dominants can continue their influence on one's psyche and life even when they move below the consciousness threshold... 'Wounded mental complexes', or simply speaking inhibited psycho-physiological contents, continue to subconsciously act on the whole psyche and are very pathogenic.

French psychiatrist Henri Baruk (1972) describes a similar phenomenon that appears under the influence of stress: "Emotion seems to be fixed in the brain and forms a pathogenic nucleus." Cognitive psychotherapy stems from the fact that stagnant excitement foci that arise in the emotional zones of the brain under the influence of the stressor lead to the formation of stable "erroneous cognitive schemes," rigid concepts which become the key cause of neurotic, anxious, or depressive responses to the environment (Beck S., 2011). Let us recall the research conducted by A. Biondi and A. Picardi (1996): if grief remains inconsolable or psychologically complicated, it becomes part of the nervous system of the grieving person, it is as if it was imprinted in their neurochemical basis, making the individual vulnerable to developing health disorders and depression. Even if this depression is hidden, it gives rise to anxiety and a sense of hopelessness with suicidal thoughts and attempts (Gindikin V. Y., 2000), that is, to autoaggressive intentions.

The formation of a new dominant in the cerebral cortex and an alternative psycho-physiological functional system on the basis of it was experimentally demonstrated in the neurosis clinic in St. Petersburg by using the model of psychogenic disorders (neurotic depression, neurotic anxiety, and neurotic asthenia, in particular). Factor analysis of the electroencephalogram in patients with such conditions revealed a disruption in the orderliness of interregional and intra-hemispheric relationships (Ivonin A. A. et al., 2008).

According to O. S. Bulgakova (2010), the formation of a traumatic adaptive dominant in the central nervous system is the result of an extended post-stress effect, which is expressed in the form of psychosomatic physiological dysfunctions. This effect is constantly reinforced by other kinds of stresses and reflects the body's state of unsatisfactory adaptation.

Psycho-oncologist Dr. Alexander Danilin (2011) also arrived at the conclusion that the formation of a pathological dominant leads to the development of cancer: "Upon being attracted to each other in the dominant, the fear of death and the desire to die become indistinguishable from each other."

This dominant can also be considered as a stable pathological condition, the concept of which was created by academician Dr. Natalia Bekhtereva (1978), the head of the brain institute in St. Petersburg. While studying the development of chronic pathological processes, she noticed that there is a state that is supported by a complex system of reactions. Its neurophysiological action mechanism makes it similar to the compensatory mechanism. However, it doesn't aim to maintain a stable state of the norm, but instead, a stable pathological state that has replaced the norm.

As for the provocation factors not related to the consequences of the loss of significant relationships, such as the provoking of unresolved intrapersonal conflicts, they probably lead to the emergence of the oncodominant in the ways that we discussed in Chapter 11. The most important of these reasons is the impossibility of living according to the desires of our Essence, which is, the lack of self-realization in life. This, according to Tom Laughlin (1999), creates a state of "suffocation." Lawrence LeShan (1977) also considers this situation: the main reason why future cancer patients lose the meaning of life is the lack of opportunities for them to be who they really are, to pursue their uniqueness. Very frequently a person, acting in accordance with the behavior learned during childhood, has to wear a mask that helps them earn love and recognition. However, by doing this the individual rejects their individuality and suppresses their real feelings. The fundamental sign of the character of such a person is the inability to go beyond the dilemma of "being yourself but lonely and unloved" or "pretending to be someone else to deserve love." Despair that develops because of the subjective insolubility of such conflicts and suffering arises in both cases and blocks the possibility of finding an alternative solution.

In another one of his books, LeShan (1989) writes that in a majority of the patients that he treated over thirty-five years, before the onset of cancer they experienced

> ...a loss of hope in ever achieving a way of life that would give real and deep satisfaction, that would provide a solid raison d'être, the kind of meaning that makes

us glad to get out of bed in the morning and glad to go to bed at night—the kind of life that makes us look forward zestfully to each day and to the future ... The problem of their unbearable existence was being solved for them by the cancer in a final, irrevocable getting rid of themselves.

Their cancer, in the words of poet W. H. Auden, can be seen as a "foiled creative fire."

These observations are confirmed by the clinical example of a patient from Taiwan, named Wang Si-Mei (2016), who was diagnosed with a rare and inoperable form of gastrointestinal cancer. The treatment methods available to her were very limited. The cancer was inoperable and the chemotherapy prospects were highly questionable. She writes: "I chose to face this devastating news of my cancer without sadness, because it seemed to me to be a release from the hardship and burdens of my unhappy life. The diagnosis gave me a sense of relief."

There is the concept of "Ikigai" in Japan, which is something that is worth living for, something that brings joy, happiness, and a sense of existence and is a primary factor in maintaining one's health. Scientists from the Aichi Cancer Center Research Institute in Nagoya spent 7.5 years observing 31,992 women between the ages of 40 and 79 years. One hundred and forty-nine of these women developed breast cancer during the monitoring and these had a significantly smaller "Ikigai" than those who did not get sick (Wakai K. et al., 2007). Consequently, the disappearance of the joy and meaning of life contributes to the emergence of a "non-dominant emptiness," which later gets filled with the dominant of self-destruction.

Thus, the "mental neoplasm," an oncological dominant, gives rise to a somatic neoplasm—cancer. According to the data reviewed, this may be due to the formation of the neurophysiological dominant in the cerebral cortex, which is the focus of excitation. It extends to the subcortical structures, primarily the limbic system, the hypothalamus, and the pituitary gland, which all together generate a state of chronic stress. On the other hand, this excitation focus can also extend to the cortical representation of a specific peripheral target organ, activating cell multiplication processes in it. This scheme as a whole is consistent with Dr. Hamer's (2000) idea that under the influence of the shock caused by psychological conflict the Special Biological Program unfolds, and this synchronously occurs at the level of the psyche, the brain, and the specific organ.

The autoregressive state of the psyche, which is caused by such a self-destruction dominant, has very similar characteristics to those of the state of the human psyche before suicide. This was already noticed in 1954 by Dr. Max Cutler, who stated that cancer can be referred to as "passive and unconscious suicide." Therefore, it seems appropriate to turn to the science of suicidology and analyze whether or not this hypothesis can be confirmed.

Chapter 17

The "Suicidal" and the "Cancer" Personality: What do They Have in Common?

The concept of avital[1] activity, which was developed by Russian psychiatrist Yuriy Vagin (2011), is the most compatible with the topic at hand. The author explains this concept as biological, psychological, and behavioral activity aimed at damaging and/or terminating one's social and biological functioning.

According to Dr. Vagin and other scientists (Yuryeva L. N, 2006; Pilyagina G. Y., 1999), suicidal activity aimed at the conscious cessation of life is one of the main phenomena of avital activity, but definitely not the only one, reflecting the autoaggressiveness of personality in this context. As I noted in Chapter 12, this also includes both internal (thoughts, attitudes, ideas, emotions), and external (substance abuse, risk behaviors, ignoring the symptoms of the disease, antisocial behavior, self-harm) methods of self-destruction.

Being the basis of suicidal behavior, avital (also called antivital) feelings appear as a result of socio-psychological maladjustment of one's personality due to the lack of compensatory mechanisms and skills in constructive coping with stress, against the background of a conflict between the actual need and the factors that prevent it from being satisfied (Sagalakova O. A. et al., 2014). This is confirmed by a well-known suicide expert, E. S. Shneidman (1998), who investigated how unmet needs are capable of provoking suicidal behavior. These unmet needs include dissatisfaction in love (including the desire for support and friendship), violation of control (the need for independence, achievement, order, and understanding), distortion of how the "I" is portrayed (the need for social support, self-justification, and avoidance of shame), the destruction of significant

---

[1] Avital—in Greek *a* is a nullifying prefix and in Latin *vita* means "life."

relationships and grief caused by loss (need for caring for a friend or loved one), excessive anger (need for domination, aggression, and opposition). As we have already discussed in previous chapters, all of this can be fully attributed to future cancer patients.

It is necessary for us to direct more of our attention to the internal forms of avital activity, many of which are not consciously recognized by the individual. Suicidology describes these in similar and sometimes contradictory terms such as "parasuicide," "indirect suicide," "half-intended suicide," "chronic suicide," "protracted suicide," "organic suicide," "partial suicide," "suicidal equivalent," "unconscious suicidal behavior," "autodestructive (self-destructive, destructive) behavior," "autoaggressive behavior," "equivalent forms of self-destructive behavior," etc. (Vagin Y. R., 2011; Pilyagina G. Y., 2013).

Avital activity emerges in the most "simple," pre-suicidal form, when the hidden and unconscious avital tendencies gradually increase and range from the waiting syndrome and chronic fatigue to the conscious unwillingness to live, but without the conscious desire to terminate one's life.

The "waiting syndrome" (unfulfilled expectations) is manifested when an individual's existence at a given moment in time deeply dissatisfies them, but they feel powerless to influence the course of the events in any way, and therefore expect something to happen in their life without their putting in any effort. There is no conscious lack of interest in life as a whole—life at the current moment is simply unappealing for the individual. However, there is still a sliver of hope that something may change for the better in the future, although this hope is exclusively associated with external circumstances that do not depend on the individual him/herself (an external locus of control) (Vagin Y. R., 2011). In my opinion, this stage corresponds to a certain period of oncological disease development, when helplessness has already developed, but not yet turned to hopelessness.

According to Yuriy Vagin, the basis of the waiting syndrome is the formation of a "congestive focus" of negative emotions, which the person cannot completely suppress or repress. This is due to the fact that the existing need cannot (for various reasons) be transformed into behavior that is directed at its satisfaction. I dare say that such a focus can be the emerging oncological dominant.

Further, asthenic conditions and fatigue from life can emerge and this occurs when the desire to live still exists, but there already is a noticeable lack of vital force. These patients feel that they live mechanically, because "everybody has to do it": they got married, gave birth to children, raised children, retired, attended their spouse's funeral—while subconsciously realizing that "soon my end will arrive and that is a good thing, because I am so tired." If nothing changes in such an individual's life, then the hope of a turn for the better fades away, followed by a decreased desire to live, and is later replaced by the feeling that "life is not worth living." This condition is especially characteristic of people who find themselves in difficult life circumstances. The author emphasizes that a person who has lost faith in the future is prone to dying from any infectious disease because of complete decline of mental and physical strength (Vagin Y. R., 2011). As we see, this pre-suicide period is very similar to the state of hopelessness and helplessness experienced by many people before the onset of cancer.

Shortly after the unwillingness to live, the desire to die emerges, and it is a logical result of the loss of meaning and purpose in life, as well as of the lack of hope for change for the better. Such anomic[1] experiences characterize the deviant (in this case suicidal) behavior that develops as a result of suffering due to unmet needs. According to the Russian suicidologist G. I. Gordon, "It is as if a spring breaks somewhere inside the person and this spring controlled the entire complex mechanism of the individual's being. The force that once gave the individual thoughts and desires, forced him to act, fight, and strive for things, to simply live, was weakened" (cited by Vagin Y. R., 2011). Thoughts about the desirability of death begin to come out of the Shadow and appear on a conscious level: "It would be good to fall asleep and not wake up," "It would be good to accidentally fall under a car or perish in some catastrophe," "People who develop severe, incurable diseases are lucky..." And the subconscious "fulfills the request" of such an individual—either by forming suicide plans (which signifies a major, conscious suicidal drive), or in the occurrence of an "unexpected" accident, or by developing a deadly disease.

The last version Dr. Vagin, following psychiatrist Karl Menninger (1956), refers to the so-called "organic suicide," which develops according to the mechanisms of psychosomatic diseases. The author classifies this type of suicide as para-suicidal activity, manifested as a person's conscious desire to limit, reduce, disrupt, or jeopardize their own biological functioning (in the form of the external self-destruction modes described above), but without the conscious desire for suicide. However, the individual has an unconscious desire to cease to exist, which manifests itself in the disease.

Reid Henson, the co-author of Carl Simonton, experienced a lot of personal problems before he was diagnosed with cancer, and his autobiographical memoirs clearly illustrate this avital condition in oncology:

> I had less and less confidence that I could cope successfully with the difficult problems I was encountering. A feeling of helplessness had emerged in my life, and with it, a feeling of hopelessness.
>
> It is important to understand that I did not consciously wish to die, even though my subconscious beliefs about guilt and punishment indicated that I did not deserve to live. In fact, I thought I was going to live for a long time.
>
> … It seems to me that deep dissatisfaction with life (often called depression, among other things) causes some sub-conscious "switches" to be flipped that

---

[1] From the French *anomie*—lawlessness, lack of normality.

prepare the body for death—which releases the person from the very troubling circumstances encountered in this dimension. My normal bodily functions were altered. Significant changes became evident over a period of time, with the eventual diagnosis of cancer (Simonton C. O., Henson R. M., 1992).

Upon exploring the nature of self-destruction in his book *Man Against Himself*, Karl Menninger (1956) draws a clear line between the apparent and the chronic forms of suicide. In the latter case, a person delays a fatal outcome and pays for this with suffering and their bodily functions being weakened. This is identical to "partial suicide," which can also be referred to as "living death." However, since destructive impulses in such individuals often keep progressing during their life, their disease, which will eventually result in death, also progresses. In such cases, the organic disease acts merely as a sign of a general disintegration of the person who is determined to destroy themselves.

Menninger believes that the bases for this are the following subconscious factors:

a) an impulse of hostility directed at an external object or subject (*which may correspond to the suppressed aggression of cancer patients*—*V. M.*);

b) an impulse to punish themselves, which is created by a sense of guilt and defines the above-mentioned hostility. According to the author, self-punishment, especially in the presence of excessive "correctness" or "rectitude," is one of the most important subconscious factors that create organic disease symptoms. Menninger uses the significant metaphor: hypertrophied, a "cancerous conscience" generates a sense of guilt, which then causes depression and, as a result—destructive actions. This definition of guilt and rigid "correctness" perfectly describes the situation that Reid Henson and other cancer patients cited above found themselves in.

c) an erotic impulse that has a masochistic sacrifice nature. This is an aspect that we have also examined before when looking at the traits of cancer personalities (researchers found the sexuality and masochism disorders to be present there). I already mentioned that Menninger views such sacrifice as a "neurotic martyrdom"—a form of self-destructive behavior based on one's unconscious desire for death.

The author also draws our attention to the lack of love experienced by suicidal individuals, stressing that its function (*libido*) normally results in the transformation of destructive tendencies into productive forms. These include the self-preservation instinct, social activity, and the formation of self-consciousness. Owing to the lack of love (*as we already know, this issue arises during childhood and has a role in the formation of a predisposition to diseases*—*V. M.*), productive factors gradually disappear, and death prevails (Menninger K., 1956).

Bernie Siegel (1989) genuinely agrees with this: "If you doubt the damage caused by the lack of self-love in our lives, you have only to look around you. Notice how many people commit suicide, overtly or otherwise, with accidents and untreated illnesses. We're so self-destructive that there have to be laws—what I call please-love-yourself laws..."

Ukrainian suicidologist, professor Galina Pilyagina (2013) has developed the concept of equivalent forms of self-destructive behavior, aimed at unconscious or conscious self-destruction. These forms are potentially disastrous and accelerate the death of a person, despite the fact that immediate suicidal or other self-damaging actions are not taken. Although such equivalents have a very low level of direct suicidal risk, they have a sufficiently high autodestructive potential, since the self-damaging effects of their presence accumulate over time, leading to both the psychic (psychological) self-destruction of the individual's personality and the physical destruction of their organism.

Dr. Pilyagina believes that the mechanism of such self-destructive behavior is an uncontrollable excess of emotions, which in turn lead to a critical increase in the level of frustration and aggression, intense anxiety and fear, prolonged psychosomatic overstrain, as well as various neurotic symptom-complexes (*as we have already seen, all of this also corresponds to a precancerous state—V. M.*). To somehow stabilize the psychosomatic state and reduce the subjectively intolerable level of mental pain, a person resorts to the form of psychological defense that we are now familiar with: a shift in intrapersonal, cognitive-emotional and external behavioral activity.

Let me remind you that shifted activity can be directed outward (expressed in external forms of autoaggression); This occurs when intense negative emotions manifest themselves clinically in the form of self-damaging or suicidal actions. Or this shifted activity can be directed inward (internal forms of autoaggression), which happens when the behavioral manifestation of intensive emotions is repressed, but their energy is expressed in the form of various bodily dysfunctions.

The emergence of shifted activity occurs at an early age and is a result of psychic traumatization and chronic dissatisfaction with the basic needs of the child, accompanied by intense feelings of guilt, resentment, protest, and psychological pain. The aggressive energy created by these feelings gets pushed back into the subconscious and this occurs because that the child is not able to adequately express them in relation to the caregiving adult in the unharmonious child–adult relationship. In addition, hostile energy becomes a platform for the formation of a hypercognitive variant of CEID. As the permanent anti-vital feelings and periodic suicidal thoughts begin to appear, this energy manifests itself clinically in the forms of self-destructive behavior as self-punishment, self-sacrifice, or a negative life balance. Since it develops over a long period of time, the process of psychological shift is constantly reinforced owing to the formation of a pathological dominant in the individual's neuropsychological activity (Pilyagina G. Y., 2013). Therefore, this is one more aspect of the formation of the dominant of self-destruction that is equivalent to the oncological dominant—as a result of the internally shifted activity.

Children's psychic traumas and subsequent pathological adaptation to life conditions become a predisposing factor in the development of autoaggressive behavior leading to suicide, similarly to mechanisms of psychosomatic diseases. Psychological violence inflicted by parents or caregivers and the conditional nature of their love (when the child can only be loved *for* something), categorical rejection of the individual needs of children, indifferent, rigid, and perfectionist parental attitudes are especially traumatic for the psyche of future suicidal individuals, as well as future cancer patients. Research shows that students who have attempted suicide have memories of emotionally "absent" parents, particularly the mother, in their childhood (de Jong M. L., 1992). A similar situation was observed during the childhoods of future cancer patients (Roe A., Siegelman M., 1963; Thomas C. B. et al., 1979; Shaffer J. et al., 1987).

Physical and sexual abuse of the child, especially if it is repeated, has a cumulative effect and makes a significant contribution to the occurrence of suicidal thoughts and attempts. It is established that the accumulated traumatic childhood experiences, such as a combination of the parents' alcoholism, rape, aggressive behavior of family members, problems with physical health, etc., cause the individual to be highly vulnerable to stressful events in adulthood and provoke suicidal feelings (Rozanov V. A. et al., 2011; Amaral A. P., Vaz Serra A., 2009; Borges G. et al., 2008).

Similarly, those having suicidal thoughts depend emotionally on their mother and have a symbiotic relationship with her. When she is authoritarian, anxious, and over-caring (a "psychosomatic mother"), they develop psychosomatic disorders. Just like future cancer patients, they experience additional psychic traumas, especially those that are associated with the suicidal individual's attempt to create a lifestyle of their own that does not coincide with the parents' opinion. Such individuals develop the sensation of an existential crisis, a feeling of unbearable loneliness, helplessness, and hopelessness (Pilyagina G. Y., 2003).

American scientists also confirm these findings: a prolonged stay of children in the "space of cruelty" triggers the phenomenon of "paradoxical self-destruction" as a way of avoiding the traumatic impact caused by the environment. In addition, it disrupts cognitive abilities, behavior patterns, interpersonal interactions, and influences the entire subsequent life of a person (Conger R. D. et al., 2003). A number of these behavior patterns are similar to those expressed by future cancer patients, such as psychological infantilism, the predominance of external control (i.e., dependence on external circumstances and belief that the surroundings should change and not the person themselves), rejection of oneself and acceptance of others (or vice versa), activation of psychological defenses in the form of repression of negative emotions, displacement and reactive formations (Pilyagina G. Y., 2003).

Avital experiences (as one of the internal forms of pre-suicidal self-aggression) emerge also as a result of an individual's perception of themselves as a non-independent, needy, incompetent, incapable of manifesting an initiative and achieving results, helpless, subordinate, dependent, and in need of care (Sagalakova O. et al., 2014). Factors that play a major role in suicidality are experiencing a high level of mental pain and at the same time containing it, that is, the accumulation of emotions in the subconscious, and not allowing them to be expressed (Haritonov S. V., 2013; Pilyagina G. Y., 2013); pronounced selfishness and overstated claims, rigidity in assessing the situation, alexithymia, a tendency to be emotionally dependent, psychological vulnerability, high anxiety, suppressed self-doubt, and dissatisfaction with the results achieved (Pilyagina G. Y., 2003). We also observe similar personality and behavior traits in cancer patients.

Edwin Shneidman (1998) comments that when we are confronted with an individual's suicide, at first glance, it appears that the individual had no reason whatsoever to take their own life, regardless of whether it was directly or indirectly. However, if we take a deeper look at the individual's character and behavior during their life, we will be able to notice subtle suicidal hints. It is necessary to examine their emotional state, their ability to endure psychic pain, and try to find other "escape paradigms" that were used by the individual. Once that is done, we will be able to understand the reason for the suicide. This is what we saw in the clinical case of Marina in the previous section.

Further psychotraumatic events that happen to a suicidal individual become provocative factors and are a starting point for a transition from internal to external forms of self-aggression, in this way creating an "irresistible desire to destroy subjectively intolerable emotions through self-destruction" (Pilyagina G. Y., 2003). This is because a mental trauma leads to instinct and affection distortions, which inevitably weaken and pervert the instinct of self-preservation (Tukaev R. D., 2003). A study was conducted where a significantly greater number of psychotraumatic events in the lives of patients with both internal forms of autoaggression and external suicidal forms were revealed, compared to the control group (Pilyagina G. Y., 2004).

According to psychiatrists from the University of Pittsburgh, complicated grief caused by the loss of a loved one provoked suicidal thoughts in 65% of people surveyed. As a result, more than half of them showed self-destructive behavior, including 9% of them who attempted suicide and 29% who showed indirect suicidal behavior (Szanto K. et al., 2006). R. D. Goldney's (1981) research demonstrated that women who attempted suicide had more often experienced the death of one or both parents, their divorce, or living apart from one of their parents during childhood, than women who made no suicide attempts. Quarrels and disagreements between parents were more often observed in families where suicidal women grew up, and their attitude to their parents' personalities and behavior was negative.

In a similar pattern to that encountered with cancer patients, the second most important factor that causes an individual to develop a desire for suicide is unresolved psychological problems—both intra- and interpersonal conflicts that engender mental pain (Sokolova E. T., Sotnikova Y. A., 2006; Starshenbaum G. V., 2005; Foster T., 2011; Koivumaa-Honkanen H. et al., 2001). Their nature contains the same unmet needs which we examined in Chapter 11. Edwin Shneidman (1998) confirms that the common stressors in suicide are frustrated psychological needs, and should these needs be satisfied, the suicide will not occur.

However, even when an individual experiences persistent suicidal thoughts (in addition to predominantly neurotic disorders), most cases of internal self-aggression do not transform into an external form and self-destruction does not occur. When it is the result of shifted activity, autoaggression, in such people, manifests in the repression of frustration and aggressive feelings, in a decrease in social activity and self-realization, and in limited interpersonal interactions, which in turn increase the severity of neurotic and somatized disorders. That is why 83.81% of patients with internal forms of self-aggression suffering a significant depletion of adaptive reserves were found to develop psychosomatic disorders (Pilyagina G. Y., 2003); one of them may be cancer.

Denial and rejection of the traumatizing situation leads to self-denial, since the need to resolve a psychogenic conflict by any means becomes more significant than one's own life. Therefore, "excluding oneself" from a difficult situation allows a person to resolve the conflict and get rid of severe psychic pain. In this manner, an internal variant of a pathological adaptation gets manifested – "I repress the desire to destroy you, so instead I destroy myself, because I cannot destroy you". As it progresses it can be transformed into an external, suicidal variant (Pilyagina G. Y., 2000, 2003), or into an internal one, which could end up being oncological. Sigmund Freud (1990) also had his own opinion about this: One can find suppressed aggression at the base of a suicidal act. It is a kind of resentment against the whole world, which a person cannot express externally on account of various circumstances, so the person transforms this into aggression directed at themselves. Let us recall the words of psycho-oncologist Alexander Danilin (2011), which can be related to this opinion: a cancer patient is "offended by the whole world."

The development of an existential crisis accompanied by high levels of helplessness and hopelessness becomes the most important cause for the autoaggressive motives that arise in people with internal forms of self-aggression, as well as in cancer patients. This is what determines the suicidal readiness of the individual and causes the internal form of autoaggression to transform into a clinically observed external disorder (Pilyagina G. Y., 2004). M. L. Farber (1968) considers suicide to be a "disease of hope." On the other hand, according to B. J. Limandri and D. W. Boyle (1978), hopelessness and the loss of the will to live can be referred to as a form of passive suicide, and when combined with desperate depression, hopelessness becomes a key factor in suicidal tendencies and serious suicide attempts (Beck A. X. et al., 1975; Kazdin A. E. et al., 1983). E. I. Tereshchuk (2012) argues that when an individual is depressed, their aggression turns against their own personality, which is the reason for the individual's desire to commit suicide. The author believes that the base for this behavior is an extremely low self-esteem and insufficient self-love, which is rooted in a lack of love by parents or caregivers.

17.1. Similar Biological Mechanisms

Modern suicidology shares the biopsychosocial approach to this pathology, making use of the same diathesis-stress concept as psychosomatic medicine does—after all, these two types of pathology have the same sources. The psycho-social model of "stress-vulnerability" created by Danuta Wasserman (2001) represents suicide as a process unfolding in time that has biological predisposition (vulnerability to stresses based on neurotransmitting and genetic factors), under the influence of risk factors, which are social and personal stressors, and dependent on stability factors—protective mechanisms (mainly social order) and the ability to cope with stress.

In his neurobiological concept of suicide diathesis, John Mann (1998) informs us of a certain predisposition to suicide, whose formation is caused by the interaction of genetic factors and acquired susceptibility. Psycho-traumatic events, mental and behavioral disorders (including those that are the result of the use of psychoactive substances), chronic diseases, etc. are referred to as acquired susceptibility by the author.

The state of physiological and neurotransmitter systems in those who are prone to suicide or have attempted it is generally associated with the fact that these systems take part in mechanisms of stress and depression. Similarly, we can also observe hyperactivity of the hypothalamic-pituitary-adrenal system, involvement of serotonergic, dopaminergic, noradrenergic, GABAergic and other brain systems, suppression of the immune system's activity, and growth of inflammatory reactions (Rozanov V. A., 2004).

As in oncology, the understanding of genetic mechanisms of suicidality is changing. In the past, the observed phenomena of a high incidence of suicide (as well as psychological pathology, especially depression) among children and relatives of individuals who committed suicide (Tsuang M. T., 1983; Baldessarini R. J., Hennen J., 2004) were associated with classical genetic conditioning (Shulsinger F. et al., 1979). Over the last decade, geneticists have come to the conclusion that family manifestations of this kind of self-aggression are closely associated with personal characteristics and the amount and intensity of stress experienced by family members (Brent D. A., Melhem N., 2008; Brezo J. et al., 2008). Genes associated with suicide are activated only in the presence of predisposing factors, which are severe damaging stress in early childhood, specific personality traits (for example, high neuroticism), and traumatic life events, in particular the loss of social status in adulthood (Caspi A. et al., 2003; Statham D. J. et al., 1998).

The role of epigenetic mechanisms in the formation of suicidal activity became evident as soon as there was sufficient scientific data (Labonte B., Turecki G., 2011; Rozanov V. A., 2015). For example, one study found that the methylation intensity of a gene that determines synthesis of a receptor to a stress hormone, cortisol, is increased in the brains of suicidal individuals if they experienced violence during their childhood. As a result, the content of this receptor in the brain decreases and the growth of cortisol goes out of control, which probably leads to hyperactivity of the hypothalamic-pituitary-adrenal system (McGowan P. O. et al., 2009).

As a result of experimental chronic stress, methylation of the nerve tissue growth factor (BDNF) gene increases, which leads to the inhibition of this nerve-cell survival regulator synthesis in certain parts of the brain (Roth T. L. et al., 2011; Tsankova N. M. et al., 2006). This in turn corresponds to an increase in the methylation of this gene in the blood of people experiencing suicidal thoughts (internal form of self-aggression) and those who have already attempted suicide (external form of self-aggression) (Kang H. et al., 2013). This also corresponds to the data gathered on the decrease in BDNF concentration in the brain and blood samples taken from suicide victims (Deveci A. et al., 2007).

The discovery made by Korean scientists in the above cited study is of particular significance to this subject matter (Kang H. J. et al., 2013) They determined that the increased methylation of the BDNF gene is associated not with the number of actual negative stressful events in a person's life but with the their thoughts about depriving themselves of life. This once again confirms the validity of the central idea of this book: All the types of pathology that occur in our bodies are the result of the erroneous functioning of our mind!

17.2. Confirmatory Observations Made by Other Authors

Similarities in the mechanisms of development of both types of pathology, as well as the individual characteristics of cancer patients and suicidal individuals, have been noticed by a number of scientists and health practitioners.

In Chapter 9.2 on the type "C" personality, I mentioned the long-term observations of medical university students conducted by Dr. Caroline Thomas and colleagues (1974). Among the individuals she examined were those who contracted cancer and those who committed suicide. The findings led her to an "astounding and unexpected" conclusion: the psychological characteristics of people who developed cancer were almost identical to the characteristics of those students who subsequently committed suicide.

Psychotherapist S. P. Semenov (2007) believes that malignant tumors, along with other serious diseases, can express one thing—anthropoptosis, which is the socially conditioned self-destruction of an individual. According to Dr. Semenov, this is a kind of suicidal act that can be the result of an aggressive attitude either toward oneself or toward one's life that is manifested in the form of suicide; or a consequence of depression or other suffering, when self-destruction becomes an appealing option for getting rid of the suffering. The author writes:

> Here is the formula of anthropoptosis: premature death occurs due to the organism's loss or deprivation of its natural purpose of existence. ... If for some reason the Alter EGO (the other 'I') becomes the enemy telling the individual: 'die!', the person then either commits suicide or dies from one of the immediately developing fatal ailments. Apparently, in most cases, it is precisely such an 'order', that has been unconsciously given by an individual to themselves in one form or another, or received in a veiled form from society, that is the main psychological mechanism of anthropoptosis.

On the basis of working with cancer patients Dr. Graham Gorman (1997) argued that, as a result of prenatal mental trauma, a person can become convinced that death is a possible way out of a situation of unbearable stress. And if such subjective stress has already been given the opportunity to form during childhood or adolescence, it can influence earlier development of avital activity. When speaking of conflicts based on mutual misunderstanding between parents and adolescents, Dr. Frederick Levenson (1985) emphasizes that the child perceives this lack of understanding as a lack of their parents' love, as a rejection by them: "This pushing away can eventually lead to totally self contained hyperirritation, which can be fatal. In adolescence it leads to suicide, which can be either conscious and direct (pills, guns, hanging, etc.) or unconscious and indirect (auto accidents, overdoses, provoked homicide, leukemia, etc.)."

Psycho-oncologist Dr. Alexander Vasyutin (2011) found that the exchange of information with the subconscious is very often disturbed in cancer patients:

> The feeling of hopelessness, helplessness, and despair that a person has already been experiencing for some period of time, eventually transforms itself into a powerful message to the subconscious: "It's impossible to live like that!" and "I do not want to live like this!" It is AT THIS MOMENT that the person gives their

subconscious a command for self-destruction, after which the subconscious closes in itself and begins to work on the extermination of the body.

Psychotherapist Francine Shapiro (2001) draws attention to the fact that the cancer patient must ultimately answer the following question for themselves: "Do I want to live?," while being ready to face any negative emotions. Indeed, at a regular appointment one of my patients, who was suffering from a tumor in the uterus, told me: "I am doing meditation, reiki, and the exercises that you taught me. I try not to lose motivation ... but something happened: I realized that I actually still haven't decided if I want to heal myself..."

Professor A. V. Gnezdilov (2002), a psychiatrist and psycho-oncologist, notes that frequently depression results in the reluctance to live on, and although consciously everyone is afraid of disease and does not want to fall ill, this subconscious reluctance to live can trigger the mechanism of disease. One such disease can be cancer. Dr. Alexander Danilin (2011) expresses a similar opinion. He writes in his book: "We do not want to die, while also wanting death to bring our torment to an end." The remarkable twentieth-century Danish philosopher, Søren Kierkegaard (1981), confirms the existence of such an experience: "Anxiety is the desire for what one fears, this is sympathetic antipathy; anxiety is an alien power which grips the individual, and yet he cannot tear himself free from it and does not want to, for one fears, but what he desires."

In his clinical psychotherapeutic practice, Antonio Meneghetti (1977) has encountered the invariably present strong (partly conscious, partly unconscious) desire in a patient that led them to develop the disease. "The appearance of the tumor is accompanied by the following internal decision: 'Either I will become who I should be, or I will die! I do not want to change anything, I do not want to adapt'."

Upon observing cancer patients, S. Grof and J. Halifax (1978) were able to notice that the number of depressive states, pronounced negative attitudes toward life, self-destructive and suicidal tendencies were stronger than it expected in the average statistical sample population. One of their patients, who was in the process of psychedelic therapy, viewed her sadness as the main theme of her life, lasting from early childhood throughout her life. She realized that she was always trying to hide it and show people what they apparently wanted to see in her: "smile," "look alive," "stop dreaming," and how much energy she wasted while pretending to be content, happy, or smiling: " I became suddenly aware that I had found a way to legitimize my lifelong sadness: to become terminally ill."

In the work conducted in the St. Petersburg Research Institute of Oncology the attitude to life of cancer patients with different types of personalities was studied. It was found that owing to the discrepancy between the desired world and reality, those with the hysteroid personality experience a hypertrophied sense of "eternal loss" and "deprivation of the possibility of further happiness," with the appropriate self-pity and the declared renunciation of life. The crisis associated with the loss of a loved one or a social situation provoked self-destructive tendencies of the "nothing to live for" type. *Cycloid* patients expressed depressive feelings with a predominantly subconscious and sometimes conscious refusal to continue living (Gnezdilov A. V., 1996).

The initial tendencies for self-destruction in women with uterine body cancer are defined as their most important psychological characteristics (Volodin B. Y., 2007), whereas Dr. M. Cutler (1954) regards the feeling of guilt in women with breast tumors as their self-punishment for their hostility. Therefore, he called for special attention to be directed to the internalized tendencies for self-destruction in cancer patients.

17.3. Manifestation of Avital Feelings: Cancer or Suicide?

The data examined above indicates that the same four factors that we identified in cancer patients are also present in the development of suicidal behavior:

- predisposition (including hereditary) that formed during the development of the organism and in childhood;

- provocation factors—acute and chronic psychic traumas and inner conflicts;

- a state of pre-illness (premorbid)—helplessness, hopelessness and depression;

- the factor of initialization—the loss of the meaning and will to live.

This allows me to confirm that at the psychological level the oncological disease is an autodestructive equivalent and is one of the internal forms of self-aggression.

Why does autoaggression (most often unconscious) that increases over the course of one's life and leads to avital experiences, depression and, eventually, the loss of the will to live, in some cases lead to suicide (an external form of self-destruction), and in others to cancer (an internal form)?

In my opinion, the answer to this question is overall the same as that to the question of the dichotomy of oncological-mental diseases, which was discussed in Chapter 12.4. It is common knowledge that the growth in frequency of suicide is equal to an individual's degree of mental ill health. Therefore, it can be assumed that the path of development of avital activity also depends on the way that an individual deals with psycho-emotional problems. Should the conflict be externalized, the process will develop in the psycho-pathological, up to suicidal direction, while the internalization of the conflict will cause the process to develop in the direction of somatic pathology, with cancer being an extreme degree of its manifestation. The formation of a dominant of self-destruction and the launch of the corresponding executive program are common to both directions.

Earlier we arrived at the conclusion that such a difference in the way of processing a traumatic conflict is associated with childhood attachment disorders. The formation of a hypercognitive CEID variant, along with the avoiding type of an attachment disorder, leads to a predominant conflict somatization, while the regressive-emotional CEID type with a basis in an anxious-ambivalent disorder of attachment leads to a predominant resolution of problems in the direction of psychopathology. On the basis of this, it can be assumed that an anxious–ambivalent disorder of attachment more often than not contributes to resolving a life crisis through suicide.

Indeed, the regressive-emotional version of CEID can lead to a disorder of adaptation, development of emotionally unstable, hysterical, mosaic, and schizotypal personality disorders, and the emergence of clinically observed forms of self-destruction that quickly progress to suicidal actions. This takes place during stressful circumstances and can occur as early as during adolescence (Pilyagina G. Y., 2013). A number of studies have also confirmed that the anxious–ambivalent attachment disorder leads to a greater likelihood of suicidal thoughts and actions when compared to the avoiding attachment disorder (Wright J. et al., 2005; Stepp S. D. et al., 2008; Grunebaum M. F. et al., 2010; Lessard J. C., Moretti M. M., 1998; Levi-Belz Y. et al., 2013). The latter is characterized by a longer development period of avital experiences and a lower frequency of suicidal thoughts. In stressful circumstances, such people are prone to severe depression and careful consideration of suicidal actions (Pilyagina G. Y., 2013).

In other words, if an individual's personality traits make it natural for them to suppress and repress their negative feelings, to express them through somatization, then it is very likely that such a powerful existential experience as the loss of the will to live will be unconsciously manifested through a severe bodily disease, such as cancer. I have already mentioned Tom Laughlin's (1999) observations that oncogenic conflicts of future cancer patient remain unknown to them, since they occur in the subconscious and the person does not realize their own suffering. The fact that many cancer patients were not aware of their state of helplessness, despair, and hopelessness prior to their diagnosis was also noted by O. V. Bukhtoyarov and A. E. Arkhangelskiy (2008). Søren Kierkegaard (2013) writes that some people experience "double despair": although they are already in despair, they are so used to deceiving themselves that they do not even suspect that they are in despair.

Alternatively, if negative experiences are commonly expressed outwardly in the form of emotional instability, then the loss of the will to live is most likely to be manifested through suicide. Consequently, the type of childhood attachment disorder, along with other predisposing factors, largely determines the direction of avital activity.

Another important aspect is the strength of the so-called anti-suicide barrier. This is understood as a combination of resources that helps a person cope with a suicidal situation: their personal characteristics, beliefs, and values (including religious ones), their possibilities and social ties, as well as other resources and circumstances that prevent the individual from choosing suicide as an option to help them resolve a crisis in a suicidogenic situation (Trunov D. G., 2013).

The author refers to the most common anti-suicide factors: "the instinct of self-preservation"; fear of death, pain, and possible suffering; fear of the unknown; physical and aesthetic rejection of the act of suicide and its consequences; the sense of owing something to their family and others; reluctance to cause loved ones to suffer; responsibility for the ongoing business and the existence of unrealized plans; the feeling of the uselessness of the suicidal act; the desire to win by all means in spite of all circumstances; religious prohibitions and ideas about the sinfulness of suicide; fear of public condemnation, of assessing suicide as a shameful act, as a manifestation of weakness or mental abnormality, etc. (Trunov D. G., 2013).

Most likely, it is precisely the specific combination of the psychosomatic "C" type personality, with its proneness to internalize conflicts and negative feelings, and an individual set of anti-suicidal factors, that makes the subconscious choose such a "civilized" method of self-destruction as cancer.

Upon examining the same question, Lawrence LeShan (1977) reports that although the probability of suicide was always present in future cancer patients, they pushed it aside or suppressed it. The author refers to Karl Menninger, who believed that in order for suicide to occur, three factors need to be present in the human psyche: the desire to die, the desire to kill, and the desire to be killed. In the case of cancer, LeShan discovered that only the first factor is present: the desire to die. He assumes that what prevents such people from committing suicide is the lack of aggression toward other people (*i.e. there is no desire to kill—V. M.*). Therefore, they simply allow the cancer to do its job.

At the same time, in my opinion, the most important anti-suicidal factor is the level of a person's spirituality, which determines whether or not there is a presence of meaning in their life.

Chapter 18

The Spiritual—Existential Crisis as the Basis of Self-Destruction

> The cause of disease is not external;
> it is in the mind—or we could say, it is the mind.
> Lama Zopa Rinpoche,
> *Ultimate Healing*

The loss of the will to live is the fundamental existential crisis for an individual, which begins to cast doubt on the presence of their Essence, or spirit, in their body. Therefore, I consider this situation to be a spiritual crisis. The founders of existential–humanistic psychology, Viktor Frankl (1984) and Irvin Yalom (1980), believe that suicidal behavior develops when unresolved existential conflicts cause a person to stop believing in the meaning of life and they appear in a state of an existential vacuum (*that is, in the non-dominant state— V. M.*).

According to E. P. Korablina et al. (2001), the crisis is a person's reaction to situations that require them to alter their way of being: their way of thinking, their lifestyle, their attitude to themselves, to the surrounding world and to their basic existential problems. This crisis occurs in response to a conflict between the old and the new, between the habitual past and the possible future, between who the person is now and who they may become. Such a crisis awakens potential opportunities for personal growth, inherent in one's primary personality (*the true personality—V. M.*), which is the desire to develop and improve.

"The call of the crisis is multifaceted," Vladimir Kozlov (2015), professor of psychology at the Yaroslavl University (Russia) writes:

The more aspects of the social body that are swept away by this majestic call, the stronger it becomes. ... This call can be embodied in sinister figures of existential anguish, feelings of loneliness and alienation, the absurdity of human existence, the excruciating question of the meaning of life. The spiritual crisis can take the form of an aching and seemingly causeless dissatisfaction in the divine, which deprives one of one's habitual interests, the small and great pleasures of life—sex, fame, power, and bodily pleasure.

The call is fate's message about the demiurgic mission of the human spirit. Deafness to the call, caused by fear that anesthetizes the curiosity, can result in the person's regretting missed opportunities, ruminating about how everything could have been different: better, stronger, deeper, brighter … And that peace that the individual once chose in the form of the usual lazily lying on the couch and watching TV can quickly transform itself into a feeling of unrealized, worthless, faded habitual existence.

During a crisis, a person is loaded with unresolved problems, is confused and embarrassed, feels hopeless and helpless, views their life as a "dead end" and their current situation as an unbearable evil. It is as if the individual's life completely collapsed into darkness, without any possibility of reversing this incident. Without inner support, the individual's previous life goals and meanings are destroyed, lose their value (so that it is equal to that of a non-dominant state), and the person loses their ties with the world and people around them. Should the crisis not be adequately resolved by the person, it will grow and enter a destructive phase, which can be solved through suicide, neuro-psychic and psychosomatic disorders, social disadaptation, post-traumatic stress disorder, criminal behavior, alcohol or drug addictions, etc. (Korablina E. P. et al., 2001). As we already know, this destructive phase can also be resolved with cancer's help.

In Chapter 11, I shared similar data collected by a number of scientists, which demonstrated that even before the development of the existential crisis, an existential vacuum was observed in many cancer patients and was expressed in the absence of the meaning of life, especially of spiritual meaning. In my opinion, the escalation of an existential vacuum into an existential-spiritual crisis is what transforms avital experiences into avital activity, be it external or internal.

What is the specific reason for the transformation of an existential vacuum into an existential-spiritual crisis? It seems to me that the main reason is the depth of the existential vacuum which reflects the spiritual incompleteness of the false personality. Since the false personality is solely composed of the basic human needs and affections —family, job, money—the desire to satisfy higher human needs (finding the meaning of life, self-knowledge, personal and spiritual development) is not developed in it. When basic values are lost during a crisis, such individuals do not have something from a higher level to support them during this difficult period of life. This is what leads to the disintegration of the subjective meaning of life, as was shown by studies conducted by psychologists from the Grodno (Belarus) State University (Karpinskiy K. V., 2011).

According to some authors, the prevalence of false ideas that happiness is exclusively based on material wealth, the egocentricity of a person, and the imbalance and disharmony of their inner spiritual state, contribute to a weakening of their social interrelations and, as a result, to an increase in suicidal manifestations (Smirnov M., 2007; Polozhiy B. S. et al., 2014). Such a spiritual deficit is especially dangerous when it is diagnosed in children and adolescents, in whom consumerism, egoism, and the competition of modern society provoke the loss of "great meanings," cause conflict between external and internal life goals and values, thereby increasing suicidal potential (Rozanov V. A., 2014).

Such a false personality with an immature (infantile) structure of the ego and the initially "weak" dominant of the life goal is not able to provide the individual with sufficient adaptive capacity to cope with complex life circumstances, and this results in an existential crisis.

Similar ideas about cancer being a somatic manifestation of the existential crisis can also be found in the works of the American psychiatrist Gotthard Booth (1973, 1979), who believed that such an inescapable crisis leads to the disintegration of the physiological systems of the organism. Italian psycho-oncologist Pierre Mario Biava (2009), a professor at the University of Trieste and president of the Foundation for the Study of Biological Cancer Therapy, refers to the same spiritual crisis in cancer patients. He regards this disease as one of the by-products of the loss of the meaning of life, as a pathology of significance: just as interpersonal relationships change with the loss of meaning, so do biological interactions—important contacts between the cell and the organism are lost. This occurs because in modern society the meaning of life increasingly gets lost as a whole.

Indeed, the activity of modern humanity resembles the behavior of a tumor: upon becoming more advanced technologically, humans dig into the planet, depleting its resources, polluting it with waste that results from their activity, and gradually destroying the Earth, just as a tumor in its development depletes and destroys the organism that gave birth to it.

Dr. S. A. Misyak (2002) believes that if the mind of a person, especially a cancer patient, is detached from spirituality, this is a sign of a personality crisis. When frustration, nihilistic moods, and cynicism have a dominant character, it becomes a crisis not only for the person, but also for society. Yuri Kuznetsov (2014), the creator of the ideo-analysis system, has a similar stance on the matter:

> If you define a person as a system of relationships, then cancer can be viewed as dying out, the necrosis of one's personality, the product of alienation, the rupture of fundamental relationships and connections in the internal and external world and the replacement of these by something that is superficially similar.

Famous American cyclist, six-time Tour de France winner Lance Armstrong, who beat cancer, realized the importance of spirituality based on his own experience. Before the illness, he neither understood, nor noticed people's daily struggle against the creeping negativism of the surrounding world. "Without belief, we would be left with nothing but an overwhelming doom, every single day. … Dispiritedness and disappointment, these were the real perils of life, not some sudden illness or cataclysmic millennium doomsday" (Armstrong L., Jenkins S., 2000).

R. A. Akhmerov (1994, 2013) found that cancer patients underestimate the productivity of life in the past, present, and future. This reflects the combination of three types of biographical crises—non-realization, devastation, and hopelessness, which in turn indicates the presence of an existential vacuum in their life. Professor of oncology Theodore Miller (1977) is even more adamant: "Cancer is the bodily expression of an existential crisis."

According to Lawrence LeShan (1977), the main reason that such patients lose the meaning of life is that they do not have opportunities to be themselves (this impossibility of self-realization Tom Laughlin (1999) calls a state of "suffocation"). However, the appearance of cancer makes the person think about the meaning of such a life and gives the individual a choice—to accept themselves or to die.

Another cause of the oncogenic crisis is the subjective intensity of negative experiences of loss. This is when a person cannot find a solution, cannot imagine their life without the object they lost, cannot replace it by finding another person or activity. The individual believes that there is no future without the given object(s) and, therefore, loses their existential meaning, their meaning of life. "Further is the darkness of absolute loneliness, and viewing things from this perspective causes such fear that one begins to wonder whether one really is better off alive or not. However, beliefs do not allow one to consciously end one's life and that is when the unconscious comes in...," psychotherapist M. Voronov (2011) writes.

This is confirmed by S. and C. Grof (1989), who noted that the onset of a spiritual crisis can take place following strong emotional experiences, such as the loss of important relationships due to the death of a close relative, the end of a romance or divorce, the loss of a job or property. At the same time, an existential crisis may arise even if the event that initiates it appears to be completely insignificant. The "last straw" principle is manifest in such cases (Korablina E. P. et al., 2001), and it is most commonly present in chronically unsolvable intrapersonal conflicts.

The crisis, which is associated with of the loss of the will to live prior to the development of cancer, is also described by other psycho-oncologists (Simonton C. et al., 1978; Laughlin T., 1999; Rusina N. A., 2010). In a certain sense, the loss of the will to live can be seen as a new occasion of distress through loss in the fate of a person and this time, it is the final one.

Such a crisis can develop both over a long period of time and instantaneously. In the case of the externalization of emotions, it can lead to psychosis or spontaneous suicide. What comes as a surprise for our modern-day understanding of the issue is the fact that when the conflict is internalized, the crisis can also quickly manifest itself in the form of cancer. One of my patients, who is 52 years old, recalled:

> On 5th December 2007 I woke up with apparently normal breasts. When I went to bed that night, I had a tumour the size of a grapefruit in my right breast, with a very red, sore and inflamed part the size of an olive, growing out of the bottom of the main tumour. A biopsy revealed that the cancer had already spread to my lymph nodes. [Despite] treatments for two years, the cancer had spread to my bones, liver, and lungs, as well as my left breast. The 6cm tumour in the left breast also appeared overnight, just like the original tumour did. I actually felt it growing!

This is how the life crisis that this woman was experiencing expressed itself.

This ability of early-stage tumors, to often grow or shrink surprisingly quickly for no apparent reason, was first described by E. V. Cowdry in 1955. Jeanne Achterberg (2002) confirms that "tumors can change as rapidly as nightblooming flowers, growing, shrinking, perhaps changing shape. People diagnosed with stage IV cancer may be living active lives with few symptoms and no pain, or they may be bedridden; and they can move from one of these conditions to the other, and back, within days."

Lawrence LeShan (1977) recalls one female patient with Hodgkin's lymphoma. Her fairly small lymph nodes significantly increased in size over the course of several days when she broke up with her fiancé. However, after reconciliation with him, the lymph nodes returned to their former state just as quickly. C. Hirshberg and M. I. Barasch (1995) describe a similar condition observed in a woman with terminal prognosis, whose kidney tumor had metastasized to her lungs. Her doctor observed that her tumors would grow and shrink based not on how the disease was progressing, but instead, depending on the ups and downs in her relationship with her physically abusive husband. In Chapter 28 we will also learn about the experience of Mr. Wright, whose tumors disappeared and reappeared over the course of several days under the influence of the placebo. And this is how powerful the human psyche is…

> The crisis can be described as the time spent inside a cocoon; sometimes you are in total darkness and loneliness, alone with your fears, disappointment, and pain. This is a time of farewell, sorrow, and rejection; a time of endless questions and endless misunderstanding. This is the time of searching for that thin line that separates submissiveness and overcoming, the will to live and hopelessness, an obstacle and a reward, a movement forward and a silent peace. This is the time when faith strengthens our spirit and opens our heart to love; this is a time that will allow you to learn to understand and accept the variability of life and life itself. A crisis is a period of time that allows the caterpillar to make a choice: to succumb to the fear of darkness and uncertainty or to become a butterfly. … The state of the crisis, thus, being a situation when one encounters the basic existential categories, provides the individual with the opportunity for growth, as well as for "giving in" to illness,

argue E. P. Korablina and colleagues (2001).

S. and C. Grof (1989) also noted that if it is necessary for one to work on the "liberation of the spirit" sometime during one's lifetime, but he or she do not

344 Vladislav Matrenitsky

consciously fulfill this responsibility, if the individual does not understand their goals and does not make significant efforts to grow, then his or her psyche can "seize the initiative" and suppress the conscious personality by means of its powerful processes, which include destructive ones. O. Serebryanaya (2006) metaphorically describes the result:

> ... It is as if a person who does not express themselves spiritually for a long time, begins to strive for physical self-expression and the body responds by growing 'fruits' in the form or tumors, with metastasis claws, using myriads of the cells that went mad.

Unfortunately, as in most intrapersonal conflicts, a person most often does not realize the existential-spiritual crisis that is reflected in their subconscious depression, helplessness, and hopelessness. As I have already written, at the external level, this crisis mainly manifests as background psychological discomfort, negative emotional perception of oneself and/or the environment, a state of dissatisfaction with life, "unreasonable" anguish. In the absence of self-awareness skills, and particularly in the presence of alexithymia, the cancer diagnosis that follows appears to be completely "out of the blue."

Søren Kierkegaard (2013) believed that when the individual understands that they are in despair, they transform it into "an attempt to reach spirituality." However, when doing this, it is necessary to get rid of one's own "I" (for it is precisely because of this "I" that despair is experienced) and replace it with some other "I," argues Kierkegaard. In my opinion, this despair is the Essence's reaction to the "suffocation" caused by a false personality, where the development of cancer is the physical expression of this protest. Understanding early on that one is going through a crisis and taking the correct path to "get rid of one's own 'I'" (which is a false personality) can allow the individual to free their Essence and allow it to grow, thereby acquiring "some other 'I'," which will heal the human body from a precancerous state.

We can say that self-actualization and self-transcendence are an expression, a function of the dominant of the higher life goal. Should it be underdeveloped or suppressed, on top of an existential vacuum, its place will be occupied by the dominant of the overvalued subject, object or need. And should it get lost, it will result in an existential and spiritual crisis that destroys the third barrier of psychic adaptation, provokes avital experiences, and provides a basis for the development of the oncological dominant.

At the physiological level, this is reflected by the transition of chronic stress to the stage of exhaustion, which corresponds to the third stage of the adaptation syndrome, according to Hans Selye. This transition takes a certain amount of time and may explain why cancer occurs at a time when it seems that a person's life has stabilized after a period of adversity, and when he feels relatively well (Valenzuela F. O., 2014).

Chapter 19

Biological Mechanisms of Cancer Initiation and their Relationship with Chronic Stress and the Oncodominant

The psychological data presented in the previous chapters seems to be very convincing to the most readers. However, it can make some readers, particularly physicians and representatives of biological sciences, skeptical, because (as I have noted myself above) psychological research can be contradictory at times and is less consistent than biological research.

I will not elaborate on the fact that the results of biomedical cancer research also do not always coincide with one another. What would be more appropriate to consider in this chapter is biological studies that confirm that the state of chronic psychophysiological distress, which develops as the result of the avital psycho-spiritual crisis, does indeed lead to the malignant transformation of cells.

19.1. The Main Stress Hormones and Cancer

We have repeatedly encountered the principal actors of the stress mechanisms: catecholamines (epinephrine and norepinephrine) and glucocorticoids (cortisol and corticosterone), as well as the negative results that are caused by their imbalance in the organism. The question at hand is, how do they cause an oncogenic effect?

19.1.1. Catecholamines

Catecholamines are synthesized in the body in the sympathetic division of the nervous system, in the adrenal medulla, and in the brain. Receptors to them are present in almost all organs and tissues and that is why the excess of catecholamines, which occurs when one experiences chronic stress, can stimulate the development of tumors anywhere. There are two main ways in which this happens: systemically, which is when catecholamines spread by means of the blood and impact the physiological systems of the body (especially the immune and nervous systems), and locally—both by direct exposure of target organ cells and by indirect influence on the surrounding cells, for example *macrophages* and vascular cells.

Scientists from the Department of Biology of Cancer at Wake Forest University, NC, found that during stress both in people with prostate tumors and in animals with an experimental tumor in the same localization, the levels of epinephrine and/or norepinephrine in the blood rise. Upon studying the oncogenic effects of chronic stress, these authors were able to discover the accumulation of precancerous lesions, which could be prevented by the beta-blocker, a drug that does not let epinephrine connect its receptors and thereby blocks its effects. In addition, stress causes the body to lose its susceptibility to a specific medicine for prostate cancer, that is, bicalutamide. However, this problem can also be solved through the use of the beta-blocker (Hassan S. et al., 2013). Similar data was obtained regarding the important role of stress and catecholamines in the development of tumors in the pancreas, colon and lungs (Schuller H. M. et al., 2011; Al-Wadei H. A. et al., 2012). These findings indicate the universality of this oncogenic mechanism.

In laboratory conditions, researchers use cell cultures, which are cells from various different tissues that are artificially grown in vials. The direct injection of stress hormones in such cultures makes it possible to determine if their damaging effect on cells occurs directly, or indirectly, through various physiological systems of the body.

By using an experimental model of the prostate cell culture, scientists treated them with a pharmacological agent that simulates the intracellular effects of catecholamines, which arise when they connect to receptors. As a result of prolonged exposure to this agent, the cells became malignant (Cox M. E. et al., 1999). As we shall see later, this catecholamine effect occurs at the genetic level (Flint M. S. et al., 2013).

Another laboratory method for studying cancer mechanisms and their relationship with cancer is the animal model. It uses the injection of preliminary isolated malignant cells in animals—a kind of "tumor inoculation." The first experiments of this kind were carried out in the 1970s at the University of Washington. Ninety-two percent of the "inoculated" mice that were subjected to severe stress developed cancer, while in another group where the animals were not stressed (control group), the disease was detected in only 7% of the mice (Riley V., 1975). In similar studies, which took place later, Japanese scientists modeled the stressful life conditions for mice, thus causing them to develop tumors. However, the administration of the beta-blocker propranolol, the drug that precludes the effect of epinephrine, prevented this process (Hasegawa H.,

Saiki I., 2002). The same result was obtained on the "inoculation" model of acute lymphoblastic leukemia. The two-week stress caused by restricting the mobility of the mice contributed to a significant progress of the disease and the development of metastases, whereas propranolol prevented this effect from occurring (Lamkin D. M. et al., 2012).

Other scientists used the inverse principle of the experiment—the effect of so-called beta-agonists (pharmacological agents that have the same effect as epinephrine) on mice that had been previously injected with ovarian tumor cells. In these experiments, both the incidence of cancer in mice and the average weight of the developed tumors increased (Thaker P. H. et al., 2006).

All this data clearly demonstrates the important role of hormones of stress catecholamines in the growth and metastasis of cancer.

19.1.2. Glucocorticoids

Glucocorticoids—cortisol (predominant in humans) and corticosterone (prevalent in rodents) are steroid hormones synthesized by the cortical part of the adrenal glands. During acute stress blood level of glucocorticoids rises rapidly as an element of the organism's adaptation to the changing situation. The hormones relocate from the blood to the surface of the cells, where they connect to their receptors and get transported into the nuclei of cells in this conjunction. There they interact with chromosomes, executing the role of a *transcription factor* and thus influence the expression rate of certain genes. Under long-term exposure to the body, glucocorticoids make use of this mechanism to suppress immunity by inhibiting the maturation and differentiation of T- and B-lymphocytes and causing their apoptosis (self-destruction), as well as inhibiting the activity of phagocytes.

As we saw in Chapter 3.2.3, chronic stress also leads to increased secretion of cortisol and suppression of immunity. It is believed that this is an important factor in the development of the precancerous state—on account of both a local change in the microenvironment of the cells and the decrease in the protective function of immune cells (Volden P. A., Conzen S. D., 2013). At the same time, blood leukocytes lose sensitivity to cortisol owing to a reduction of the number of receptors on the cell surface (phenomenon of desensitization), and for this reason they become unable to withstand inflammatory signals (Miller G. E. et al., 2002). This leads to the activation of the inflammatory process in the body, which, as we will learn below, is one of the factors of tumor growth.

Just as catecholamines in the cultures of tumor cells stimulate their reproduction, glucocorticoids have a similar function and this is shown in the cultures of breast tumor cells (Simon W. E. et al., 1984) and prostate (Zhao X. Y. et al., 2000). In addition, cortisol in the epithelial cells of breast cancer affects the special genes of cell "survival," and this suppresses their ability for self-destruction and enhances tumor growth. Moreover, the hormone protects cancer cells from the chemotherapeutic drug (Wu W. et al., 2004), which may explain why chemotherapy is less effective against a background of distress (Zorzet S. et al., 1998). In the experiments conducted by other scientists, it was found that an excess of glucocorticoids inhibits the activity of the BRCA1 gene, which functions as a suppressor of breast cancer, and its mutations are found in hereditary cancer (Antonova L., Mueller C. R., 2008).

The relationship between psychological stress in animals and humans, glucocorticoids, and breast cancer has also been investigated by scientists from the Center for Interdisciplinary Health Disparities Research (CIHDR) of the University of Chicago.

Rats that were genetically predisposed to the development of breast tumors were taken from the groups in which they usually live and placed in solitary cages. After a while, they began to manifest behavioral and physiological changes, indicating the development of stress. Unlike their relatives living in the group and usually actively studying new objects placed in their cages, isolated rats demonstrated the so-called "vigilant behavior": they stayed put in one place for prolonged periods of time and constantly looked around. In an interview with the prestigious journal of the National Cancer Institute, CIHDR lead researcher Sarah Gelert noted that although it is difficult to assess the feelings that rodents' experience, their appearance is akin to the vegetative symptoms of human depression. Changes in the content of glucocorticoids in response to stress were also observed in isolated rats, which were similar to those observed in humans during stress. Rats confined to solitary cages developed breast tumors with much greater frequency and at a younger age than those who were kept in the group, and these tumors were larger and more aggressive in their development.

These experiments served as the basis for further study of the relationship between the stress caused by social exclusion and breast cancer in African-American women from Southern Chicago. Dr. Gelert carefully studied their social situation on the basis of interviews and statistics about their place of residence, income, access to medical care, etc. Simultaneously, their level of glucocorticoids was determined, and it was noticeably impaired in women who experienced high levels of social isolation. This study confirmed the obvious relationship between chronic stress and cancer (Ross K., 2008).

Constantly elevated levels of cortisol lead to disorders in the other main area of activity of this hormone—the regulation of the carbohydrate metabolism. This also contributes to the development of the tumor (Sapolsky R. M., Donnelly T. M., 1985), since an increased sugar intake is one of the main ways that cancer cells obtain their energy.

An important feature of the activity of glucocorticoids in the body is their ability to interact with the adrenergic (catecholamine) system. They increase the sensitivity of the cardiac muscle and vessel walls to catecholamines and prevent the desensitization of their receptors (i.e. decrease in receptors number when there is a high level of catecholamines). This may explain why during an oncogenic distress the adaptive protection of the body to an increased level of epinephrine is not being developed, and this contributes to the malignant transformation of the cells. Indeed, scientists from the laboratory of physiological and pharmacological studies of the National Institute of Health in the USA have shown that catecholamines and glucocorticoids "cooperate" in the development of cancer. In particular, cortisol activates an epinephrine-induced increase in the quantity of epinephrine receptors on the surface of a cancer cell and parallelly enhances the inflammatory functions of regulatory cytokine-interleukins IL-1α, IL-1β cytokine and TNF-α (Nakane T. et al., 1990).

For an individual to have good health, what matters is not only the absolute content of cortisol in the blood, but also its daily fluctuations—the circadian rhythm. It was found that this rhythm depends on the stress experienced by humans and is disrupted in cancer patients with tumors in different locations, which adversely affects the course of the disease (Touitou Y. et al., 1996; Mormont C. M., Levi F., 1997; Sephton S. E. et al., 2000, 2013). Patients with metastatic breast cancer experience much more "flattened" daily fluctuations in their cortisol content (i.e. the amount does not change much throughout the day). This can be observed in both highly anxious patients and those who suppressed their emotions, but not in those who do not have such personal traits. However, the mean cortisol content of all these groups did not differ (Giese-Davis J. et al., 2004).

Such data is beginning to attract more and more of scientists' attention to the role of stress hormones in the development of cancer and makes this one of the priority research areas in psychoneuroendocrinology (Powell N. D. et al., 2013).

19.2. Other Hormones Involved in the Mechanisms of Chronic Oncogenic Stress

It is obvious that chronic stress affects the entire body, and is reflected in the imbalance of most, if not all, hormonal systems. Although the pathophysiological effects of the main stress mediators, epinephrine and cortisol, are best studied today, data is gradually being accumulated about the role of other hormones in oncogenic distress (Antoni M. et al., 2006). We will consider only a few of these hormones: prolactin, oxytocin, insulin, dopamine, and estrogens.

Prolactin and oxytocin are called "behaviorally sensitive neuropeptides," because they participate in both the biological and psychological aspects of relationships between the sexes, including the birth and the feeding of children.

Prolactin normally participates in the pregnancy process, by stimulating the growth and development of mammary glands and the formation of milk in them.

However, prolactin receptors are also present in many other organs, including immune cells and many cell cultures of breast cancer. It is interesting that this hormone is even produced in lymphocytes, where its concentration increases with the activation of immunity and inflammatory processes. The synthesis of prolactin is noticeably increased during stressful conditions and associated anxiety, depression, and trauma. According to experiments, prolactin stimulates the growth of cancer cells and the survival of breast tumor cells and other malignant tumors. As a result of epidemiological studies, it was confirmed that there is a link between the level of prolactin and cancer risk factors such as the age at which a woman has her first menstruation and the number of times that she gives birth. In addition, the hormone stimulates the proliferation of prostate and uterine tumor cells (Antoni M. H. et al., 2006). On the other hand, after the onset of menopause, the risk of morbidity in women with breast cancer is reduced owing to an age-related decrease in the synthesis of prolactin.

Oxytocin is produced in the hypothalamic region of the brain and its main role is to contract muscle fibers around the breast ducts, which makes it possible for the milk produced by prolactin to be released from the breast. In addition, oxytocin is able to increase the frequency and strength of uterine contractions, and in this manner participates in the delivery process. Receptors for oxytocin are also present in the heart, brain, kidneys, thymus, and even in male testicles, prostate, and vas deferens, which indicates that this hormone has a wider range of functions in the body. What is especially important is the fact that oxytocin impacts the areas of our brain that influence our behavior, reducing feelings of fear and anxiety and creating a sense of satisfaction and tranquility. Oxytocin is even nicknamed the "hormone of unity, caring and affection."

For example, when a baby mouse was placed into a cage with an adult male for just ten minutes, the adult male, who had no previous experiences with children or females, approached the baby and began taking care of him, after a certain period of time. This experiment was conducted by scientists from the Brain and Body Center at the University of Illinois in Chicago, who found that the level of oxytocin in the blood of males increased after such an experience, whereas the level of the corticosterone stress hormone decreased, compared with the males in the control group, who were not exposed to baby mice. It is worth mentioning that the males that were more involved in caring for the baby mice had a higher content of oxytocin and less corticosterone (Kenkel W. et al., 2012). This shows that oxytocin is clearly involved in reducing stress, and those who have to deal with a significant amount of stress would benefit from spending more time with children. These findings are confirmed by other studies that directly demonstrated a decrease in the level of oxytocin during chronic stress (Young W. S., Lightman S. L., 1992).

Therefore, the data on how oxytocin is able to prevent the growth of epithelial cells of breast and endometrial tumors, as well as tumors of the nervous and bone tissues, is fairly believable. On the other hand, however, this hormone stimulates the multiplication of tumor cells originating from the trophoblasts[1] and the endothelium (Cassoni P. et al., 2001; Strunecka A. et al., 2009). This once again shows us that everything has dual properties in the body, just as in nature as a whole; duality is prevalent, starting from an electron capable of manifesting the properties of both waves and particles, and ending with a mind that is capable of creating health and disease.

Estrogen hormones (estradiol, estriol, and estrone) are predominantly synthesized in the ovaries in women, as well as in small amounts in male testicles and in the adrenal cortex in both sexes. Estrogens are responsible for the development of the female reproductive system and the secondary sexual features of women, as well as for the menstrual cycle. Both in women and men, estrogens play a role in the regulation of the thyroid hormone thyroxine, as well as lipids, cholesterol, sodium, water, iron, and copper.

Maintaining a normal level of estrogen is important for the proper functioning of the brain; this makes it easier to tolerate chronic stress, reduce anxiety, and solve problems more effectively (Bowman R. E. et al., 2002). I have already mentioned that chronic stress causes damage to the middle part of the prefrontal cortex, which is involved in cognitive and behavioral functions, emotions, and abstract thinking (Cook S. C., Wellman C. L., 2004). Estrogens also play a role in stress-related disorders, as was confirmed by experiments conducted on rats: the removal of the ovaries in females prevented damage to neurons, and the subsequent administration of elevated doses of estradiol created conditions for damage (Garrett J. E., Wellman C. L., 2009).

The reason for such damage may be the fact that a high level of estrogen makes the brain more sensitive to stress. This effect of estrogens was determined by scientists from the School of Medicine at Yale University. They exposed male and female rats to stress of varying intensity, and then tested their short-term memory. Prior to being exposed to stress, males and females had the same memorization level. After being exposed to intense stress, both sexes had significant memory issues. However, after exposure to moderate stress, memory was disturbed only in female rats, whereas the males were capable of remembering just as well as before the exposure. Further experiments allowed the researchers to conclude that this effect in females is due to estrogen, since the removal of their ovaries prevented memory impairment (Shansky R. M. et al., 2004). This suggests that females are more sensitive to stress, with the result that women, according to the statistics, are twice as likely to develop a depressive disorder, as are men.

----

[1] Trophoblasts are the specialized cells of the placenta which provide nutrients to the embryo.

In addition, chronic stress in female rats increases the estrogen content in their blood and blocks the onset of pregnancy (MacNiven E., Younglai E. V., 1992). Clinicians are aware that an increase in the concentration of estrogen in women due to an impaired metabolism is manifested through the development of diseases such as endometriosis, endometrial polyps, cervical dysplasia, fibrocystic mastopathy, uterine fibroids, etc. When there is a pathological increase of the estrogen level in the body (hyperestrogenemia), there is a high probability of development of malignant tumors in the mammary glands and ovaries, as well as endometrial and cervical cancer (Key T. J. et al., 2003; Helgesson O. et al., 2003). On the other hand, a decrease in the estrogen content in women's bodies after menopause is accompanied by a deterioration of adaptive reactions and a more pronounced body reaction to stress, which also increases the risk of morbidity (Lindheim S. R. et al., 1992).

Estrogens are also involved in stress mechanisms by impacting the content of the main stress hormones, the catecholamines (Serova L. I. et al., 2005) and glucocorticoids (Figueiredo H. F. et al., 2007).

Dopamine is a hormone that belongs to the catecholamine family. It is synthesized in the cerebral part of the adrenal gland and is a precursor of epinephrine and norepinephrine, but also exerts various effects on the body as an independent hormone. Dopamine is also produced in the brain, serves as a neurotransmitter (mediator) between neurons, and is capable of inducing both excitation and inhibition in them. Its main function in the brain is to create a good mood. Therefore, dopamine is part of the reward mechanism in the central nervous system and is responsible for feelings of pleasure when we do things that we like, such as eat or have sex. Dopamine called the "hormone of love and tenderness," because it is produced in the human body when one falls in love and creates the so-called "dopamine addiction."

During acute stress, as well as during pain attacks, anxiety, and fear, the level of dopamine increases sharply, which helps to speed up the body's reaction to a dangerous situation. When it comes to more prolonged stress, if the body is able to adapt to repeated exposures to it, the content and the reserve possibilities of dopamine synthesis in the brain are increased (Anokhina I. P. et al., 1985; Kvetnansky R. et al., 1975). However, when the stress enters a chronic phase or becomes distress, the hormone content falls (Imperato A. et al., 1992). This phenomenon most likely occurs owing to the influence of glucocorticoids, since they have the ability of suppressing the synthesis of dopamine and reducing its inhibitory effect on the synthesis of prolactin (Lavin N., 1999). Reduction in dopamine content may be one of the causes of impaired immunity during chronic stress, since T-cells have receptors for dopamine. Experimental suppression of dopamine synthesis in mice inhibits the protective response of T-lymphocytes and activates tumor growth (Basu S. et al., 1995).

In contrast to its "relatives," the catecholamines, dopamine exhibits inhibitory properties in relation to tumor growth. Scientists from the School of Medicine at the University of Washington found that if the dopamine system is hyperactive, then the size of the tumor decreases. Such suppression has been demonstrated in cancer cells of various origins, including neuroblastoma, melanoma, breast and neck tumors (Thaker P. H., Sood A. K., 2008). The mechanism of the anti-cancer effect of dopamine is associated with the activation of apoptosis (self-destruction) of tumor cells (Moreno-Smith M. et al., 2011), blocking the development of blood vessels in them, suppressing metastasis and the development of ascites (accumulation of fluid in the abdominal cavity) in the animals that experiments have been conducted on (Basu S. et al., 2001; Teunis M. A. et al., 2002).

Another important aspect of dopamine involvement in the cancer mechanisms is that a decrease in its content provokes depression (as opposed to pleasure when the hormone content increases). As we already know, depression is one of the critical precancerous states of the psyche.

Insulin is the main hormone responsible for transferring sugar (or rather, glucose) from the blood to its storage locations, the liver and muscles. Both acute and chronic stress and the depression that occurs as a result lead to a decrease in the sensitivity of cells to insulin, and consequently, the levels of insulin and blood glucose increase (Depke M. et al., 2008; Li L. et al., 2013). High glucocorticoid content and systemic inflammation play an important role in such insulin resistance (decreased sensitivity) (Goldberg R. B., 2009; Bardini G. et al., 2010; Solomon S. S. et al., 2010). In turn, an increase in the level of insulin in the blood is accompanied by an increase in the activity of the sympathetic nervous system, which plays an important role when it comes to responses to stress (Dedov I. I., Melnichenko G. A., 2004). When insulin is present in the brain in high quantities, it disrupts the mechanisms that control food intake, body weight, learning, and memory (Zhao W. Q. et al., 2004), and in this manner creates a vicious cycle of increasing distress.

Insulin resistance is considered to be a precursor of clinical symptoms of obesity and type 2 diabetes mellitus. This type of diabetes, also called insulin-independent (in contrast to insulin-dependent type 1 diabetes, which is treated by injection of external insulin), is a metabolic disease accompanied by a chronic increase of glucose in the blood, which occurs owing to a decrease in the sensitivity of cells to insulin. For our analysis, it is important to note that insulin resistance may also indicate a latent development of a tumor process. This is because an excess of sugar is one of the most important conditions that must be met for the development and metastasis of tumors: cancer cells consume glucose ten to thirty times more actively than healthy cells. Glucose is consumed by cancer cells faster than the rate at which it comes to cells, as if it were pumping it from the host's body. Reduced sensitivity of cells to insulin is considered a risk factor for the development of breast cancer and an unfavorable prognosis of the disease (Rose D. P. et al., 2004). Therefore it is not surprising that type 2 diabetes itself is strongly associated with the development cancers of the breast, rectum, pancreas, and uterus (Kravchun N. A., 2010).

Moreover, since insulin and insulin-like growth factors (that regulate the growth, development, and differentiation of cells and tissues of the body) increase the proliferative activity of cells, that is, the rate of their multiplication (Yam D. et al., 1996; Lavin N., 1999), they also act as factors that stimulate carcinogenesis (Bershteyn L. M., 2000).

In addition to supplying tumor cells with "food" and directly stimulating their growth, glucose and insulin also activate the synthesis of inflammatory cytokines (Jagannathan-Bogdan M. et al., 2011; Kologrivova I. V. et al., 2013), and this, as we shall see shortly, leads to the development of inflammation—another important condition for tumor growth.

In the process of its further development, the tumor continues to "take control of the sugar" (similarly to the situation with immunity, as we will learn below). Scientists from the University of Southern California found that most types of malignant tumors cause insulin resistance in the muscles, liver, and adipose tissue of the patient in parallel with an increase in the level of the pro-inflammatory cytokine TNF-α (Orgel E., Mittelman S. D., 2013). This is how the tumor achieves more favorable conditions to grow, at the expense of the normal functioning of healthy organs and tissues.

Much as beta-blocker drugs suppress the effect of epinephrine on cells, thus reducing the incidence of cancer, metformin, which is a drug used to treat type 2 diabetes, can reduce the risk of cancer and improve the prognosis of the disease. Scientists from McGill University in Montreal arrived at this conclusion when they found that metformin significantly inhibits the growth of cancerous epithelial cells in the ovaries. The preclinical studies that followed these experiments confirmed the efficacy of metformin in treating ovarian cancer (Gotlieb W. H. et al., 2008). The same conclusion was reached at the Institute of Endocrine Pathology Problems of the Academy of Medical Sciences of Ukraine, named after V. Y. Danilevsky, based on the analysis of 194 cases of patients with type 2 diabetes. Cancer was not diagnosed in any of the patients who had taken metformin for an average of five years prior to the study (Kravchun N. A., 2010).

19.3. The Immune System

In Chapter 3.2.3 we have seen a lot of data confirming that chronic stress suppresses the activity of the immune system. In clinical settings it was noticed a long time ago that patients with suppressed immunity, caused by pharmacological agents or immunodeficiency diseases, for example AIDS, have an increased risk of developing cancer (Cohen S., Rabin B. S. 1998). Studies conducted by other scientists confirmed that in patients with penetrating breast cancer that regularly deal with a high level of stress, the ability of NK ("killer")-lymphocytes to destroy tumor cells is significantly reduced (Andersen B. L. et al., 1998). In contrast, when women with first and second stages of breast cancer were observed at the Cancer Institute in Pittsburgh it was discovered that those patients who received significant emotional support from their spouse, family, and attending physician, and actively interacted with other patients, had more active NK-lymphocytes (Levy S. M. et al., 1990). Similar data on the reduced activity of NK cells during periods of high levels of stress was obtained by examining forty-two patients with epithelial ovarian cancer (Lutgendorf S. K. et al., 2005), 108 patients with cancer of the digestive system in various locations (Nan K. J. et al., 2004) and sixty-one men with prostate tumors (Penedo F. J. et al., 2006).

Women with high levels of everyday stress have a reduced immune response to the HPV16 papilloma virus, which makes them more vulnerable to developing cervical cancer (Fang C. Y. et al., 2008). A comprehensive study of the quantitative and functional parameters of the immunity of cancer patients, conducted at the Research Institute of Clinical Immunology in Novosibirsk (Russia), revealed that there is a close correlation with the mental state, types of psychological defense, and the quality of patients' lives. This confirms the relationship of the functions of the nervous and immune systems in the development of the tumor process (Bukhtoyarov O. V., Arkhangelskiy A. E., 2008).

Readers may argue that stress in cancer patients is the result of the diagnosis, living with the disease and the associated fear of death. This aspect is undoubtedly present and, as discussed below, contributes to the progression of the disease. However, the data discussed earlier on the negative effect of stress on immunity demonstrates that it can be a primary factor in reducing the activity of this system.

This point has been already confirmed through experiments. A number of studies have been conducted in which animals were first exposed to chemical carcinogens or irradiated, and then subjected to various stresses—electrical shock, bright light, restriction of mobility, isolation, or confrontation with other animals. In most cases, the decline in immunity followed by the development of tumors was more prominent in the animals that were subjected to stress, than in those who did not undergo stress (Glaser R. et al., 1985; Parker J. et al., 2004; Adachi S. et al., 1993). However, even without prior carcinogenic effects, stress can cause the disease: for example, mice experiencing the stress of social isolation (loneliness) had reduced macrophage activity and an increased incidence of cancer (Palermo-Neto J. et al., 2003).

It has been proven that catecholamines and glucocorticoids, which are stress agents, make it possible for tumor cells to avoid being destroyed by the guards of the immune system (Antoni M. H. et al., 2006). Consider another model of chronic stress in mice that is popular among researchers: repeated social defeat. The rodent is placed in a cage with an unfamiliar group of mice, where it is often forced, generally unsuccessfully, to fight to defend its position (does this situation remind one of the arrival of a new employee into a new unfriendly workplace?). Upon studying the immune cells of mice in this stress model, scientists from the University of Ohio found that these cells lose the ability of apoptosis (natural death) and cease to react to anti-inflammatory agents. However, if the mice were given a certain drug prior to being exposed to stress, a drug that we are already familiar with: a beta-blocker that prevents epinephrine's effect on cells, then their immune functions did not get disrupted.

In addition, the researchers found that following repeated social defeat, the bone marrow of a mouse increases its production of immature immune cells (precursors of differentiated cells) of *myeloid* origin and their migration is activated to the peripheral tissues, which then promote tumor growth through the development of local inflammation. Furthermore, these immature immune cells affect the central nervous system, where they can increase stress and cause a state of anxiety as a result. This adds an additional imbalance to the already broken connection between the neuroendocrine and immune systems (Powell N. D. et al., 2013a).

It is known that the developing tumor is able to use immune cells that penetrate into its tissue, transforming them from enemies into allies, which causes the immune cells to no longer recognize cancer cells as pathogenic ones and in this manner to enhance tumor growth. These features of the cancer cell are one of the most important mechanisms of carcinogenesis and the reason for tumor survival in the body. At the same time suppressor cells of myeloid origin, that are normally responsible for the effectiveness of the immune system functioning (for example, not allowing it to negatively affect the body), begin to put down the antitumor reactions of tissues. This plays a significant role in the abnormal behavior of the immune system, contributing to the development of the tumor. Studies that show the relationship of this process with stress hormones underline the importance of the complex connections between our stress-inducing behavior and the major systems of the body—nervous, endocrine, and immune (Powell N. D. et al., 2013).

19.3.1. The Inflammatory Process

Inflammation is a product of the activity of the immune system, its initial response to an aggressive external intervention. It is an innate, automatic, and nonspecific reaction of the organism that occurs when antigens (substances alien to the host) get into the body. Inflammation promotes neutralization and destruction of various pathogens and initiates wound healing, allowing the body to cope with pathological processes—from viral infections to allergic reactions. Cytokines play the main role in the mechanism of inflammation and these are small informational peptides (proteins) that transmit intercellular signals in order to attract and activate other immune cells in the affected area of the body. Some types of cytokines can activate inflammation (interleukins IL-1, IL-2, IL-6, IL-8, TNFα, and interferon γ), while others inhibit it (interleukins IL-4, IL-10, and TGFβ), as well as regulating other aspects of immunity.

Cytokines IL-6 and TNFα are of particular interest to us, since these are known as the mediators of both stress and inflammation.

Interleukin 6 (IL-6) is a cytokine synthesized by activated macrophages and T-cells that activates immune reaction. The uniqueness of its function is that, depending on the circumstances, it can both stimulate and suppress inflammatory processes. During acute and chronic stress, and during depression, the IL-6 content increases, which leads to the activation of inflammatory processes (Kiecolt-Glaser J. K. et al., 2003; Costanzo E. S. et al., 2011). For example, people caring for a spouse with senile dementia have increased levels of IL-6 due to chronic stress (Kiecolt-Glaser J. K. et al., 2003). Increased IL-6 in women with ovarian cancer is a poor prognosticator for the survival of these patients, but those receiving better social support have lower levels of IL-6 (Kiecolt-Glaser J. K. et al., 2003, Costanzo E. S. et al., 2005).

Chronic subfebrile inflammation (a prolonged rise in body temperature between 0.5 °C and 1°C) is one of the main pathophysiological processes that contribute to the development of various diseases, including cancer. Rudolf Virchow, an outstanding German physician of the nineteenth century, the founder of the theory of cellular pathology in medicine, suggested that chronic inflammation is the main cause of cancer. And although it is now clear that this is only partially true, a deep interconnection exists between these two phenomena.

During a two-week follow-up observation period of people who have experienced strong interpersonal stress, it was found that the level of the C-reactive protein (indicator of inflammation) remained high in their blood (Fuligni A. J. et al., 2009). Researchers from the University of Ohio conducted an experiment on mice by modeling the stress caused by the destruction of the social hierarchy in the group. A new aggressive male was temporarily inserted into a group of male mice living together, which resulted in fights for dominance. This led to a significant increase in the inflammatory process in the lungs of the mice (Curry J. M. et al., 2010). The same stress model was also used to detect the migration of immature myeloid cells to the spleen and other peripheral organs, where they produce increased amounts of inflammatory cytokines (Powell N. D. et al., 2013a) and thereby create a predisposition to cancer.

Since catecholamines directly participate in the body's reaction to stress, it is natural that norepinephrine enhances the synthesis of inflammatory cytokines by activating the corresponding gene (Bierhaus A. et al., 2003; Straub R., Harle P., 2005). In the ovarian cancer model, the injection of norepinephrine leads to an increase in the concentration of IL-6, increased inflammation, and activation of tumor progression mechanisms (Nilsson M. B. et al., 2007).

Over the past decade, plenty of evidence has accumulated confirming that chronic inflammation is a precursor of the development of tumors, metastases, and the recurrence of cancer, and the level of circulating cytokine can be used as an indicator of survival and the predictor of metastases in cancer patients (Chung Y. C., Chang Y. F., 2003; Pierce B. L. et al., 2009; Salgado R. et al., 2003). Chronic inflammatory diseases such as erosive colitis, hepatitis, and infection with the Epstein-Barr virus create a high probability of colon cancer, hepatocellular carcinoma, and nasopharyngeal cancer, respectively (Lu H. et al., 2006). I already mentioned that during the process of its development, the tumor "reprograms" immune cells which have been attracted into the tumor microenvironment. As a result, these cells (macrophages) begin to release inflammatory cytokines and provoke the appearance of factors that stimulate the formation of new blood vessels. In this way local inflammation is activated and further tumor growth is stimulated (Cohen T. et al., 1996; Costanzo E. S. et al., 2011).

TNF-a (tumor necrosis factor) is another multifunctional cytokine produced mainly in *monocytes* and *macrophages*, as well as in the liver, adipose tissue, and spleen. TNF-a is an important mediator of insulin resistance, a regulator of energy metabolism in the body that coordinates the functional relationships between fat tissue and insulin-sensitive organs.

This kind of cytokine received its specific name in the process of its discovery: the serum of mice that were injected with bacterial products was able to induce necrosis and a decrease in the sizes of "grafted" tumors in other rodents. However, TNF-a failed to become a therapeutic drug because of its high toxicity. This cytokine also stimulates inflammation by activating the synthesis of other interleukin-cytokines, including IL-6. Subsequently, it was found that, like many other hormones and mediators, depending on the situation in the body and its concentration, TNF-a may have opposite effects: for some tumors, this cytokine serves as a factor that contributes to metastasis (Malik S. T. et al., 1990). That is why during the acute phase of stress, catecholamines and glucocorticoids can inhibit the synthesis of TNF-a, and during the chronic phase, they can activate it, creating a pro-cancer inflammation (Nakane T. et al., 1990; Elenkov I. j., Chrousos G. P., 2002).

As we have learned in the previous sections, the immune and central nervous systems constantly influence each other. Therefore, inflammation, as a component of the immune function, is given a key physiological significance in mediating the effect of negative emotions and stress on health. For example, cortisol, one of the most important stress agents, enhances the function of cytokines-IL-1α and IL-1β-interleukins, resulting in inflammation in the tumor and stimulating its development (Nakane T. et al., 1990), whereas upon penetrating the brain, IL-1α cytokines and IL-1β affect one of its central loci—the hypothalamus, provoking synthesis of two hormonal mediators—corticoliberin and ACTH. As a result of these changes in the adrenal glands, the production of cortisol is enhanced (Turnbull A. V., Rivier C. L., 1999). The described processes lead to a situation where the mechanism of stress "gets stuck," which intensifies its pathogenicity and causes distress.

Consequently, the relationship between the tumor and the brain is two-sided: on one hand, the brain initiates the production of a cascade of hormones that directly affect the growth of the tumor. On the other hand, biologically active molecules, such as pro-inflammatory cytokines, that are synthesized by the tumor and by attracted immune cells, affect the brain, thereby conditioning the psychological states and behavior of cancer patients (Dantzer R. et al., 2008). Along with the already existing chronic stress, all these processes aggravate the clinical picture of the disease. Psychological conditions caused by pro-inflammatory cytokines include fatigue, depression, lack of appetite, impaired mental concentration, hypersensitivity to pain, sleep disturbances, and lack of mobility (Khasraw M., Posner J. B., 2010; Costanzo E. S. et al., 2011).

In general, today there is no doubt that inflammation is the link between chronic stress, interpersonal relationships, depression, and health (Black P. H., 2002; Kiecolt-Glaser J. K. et al., 2010). For example, loneliness in the elderly is an important component of everyday stress and acts as an increased mortality factor (Tilvis R. S. et al., 2011). The additional acute stressful situation, which arises against the background of loneliness, leads to a significant increase in the synthesis of cytokines TNF-α and IL-6 and, consequently, to the growth of inflammation. A similar increase in inflammation in response to stress was also observed in patients at the end of treatment for breast cancer, although the inflammatory markers this time were cytokines IL-6 and IL-1β (Jaremka L. M. et al., 2013). As we see, as a precursor of depression, loneliness can be an important psychosocial factor in the onset of cancer.

However, depression and anxiety on their own, as I have already noted above, lead to an increase in the content of IL-6 and TNF-α cytokines, which form a pro-inflammatory state in the body and contribute to the development of cancer, cardiovascular diseases, arthritis, type 2 diabetes, and osteoporosis (Raison C. L. et al., 2006). If, on top of depression, there is additional acute stress, then the level of IL-6 increases more and lasts longer than in people without depression (Fagundes C. P. et al., 2013). In Chapter 14 the reader was introduced to scientific evidence of the role of depression in the development of cancer and of the aggravation of the course of the disease. For example, the severity of depressive symptoms and the level of cortisol are directly related to unfavorable prognoses of the survival of patients with metastatic kidney cancer (Cohen L. et al., 2012). On the other hand, depressive women suffering from breast cancer, who underwent a program of rehabilitation and stress management developed by the Department of Psychology at the University of Ohio, were not only able to improve their mood and quality of life, but also a reduced content of inflammation markers was observed in their blood (Thornton L. M. et al., 2009).

Just as beta-blockers and antidiabetic drugs counteract the development of cancer, so do drugs that have anti-inflammatory properties. Regular use of nonsteroidal drugs (ibuprofen and aspirin) by patients with chronic inflammatory diseases leads to a lower incidence of breast cancer in these patients (50% and 40% decrease, respectively) compared with those who do not take such drugs (Harris R. E. et al., 1999).

19.4. Oxidative Intracellular Stress

Not only does the body as a whole experience stress, but there is also a local type of stress, called the oxidative, which occurs in the cell and is associated with an energy metabolism disorder. Normally, there is a certain level of oxidation-reduction reactions in the cell, and these ensure the production of energy and proper metabolism, and are regulated by specialized enzymes of the antioxidant system. When there are various pathological conditions of the body, there is a failure in this regulation, which is followed by the appearance of active forms of oxidants (in another term, reactive oxygen and nitrogen species, RONS, or free radicals) in the cell— superoxide anions, hydroxyl radicals and hydrogen peroxide. As is usually the case in the body, a small quantity of these metabolic products is used as a protective mechanism. For example, these metabolic products get utilized in the immune system and in the process of cell repair. However, an excessive amount of active forms of oxidants causes damage to DNA, as well as to lipids that make up the cell membrane. This in turn results in a risk of developing cardiovascular, endocrinological, and autoimmune diseases, Alzheimer's disease, diabetes, and cancer.

Psychological stress contributes to the activation of oxidative stress in cells at various levels. In particular, oxidative stress activates in the blood plasma, spleen, and thymus of rats under the influence of a two-week noise stress, and lipid peroxidation increases, as it does also in the brain tissue of rats suffering from the stress of fear of electric shocks (Matsumoto K. et al., 1999; Srikumar R. et al., 2006).

The longer stress persists in the lives of women caring for sick children, the greater the oxidative stress in their leukocytes (Epel E. S. et al., 2004). A similar result was found by scientists from the University of California when studying women who were experiencing chronic stress, which resulted from caring for husbands with senile dementia. Compared to the control group of women with healthy husbands, the level of oxidative stress and damage to RNA was increased in the cells of their saliva, accompanied by a higher content of cortisol (Aschbacher K. et al., 2013). One of the most dangerous consequences of chronic stress is that the oxidative cellular stress which it generates causes DNA damage.[1] This was experimentally observed in the blood plasma of students on the day of an exam, compared to the non-examination period. They had an increase in oxidative DNA damage and membrane lipid peroxidation, while the antioxidant protection level was decreasing (Sivonova M., Zitnanova I. et al., 2004).

This stimulating effect of psychological stress on oxidative stress is due to the effect of stress agents—hormones. For example, glucocorticoids have been shown to produce such an effect in the rat nerve cell culture (McIntosh L. J., Sapolsky R. M., 1996). A similar result was obtained using laboratory rats: the injection of glucocorticoids led to a decrease in antioxidant protection due to the disruption of the activity of the superoxide dismutase enzyme, whose function is to neutralize free radicals (Orzechowski A. et al., 2002). Prolonged administration of norepinephrine (*which can be regarded as a model of chronic stress—V. M.*) to rats also leads to an increase of the quantity of oxidative stress markers in their blood plasma (Aizawa T. et al., 2002). The mechanism of the formation of free radicals under a stress-induced increase in epinephrine content is shown to be a result of epinephrine breaking down into adrenochrome as a result of oxidation (Hoffer A., 1994).

Based on the data presented, it is clear why scientists today assign a major role to oxidative stress in the processes of aging and cancer (Khansari N. et al., 2009). It is known that many carcinogens and radioactive radiation contribute to the appearance of oxidative damage in cells. In addition, oxidative stress actively stimulates the process of inflammation (Weitzman S. A., Gordon L. I., 1990) and activates more than 500 different genes, including the genes of pro-inflammatory cytokines, cell cycle regulators, and tissue growth factors (Reuter S. et al., 2010).

Also, chromosome damage and DNA mutations occur during oxidative stress, and this leads to genome instability and cell division activation (Epel E. S. et al., 2004; Visconti R., Grieco D., 2009). The hydrogen peroxide oxidation agent also has an epigenetic effect, activating DNA methylation and histone acetylation enzymes. This has the effect of suppressing the RUNX3 tumor growth suppressor gene and thus contributing to the active division of tumor cells (Kang K. A. et al., 2012).

The above factors contribute to the progress of tumor growth: for example, the content of specific markers of general oxidative stress (8-oxo-G or 8-OHdG)

---

[1] In particular, there is a reduction in their telomeres (discussed in the next section).

is increased in the urine of patients with different types of cancer (Kryston T. B. et al., 2011).

19.5. Mutations and Disorders of Gene Regulation

The mutational theory claims that at the molecular level, cancer is caused by disturbances in the structure, function, and regulation of the genetic apparatus. Such disorders are constantly present in the body owing to the natural influence of the external environment—ultraviolet radiation of the sun, ionizing radiation, viruses, and technogenic effects of radiation and chemical carcinogens. In addition, some products of normal metabolism in the body, such as free oxygen radicals, may also have a damaging effect. The possibility of spontaneous (random) mutations of the genome is also recognized.

In a healthy organism, these damages of the genetic apparatus are monitored by the repair (recovery) systems; however, it is possible for their effectiveness to decrease and, as a result, various problems may arise. Some examples of these problems are: chromosomal rearrangement—a change in the primary structure of the chromosome, amplification—multiple repetition of any of its parts, and chromosomal deletion—loss of part of a chromosome. Especially dangerous are mutations—stable (able to be inherited) changes in the structure of genes, which cause disruption of the body's functions and a decrease in its adaptability to changes in the external environment (to stress, for example). All these disorders lead to the situation where some normal "dormant" genes—proto-oncogenes, that were previously involved in the natural processes of cell division, growth, and differentiation, get activated again and become oncogenes. Hyperexpression (overactive functioning) of oncogenes and inhibition of expression of anti-oncogenes constitute one of the main causes of cancer initiation. It is the oncogenes that begin to synthesize nuclear and other oncoproteins that stimulate the development of the tumor.

Until recently, the causes of the described disorders were considered to be purely physical, personality-independent carcinogenic factors. The discoveries of the last decade have noticeably shaken this "physical" paradigm. Researchers working in the field of epigenetics, as well as in psychoneuroimmunology and psychoneuroendocrinology, began to talk about the so-called "social signal transduction." Under the influence of changing social conditions, neuronal impulses arise in the brain, are transferred to the nucleus of the cell and then to the genes through the sympathetic nervous system and its mediators, catecholamines, as well as the HPA axis (the hypothalamic-pituitary-adrenal gland chain) with its glucocorticoid mediators (Cole S. W., 2009). Now scientists understand the role played by the subjective psychological perception of what is happening in the regulation of certain genes (Chen E. E. et al., 2009; Irwin M. R., Cole S. W., 2011).

The researchers went deep into studying the genetic apparatus of cancer cells to find out how stress hormones work to initiate malignant transformation. General biology taught us that the connection of catecholamine molecules and glucocorticoids to the corresponding receptors on the cell membrane triggers a complex chain of intracellular reactions, resulting in gene activity changes and subsequent synthesis of different substances that are necessary for the response of cells and organs to hormonal stimuli.

We can see how this mechanism works by using transcription factors as an example. One such transcription factor is the CREB protein. When the sympathetic nervous system releases norepinephrine during a stress reaction, it connects to the receptor on the target cells and initiates multiple processes during which CREB enters the nucleus, connects to DNA, and activates the synthesis of hundreds of different genes (Zhang X. et al., 2005). Other such proteins are transcription factors of the CTRA group, characteristic of the reaction of leukocytes to unfavorable stress conditions.

In psychological states such as grief due to the loss of a loved one, a post-traumatic stress disorder, chronic loneliness, other severe adversities in life, and low socioeconomic status, transcription factors increase the activity of pro-inflammatory genes (in particular those that regulate the synthesis of cytokines) and inhibit the activity of those genes that regulate the immune response—antiviral reactions and the production of immunoglobulin G (Cole S. W., 2012; Antoni M. H. et al., 2012). Upon investigating the functions of CTRA transcription factors, the researchers found that their activation depends more on the individual, subjective perception of the social threat than on the objective characteristics of the social environment. Inhibition of their activity can be achieved by psychological and meditative practices that reduce the significance of perceived threats, and also reduce social exclusion feelings (Antoni M. H. et al., 2016; Creswell J. D. et al., 2012).

Negative changes in the activity of genes in leukocytes last for several months when a person experiences social instability (Cole S. W. et al., 2012), whereas psychological practices and positive personality changes restore CTRA activity to normal levels in eight weeks (Creswell J. D. et al., 2012), and this stabilization persists for the duration of the following year (Antoni M. H. et al., 2016).

It is believed that transcription factors such as CTRA emerged over the course of evolution as elements of the organism's adaptation at the molecular level, to protect against those periodic and ongoing threats that were characteristic of our ancestors' lives. However, in modern human social ecology, chronic activation of these transcriptional defense systems of the genome occurs mainly because of symbolic or imaginary threats. This overactivity leads to a deterioration in health both on account of the increased inflammation processes underlying the chronic pathology (for example, type II diabetes, atherosclerosis, neurodegenerative and oncological diseases), and through a reduction of the body's resistance to viral infections (Cole S. W., 2014).

19.5.1. Oncogenes and Oncoproteins

Special transcription factors, called nuclear oncoproteins, are also found in the cancer cells. For example, oncoproteins such as fos, myc, jun, erbA, myb, alter the expression of certain sections of genes, and this is followed by the synthesis of proteins that are abnormal for the particular cell, which results in pathological hormonal or antigenic activity.

At the same time, some proto-oncogenes play a role in the regulation of normal immunity. This mechanism was studied at the laboratory of a well-known psychoneuroimmunologist, Professor Ronald Glaser, director of the Institute for Behavioral Medicine Research at the University of Ohio. The genetic apparatus of the medical university students' immune cells was observed when they were under stress during exams and one month prior to the exams. It turned out that two proto-oncogenes, the c-myc and c-myb, in the leukocytes of their peripheral blood were significantly less prominently expressed during exam stress than before it, which resulted in reduced activation and reproduction of T-lymphocytes by specific mitogen agents. This indicates a genome-mediated decrease in immunity under the influence of stress (Glaser R. et al., 1993).

How do these mechanisms promote oncogenesis?

According to the Institute of Cancer Research at the University of Pittsburgh, PA, psychological stress, accompanied by an increase in epinephrine, norepinephrine, and cortisol, causes DNA damage. This is determined by the corresponding increase in the activity of the special enzymes (protein kinases Chk1 and Chk2), whose function is to find DNA damage, and in the raised function of the proto-oncogene CDC25A, which is how this damage is expressed. Such abnormalities in DNA lead to an increased risk of malignant cell transformation (Flint M. S. et al., 2007). The same group of scientists found that a long-term epinephrine or norepinephrine influence on the cell culture results in significant and permanent DNA damage, which is what causes further mutations and malignancy of the cells (Flint M. S. et al., 2013).

Scientists from the University of Ohio studied the mechanisms of stress caused by the disruption of the social hierarchy in a group of mice. The increase in rodents' anxiety coincided with the activation of the proto-oncogene c-Fos in the brain regions responsible for fear and perception of a threat, such as the amygdala, hippocampus, prefrontal cortex, and some others. At the same time, in most of these regions degeneration and signs of inflammation increased in the microglia, which are specialized brain cells that provide local immune functions aimed to destroy pathogenic agents. There was also transfer of macrophages into the brain, where they produced pro-inflammatory cytokines in nerve cells, which further activated the inflammatory process. Since all these phenomena were prevented by the beta-blocker propranolol, the role of catecholamine stress hormones became apparent (Wohleb E. S. et al., 2011).

Professor Suzanne Lutgendorf of the University of Iowa (2009, 2011), author of many important discoveries in the field of oncogenic distress, together with her coworkers studied the activity of genes in early-stage ovarian tumors. Patients who showed signs of severe stress, who were deeply depressed, and had weak social support, had an impaired expression of 266 genes corresponding to the class and stage of the tumor—compared with patients who were in a more balanced psychological state. In addition, the level of norepinephrine and the activity of the associated transcription factors of the CREB family and other families were higher in the tumors of patients experiencing stress.

Along with a large group of scientists from the universities of Texas and Los Angeles, laboratories from New York, Puerto Rico, and Germany, Professor Lutgendorf carried out further large-scale studies of the relationship of stress to ovarian cancer in cell cultures of experimental animals and human tumors. When cells in the culture were stimulated with norepinephrine, the genes responsible for the synthesis of the cytoplasmic enzyme Src kinase were activated. This enzyme plays a significant role in intercellular signaling and intracellular rearrangements, as well as in the development of cancer and its metastasis. The level of Src kinase increases not only in ovarian tumors, but also in tumors of many other human organs and tissues.

An increase in the Src-kinase content also occurs in ovarian tumor tissue in mice subjected to mobility stress, and their tumor growth was more active than in rodents without stress. In the final experiments, scientists found a significant increase in the level of Src-kinase content and norepinephrine concentration in tissues of human ovarian tumors. The level of Src-kinase content was correspondingly higher in patients with deeper depression, and the survival prognosis was worse than in patients with less severe depression. The authors conclude that a new mechanism has been discovered, through which neuroendocrine stress can directly affect the growth and metastasis of tumors (Armaiz-Pena G. N. et al., 2013).

19.5.2. Anti-oncogenes and Anti-oncoproteins

In most cases, oncogene activation only is not enough to trigger the malignant transformation of cells: uncontrolled cell division is hampered by the so-called suppressor genes or anti-oncogenes, and their products, respectively, are suppressor proteins, or anti-oncoproteins.

The p53 protein, which is the product of the activity of the TP53 anti-oncogene, is one of the most researched anti-oncoproteins to date. At its core, it is a transcription factor that regulates cell division. In malignant tumors, the p53 protein acts as a suppressor of unrestricted cell reproduction and that is why it is called the "guardian of the genome." When mutations of the anti-oncogene TP53 occur (this is observed in almost half of all malignant tumors), the synthesis of the p53 protein is disrupted, and it can no longer perform its restraining division functions. The p53 protein also participates in the processes of repairing DNA from damage caused by various carcinogens, and as a result, reducing its content increases the intensity of the dangerous genome mutations (Adimoolam S., Ford J. M., 2003).

In a joint study by scientists from the medical universities of New Jersey and Harbin, mice of a special line were injected ("grafted") with human tumor cells and afterward underwent stressful mobility limitation for a week (six hours a day). Then the mice were subjected to ionizing irradiation, which resulted in an active development of tumors. It turned out that the rodents that were under the influence of stress developed cancer much more actively, and the p53 content and function decreased more severely than in control mice that were not exposed to stress. The reason for these disruptions in p53 activity is due to the glucocorticoids that activate the SGK1 gene under stress. This gene, in turn, encodes the synthesis of subsequent enzymes that inhibit the synthesis of p53 (Feng Z. et al., 2012).

Another effect of the p53 protein was discovered by researchers from the Montreal and Sherbrooke universities in Canada while studying another protein, SOCS1, which suppresses the activity of pro-inflammatory cytokines. As we already know, their content grows under stress and creates an inflammatory "field" for tumor growth. SOCS1 happened to be the direct regulator of the TP53 gene and activates the synthesis of the p53 protein: in its absence, p53 cannot perform its functions of suppressing the proliferation of tumor cells, and this is often observed in cancer patients. However, the introduction of the SOCS1 protein into tumor cells resumed the suppression of cell division. According to the project manager, professor of biochemistry Gerardo Ferbeyre, this discovery gives hope for the development of a new treatment method that can activate the body's natural anti-cancer defense mechanism (Mallette F. A. et al., 2010). Other scientists were also successful when using this method: by restoring the initial level of the p53 protein synthesis in cells they achieved the regression of lymphomas and sarcomas in mice without side effects on normal tissues (Ventura A. et al., 2007).

One more mechanism of reduction of the p53 protein content in tumors was discovered by scientists from the medical center of Duke University, NC. They injected a drug that simulates the activity of epinephrine into lab mice for a duration of four weeks. This led to a prolonged activation of the specific beta-adrenergic receptor of the cell and a subsequent decrease of the p53 protein level in it. The head of the laboratory where the study was conducted, Dr. Robert

Lefkowitz, believes that the mechanism found will help to understand how humans' stress leads to health problems—up until the onset of cancer. The model of chronic stress used by scientists in the experiment showed that the content of p53 remains at a low level for a long time, and this explains the cause of the DNA functions disorders (Hara M. R. et al., 2011).

The BRCA1 and BRCA2 anti-oncogenes regulate the adequacy of the growth of the mammary gland cells, protecting the body from altered cells that result in the appearance of neoplastic tumors. Mutations of these genes bring a high risk of developing hereditary breast cancer and ovarian cancer. In the normal state of the organism, by binding to its receptor, cortisol stimulates its function as a transcription factor that interacts with the BRCA1 gene and activates its expression (i.e., this complex acts as an anti-oncoprotein). Studies have shown that under stress, an excessive amount of cortisol binds to a large number of receptors and in this manner blocks their activities as transcription factors and can inhibit the work of the BRCA1 gene, thus increasing the risk of breast cancer (Ritter H. D. et al., 2012).

19.5.3. DNA Damage and Repair

Cell culture studies showed us that just ten minutes after the stress hormone content is increased, DNA damage begins to occur (Flint M. S. et al., 2007). Daily addition of catecholamines to the culture of 3T3 cells (which proved to be a sensitive model for the detection of potential carcinogens and mutagens) caused an increase in DNA mutations and a change in the cellular phenotype, which stimulated accelerated division. In addition, these cells caused a more aggressive development of cancer after being "grafted" to a special line of mice (Flint M. S. et al., 2013). The relationships of chronic stress and DNA damage were also studied in the Institute of Biology at the University of Athens in Greece. Lymphocytes isolated from the blood of people experiencing stress were subjected to X-ray irradiation, which, as we know, causes DNA damage. Stress led to an increase in the vulnerability of DNA: the number of ruptures and residual lesions in these people's genome was greater than in those of people without stress (Dimitroglou E. et al., 2003).

An important way in which stress hormones cause damage to the genome is through the activation of the intracellular oxidative stress, which was discussed in Section 19.4. In particular, the level of oxidative damage of nuclear DNA increases in rats subjected to psychological stress (Adachi S. et al., 1993).

According to the Department of Mental Health of the University of Tokyo, the number of oxidative damage in DNA is increased in healthy Japanese workers that are experiencing stress due to an excessive workload (Inoue A. et al., 2009). Other Japanese scientists found that the intensity of oxidative DNA damage in women corresponds to their stress, which is manifested as tension, anxiety, depressiveness, anger, hostility, fatigue, and reduced ability to cope with complex life situations. For men, more typical types of stress reflected in DNA damage were negative reactions to an excessive workload, self-criticism, and the recent loss of a loved one. The authors conclude that it is obvious that psychological factors influence the development of cancer (Irie M. et al., 2001).

The same team of Japanese researchers revealed that the more parents are psychologically distanced from their child, the more intense DNA damage the child will have during in adulthood. The level of damage is especially high in individuals who experienced the death of a loved within three years before the experiments (Irie M. et al., 2002). This data once again confirms the diathesis–stress concept of cancer.

Throughout the process of evolution, the human body has developed ways of protecting itself against damage to and mutation of the genetic apparatus. These are immune cells and enzymes that destroy carcinogens and other foreign substances, as well as special enzymes that determine where DNA damage has occurred. They either repair it, or destroy the cells where DNA is damaged to a point where it can no longer be repaired. Disorders of the DNA repair system constitute another important factor in the development of cancer.

Scientists at the School of Medicine at the Ohio University have investigated the relationship between psycho-emotional stress and the restoration of DNA in blood samples obtained from patients admitted to a psychiatric hospital (without a state of psychosis or drug abuse), which can be considered a stress factor. These blood samples, together with the corresponding control samples from the blood bank, were subjected to X-ray radiation, after which the state of DNA repair was studied in the lymphocytes isolated from the blood. In hospitalized patients, the level of DNA repair was lower than that seen in the blood of people from the control group. In addition, the DNA of patients who were deeply depressed was recovering at even slower rates (Kiecolt-Glaser J. K. et al., 1985).

These scientists further carried out a series of experiments on rats. The rodents were exposed to the carcinogen dimethylnitrosamine and afterward divided into two equal groups. One group was stressed by prolonged rotation. As a result, the level of the methyltransferase enzyme, which plays an important role in DNA repair in response to external intrusions, was significantly reduced in the lymphocytes of rats in the stressed group compared to those in the control group (Glaser R. et al., 1985). Another team of researchers studied the level of stress and the ability of DNA to be repaired in students. The experiments were conducted on the third day of a five-day examination session and three weeks after vacation. The result showed that students with a higher subjective level of stress also have a higher level of DNA damage, which is defined by the activity of its recovery process. After the break, when students had rested, the level of DNA damage was normalized (Cohen L. et al., 2000).

As I reported in Chapter 3.2, chronic stress also causes epigenetic modifications of the genome, in particular, the enhancement of the DNA methylation. This modification makes it difficult to unpack the chromosomes, which hinders the repair enzymes' ability to access the DNA, and thereby increases the risk of mutation accumulation and the development of cancer (Lahtz C., Pfeifer G. P., 2011). In addition, the hypermethylation of DNA lowers the activity of tumor suppressor genes and this, according to B. Tycko (2000), happens even more often than when it occurs as a result of mutations in these genes.

Dr. Frank Jenkins of the Institute of Cancer at the University of Pittsburgh, PA, formulated the following concept, based on the research done in his laboratory and the experiments of other scientists. On account of the fact that during psychological stress the cells of the body are actively influenced by catecholamines, a chain of related reactions leads to two main consequences: a) the development of oxidative stress and the accumulation of its products—reactive oxygen formations that damages DNA; and b) changes in the mechanisms of the p53 protein regulation, which result in the loss of its ability to restore DNA and inhibit the dangerous multiplication of cells (Jenkins F. J. et al., 2014). Glucocorticoids have the same effects (McIntosh L. J., Sapolsky R. M., 1996; Orzechowski A. et al., 2002; Jenkins F. J. et al., 2014).

19.5.4. Disorders at the Chromosome Level

The chromosome, in simplified terms, is a long-lived complex of DNA and proteins that supports the folded DNA structure and is responsible for proper gene activity and cell division. In unfavorable conditions, chromosomes can undergo various mutations that disrupt their structure and functions. Cancer is often accompanied by breaks in chromosomes and translocations of their fragments, their doubling, loss, wrong location, etc.

One of the mechanisms supporting the vital activity of the chromosomes is the sister chromatid exchange (SCE), which is the exchange of sites (fragments) between the sister chromatids ("legs") of one chromosome. This process occurs periodically during normal cell division and can be associated with DNA repair, while under the influence of damaging agents, the frequency of SCE can increase substantially.

One of the factors that damages chromosomes is stress. Scientists from the Department of Medical Genetics of the New York Psychiatric Institute used various types of stress (swimming, white noise, and electrical irritation) in an experiment on rats. They found that any type of stress increases the frequency of SCE and chromosomal aberrations (mutations that break the structure of chromosomes) in the rodents' bone marrow cells (Fischman H. K. et al., 1996). Given these results, data on the increase in the incidence of SCE in patients with cancer of the prostate (Dhillon V. S., Dhillon I. K., 1998), nasopharynx (Li G. Y. et al., 1989) and bladder (Guo G. et al., 2013) appear to be logical.

Another important mechanism responsible for cell division in general that also contributes to the frequency of this process in cancer cells (and makes them potentially immortal) is the high activity of the chromosomal enzyme telomerase. During the division of any cell, the chromosome undergoes its duplication process, which is very complex and fraught with the loss of genes. The latter leads to instability of the genetic apparatus, mutations, and pathological processes in the body. After division, the length of telomeres (end sections of chromosomes) is reduced and that is why the cell needs telomerase. Its function is to restore the original length of the telomeres after DNA replication is complete. Normally, telomerase is active in continuously dividing embryonic cells that form tissues and organs. As the organism matures and once the terminal differentiation of cells has occurred, the telomerase synthesis in them ceases, and remains in only those cells that continue to divide: for example, in cells of the outer layer of the skin, bone marrow, sexual and immune systems, intestinal epithelium. With age, the length of telomeres in cells gradually decreases, which is considered to be one of the most important mechanisms of aging (Frenck R. W. Jr et al., 1998). A more active shortening of telomeres reflects chromosomal instability, which increases the likelihood of mutations. This is a risk factor for cancer, cardiovascular and infectious diseases, their further progression, and premature death (Ornish D. et al., 2008; Calado R. T., Young N. S., 2009).

A significant number of studies have shown the shortening of telomeres in both pre-tumor epithelial tissues (the bladder, esophagus, large intestine, oral cavity, cervix uteri—Meeker A. K. et al., 2004), and in developed cancer tissues and blood cells. Telomere shortening is currently considered to be a diagnostic sign of the onset and progression of an oncological disease, regardless of its localization (Kondo T. et al., 2004; Ornish D. et al., 2008; Willeit P. et al., 2010; Wentzensen I. et al., 2011). In addition, the length of telomeres decreases with chronic stress, which indicates the common mechanisms of both pathological conditions.

Stress-induced shortening of telomeres may begin as soon as during the early stages of human development, which demonstrates the deep genetic level of the formation of psychosomatic predisposition. I have already reported a reduction in the lengths of telomeres in young people whose mothers experienced severe stress during pregnancy (Entringer S. et al., 2011). Similarly, nine-year-old children from dysfunctional families had telomeres that were an average of 19% shorter than those of their peers from privileged families (Mitchell C. et al., 2014). This shortening of telomeres also persists during adulthood: the meta-analysis of scientific data, including twenty-seven samples and 16,238 participants, revealed a significant relationship between a higher level of childhood stressors and a shorter telomere length at the mean age of forty-two (Hanssen L. M. et al., 2017).

Researchers from the University of California studied white blood cell chromosomes of women who had been in a state of chronic stress while caring for sick children for between one and twelve years. It was found that the longer the period of stress, the smaller was the length of telomeres and the more sharply decreased the activity of telomerase, and in addition the greater the oxidative stress in cells. Of particular interest is another observation made in these experiments: the degree of the reduction in the length of telomeres depends not only on the stress actually existing in the life of women, but also on their subjective evaluation of this stress. Women in the control group who did not have sick children to care for, but claimed to be experiencing a high level of everyday stress during preliminary psychological testing, had a similar decrease in the length of telomeres to those of the women who actually were caring for sick children. The authors of the experiment suggest that women with longer telomeres may have greater psychological resistance to stressors than women with reduced telomeres (Epel E. S. et al., 2004).

In further studies, these scientists found that chronic stress in women, when accompanied by an increase in the nighttime level of epinephrine, corresponds to low activity levels of leukocyte telomerase and an increased risk of cardiovascular disease. In addition, the higher the urinary content of all major stress hormones—epinephrine, norepinephrine, and cortisol, the greater is the shortening of telomeres (Epel E. S. et al., 2006). A similar pattern was found in patients with depression: the longer the history of the disease, the smaller the length of their telomeres (Wolkowitz O. M. et al., 2011).

Cell culture studies also demonstrated that exposing T-lymphocytes to high doses of cortisol leads to a decrease in their telomerase levels, which can persist for three days after the experiment (Choi J. et al., 2008). As mentioned in the previous section, this effect of stress hormones on telomeres, among other mechanisms, is mediated by oxidative stress. Agents of the latter (for example, free oxygen radicals) are able to damage the genetic apparatus directly, while repair in telomeres is generally worse than in the rest of the chromosomes (von Zglinicki T., 2002; Epel E. S. et al., 2004).

The decrease in the length of telomeres in leukocytes also occurs in people who experience chronic stress when caring for patients with Alzheimer's disease (along with a decrease in their immunity) (Damjanovic A. K. et al., 2007), those in a state of depression (Lung F. W. et al., 2007), loneliness (Mainous A. G. et al., 2011) and in an unsatisfactory socioeconomic situation (Steptoe A. et al., 2011). One of the studies found a shortening of telomeres in patients with gastric cancer prior to surgery, which, undoubtedly, is a stressful event. Scientists have determined the length of telomeres in T-helper and T-killer lymphocytes, which can help to reveal one of the mechanisms of reduced immunity during cancer (Bukhtoyarov O. V., Arkhangelskiy A. E., 2008).

However, the good news is that the disturbances in telomere length and telomerase activity are reversible. Meditation practices aimed at reducing stress lead to an increase in telomerase activity in both healthy individuals and cancer patients (Falus A. et al., 2011; Lengacher C. A. et al., 2014). The increase in telomerase activity in immune cells also occurred during a three-month program with the objective of changing the lifestyle of prostate cancer patients (includes diet correction, exercises, stress management, and social support) (Ornish D. et al., 2008), and after a nine-week course of hypnotherapy and autosuggestion in patients with stomach cancer (Bukhtoyarov O. V., Arkhangelskiy A. E., 2008). Such programs (we will discuss them in more detail in Chapter 32) lead to an increase in the survival rate of cancer patients.

All of this data once again demonstrates the paramount importance of how our mind interprets everything that happens in our lives. Indeed, it is our mind that creates our body: by managing stress, we change epigenetic modifications and control telomerases, thereby impacting gene activity and the state of our health!

Chapter 20

Under What Conditions do Carcinogens Become Dangerous?

Despite the fact that it has long been confirmed that carcinogens play a role in the development of cancer, there is one important fact that has not received the attention it deserves: the vast majority of people who have been exposed to background carcinogenic substances remain healthy. With the rare exception of work hazards, poisonings, or catastrophes such as the Chernobyl disaster, those that develop cancer and the rest of the population are exposed to the same amounts of carcinogens. Moreover, as is known, cancer often affects those people who have fairly favorable life conditions: a good ecology, high-quality nutrition and no bad habits. Therefore, what matters is not so much the presence of carcinogens, but how effectively the body is able to defend itself against them. An increasing number of studies confirm that psychosocial stressors, for example noise, poverty, and exposure to violence, may alter human susceptibility to environmental chemical exposures (Clougherty J. E., Levy J. I., 2018).

Scientists have identified the three main classes of carcinogens:

- Chemical. Some examples are asbestos, aniline dyes, pesticides, and components of tobacco smoke. It is worth mentioning that some substances used for the production of food, beverages, household chemicals, and cosmetics may be carcinogenic as well.

- Biological. The main representatives of this group are viruses.

- Physical: ionizing, ultraviolet, and electromagnetic radiation, temperature effects and injuries.

All these types of carcinogens cause different damages, which was discussed in the previous chapter—a mutation or disruption of the genetic apparatus, which results in the activation of oncogenes and the deactivation of suppressor genes. We now know that the degree of the damaging effect of carcinogens depends on the state of the antitumor defense systems of the body—its anticancer resistance. The main defense systems include the immune system, the DNA recovery system, and the anti-oncogene system. In turn, as the information presented above shows, the state of the antitumor protection depends on the depth of the organism's chronic stress. If the antitumor defense system is significantly weakened, then, any carcinogen prevailing in the environment around the person can indeed cause oncogenic mutations; neither its class nor its specificity will any longer make a difference (Armaiz-Pena G. N. et al., 2009).

20.1. Physical and Chemical Carcinogens

Studies conducted on animals demonstrate that chronic stress significantly increases the carcinogenic effect of radiation. In particular, chronic stress that is the result of mobility restriction leads to an increase in the sensitivity of mice to the oncogenic effect of ionizing radiation, which has a toxic effect on their hematopoietic system and increases the frequency of chromosomal aberrations in their spleen cells (Wang B. et al., 2016). Other experiments have shown that mice that are chronically stressed suffer from an increased frequency of squamous cell carcinoma of the skin when exposed to ultraviolet irradiation (Saul A. N. et al., 2005; Parker J. et al., 2004), and the growth of tumors (predominantly lymphomas), caused by ionizing radiation, is activated (Feng Z. et al., 2012). It is also believed that when one is undergoing psychological distress, even low-level environmental radiation can cause mutations in oncogenes and impair the restoration of DNA, leading to the initiation of malignant growth (Cwikel J. G. et al., 2010). Earlier, I also cited data from Greek researchers who found that X-ray irradiation on blood lymphocytes significantly increases the amount of DNA damage in patients that are in a state of stress (Dimitroglou E. et al., 2003).

At the same time, the negative health consequences of technogenic catastrophes such as the Chernobyl nuclear power plant meltdown are not solely caused by the radiation itself. Thus, upon examining the consequences of this accident, experts from the League of the Red Cross and Red Crescent Societies came to the conclusion that many of the identified public health problems, which according to the public and physicians were due to irradiation, are not in fact connected to it. The data obtained allows to assume that psycho-emotional stress, age, labor intensity, and other factors that were not directly related to radiation had a greater impact on the health of veterans of special risk units and civilians residing in areas contaminated by radiation (Nikiforov A. M., 1994; Moroz B. B., Deshevoy Y. B., 1999). It can be concluded that the state of high anxiety and fear which was the basis for the stress experienced by these people distorted their health in general and increased their vulnerability to irradiation.

Putting animals into a state of chronic stress while treating them with chemical carcinogens has the same stimulating effect on the development of the tumor process as exposure to radiation. For example, after the application of urethane, mice that were exposed to chronic stress had an increase in the incidence of lung tumors in comparison with rodents that only got the chemical (Adachi S. et al., 1993). Similarly, when the carcinogen dimethylbenzanthracene (DMBA) was applied to the skin of stressed mice, the incidence and intensity of their skin tumors increased (Suhail N. et al., 2015).

Rats that were injected with another carcinogen—diethylnitrosamine—and at the same time subjected to the stress of mobility restriction had an increased frequency and size of liver tumors (Laconi E. et al., 2000). Experimental neurosis in these rodents promoted a growth in the incidence of gastric cancer when they were exposed to carcinogenic hydrocarbons (Arkhipov G. N., 1971), while the stressful influence of constant illumination upon administration of DMBA intensified the development of breast cancer (Haetskiy I. K., 1965). R. Glaser and colleagues (1985) determined one of the mechanisms of this carcinogenesis: in a similar situation (administration of dimethylnitrosamine to rats under stress caused by prolonged rotation), the level of the methyltransferase enzyme in the lymphocytes, which plays an important role in DNA repair in response to external injuries, was significantly reduced.

The data obtained in animal experiments is confirmed by studies on the role of stress in the relationship between tobacco smoking and lung cancer in humans.

Between the 1960s and the 1980s, a team led by the famous German-British psychologist Hans Eysenck conducted research on the relationship between smoking cigarettes and the suppression of emotions. Scientists found that smokers who were not able to express emotions were five times more likely to develop cancer than those who freely expressed their feelings. The more a person suppresses their emotions, the smaller the total number of cigarettes they need to smoke to increase the risk of developing cancer (*i.e. the person's sensitivity to carcinogens is increasing—V. M.*). Smoking is a carcinogenic risk factor only when it is combined with psychosocial factors, which are stress and the suppression of anger (Kissen D. M., Eysenck H. J., 1962; Grossarth-Maticek R. et al., 1985). This was the basis that Eysenck (2000) used when he wrote that cancer is not caused by cigarettes or by one's goofy life; what matters is whether or not one's personality type is prone to the disease, that is to say characterized by the inability to express emotions, inappropriate reaction to stress, pressure of hopelessness, helplessness, and depression.

20.2. Biological Carcinogens—Oncoviruses

The viral-genetic theory of cancer was formulated by the eminent Soviet virologist L. A. Zilber in 1948. He believed that although viruses cause cancer, the disease itself develops as a noncontagious and pathological process, unlike other viral diseases. Today, it is believed that about 15% of all the cancers in the world are caused by viral infections (zur Hausen H., 1991).

The main difference between oncogenic viruses and common infectious viruses is a significant similarity between the structure and composition of some parts of their DNA (the so-called viral oncogenes) and certain DNA regions (proto-oncogenes) in the host's cells which these viruses penetrate. Therefore, viral DNA can partially or completely integrate itself into the host's cell DNA as a fragment and become a full-pledge part of the cellular genome. After intrusion, the viral genes begin to activate local proto-oncogenes, cause chromosomal mutations and the synthesis of nuclear proteins, which work as transcription factors that disrupt the regulation of the host's cell cycle. In essence, oncogenic viruses cause the same basic disorders of the genetic apparatus that we discussed in the previous chapter.

The oncovirus family includes a number of viruses, which, when they affect humans, generally cause diseases that are less dangerous than cancer, including hepatitis B and C viruses, the human papilloma virus, the Epstein-Barr virus, the cytomegalovirus and others, including one seemingly harmless virus—the human herpesvirus (HHV-8). Nowadays, a large number of people are carriers of inactive forms of many of these viruses, especially the herpesvirus, cytomegalovirus, and the Epstein-Barr virus, which over 90% of adults carry (Glaser R., Kiecolt-Glaser J. K., 1994). As a general rule, a healthy organism has full control over these viruses and they manifest their oncogenic properties only under special conditions that are yet to be understood by modern oncology. According to L. A. Zilber (1948),

> Regardless of how the tumor virus gets inside the human body, it does not manifest itself for a prolonged amount of time. There is nothing to be surprised about here. It has a weak pathogenic power. It needs special conditions to manifest itself as a disease, and as long as these conditions do not exist, the virus is completely harmless.

What are these special conditions? Modern research suggests that these conditions are the suppression of the protective potential of the body, caused by chronic stress.

All major human oncoviruses are sensitive to intracellular signaling pathways, which are activated by stress hormones. These mediators can reactivate "sleeping" oncoviruses, stimulate the expression of oncogenes, and suppress the antiviral response of the organism. Studies have demonstrated the accelerated growth of virus-induced tumors in animals that are exposed to stress (Justice A., 1985; Riley V., 1981).

In humans, owing to a disruption of the ability of the immune system to control the latent (inactive) state of viruses, chronic psychological stress and depression activate the multiplication of oncoviruses such as cytomegalovirus, herpesvirus, and the Epstein-Barr virus. In addition, an increased amount of stress means that the herpesviral infectious disease will be more active and will last for longer (Glaser R., Kiecolt-Glaser J. K., 1994; Godbout J. P., Glaser R., 2006). Childhood adversities that reduce immune protection play their own role in the degree of activity of viruses: the activity levels of cytomegalovirus and the Epstein-Barr virus were higher in women with breast cancer who had more negative experiences during their childhoods than in patients with fewer negative childhood experiences (Fagundes C. P. et al., 2013).

Loneliness is also a factor in chronic stress: lonely students develop more antibodies to the Epstein-Barr virus (hence, the virus is more active in them) than those who do not consider themselves to be lonely (Glaser R. et al., 1985). The same situation is observed in those students who suppress their emotions and do not allow themselves to share their experiences with other people (Esterling B. A. et al., 1990). The herpes simplex virus and the Epstein-Barr virus are also activated in students that are going through examination stress (Glaser R. et al., 1993a, 1994) and in those that are overall not satisfied with their socioeconomic situation (Stowe R. P. et al., 2010), which can also be regarded as a factor of chronic stress.

An interesting experiment, once again demonstrating the important role of consciousness in the development and control of cancer, was conducted at the Ohio University's Institute for Behavioral Medicine Research. Two hundred twenty-four women under the stress of a recent diagnosis of breast cancer were examined for the activity of herpes simplex and Epstein-Barr viruses, in parallel with determining the levels of their socioeconomic status and support received. Women with higher status, level of education, and levels of support from friends had lower levels of antibodies to the Epstein-Barr virus (i.e., the virus was less active, which indicates better protective functions of the immune system) than women with lower socioeconomic status (Fagundes C. P. et al., 2012a).

Human papilloma virus is one of the main causes of cervical cancer. Women experiencing chronic stress have a decreased immune response to the HPV16 papilloma virus, which makes them more vulnerable to cancer (Fang C. et al., 2008). Stressful events in the personal lives of women (divorce, infidelity of a spouse, frequent conflicts, psychological and physical aggression of the husband or partner) that occurred five years before the examination, lead to cervical dysplasia, which is a precancerous condition that is accompanied by the activation of the papilloma virus (Coker A. et al., 2003).

In experiments conducted on animals, it was observed that chronic stress activates the development of viral tumors in the same way that physical and chemical carcinogens do (Justice A., 1985).

We already know that one of the main mechanisms of stress is the release of specific hormones into the bloodstream. That is why there is a possibility that they play a role in the distortion of the body's ability to control the state of oncogenic viruses. Indeed, under experimental conditions, glucocorticoids are able to activate oncogenic viruses, such as the human papilloma virus (Mittal R. et al., 1993) and the Epstein-Barr virus (Cacioppo J. T. et al., 2002). Scientists of the University of Texas, in collaboration with NASA, measured the level of epinephrine and norepinephrine in the urine of astronauts and the activity of the Epstein-Barr virus in their organisms prior to going into space, ten days before landing, on the day of landing, and three days after landing. It turned out that in the 40% of the astronauts who had an increase in the level of catecholamine from ten days before landing (that is, these astronauts experienced stronger landing-related stress), the virus was activated (Stowe R. P. et al., 2001).

Catecholamines can also promote the reproduction of the human immunodeficiency virus (HIV1) by increasing the cellular susceptibility to this infection, activating the gene of viral transcription (Cole S. W. et al., 2001), and suppressing the activity of antiviral cytokines (Cole S. W. et al., 1998). Therefore, HIV-infected people with increased autonomic nervous system activity (which occurs under stress) have an increased virus blood plasma content and worse results during specific antiretroviral therapy (Cole S. W. et al., 2001). This, in turn, increases the risk of non-Hodgkin's lymphoma, which is an oncological disease typically found in AIDS patients (Killebrew D., Shiramizu B., 2004).

* * *

The studies presented allow us to conclude that in most cases, external carcinogenic factors (outside extreme situations) are able to trigger disease only when the organism has already developed a precancerous state because of chronic stress.

Buddhist master Lama Zopa Rinpoche (2001) describes the influence of carcinogens from the point of view of Tibetan medicine:

> Exposure to sunlight is a condition for skin cancer but not its main cause. The main cause of skin cancer is internal, not external. The main cause is the mind. For people who have the cause of skin cancer in their mind, exposure to the sun does become a condition for the development of skin cancer. For those who don't have the internal cause, however, exposure to sunlight won't become a condition for them to develop skin cancer.

Chapter 21

Why is Aging a Particular Risk Factor for Cancer?

Stress is a catalyst that speeds up almost every one
of the known mechanisms of aging.
I. N. Todorov, G. I. Todorov,
Stress, Aging, and its Biochemical Correction

Although oncologists usually consider aging to be a predisposing factor, this study analyzes the development of cancer over the course of human life (ontogeny). Therefore, it will be logical to pay special attention to aging in this part of the book.

According to statistics, the risk of cancer increases with aging, with three quarters of all patients being over fifty-five when first diagnosed with the disease. Between the ages of sixty and eighty, every third man and every fourth woman gets cancer (Jemal A. et al., 2008; Belyalova N. S., Belyalov F. I., 2005). And because of this, I cannot ignore this topic for the purpose of this book and must analyze it from the standpoint of the diathesis–stress model of diseases.

Medical science explains the age-related increase in cancer morbidity by both the duration of the action of external oncogenic factors (the accumulation of their effects) and the age-related decrease in the antitumor resistance of the organism (Novitskiy V. V. et al., 2009). But why does this resistance weaken with age?

Back in 1905, Sigmund Freud noted that strong emotional experiences can reduce one's resistance or increase the body's susceptibility to infectious diseases and even contribute to a reduction in life expectancy (Freud S., 1953). In 1928, Professor G. B. Bykhovskiy from Kiev reported studies conducted by colleagues, which showed that during the First World War and the Communist revolution, many young people who were under the influence of "soul worries" and "nervous mental trauma" had premature gray hair and atherosclerosis.

In the forties, M. K. Petrova (1946) obtained similar data in experiments conducted on animals in the laboratory of Ivan Pavlov. When in a state of chronic stress, dogs gradually acquired a decrepit appearance, looked older than their age, had gray hair in their wool and dystrophic manifestations on their skin. They lost teeth, the lenses of their eyes became cloudy, muscle tone and sexual arousal were lost, and, as I mentioned above, they often suffered from a tumor disease. At the same time, those dogs who were not stressed looked significantly younger than their age.

Hans Selye (1975), the founder of the doctrine of stress, wrote that

> Each period of stress, especially if it results from frustrating, unsuccessful struggles, leaves some irreversible chemical scars which accumulate to constitute the signs of tissue aging. Many authors still use my earlier definition of biological stress as 'the wear and tear' in the machinery of a living being, but this is actually the result of stress, and the accumulation of the irreparable part of this attrition is aging. ... Aging results from the sum of all the stresses to which the body has been exposed during a lifetime and apparently corresponds to the 'stage of exhaustion' of the G.A.S., which is, in a sense, an accelerated version of normal aging.

Selye (1952) found that morphological changes in the organs of animals that died at the stage of depletion of the general adaptation syndrome in many ways resemble senile degenerative changes.

Gerontologists I. N. and G. I. Todorov (2003) state that most of our organ functions deteriorate with age and it would be natural to expect that the intensity and strength of stress reactions will likewise decrease with age. However, in reality, the opposite happens: a number of major stress manifestations become more pronounced with age. Therefore, the same stressor usually causes a more intense stress reaction in old people or animals than in young people. "Often, older individuals show an elevated level of certain stress hormones even in the absence of any stress factors, which is actually equivalent to a state of constant chronic stress. So, obviously a vicious circle develops: stress speeds up aging, and aging increases the body's response to stressful factors," the authors note.

The reasons for this paradox were thoroughly investigated at the Research Institute of Gerontology of the Academy of Medical Sciences of Ukraine, where I had the pleasure of working in the early 1990s under the guidance of an outstanding scientist, one of the leading gerontologists of the USSR, academician Vladimir Frolkis, the founder of the Ukrainian scientific school of the biology of aging. Researchers of our institute found that with aging, a complex of hormonal, metabolic, tissue, and cellular changes typical of the general adaptation syndrome develops, which V. V. Frolkis (1991) named as the "stress-age-syndrome."

This syndrome, as well as chronic stress in general, is characterized by an uneven change in the excitability of hypothalamic centers and their sensitivity to hormones, a distortion of the balance of positive and negative emotions, an increase in the blood concentration of epinephrine, cortisol, vasopressin, ACTH, cholesterol, and free radicals that damage the cells. At the same time, the levels of thyroxine, testosterone, and the P substance decrease in the blood, tolerance of carbohydrates decreases, cardiac and vascular reactivity changes, hypercoagulation and immunosuppression develop. These changes, despite the fact that they generally perform adaptive tasks during aging, nevertheless limit the ability of the aging organism to fully react to the stresses of life and contribute to the onset of age-related diseases (Frolkis V. V., 1991).

Of particular interest is the data obtained in the institute on the topic of the shift of the emotional balance toward negative manifestations that occurs at old age. The results of the experiments performed there showed that in old rats the "behavior of despair" developed more often than in adults while experiencing the stress caused by prolonged swimming. It was determined by the duration of periods of torpidity during the first minutes of swimming when the animal was not yet tired (Frolkis V. V., 1991).

Another prominent Soviet gerontologist, Professor Vladimir Dilman (1986), developed the concept of hyperadaptosis. According to it, the body's adaptive systems create an excessive response to stress when an organism reaches old age. In this case, a prolonged increase in the blood concentration of stress hormones occurs due to the age-related increase in the hypothalamic threshold to inhibition (i.e., inadequate homeostatic inhibition). In this way, while defending itself from different distresses (external causes of death), the body must pay for this possibility by developing adaptation illnesses and thereby accelerates the natural process of aging.

"Thus, adversity and sorrow diminish one's days of life," writes Dilman (1986).—"While aging, a person begins to live as if in a state of chronic stress, and therefore becomes more and more defenseless when actual stress takes its toll on the body. Time is a universal stressor."

A similar conclusion was reached by the research team of the Rostov Research Institute of Oncology (Russia):

> During the prevalence of stress, especially the severe stress of low levels of [body] reactivity, there is a deviation of homeostasis, which in turn leads to rapid aging. We believe that the system of nonspecific adaptive reactions has a direct relationship to the mechanisms of aging, and to the mechanisms of anti-aging (Garkavi L. H. et al., 1990).

Scientists from the University of Iowa determined that, when under the influence of stress, age-related changes in the brain are activated; that is, because of stress, the brain ages faster. This is due to a decrease in the number of neural connections in the prefrontal cortex—the part of the brain that is responsible for emotions, thinking, and control over movements (Anderson R. M. et al., 2014). Another cause of age-related disorders of the nervous system was found by the Danish researcher A. Jørgensen (2013). As we already know, oxidative damage to DNA increases as a result of chronic stress. The scientist confirmed the role of elevated cortisol in these oxidative lesions and showed that they activate the aging process. Likewise, chronic stress accelerates the aging of the immune system (Bennett J. M. et al., 2013); so after the age of fifty-five the acute stressful events are accompanied by an insufficiently active immune response (Segerstrom S. C., Miller G. E., 2004).

An important discovery was made by researchers at the Medical Department of the University of Indianapolis. They studied genes that are simultaneously involved in the processes of stress, mood regulation, and life expectancy. As it turned out, the activity of these genes, which is known to change with age, gets even more disrupted by stress and a negative emotional state (which can even lead to suicide), eventually contributing to accelerating aging and reducing an individual's life expectancy (Rangaraju S. et al., 2016).

Thus, over the course of the last decade (since 2008), an understanding has begun to form in the field of medical science stating that a decrease in the body's resistance in response to stressful effects is the universal and most important manifestation of aging from the point of analysis of morbidity and mortality (Anisimov V. N., 2008).

21.1. Common Epigenetic Mechanisms of Stress, Aging, and Cancer

Gerontologists' research has traditionally been focused on just the period of aging, and few believed that the period of development affects aging. However, at the present moment, these views are being revised, since the achievements of epigenetics and psychoneuroendocrinology convincingly attest to the crucial contribution of the early stages of development to the formation of life expectancy (Vayserman A. M., 2008). In fact, all the stresses of the early period of development and childhood, which I summarized above, when considered as cancer predisposition factors, not only have a negative impact on health, but also accelerate the aging process. Scientists believe that the stresses of both early and adult age lead to increased vulnerability and reduced brain resistance to stress in old age, as well as metabolic changes that disrupt the process of natural aging (Garrido P., 2014).

In particular, the decrease in methylation of the human genome, which begins during childhood consequent on experiencing psychic trauma or attachment disorders and continues into adulthood due to persistent stress, accelerates even more with aging (Vayserman A. M. et al., 2011), although it can follow a different direction, depending on the organ (Anisimov V. N., 2008). This effect of the accumulation of life stresses is considered to be one of the major epigenetic mechanisms that accelerate aging and increase the risk of age-related diseases (Zannas A. S. et al., 2015). For example, methylation of a number of genes in blood cells increases with age, and these genes also show an increased level of methylation in the tissues of seven different types of tumors. The study's authors suggest that the age-related change in methylation may result in a decrease of the expression of certain genes and this is associated with the transition of cells to a malignant state (Xu Z., Taylor J. A., 2014).

An important consequence of early stresses is, as I have already noted, the formation of a "pro-inflammatory phenotype" of an adult organism, that is, its increased propensity to inflammatory diseases (Miller G. E. et al., 2011). Because of the accumulation of life stresses, these inflammatory reactions are reinforced in old age according to epigenetic mechanisms (Christian L. M. et al., 2011; Zannas A. S. et al., 2016), stimulating the development of age-related diseases such as cardiovascular, parkinsonism, and depression (de Pablos R. M. et al., 2014; Akil H. et al., 1993). In turn, this age-related depression further accelerates the aging process (Wolkowitz O. M. et al., 2011). "The relationship between aging and depression is that the aging process contributes to the development of depression, and vice versa: depression seems to accelerate aging.... physiological changes in depression have a similarity with changes that occur when one is experiencing chronic stress," write I. N. and G. I. Todorov (2003); and depression, as we have already seen, along with inflammation becomes one of the significant factors in the development of cancer.

Another epigenetic mechanism, discussed above in connection with chronic stress and cancer, is the reduction of chromosome telomeres, which are also considered to be among the most important factors of aging. For example, the studies done by Elissa Epel and coworkers (2004) showed that the degree of decrease in telomere length in women with a high level of stress corresponds to the acceleration of their biological aging by about ten years. In addition, age-related depression and pessimism are also accompanied by a reduction in the size of telomeres, and the greater the depression, the more telomeres shorten (Wolkowitz O. M. et al., 2011; Verhoeven J. et al., 2014; O'Donovan A. et al., 2009). However, the most obvious confirmation of how our mind accelerates aging, "inventing" stress, was also obtained by E. Epel and her colleagues from the universities of California and New Jersey. Having examined elderly women caring for husbands with dementia, the researchers found that the degree of shortening of women's telomeres corresponds to the degree of their worries about their abilities to cope with the expected difficulties (O'Donovan A. et al., 2012), that is, to ideas subjectively created by their mind.

One of the universal sources of chronic stress is low socioeconomic status. The psychological state associated with it also results in the shortening of the chromosomal telomeres, contributing to an acceleration in the organism's aging (Cherkas L. F. et al., 2006). This may partly explain why in many post-Soviet countries, where the pensions of the majority of elderly people are at the level of the subsistence minimum, the morbidity among this age group is so high.

We already know that stress not only causes a variety of types of DNA damage, but also complicates the restoration of the DNA's damaged areas. It was determined that DNA in the telomere region is especially sensitive to stress and damages in this area are almost never repaired, which therefore causes them to accumulate with age. This discovery, made at the University of Newcastle, helps to understand why body cells lose their ability to regenerate as they age (Hewitt G. et al., 2012).

I am pleased to recall that back in the late 1980s, as a graduate student at the Kiev Institute of Gerontology, when epigenetics in its modern form was in the making and data on the relationship between the modifications of DNA and nuclear histone proteins with gene expression was just accumulating, I was able to understand the major role of the main modifications of chromosome proteins (acetylation, methylation, and phosphorylation) in the mechanisms of aging. In my review study, published in the leading Soviet journal, *Success of Modern Biology*, among other things I concluded that during aging, the way through which signals from catecholamines, connecting to the cell, are passed to the genes, is disrupted. As a result, the histone-modifying process changes, the degree of chromatin compaction increases, and disturbances occur in the functions of the genome (Matrenitsky V. L., 1989).

In other words, just as with age the whole organism often "shrinks" and becomes more compact, losing its functions, our chromosomes also change in a similar way. Because of this increase in chromatin compactness, access to the DNA of the enzymes that restore it after damage is hampered. This can be one of the causes of the increase in mutations that leads to malignant transformation of cells. The fact that DNA restoration is disrupted in old age owing to exposure to radiation and other damaging agents is also confirmed by gerontologists (Plesko M. M., Richardson A., 1984).

Modern studies show that chromatin modifications are directly and indirectly interrelated with DNA methylation processes and subsequent changes in the activity of key genes, which occur both in connection with aging and in connection with malignant tumor growth. For example, the character of acetylation and methylation of histones influences the progression of the prostate tumor (Seligson D. B. et al., 2005). In turn, chronic stress is considered to be one of the major factors that affect the degree of chromatin compactness (Johnstone S. E., Baylin S. B., 2010).

When working on my Ph.D. thesis, I studied how in the course of aging the reaction of the organism's central part—the heart—changes as a result of the long-term effects of epinephrine. This situation can be considered as a model of the distress process.

My attention was centered on the desensitization reaction—the adaptive mechanism of the cell, which consists in reducing the number of receptors to epinephrine on the surface of the membrane, thus limiting its damaging effect. This mechanism refers to the general adaptation syndrome and reflects the unified principle of the neuroendocrine system function—the "feedback" principle: the higher the level of catecholamines in the blood, the fewer receptors are on the cell membranes. It gives the body an opportunity to withstand the stressful and damaging effects of the environment. As I discovered over the course of my research, during old age the mechanism of desensitization is disrupted: it is less pronounced and requires more time for its development (Matrenitsky V. L., 1992). Because of this, catecholamines have a longer-lasting, and therefore more damaging, effect on the cells. The results obtained in these experiments confirm the data of the researchers cited above showing that the stresses experienced in old age have a more protracted character, and therefore contribute to the development of a diverse pathology, including the cancer.

A similar dynamics is observed for the second major stress hormone—cortisol. Scientists from the Salk Institute for Biological Studies in California have determined that in older rats the elevated cortisol content in the blood persists longer than in young rats following a stressful situation. If rodents of both age groups were "grafted" with tumor cells, then in old animals the cancer developed significantly more actively than in young animals (Sapolsky R. M., Donnelly T. M., 1985). This data reflects the general trend observed in animal experiments, according to which the sensitivity of cells to the effects of carcinogenic substances and the frequency of development of transplanted tumors increase with age as a whole (Anisimov V. N., 2008).

As reported in Chapter 19.4, one of the ways in which chronic stress contributes to the malignant transformation of cells is by the activation of oxidative intracellular stress that damages the membrane, DNA, and other cellular elements. In the 1950s, the important contribution of reactive oxygen and nitrogen species accumulation to aging was discovered and there was even the development of a 'free-radical theory' of ageing (Harman D., 1957). Today, significant evidence exists indicating that generation of ROS and the corresponding response to oxidative stress are key factors determining longevity and the onset of age-related diseases (Liguori I. et al., 2018). According to Thomas Jefferson University, PA, during aging damage caused by oxidative stress also accumulates in the mitochondria—the "power stations" of the cell. Because of this, the cell begins to get rid of the mitochondria, resulting in an anoxic (anaerobic) pathway for the breakdown of nutrients. This is exactly what is necessary for the reproduction of cancer cells. Thus, aging cells seem to "feed" the tumor, helping it to grow and metastasize (Balliet R. M. et al., 2011).

According to the works of Professor Vladimir Dilman (1986), age-related hyperadaptosis, which increases the level of chronic stress in the body via a compensatory enhancement of the activity of peripheral endocrine glands, leads to immunodepression and the disruption of metabolic processes in the body. This specific state of an individual's metabolism, which the author referred to as cancrophilia, contributes to raising the sensitivity threshold of tissues and cells to various types of carcinogenic substances and increases the likelihood of their malignant transformation.

All the above data from biological studies indicates that a high incidence of cancer during old age is a natural result of the accumulation of consequences of life stresses and an increase in the sensitivity of the organism to both stressors and carcinogens. But what do the observations made by psychologists and sociologists say about the relationship between aging and stress?

21.2. How You Respond to Stress Determines Your Health in Old Age

Between 1939 and 1942, a long-term study was launched in the United States, which became known as the Grant experiment. Scientists surveyed 268 of the most healthy and promising graduates of Harvard University at the age of about twenty years. Then, once or twice a year they conducted polls or interviews with these young people. When the examinees reached adulthood, the results of the study were collected. It turned out that a healthy psyche prevents the deterioration of physical health in the second half of life. Among the fifty-nine people with the best mental state during their youth, only two had chronic illnesses or died before fifty-three years of age, while eighteen out of forty-eight people with the poorest mental states developed chronic diseases and several died before the age of forty-three (Vaillant G. E., 1977).

I have also quoted the data collected by scientists from the University of Pennsylvania who found that the way a person responds to adversities in life predicts the occurrence of chronic diseases ten years ahead, regardless of their current state of health and future stresses (Piazza J. R. et al., 2013). According to studies conducted at the Gerontological Center of the University of Jyväskylä in Finland, the stress that a middle-aged person experiences at work determines their functional limitations and disability in old age. Observing more than 5,000 people for almost thirty years, from forty-four to fifty-eight years old at baseline until their retirement, scientists have identified four different types of responses to stress related to the type of their professional activity. These are emotionally negative manifestations and depressiveness, deterioration of cognitive abilities, sleep disorders, and somatic symptoms. A clear gradient of increasing severity of disability in old age for increasing intensity of midlife stress symptoms was shown, i.e. those who complained about such long-term symptoms of stress in middle age faced significant difficulties in basic activities in daily life by the age of eighty (Kulmala J. et al., 2013).

So, what are the characteristics of centenarians, then? T. N. Berezina (2013), upon investigating this issue in a review of scientific literature, came to the conclusion that, along with genes, the individual life expectancy is influenced by environmental factors and genetic–environmental interaction factors; in other words, personal factors. Among them, the researcher would like to point out: optimism, sense of humor, stress-resistance, diligence, general activity, altruism and helping other people, intellect and creativity, optimal organization of one's life, self-development.

Scientists from the University of Bordeaux, having examined about four thousand elderly people, found that the main factor statistically associated with their longevity is the predominance of positive emotions in the mood (Gana K. et al., 2016). Jane-Ling Wang (2016), Distinguished Professor from the University of California, talks about the French woman Jeanne Calment, who lived to 122 years. She never did anything special to achieve longevity—she just laughed a lot and did not worry about stresses. Jeanne said: "If you can do nothing about it, do not worry about it!"

The Chinese county of Bama in Guangxi Province is famous for its centenarians. Local residents explain this phenomenon by their calmness and physical activity (Zotov G., 2014):

> People live long because they do not envy neighbors, they do not compete with those who have a more beautiful car or house. They were quite satisfied with having rice for lunch, as well as with reverence from children and grandchildren. Air and water of course influence [health] as well. But in general, we do not have any miracles. Just be calm, sleep and eat vegetables - that's the recipe for eternal youth.

109-year-old grandmother Juan Makan shares her experience:

> If you are lazy, your body will cease to function, the body will become bored, and it will weaken. I am always in a good mood, I'm an optimist by nature. I do not understand why people are upset because of bad weather—so what, tomorrow it will be good! Do not tear your heart. We always live with large families in the same house, we help each other with advice and actions. I have never been ill or caught cold—in general, I sincerely hope to live to 150 years!

The centenarians from the Japanese island of Okinawa, who live according to the principle "Ikigai—have something you care about to get out of bed for," reveal similar secrets. They are satisfied with the small things, they feed on what they grow themselves, accustomed to work in old age physically and helping each other. This lifestyle also corresponds to the local concept of "yuimaru," which can be translated as a "kind and friendly joint effort." The atmosphere of mutual assistance contributes to the development of peace of mind and optimism in centenarians, which is so necessary to enjoy life in old age (Dmitriev A., 2014).

Dan Buettner (2008) is a longevity expert and National Geographic Explorer of health and aging in extraordinarily long-lived communities around the globe. For example, he wrote about the inhabitants of the island of Sardinia, whose most important secret of longevity is their unique worldview, including a great sense of humor, unconditional devotion to the family, an inescapable desire to work, and a love of contemplation of nature. Another example is the Nicoya centenarians of Costa Rica: it is obligatory for them to have a meaning for life, they feel themselves to be needed and strive to do good, maintain strong ties with their family, happily communicate with people, know how to listen, laugh, and value something that they have, and also work a lot throughout their lives, finding pleasure in doing their daily work.

And though these observations were not made by scientists, but by journalists, I decided to mention them here since they are fully confirmed by all the scientific data we examined above. In particular, I. N. and G. I. Todorov (2003) note that "... centenarians tend to have a higher (than average) ability to overcome difficulties and quickly and successfully overcome psychological stress ... A low level of stress, as we are sure, serves as a magic key to the secret of longevity."

We also see that the aspiration to harmony of the mind and the search for the meaning of life does not only support the pursuit of the task of being free from cancer or other diseases—finding meaning in life prolongs our life and makes it happy. Viktor Frankl (1991) wrote that what matters isn't whether a man is young or old, but much more importantly whether his time and soul are filled with activities to which he can devote his life now. The main issue is whether this activity awakens in a person, despite advanced age, a strong desire to be—to be for someone or for something.

Otherwise, the existential emptiness in old age will increase, poisoning a person's existence and forcing them to bitterly regret a life lived in vain. There is a "psychological situation of a person who has devoted many years of his life to pursuing certain ideals and goals and eventually clearly realized or vaguely felt that the ideals are false, and the goals are false and do not coincide with what is truly valuable for the person. Such insight is usually accompanied by negative, subjectively painful experiences, typical of the life-meaning crisis: disappointment, despair, dissatisfaction, alienation, apathy, regret about lost time, meaninglessness of habitual concepts, etc." (Karpinskiy K. V., 2011). This is another source of chronic psychosocial stress, increasing the likelihood of age-related cancer.

The meaning of life, as we saw above, is closely related to spirituality. It is not surprising that this relationship becomes particularly acute for the elderly. V. D. Troshin (2009a) notes that in gerontology the role of spirituality in generating stresses contributing to the aging process is not sufficiently taken into account. Meanwhile, each person's own dynamic spiritual and genetic stereotype, developed over the course of their life, forms a spiritual dominant, the loss of which leads to the development of pathological conditions and activates the aging of the organism.

On the other hand, in concord with the observations made by the journalists above, scientific research shows that what contributes to good health in old age and longevity is an active social position, spirituality, and religion (Mantovani F. M., Mendes F. R. P., 2010), a high level of life satisfaction, an increase in the religious meaning of life and the ability to forgive, reduced "spiritual struggle" (Park C. L., 2008), a high level of religiosity, successful adaptation to and coping with difficulties, a significant level of life satisfaction (Archer S. et al., 2005). Also, existential and spiritual well-being promote the psychological well-being of the elderly (Lawler-Row K. A., Elliott J., 2009). In general, this topic is becoming increasingly important in our time, as evidenced by publications in the scientific *Journal of religion, spirituality and aging* established in 2005 in the UK.

All of the above, in my opinion, convincingly suggests that the chronic psychosocial stress that increases toward old age, along with the increase in the tendency toward depression and the existential vacuum, is actually the mysterious link that is responsible for the increase in the incidence of cancer with age. Those who have become centenarians are people who since childhood most probably have been raised in harmonious conditions, have learned to cope with the stresses of life adequately, and have a spiritual meaning for life. For such people, life's difficulties and upheavals do not bring destruction but training, strengthening their health.

As Hans Selye (1975) writes, successful activity, even intense, leaves relatively few "chemical scars." It causes stress but usually not distress. Even in old age, it gives an invigorating feeling of youth and strength. Work exhausts an individual mainly through frustrating failures. Many outstanding workers in almost all fields of activity have lived long lives and overcome the inevitable failures, so their advantage was always on the side of success. These people continued to achieve success and happiness even when they were over seventy and beyond. They did not "work," in the sense of having to do a boring job for the sake of a piece of bread. Despite the long years of hard work, their life was a real leisure as they always did what they enjoyed.

This observation is supported by the research showing that soft, "training" stress can both prolong the life of animals under experimental conditions and protect them from the occurrence of cancer (Garkavi L. H. et al., 1990; Frolkis V. V., 1991), once again confirming the generality of the biological mechanisms involved in both processes. What is interesting in this connection is the observation of O. V. Bukhtoyarov and A. E. Arkhangelskiy (2008) who used a special course of hypnotherapy to activate the immunity and healing resources of cancer patients to promote their remission. They also noted signs of a decrease in the biological age of patients: a reduction of gray hair, increased visual acuity, vitality and motor activity. These changes were associated with an increase in the content of stem cells (precursors of immune cells) and an increase in the length of chromosomal telomeres in lymphocytes, which, as we saw above, is usually reduced during chronic stress, aging, and cancer.

So where there is longevity, there is freedom from cancer!

Conclusion

The data presented in this part convincingly testifies to the fact that the state of chronic psychophysiological stress caused by unmet needs, long-standing unresolved conflicts, or psychic trauma can gradually cause an individual to experience feelings of helplessness, hopelessness, and subconscious depression up to avital experiences, subconscious loss of the will to live, and the formation of a cancer dominant in the psyche and the brain.

Chronic stress becomes as if a bodily "executor" or "contractor" of the pathogenic state of mind. It is this state of mind, progressing from unresolved conflict and/or psychic trauma, through an existential crisis to an oncodominant, that ultimately leads the body to an oncological disease.

At the physiological level, the initialization stage is reflected in significant disturbances in the adaptive capacity of the organism and depletion of its protective resources. The function of the immune system and the DNA repair system is significantly reduced, the increase in intracellular oxidative stress is progressing, and the hormonal balance is distorted. As a result, the threshold of vulnerability to internal (metabolic products of some hormones and oxidative stress) and external carcinogens is decreased, the number of mutations and disorders resulting from epigenetic regulation of the genome is increasing, oncogenes are activated and anti-oncogenes are deactivated. This is followed by a growing number of atypical, malignantly transformed cells, which the immune system is no longer able to eliminate effectively. In this way, in the most general terms, the beginning of the tumor growth is triggered, and aging significantly contributes to all these processes.

However, how can we explain why cancer develops in animals that lack mental activity and clearly cannot experience a suppression of anger, a spiritual crisis, and an unconscious desire for death? The answer, it seems to me, is that the type of chronic distress does not make a difference for the organism: it can be caused by prolonged noise stimulus, or repeated social defeat, or limitation of mobility, etc. in animals, or by conflicts of unrealized needs and an existential crisis in human. The only thing that matters is the depth of distress and the level to which the anticancer defenses of the organism fall.

From this position, the theory of Dr. Ryke Hamer (2000) that any human's psychological conflict has its analogy in the animal world seems correct. However, animals experience conflicts literally—for example, when they lose their partner or offspring, lose their nest or territory, are attacked by predators, or threatened by hunger or death. Humans, by virtue of the psychological origin of most modern conflicts, experience many of them at a symbolic level (we discussed the connection between this ability that humans have and how cancer "chooses" targets in chapter 12.3) and for much longer. For example, for a human, the animal's "loss of territory" is analogous to the loss of a house or property, the "threat of hunger" is experienced when an individual loses their business, the psychic trauma of "attack" may occur when another person's words are perceived as insults, "conflict due to abandonment" occurs when one loses one's partner or team (Markolin C., 2007).

At the same time, a data has been obtained indicating that in animals, "psychological experiences" can also contribute to the appearance of potentially oncogenic mutations. Japanese scientists placed rats in a cage adjacent to the one where their relatives were exposed to electric shock. Thus, these rodents were forced to watch the torments of others for two to four hours. As a result of being forced to be in the presence of other beings' sufferings, the "observer" rats had levels of oxidative DNA damage in their livers significantly higher than in animals not exposed to such stress (Adachi S. et al., 1993). However, in the wild, there are almost no such situations.

Although the human oncogenic conflict—or rather crisis—is much more complicated and multilayered, involves various unrealized needs, intertwines the conflicts of fear, dependence, subordination, "suffocation," suppression of one's interests and emotions, helplessness, and hopelessness, it seems that the basic, ultimate biological mechanisms of oncogenic distress and the activation of the cancer process are the same for all living things. For millions of years of evolution in nature, there was no need to adapt organisms to the state of chronic stress, because originally it was not characteristic of living beings. It was relatively rare and has only begun to advance in humans over the last several hundred years—which has been reflected in the growth of chronic diseases. Therefore, animal and human organisms do not yet have such an effective system of protection from chronic stress as the one that we have for fighting infections with our immune system. From this viewpoint, the cancer may act as a factor of natural selection according to Darwin's theory, removing those individuals who cannot cope with chronic stress from the human population. Although this statement may seem cruel at first glance, for the evolution of humanity as a species, such individuals are not needed, because, by transferring their psycho-epigenetic limitations and disorders to children, they hamper the progress of mankind ... Fortunately, a human has a mind not only to create a crisis but to understand all of what is mentioned above and to change!

Steven Cole, a professor of medicine, psychiatry, and behavioral sciences at the Department of Oncology-Hematology School of Medicine, University of Los Angeles, is one of the world's leading researchers on oncogenic distress. He authoritatively argues that the study of biological pathways through which the social and psychological characteristics of cancer patients at the level of the genetic apparatus affect the emergence, development, and treatment of cancer, today is a revolutionary way to understand this disease (Cole S. W., 2013). Prof. Mardi Crane-Godreau of the Geisel School of Medicine in Dartmouth, NH, also agrees with this view: "Stress is a recognized factor in predisposing people to cancer and in adversely impacting treatment and recovery" (Lebanon N., 2015).

The reader may have a question: if it is our mind that creates cancer through stress and the desire for death, then should patients be the ones blamed for getting sick?

My position is: although in most cases the patients themselves create cancer in their bodies, it is not their fault—after all, we are not taught to manage ourselves, manage our emotions, and cope with stresses. We behave in accordance with the programs of life that have been inherent in us since childhood, and if these programs are not effective enough, the results are diseases. Dr. Lydia Temoshok, who studied the features of the personalities of cancer patients, says that people do not create cancer in themselves. They do not choose to behave according to the type "C" personality characteristics and to preserve it without their conscious approval. Since one does not know about relationship of the type "C" personality and cancer, how can one understand that their behavior can affect their cancer defense system at the molecular level? (Temoshok L., Dreher H., 1993).

Understanding of the psychological mechanisms underlying the formation of oncogenic distress provides a base for the targeted psychotherapeutic influence on those factors, which lead to hopelessness, depression, and avital feelings. What is especially important is the fact of detecting the hidden desire for suicide in the occurrence of cancer, as it allows us to bring the knowledge and experience gained in the psychotherapy of suicides into psycho-oncology. This, in my opinion, will significantly increase the effectiveness of antitumor therapy and reduce the percentage of cancer recurrences after therapy, since it will eliminate the deep desire of the person for death.

Of considerable interest is the question of whether the avital experiences and the unconscious desire for death are unique characteristics of future cancer patients exclusively. As we saw above, most of the personal and social characteristics of cancer patients and their internal conflicts are similar to those occurring in other psychosomatic diseases. I also wrote about the works of Karl Menninger (1956) and Yuri Vagin (2011), who believe that the desire for "organic suicide" is common to psychosomatic diseases. Obviously, only broad prospective studies that determine avital experiences in people without clinically visible pathology, and subsequent long-term observation of the nature of pathology developing in them will be able to provide an answer to this question. In addition, if antisuicidal psychotherapy proves to be effective in improving the results of medical therapy and preventing relapses of cancer, this will confirm the correctness of my reasoning.

Summing up this part, I want to express my hope that as a result of the development of the biopsychosocial-spiritual trend in medicine, the work of the psychotherapist will become just as important in oncological clinics as the work of the physician-oncologist, and next to biomedical diagnoses we will be able to see a psychological diagnosis similar to the following: "Avital state. Somatic-equivalent form of nonsuicidal autodestruction: oncological disease. Source: unresolved intrapsychic conflict (or psychic trauma). The nature of the conflict: unmet need in ... ".

Part VI

Will a Tumor Develop or Degrade? Promotion and Progression as a Result of Distress Activation

Once upon a time a traveler came to a fork in the road.
In front of him there stood a large stone,
and the stone was shaped just like a brain.
Written on this stone were the words:
Go straight on, and you will get promotion.
To the left, you will find dormant remission.
To the right, you will find spontaneous regression.
(Taken from a folk tale)

The next phase in the development of the disease is tumor promotion (progression, acceleration). When this phase occurs, those initiated cells that are already capable of unlimited division need an additional stimulus to begin intensive reproduction, which results in the formation of a primary tumor. Such division stimulators are called promoters and they are chemicals that, as a rule, do not cause DNA damage, i.e. are non-direct carcinogens. However, following prolonged exposure to the initiated cells, these promoters trigger tumor growth. Hormones, drugs, plant products, and other substances that interact with the cell at various levels—with its membrane, receptor structures in the nucleus, or cytoplasm—can be promoters and induce division (Zubarev P. N., Bryusov P. G., 2017; Kutsenko S. A., 2002).

Taking into consideration the data on the stimulating effects of stress hormones on cell growth, which were discussed in the previous parts, it is quite likely that these hormones can act not only as initiators, but also as promoters of malignant cell multiplication, when the chronic psychosocial stress aggravated by avital feelings and the loss of the will to live gets deeper. These chronic stress agents best fit the description of promoters provided by oncologists: "For tumor induction to occur, a long and relatively continuous impact of promoters is necessary" (Zubarev P. N., Bryusov P. G., 2017).

Data from the leading American center for cancer research, MD Anderson at the University of Texas, is in line with these findings: studying the biopsy material of the early-stage human ovarian tumor, scientists were able to find that patients with a high psychosocial risk (in other words, with an increased stress level) had a significantly higher content of norepinephrine in their tumor tissue and this corresponded to the activity of the tumor genes. However, those patients who had better social support (care from family, friends, etc.), had a significantly lower level of norepinephrine in their tumor (Lutgendorf S. K. et al., 2009, 2011).

As a result of the promotion process, an initial tumor nodule is formed, which is equivalent to cancer in the first stage. Here we are faced with another extremely interesting question. If we consider the theory, proposed by Dr. Ryke Hamer (2000), that the onset of an early-stage tumor is due to acute stress ("conflict shock") and is a biological auxiliary program rather than pathology, then what causes initiation and promotion following chronic stress based on inner conflicts, when there is no strong "conflict shock"? The only explanation I can give at the moment comes from the concept of accumulation of experienced stress—the "accumulated trauma" discussed in Chapter 11. In this case, the succeeding and even insignificant acute stress in the life of a person who has an established oncodominant and avital experiences can trigger a primary tumor formation mechanism.

The further fate of the initial tumor, as in the case of acute psychic trauma, will depend on changes in the psychological state of the person. If there is no improvement (which is most likely the case in a situation of hopelessness, latent depression, and suicidality), then the initial tumor will develop and move on to the next stage, progression.

If, at such a moment, a person becomes aware of their psychological state and resorts to professional psychotherapeutic help, or goes through a spontaneous spiritual awakening, and also has good social support (understanding and help from family and friends), there are quite high chances of stopping tumor growth and its degradation, possibly according to the mechanisms proposed by Dr. Hamer. There is currently quite a significant data that confirms this outcome.

Chapter 22

The Phenomenon of Spontaneous Inhibition of Growth and Degradation of Early–Stage Tumors

As early as in 1952 some clinicians noted that self-healing of breast tumors is not so rare (Gatch W. D., Culbertson C. G., 1952) and that some small mammary gland tumors may spontaneously disappear (Stewart F. W., 1952). In 1954, Dr. P. M. West published the results of observations showing that 80% of all carcinomas in situ (malignant tumors in the initial stages of development without penetration of the underlying tissue) disappeared by themselves during the observation period without any treatment. Upon analyzing the data available at that time, E. V. Cowdry (1955) came to the conclusion that some small tumors that are found by chance in the uterus, prostate, and mammary glands can remain "dormant" for many years, not developing at all, or even regress (dissolve) under the influence of natural physiological mechanisms.

London oncologists, when studying the autopsy results of 2,238 elderly patients who died of general pathology, revealed that 1,152 of them had malignant tumors; but 314 (almost 27%) were not diagnosed with cancer during their lifetime and they did not show any clinical signs of a tumor (Fentiman I. S. et al., 1990). Academician V. F. Chekhun (2013), director of the Kiev Research Institute of Experimental Pathology, Oncology and Radiobiology (Ukraine), achieved similar results: when the histological sections of various organs and tissues of patients aged 50-70 years who died between 2004 and 2009 from various non-cancer-related causes were studied, isolated groups of tumor cells were found in almost 100% of cases, however, only 0.1% of these people had been diagnosed with cancer. The New Hampshire Veterans Medical Center (USA) also reported a significant number of women who died from non-cancer diseases and did not know that they had a tumor in the mammary gland. The majority of these tumors were in early-stage—carcinomas in situ (Welch H. G., Black W. C., 1997).

"Cancer cells and precancerous cells are so common that nearly everyone by middle age or old age is riddled with them," says Tea Tlsti, professor of pathology at the University of California. This fact was established at the autopsies of people who died from other causes and did not suspect that they had cancer cells or precancerous cells. They did not have large tumors or cancer symptoms. "The really interesting question," continues Professor Tlsti, "is not so much why we get cancer as why don't we get cancer?" (Kolata G., 2009). In an interview with Newsweek newspaper, Dr. Otis Brawley, head of the American Cancer Society, acknowledged that somewhere between 25% and 30% of some types of cancer tumors stop their development at some stage (Wingert P., 2009).

The Norwegian Institute of Health confirmed that even invasive breast tumors can resolve spontaneously. This conclusion was drawn following the observation of women aged fifty to sixty-four years who were diagnosed with many small tumors during the mammography. By repeating mammograms over the next six years researchers supposed that there would at least be the same number of tumors in this group, if not more. However, in reality, the twenty-two percent fewer tumors were detected (Zahl P. H. et al., 2008).

F. W. Stewart (1952) cites four-year clinical statistics: although the initial uterine carcinomas were detected in 25% of women examined, developed cervical tumors in this group were found to be only 3.7%. This suggests that many carcinomas in situ either disappear or do not develop into cancer. Scientists from the University of California arrived at a similar conclusion more recently: 60% of precancerous cervical cells detected by the pap test in young women became normalized within a year after diagnosis, and within three years of the initial observation 90% of the precancerous cells returned to normal (Moscicki A. B. et al., 2004). A spontaneous remissions of metastatic renal-cell carcinoma was discovered by scientists at a university hospital in British Columbia (Gleave M. E. et al., 1998).

A high survival rate without surgery is also observed for prostate tumors (Chodak G. W. et al., 1994), and according to Swedish scientists, a ten-year survival rate for early prostate cancer is equally high (about 87%) both after surgical treatment and without therapy in general (Johansson J. E. et al., 1992). Again, this discovery is not new: in the middle of the last century, it was noted that although more than 25% of older men have small prostate tumors, the mortality from this disease is much lower than 25% (Stewart F., 1952).

"The old view is that cancer is a linear process," like "an arrow that moved in one direction," said Dr. Barnett Kramer, associate director of the cancer prevention division at the USA National Institute of Health. The cell undergoes mutations and gradually the number of mutations increases. It was assumed that mutations cannot reverse spontaneously. However, it is now becoming increasingly clear that the development of cancer requires more than just mutations. Cancer cells need interaction with surrounding cells and even with the whole organism, with a person, whose immune and hormonal systems, for example, can destroy or nourish a tumor (Kolata G., 2009).

Accumulation of this kind of data has prompted a number of scientists to raise the question of the advisability of operating on all patients with early-stage tumors of the mammary gland, prostate, thyroid, and kidneys, since the blind belief in the need for the complete removal of all tumors sentences patients to unnecessary and dangerous treatment. In 2012, for example, the Central Oregon Quality Department of the St. Charles Health System revealed that over the past thirty years, more than 1.3 million women in the United States have become victims of breast cancer overdiagnosis. During mammography, they had tumor-like formations, which subsequently did not show any clinical symptoms (Bleyer A., Welch H., 2012), followed by excessive therapy. Overdiagnosis and overtherapy are also noted in cases of prostate, lung, and thyroid tumors (Esserman L. J. et al., 2013).

Russian oncologists also note that in health clinics and hospitals cancer patients are often diagnosed incorrectly. As a result, in 65% of cases, inadequate and sometimes harmful and dangerous treatment is carried out, which worsens the prognosis of the disease and complicates further antitumor therapy (Korzhikov A. V., 1999).

The problem of cancer misdiagnosis has become so serious that in March of 2012, the US National Cancer Institute held a meeting to assess the threat posed by the "overdiagnosis" of tumors that do not lead to clinical manifestations and death. It was noted that diagnostic procedures, including mammography, can damage an inactive tumor and result in its progression. They argue that it is necessary to abolish the use of the diagnosis "cancer" in cases of early-stage breast tumors (noninvasive ductal carcinoma) and prostate (intraepithelial neoplasia) tumors, and that a new term, "indolent lesions of epithelial origin," should be introduced instead (Esserman L. J. et al., 2013).

In April 2016, the prestigious medical journal *JAMA Oncology* published the results of a large-scale study conducted by an international group of physicians. A disease that was previously referred to as early-stage thyroid cancer (a formal diagnosis of which shows it as an encapsulated follicular variant of papillary thyroid carcinoma) is the most common cause of thyroid removal and radioactive iodine treatment, followed by lifelong use of synthesized hormones. According to the report, this pathology should no longer be considered a malignant neoplasm (Nikiforov Y. E. et al., 2016). On this basis, official advice was to change the classification of this disease to a benign one, and it is now called "noninvasive follicular thyroid neoplasm with papillary-like nuclear features." On this note, Dr. Barnett Krammer expressed great concern about how the terms that are used in medicine do not correspond to the modern understanding of cancer biology. "Calling lesions cancer when they are not leads to unnecessary and harmful treatment," said this leading manager of the US National Institute of Health (Kolata G., 2016).

Following these changes in medicine, programs of so-called "active surveillance" have appeared, where, instead of standard therapy, the behavior of the tumor is carefully monitored. In many cases, this prevents surgeries (Crispen P. L. et al., 2008; Tosoian J. J. et al., 2011).

In her comments on cases of spontaneous regression of melanomas (malignant tumors from skin pigment cells) in their early stages, Dr. Lydia Temoshok, one of the pioneers of psycho-oncology, wrote that patients with a tumor at an early stage were identified only because they underwent a thorough physical examination. She believes that, in most cases, their own immune defenses would keep the tumors under control or even eliminate them. If everyone in their city had been tested from head to toe for the presence of early melanomas, they most likely would have found more than expected. The point, according to this researcher, is that we all have the innate ability to control some tumors, especially if they are small and localized (Temoshok L., Dreher, H., 1993).

As we see, the data presented confirms Dr. Hamer's point of view that if tumors that appear in the active phase of a conflict fulfill their special mission, then they are eliminated or encapsulated by the body and do not develop further.

It is very likely that the phenomenon of such spontaneous regression of tumors is based on the activation of the natural mechanisms of controlled destruction of unnecessary and defective cells—apoptosis, which we will look at in the next chapter.

Chapter 23

Disease Activation and Metastasizing under Chronic Stress

If a tumor goes into the progression stage, then it begins to change qualitatively, acquiring previously absent properties—greater autonomy (independence from the regulatory influences of the body), destructive growth, invasiveness (penetration into the surrounding tissues), the ability to form metastases (to spread tumor cells throughout the body to form daughter tumors), and adaptability to changing conditions of existence (Zubarev P. N., Bryusov P. G., 2017). As a general rule, this corresponds to the period of clinical manifestation of the disease.

Studies show that at least the three main pathophysiological mechanisms involved in tumor progression are significantly stimulated by chronic stress, which is still experienced by a person at this stage of the disease. These are angiogenesis (the formation of new blood vessels in the affected organ or tissue), the inhibition of apoptosis (the universal mechanism of cell death), and metastasis. Undoubtedly, the continuing suppression of the immune system caused by stress also plays a huge role—this mechanism was discussed in the previous section.

Conditionally, I attribute the course of these three processes to the initial, preclinical period, when a person does not yet know about their diagnosis. Although the same processes continue after diagnosis, the colossal distress that occurs in the patient at the time of establishing the diagnosis, in addition to the initial chronic stress, significantly worsens the psycho-physiological state of the person and activates the course of the disease. We will discuss the consequences of such a psychic trauma in the next chapter.

23.1. Angiogenesis

A healthy organism needs new blood vessels during growth and development, as well as for restoring damaged tissue and scar formation at the sites of damage, healing of inflammatory foci, and other regeneration processes.

However, angiogenesis also occurs actively and constantly in a tumor, to make it well supplied with blood and to provide it with many more nutrients than the surrounding healthy tissue. This becomes one of the factors behind the rapid growth of malignant tumors and subsequent metastasis, since tumor cells are able to use new blood vessels and thus spread throughout the body. In order to create new vessels, the tumor releases special substances—the vascular endothelial growth factor (VEGF) and cytokines—IL-8 and IL-6, which we have already learned about, which play an important role in inflammation process (Hanahan D., Weinberg R. A., 2000). These angiogenesis mechanisms are also stimulated by stress hormones.

In one of the leading laboratories of the world, at the University of Iowa, joint studies by the departments of psychology, obstetrics, and cancer, conducted on models of nasopharyngeal, melanoma, and myeloma cancer cell lines, found that their exposure to both types of stress hormones—epinephrine and cortisol—stimulates the synthesis of the vascular growth factor VEGF. At the same time, the effect of catecholamines is blocked by the beta-blocker propranolol (Yang E. V. et al., 2006, 2009).

In clinical conditions, these scientists found that women suffering from ovarian cancer and experiencing greater social isolation (*and consequently, experiencing a higher level of stress—V. M.*), had higher levels of VEGF, both in the blood and in the tumor tissue removed during surgery, than women with good social support (Lutgendorf S. K. et al., 2002, 2008). Similar data was received when men with tumors of the oral cavity, larynx, and oropharynx were examined: those who experienced more stress and depression prior to the surgery, even despite the early stage of the disease, had an elevated VEGF content in the tumor tissue, which is associated with a worse prognosis (Fang C. Y. et al., 2014).

In another series of experiments, mice were subjected to chronic stress by daily mobility restriction. Then they were "inoculated" with human ovarian cancer cells, which were injected into the abdominal cavity. As a result, tumors that developed in the stressed mice had a higher concentration of catecholamines and VEGF growth factor, and greater density of blood vessels than tumors in the mice that didn't experience stress. Also, such tumors showed a more aggressive growth and spread in the body, which could be due to a high concentration of MMP-2 and MMP-9 enzymes, which contribute to the release of cancer cells from their source tumor. These effects of stress were also prevented by propranolol. The researchers concluded that stress, accompanied by an increase in catecholamine synthesis by the sympathetic nervous system, leads to the activation of angiogenesis and the progression of cancer development (Thaker P. H. et al., 2006).

As I previously mentioned, the "antistress" hormone dopamine has an effect opposite to that of angiogenesis. It blocks the ability of the vascular growth factor VEGF to perform its function by eliminating its receptors. In their absence, the growth factor can no longer activate the formation of new vessels in the tumor (Basu S. et al., 2001; Chakroborty D. et al., 2009). This may be one of the mechanisms of the protective influence of good social support.

23.2. Apoptosis and Anoikis

During the embryonic development of the organism, a huge number of various cells emerge and die. At certain stages, the so-called temporary organs appear and then completely disappear. Formation of permanent organs occurs owing to the production of an excessive number of cells, and then the elimination of everything unnecessary. This is how morphogenesis occurs—the process of the emergence of new forms and structures of the developing organism.

The mechanism for the controlled destruction of unwanted cells is called apoptosis. It works not only in embryogenesis, but also in an adult organism throughout its life, becoming an important element in protecting the body against the accumulation of damaged, weakened, virus-afflicted, mutated, and autoimmune cells, for tissue renewal, as well as for the involution of tissues during aging. This is a kind of "cell suicide"—a process of genetically programmed destruction of the cellular structure and DNA. As result, the damaged cell becomes unable to divide, to perform its functions, and undergoes self-disintegration.

It is believed that the cellular mass of an organism that undergoes apoptosis during one year of its life is equal to the mass of the body. Every day, some cells of our body die through apoptosis. The body then restores this number by producing new, viable cells, thereby controlling the size of the organs. Should apoptosis decrease, the accumulation of cells in tissues will begin, and may result in, for example, tumor growth. If apoptosis increases for some reason, then there is a progressive decrease in the number of cells in the tissue, as exemplified by atrophy. The mechanisms of apoptosis are also violated in autoimmune diseases, pathology of the blood system, atrophic diseases of the nervous system, myocardial infarction.

At the Ohio State University Medical Center the ability of leukocytes, taken from the blood of medical university students who were under exam stress, to undergo apoptosis was studied. The isolated leukocytes were exposed to a chemical carcinogen or radiation. It was found that stress reduces the ability of damaged cells to self-destruct, thereby increasing the number of potentially cancerous cells in the body (Tomei L. D. et al., 1990).

In the experiments done by other scientists, it was directly demonstrated that by connecting to its receptor on the cell surface, the stress hormone epinephrine triggers a chain of intracellular reactions that protect the prostate and breast cancer cells from apoptosis (Sastry K. S. et al., 2007). According to Associate Professor George Kulik, the head of the research group at the Wake Forest University School of Medicine, where these experiments were conducted, such evidence suggests that emotional stress is involved in the development of cancer and may reduce the effectiveness of anti-cancer therapy.

In order for a damaged cell to successfully undergo a process of natural apoptosis, it must detach itself from the extracellular matrix—a special intercellular substance that keeps it attached to other cells of any tissue. This process, the precursor of apoptosis, is called anoikis. It turns out that it is also affected by stress.

Having studied the cells of ovarian cancer, the researchers found that the depressive state in patients is associated with an increased content of norepinephrine in the tumor tissue and with a high activity level of the enzyme FAK (focal adhesion kinase), which participates in anoikis and promotes the release of cancer cells from their location. This is an unfavorable factor for the survival of patients, since it allows cells to move in the body and create metastases (Sood A. K., Lutgendorf S. K., 2011). On the other hand, as revealed in the research done on breast tumor cells, if this enzyme is blocked, the cells become less mobile and, therefore, less able to metastasize (Chan K. T. et al., 2009). Another mechanism that gets activated by stress hormones is the synthesis of other enzymes in the tumor cells, which is called metallopeptidases MMP-9 and MMP-2. These enzymes also destroy the extracellular matrix, contributing to the release of cells (Sood A. K. et al., 2006).

23.3. Metastasis

Metastasis—the formation of a secondary tumor in various organs, tissues and lymph nodes—is the most important indicator of the malignancy of a tumor process that affects the course of the disease.

Most often, this complication occurs in the later stages of cancer, but in some cases, tumors create microscopic metastases in neighboring or distant lymph nodes or organs during an early stage. The movement of tumor cells does not necessarily lead to the development of a metastatic tumor: it is restrained by local tissue resistance, immune defense, and the general state of the body.

To date, a large amount of data has been accumulated indicating the ability of both acute and chronic stress to significantly activate the process of metastasis. For example, the intensity of metastasis increased 2.59 times in women with breast cancer who had a negative life event within eighteen months after diagnosis (Dourado de Souza C. et al., 2018), and another study of the same type of tumor found that this process is based on the catecholamine stimulation of its receptors (Choy C. et al., 2016).

As it became clear, stress affects metastasis at all its phases (Moreno-Smith M. et al., 2010; Li S. et al., 2013; Giraldi T. et al., 1994). The first phase, the activation of anoikis and the release of tumor cells from the primary tumor, has been considered above. Chronic stress also rebuilds the lymphatic network in and around the tumor. This causes the lymph flow to expand, which facilitates the migration of tumor cells into the general lymphatic system (Le C. P. et al., 2016).

Upon leaving its place of origin, the released cell moves through the lymphatic or blood vessels, "searching" for the place of attachment, where it can expand its activity in the formation of metastases (embolism phase). Ukrainian scientists have found that stress has a damaging effect on both the endothelium (cellular layer of the inner surface) of the vessels and the underlying subendothelial layer, and also activates the processes of parietal vessel thrombus formation (Balitskiy K. P., Shmalko Y. P., 1987). This increases the permeability of blood vessels for migrating tumor cells and causes a pronounced stimulation of metastasis.

In the next phase, when cancer cells get fixated in a new place, anoikis is also involved. It's not so easy for a tumor cell to penetrate into healthy tissue—local cells usually defend against uninvited guests quite successfully. The aggressive cell needs some external help to weaken local resistance, and once again this help comes in the form of the stress hormones, catecholamines. They also trigger the activation of the metallopeptidase enzyme synthesis that violates the structure of the extracellular matrix and this creates gaps in the protective rows of local cells. It is via these holes that the invasive cancer cells penetrate healthy cells.

Such a mechanism for the intrusion of a cancer cell into healthy tissue was found in the research on both rectal cancer cells and the livers of mice subjected to the stress of isolation, and in ovarian cancer cell cultures under the direct influence of norepinephrine. Moreover, its effect was again blocked by the beta-blocker propranolol (Wu W. et al., 1999; Sood A. K. et al., 2006). The same effects of norepinephrine are found on nasopharyngeal cancer cells. In this case, what was increased was not only the content of metallopeptidase enzymes, but also of the vascular growth factor VEGF. This, as we saw above, is one of the most important conditions for tumor growth and metastasis (Yang E. V. et al., 2006).

Having penetrated into a new place (the fourth phase), cancer cells must be fixed in it in the same way as in the original tumor in order to receive nutrients and multiply. To do this, they must adhere—connect with laminin and fibronectin, the main components of the extracellular matrix. And the stressful state of the organism helps them again because catecholamines increase the adhesion of cancer cells to the matrix (Bos J. L., 2006).

For the further development of metastasis, the entrenched cells need nourishment—and they receive it by activating the formation of new blood vessels according to the mechanisms described above. Experiments revealed that chronic stress promotes angiogenesis in intra-abdominal metastases through the activation of VEGF synthesis (Thaker P. H. et al., 2006). Also, an inflammatory process is needed for the growth of metastases (Wu Y., Zhou B. P., 2009), which is activated, as noted above, by chronic stress.

There is no doubt that all the processes described could not proceed effectively under the efficiently functioning immune system. However, we already know that its functions are seriously suppressed under chronic stress. Experiments conducted jointly by Israeli and American scientists have directly confirmed that various types of stress activate metastasis by reducing the activity of the immune system (Ben-Eliyahu S. et al., 1991; 1999). In particular, the stronger the intensity of stress, the less the immune system is able to control the spread of metastases to the lungs (Jones H. P. et al., 2017).

The impact of stress on metastasis development has been clearly demonstrated by researchers at the University of Los Angeles. Over the course of the experiment, mice were subjected to chronic stress of limited mobility for two hours a day for twenty days. During this period, they got injections of breast cancer cells and then were examined for the appearance of cancer and metastasis. It turned out that the development of metastases in mice that underwent the stress was thirty times more active than in mice in the control group (not subjected to stress). In addition, genetic changes occurred in the cells of their immune system (specific tumor-associated macrophages) under the influence of catecholamines, which led to an increase in the ability of injected cancer cells to enter the bloodstream and spread throughout the body. These catecholamine effects were blocked by the beta-blocker propranolol (Sloan E. K. et al., 2010). An activation of metastasis in the skeletal system was found on a similar stress model, and this effect was modeled by the injection of a beta-adrenergic agonist, isoproterenol (catecholamine simulator), and inhibited by propranolol (Campbell J. P. et al., 2012).

An increase in the number of lung metastases was obtained also by the "inoculation" of tumor cells in rats, experiencing confrontational stress during the day. The rodent was placed in a cage with an "established" group of twenty-one rats who actively attacked the novice. Under these conditions, metastases developed more vigorously in newbies who demonstrated defeatist, subservient behavior (Stefanski V., Ben-Eliyahu S., 1996), which confirms the validity of my attribution of this behavior to important factors provoking oncogenesis. A direct effect of catecholamines on cells of mammary gland and prostate tumors in tissue culture also stimulates cell migration (Lang K. et al., 2004). In addition, the administration of norepinephrine activates the development of metastases in mice with "grafted" tumors of the same origin (Palm D. et al., 2006). In all three studies, these catecholamine effects were blocked by beta blockers.

Examinations of patients with metastatic breast and ovarian cancer showed a disorder of their natural daily rhythm of cortisol release: instead of decreasing after the morning surge, the level of the hormone in the blood of patients remained high during the day (Touitou Y. et al., 1996).

Thus, stress affects virtually "every step" in the path of metastasis development. In my opinion, it is the degree of intensity of chronic stress experienced that determines how soon and in what quantity metastases will occur in a particular patient.

Chapter 24

The Psychic Trauma of Diagnosis Results in the Activation of Distress and the Progression of the Disease

Even suspecting cancer and waiting for examination results cause a person to experience acute stress (Green B. L. et al., 1998; Montgomery M., McCrone S. H., 2010). The announcement of an oncological diagnosis, which patients perceive as a "death message," leads to a powerful distress—a massive psychic trauma from the diagnosis, defined as an acute stress disorder that can cause reactive mental disorders (Tarabrina N. V. et al.., 2010; Peseschkian N., 1991; McGarvey E. L. et al., 1998; Green B. L. et al., 1998; Lowden B., 1998; Vorona O. A., 2005; Bukhtoyarov O. V., Arkhangelskiy A. E., 2008; Tjemsland L. et al., 1996; Montgomery M., McCrone S. H., 2010). The Karolinska Medical Institute in Sweden conducted a large-scale statistical study on the records of more than 500,000 cancer patients from 1991 to 2006. It was found that during the first week after diagnosis, the number of suicides among newly diagnosed patients increased by sixteen times, and the mortality rate due to cardiac abnormalities increased by 26.9 times (Fang F. et al., 2012).

The threat to life, the perspective of physical mutilation, the expectation of pain and suffering, which are associated with the disease, the danger and complications of treatment, the possibilities of disability, loss of work and social status, forthcoming financial expense, lack of confidence in full recovery—all of these factors cause the majority of newly diagnosed patients to experience a strong fear for their life and the future, anxiety, self-doubt, loss of control over life, internal tensions, helplessness, and even horror (Green B. L. et al., 1997; Holland J. C., Rowland J. H., 1989; Koneva O. B., Kostichenko I. V., 2004). As a result, 53% of patients with acute stress disorder caused by a diagnosis develop

PTSD within six months; however, 36% of those without an acute disorder develop PTSD as well (Kangas M. et al., 2005).

Acute stress disorders of this kind develop according to the same psycho-physiological laws that we considered in Chapter 10, when an acute psychic trauma of loss occurs in an individual's life. Let me remind you that during this period the sympathetic nervous system and the hypothalamic-pituitary-adrenal system are activated, which entails the release of epinephrine, norepinephrine, and cortisol. Contrary to the adaptive action, should there be an excess of them, these substances can lead to DNA damage within ten minutes. There are mutations that violate the structure of chromosomes, cause a decrease in telomerase activity, activate the genes associated with cell division and those that take part in cancer mechanisms, and affect the survival of cells in the hippocampus.

However, the fundamental difference in the newly emerged stressful situation is that it not only happens on top of present chronic stress, but also on top of a developing cancer. New intense distress stimulates the disease, just like oil poured on to a fire.

Studies show that if a person is already in a state of chronic stress, the onset of a new acute stressful event may have an even greater effect on the body. For example, in response to additional acute stress the organisms of people who negatively experience loneliness (*which creates a subjective state of chronic stress—V. M.*), synthesize a greater number of cytokines TNF-α and IL-6, which stimulates the development of the inflammatory process, than do people without pre-existing stress. A similar reaction is observed in the organisms of lonely patients who have received cancer treatment (Jaremka L. M. et al., 2013a). Under the influence of the stress hormone cortisol, the concentration of the cytokines-interleukins IL-1α and IL-1β increases, followed by an increase of inflammation in the tumor and the stimulation of its development (Nakane T. et al., 1990). In other experiments, the effects of acute laboratory stress on *mononuclear* blood cells of women caring for spouses with dementia were examined. It was determined that under the influence of a higher content of cortisol in the blood of these women, there is a greater reduction in the length of chromosomal telomeres than in the control group (Tomiyama A. J. et al., 2012). Consequently, the immune system suffers even more.

The effect of the "accumulated trauma" also contributes to the consequences of the stress of diagnosis: previously experienced psychic trauma reduces stress resistance, and as a result, in the early stages of the disease, the cancer patient responds more strongly to new trauma (Andrykowski M. A., Cordova M. J., 1998; Green B. L. et al., 2000; Vorona O. A., 2005). Scientists from the Kiev Research Institute of Oncology Problems (Ukraine) have found that, at the time of tumor development, additional excessive stress effects (*this can be the psychological trauma of the diagnosis as well—V. M.*) lead to the inability of the brain's protective mechanisms to limit the intensity of the stress response. As a result, stress becomes anomalous, causing even greater damage to the body (Balitskiy K. P., Shmalko Y. P., 1987).

Under laboratory conditions, stress hormones (especially norepinephrine) can increase the ability of ovarian cancer cells to penetrate adjacent tissues by almost 200% and significantly activate tumor progression (Sood A. K. et al., 2006). Similar data was obtained in the study of melanoma cells, multiple myeloma, and nasopharyngeal carcinoma: their exposure to norepinephrine (which can be equated to the stress of diagnosis) results in the activation of the synthesis of both the VEGF (vascular growth factor) and interleukins 6 and 8 (Yang E. V. et al., 2006, 2009). This, as we saw above, is an important mechanism for tumor growth. Experts from the University of Illinois conducted a study on about a thousand women diagnosed with breast cancer in the period from two to three months after their diagnosis. The higher that the intensity of stress experienced by these women was, accompanied by the prevailing emotions of fear, anxiety, and isolation, the more aggressively the disease proceeded (Rauscher G. H. et al., 2011).

The joint study conducted by Texas and Pittsburgh universities explored the mechanisms of distress caused by a diagnosis of breast cancer. In addition to a significant decrease in the mood and quality of the patient's life, their blood lymphocyte counts decreased, which indicates a decline in the activity of the immune system, while the neutrophil content increased, indicating the activation of the inflammatory response (Kang D. H. et al., 2012).

Specialists at the University of Chicago investigated the psychological, immunological, and biochemical parameters of women scheduled for a breast biopsy—on the day of the examination and one and four months after the biopsy and therapy. The state of stress, anxiety, and mood disorders that occurred after being referred for a biopsy remained elevated throughout the whole subsequent observation period. In parallel with this, even before the biopsy, the activity of the immune system decreased and the content of interleukins-4, -6, and -10 grew. These changes persisted for a month after the examination. The revealed results did not depend on whether the tumor was benign or malignant, which confirms the mental primacy of the detected changes in the body (Witek-Janusek L. et al., 2007). Further studies carried out by this team determined that immunity disorders are associated with epigenetic mechanisms (*which confirms their dependence on the psyche—V. M.*): acetylation and phosphorylation of structural proteins (histones) of chromosomes in peripheral mononuclear cells decreased at the diagnostic stage but were restored by the fourth month of the observation (Mathews H. L. et al., 2011).

The psychic trauma of the diagnosis can also become the impetus mechanism for the process of metastasis: this conclusion is based on the results of experiments conducted on rats that underwent acute stress. Following this, scientists measured the activity of their immune killer cells in relation to the destruction of external tumor cells (in vitro—outside the body) and determined that it was significantly reduced. When the same tumor cells were injected into the blood of the animals ("inoculated") after they had experienced stress, the number of metastases in their lungs was twice as high as in non-stressed rats (Ben-Eliyahu S. et al., 1991).

All this data suggest that distress caused by the diagnosis activates the progress of the cancer process. Other scientists (Bukhtoyarov O. V., Arkhangelskiy A. E., 2008; Hassan S. et al., 2013; Spiegel D., 2001) also share this opinion. A clinical example is the story of the development of testicular cancer, described by Lance Armstrong (2000, with S. Jenkins) in his autobiography. After the announcement of the diagnosis, he was in a state of deep distress for a while, mourning the collapse of his sports career and thinking about the proposed treatment options. When he returned to the hospital to be examined before starting therapy, his blood markers showed that the cancer had made a sharp jump in development over the previous day. "The cancer was not just spreading, it was galloping," Armstrong writes, "and Youman (*attending oncologist—V. M.)* no longer thought I could afford to wait a week for chemo. I should begin treatment directly, because if the cancer was moving that quickly, every day might count."

Other factors affecting the intensity of the psychic trauma of the diagnosis and the further development of the disease include the type of personality that one has, protective psychological mechanisms, and skills of coping with stress developed by a person at the time of diagnosis. The adverse effects are also caused by an anxious type of character, previous diseases, a low level of education (Montgomery M., McCrone S. H., 2010; Vorona O. A., 2005), a tendency to depressive reactions, manifestations of helplessness and hopelessness (Reiche E. M. et al., 2004), insufficient social support (Andrykowski M. A., Cordova M. J., 1998), an unsatisfactory level of communication with health servants, insufficient awareness and understanding of one's condition, stage of illness, and its prognosis (Naidich J. B., Motta R. W., 2000; Hampton M. R., Frombach I., 2000; Mills M. E., Sullivan K., 1999).

Strong negative emotions experienced by patients in the initial period of the disease can destroy the most important stereotypes of their behavior and attitudes, developed during their whole preceding life. Their psychological problems are growing—anxiety, insomnia, demoralization, depression, sharpening of personal qualities, behavioral deviations. The habitual pattern of a patient's life and their social status is changing, their social circle gets narrowed, personal and family plans are violated, and achieving the majority of them becomes impossible. Because of the disease, the objective place a person occupies in life is lost, together with their "inner position" in relation to all the circumstances of life (Kukina M., 2009). Their self-image as the owner of their

Vladislav Matrenitsky

own life, one that is strong, independent, self-sufficient, effective, is destroyed and self-esteem is lowered. The patient often "gives in" to the illness and develops a dependence on health workers and family members (Filipp S. H., 1992; Koneva O. B., Kostichenko I. V., 2004), which can be also based on the infantilism traits discussed above. As a result, the personality structure of such patients is significantly transformed and often autistic traits arise, which were not previously characteristic of them (Tkachenko G. A., Shestopalova I. M., 2007).

Chapter 25

Deepening of the Spiritual–Existential Crisis

I f, before the diagnosis is announced, a person does not yet realize that they are in a state of existential crisis, then, after diagnosis, the crisis not only manifests itself, but also substantially deepens. In the process of transition through the illness, perhaps for the first time in the person's life, deep spiritual questions arise concerning self-identity, the meaning of life, suffering, and the inevitability of death (Jim H. S. et al., 2006; Edwards A. et al., 2010).

Whenever or however that line from health to illness is crossed, we enter this realm of soul. Illness is both soul shaking and soul evoking for the patient and for all others for whom the patient matters. We lose an innocence, we know vulnerability, we are no longer who we were before this event and we will never be the same. We are in uncharted terrain, and there is no turning back. Illness is a profound soul event, and yet this is virtually ignored and unaddressed. Everything seems to be focused on the part of the body that is sick, damaged, failing, or out of control, instead,

– writes Dr. Jean Bolen (2016), who works with seriously ill patients.

Studies show that 91%–96% of severely sick cancer patients have spiritual needs that directly determine the level of their depression. Among these is the need to cope with stressful spiritual suffering and the need for help in a spiritual search, in particular, in achieving forgiveness and understanding the meaning of life (Pearce M. J. et al., 2012; Mako C. et al., 2006). An oncological disease encourages a person to look for answers to existential questions, to accept a situation that is beyond the scope of their everyday understanding, to reveal positive spiritual meaning in their illness, to confirm that aspect of its significance that goes beyond the limits of physical injury and death, and to experience spiritual relationships that surpass mortal existence (Cole B., 2005).

The existential crisis that is experienced by cancer patients includes: an acute awareness of one's own finiteness; increase in thoughts about life and death; feeling that one's life is being threatened; dissolving the future; loss of the meaning of life; severe emotional distress (fear, anxiety, loss of control; obscurity, panic, despair); loneliness; weakness; identity crisis. At the same time, a certain number of patients try not to show that they are worried about these topics [*probably owing to their habit of avoiding the negative emotions—V. M.*], which undoubtedly increases the distress they are experiencing (Weisman A. D., Worden J. W., 1977; Yang W. et al., 2012).

The confusion and distress associated with spiritual issues, and especially the feeling of being "abandoned by God," negatively affect a patient's resistance to cancer and lower their prognosis for survival. In a study conducted on 100 patients with advanced stages of the disease who consider themselves spiritual or religious, it was revealed that most of them were experiencing spiritual suffering due to a "lack of faith," which was reflected in the reduced quality of their life (Delgado-Guay M. O. et al., 2011).

The general level of an individual's spirituality, their value-semantic sphere plays a major role in helping them successfully pass through such an existential crisis. Erich Fromm writes that the fear of death is the most burdensome for those who are self-centered and focused only on themselves. The more a person feels the emptiness of the life they have lived, the more they realize that their being is joyless and meaningless, the more they are afraid of death. A person who truly identifies with their inner being, whose inner world actively responds to the challenges of the outer world and enables the individual to feel their wholeness, does not fear death (Fromm E., 2016). The predominantly false personality of a person who is focused on everyday material values is not ready to face the threat of death, because in this person's picture of the world there is no place for the meaning of death, along with the meaning of life.

According to David Kissane, a leading researcher at the Center for Palliative Medicine of the University of Melbourne, the inability to resolve these spiritual issues leads patients into a state of "existential distress." This is often accompanied by feelings of regret, powerlessness, futility, and meaninglessness regarding the continuation of life. Dr. Kissane (2000) believes that for these cancer patients, topics such as death, meaning, grief, loneliness, freedom, and dignity are key existential issues that require understanding in their lives.

There is no doubt that such existential distress contributes to the psychic trauma of the diagnosis, increases the psycho-physiological distress, and can activate tumor growth. If answers to the existential questions are not found, the will to live is not revived, and therefore there is no motivation for inner healing. For example, the existential questions of Norwegian breast cancer patients, such as expectations for their life, struggle with death, image of the future, religious views, and awareness of life values, are closely related to the main, pivotal aspect—the will to live, which determines the success of treatment and survival (Landmark B. T. et al., 2001). This data once again confirm the important relationship that the loss of will to live has with the mechanisms of cancer.

"In many cases, these were people whose medical prognosis indicated that, with treatment, they could look forward to many more years of life," write C. Simonton and co-authors (1978).—"Yet while they affirmed again and again that they had countless reasons to live, these patients showed a greater apathy, depression and attitude of giving up than did a number of others diagnosed with terminal disease."

David Kissane and his colleagues (2004a) also concluded that if a patient moves far beyond despondency, into a state that can be called "surrendering"— when there is a loss of meaning and purpose in life, along with the helplessness and subjective incapacity that accompany it—there may be a desire for death to come sooner.

On the other hand, the awareness of one's mortality can lead to a reappraisal of life values, a shift in the priorities of the cancer patient towards sense-making, spiritual and religious direction. As we will see later, the help offered by specialists during this period is extremely important (Motenko J. S., 2012).

An encounter with death becomes the culmination of a person's experience of a previous existential crisis. There is a ruthless destruction of the former significant supports and foundations in human life. The shock intensity of the crisis is connected with its impact on the basic constructions of the personality— the image of I, the integrative status, existential values, the content of the Ego. These constructions are forced to die—but at the same time make room for the emergence of new values, for the revival of the soul.

> The crisis state also involves the destruction of everything external, unrooted, all that is superficially situated in a person. And at the same time, it is an expression of the inner, rooted, truly personal things. This destruction of the external and manifestation of the internal is important, first of all, for the true maturation of the personality, the formation of Man. Everything external comes out during the crisis, and a person begins to realize their external qualities. If the individual also refuses this external shell, then there is a purification of consciousness, contact with the true existential depth of human existence,

says Vladimir Kozlov (2015).

Such finding of a new meaning of life by a sick person, discovering their most important landmarks and values, is impossible without a radical reconstruction of the personality, turning to self-knowledge and the spiritual side of life. This creates a dominant of self-actualization and self-transcendence—the dominant of the highest order. Alexey Ukhtomskiy (2000) spoke about the existence of the most important dominant of a person, the goal-forming dominant: "It holds in its power the whole field of spiritual life, defines 'spiritual anatomy' and the vector of human existence; it is a dominating need, it is a practical motivational dominant." In my opinion, it is this spiritual dominant, that can activate the healing reserves of the human body.

How to help an individual realize this and what then happens with the disease, will be discussed in Chapter 32.

Chapter 26

Stress and Complications of Medical Interventions

Following the psychic trauma and distress caused by a diagnosis, the expectation of treatment, especially surgery, as well as the subsequent treatment itself, become additional powerful iatrogenic (caused by doctors) stress factors that deepen the distress (Green B. L. et al., 1998; Baum A., Posluszny D. M., 2001; Ben-Eliyahu S., 2003). During this period, patients showed a significant decline in mood, insomnia, fatigue, loss of concentration, and cognitive impairment (Cimprich B., 1999).

Patients experience fear and anxiety due to the process of the operation and its result, anticipation of possible complications and crippling consequences, side effects of the upcoming chemotherapy, and the absence of any guarantee of complete recovery. This further weakens their adaptive capacity, and leads to increased impairment of neuroendocrine and immune functions and the growth of the inflammatory process which activates tumor growth (Dudnichenko A. S. et al., 2003; Antoni M. H., 2013). In particular, it is shown that the higher the levels of anxiety and restlessness that the patient experiences on the day before the operation, the greater the likelihood of depression and a decrease in immunity during the week following the operation (Tjemsland T. et al., 1997). Similar data was received in the psychology department of the University of Ohio: the higher the level of subjective stress during the diagnosis of breast cancer and the subsequent operation, the more the individual's immune defense decreases. And the sooner the stress level goes down, the more effectively and faster the immune system gets restored (Thornton L. M. et al., 2007). I have already cited evidence confirming that there is increased content of the vascular growth factor in the tumor tissue in those patients who are more heavily impacted by the preoperative period than others. This indicates its active growth (Fang C. Y. et al., 2014).

In addition to this psychological stress, medical procedures themselves create physiological stress in the body, and cause significant complications.

In the 1980s scientists at the Ukrainian Research Institute of Oncology Problems found that, in an oncological clinic, many factors (staying in hospital, surgical treatment, chemotherapy, etc.) can be regarded as stressful. The resulting damage to the body and disorders of its protective and regulatory mechanisms, especially under the summation of the effects of various stressors, were considered to be complicating the course of the disease and stimulating metastasis (Balitskiy K. P., Shmalko Y. P., 1987).

26.1. Surgical Intervention

The physiological stress that occurs in the body during the operative and near-operative periods, as well as in response to damage to the function of the operated organ, manifests itself in profound changes of the neuroendocrine and metabolic systems (Bessey P. Q., 1995).

According to experiments on animals and studies done on humans, surgical procedures lead to impaired immune defenses. This is due to a decrease in the activity of natural killer cells, in the production of T-helper cells, and in their secretion of the TH1 and TH2 cytokines (Ben-Eliyahu S. et al., 1999; Pollock R. E. et al., 1991; Lutgendorf S. K. et al., 2005; Andersen B. L. et al., 1998).

Ukrainian researchers have found that both the tumor process itself and its treatment, on top of the expressed psycho-emotional tension, cause extremely severe stress. It is accompanied by intense neuroendocrine reactions, which have a direct stimulating effect on the mechanisms of metastasis and its regulation factors. At the same time, the intensity of the metastasis process quite strictly corresponds to the intensity of the stress response, accompanied by a significant increase in the concentration of catecholamines and glucocorticoids. As a result of stress, the adaptive activity of the organism, which is depleted by the tumor process, is disturbed, and this in turn leads to a general *anergy*. This is reflected in the suppressed state of antitumor and antimetastatic resistance, especially of antitumor immunity, and has a stimulating effect on the metastasis of tumors (Balitskiy K. P., Shmalko Y. P., 1987).

These observations are confirmed by the University of Tel Aviv. Shamgar Ben-Eliyahu, professor from the psychology department, and his colleagues conducted a lot of research that convincingly demonstrated the pathogenic effect of operative stress. According to their data, the suppression of the activity of immune killer cells which occurs as a result of such stress is associated with the release of catecholamines and prostaglandins. Moreover, due to a drop in immune protection, as well as to the activation of the synthesis of growth factors and angiogenesis, there is an increase in the risk of metastasis (Ben-Eliyahu S., 2003; Ben-Eliyahu S. et al., 2007; Neeman E., Ben-Eliyahu S., 2013). The reason for this is that following the operation, regardless of how carefully the main tumor has been removed, as a general rule, a number of freely circulating cancer cells remain in the blood, which are capable of giving rise to metastases, especially when the body's defense is thus weakened. The release of cancer cells into the blood during surgical manipulations is one of the main postoperative complications today (Eschwege P. et al., 1995; Yamaguchi K. et al., 2000).

The specific mechanism of this phenomenon was discovered by Japanese scientists. The intensity of stress that develops during surgery was found to be proportional to the number of consecutive surgical procedures. The cause of metastasis is the increased activity of the MMP-9 metallopeptidase enzyme of the cell membrane (we have talked about it in Chapter 23.2), which contributes to the release of cells (Tsuchiya Y. et al., 2003). Another mechanism was revealed by researchers from the University of Ottawa in Canada: surgical stress leads to an increase in blood clotting. As a result, thrombus-shaped clots composed of fibrin and platelets form around circulating tumor cells. They impede the destruction of cancer cells by immune killer cells (Seth R. et al., 2013), whose activity is already reduced owing to chronic background stress.

Near-surgical interventions, such as anesthesia and blood transfusion, as well as the pain associated with these manipulations, also contributes to the suppression of the immune response and stimulation of metastasis (Neeman E., Ben-Eliyahu S., 2013).

Another complication which results from operational stress is the activation of the opportunistic bacterium, Pseudomonas aeruginosa. It lives in the human respiratory tract, the colon, the external auditory canal, and on the skin surface in the fold area. Normally, the bacterium is retained under the control of the immune system, but when immune activity decreases under the influence of stress, it can lead to the development of deadly sepsis (Wu L. et al., 2003).

Ukrainian researchers also found that when the surgical removal of a tumor is combined with additional stressors, (*which are abundant in a patient during this period of life—V. M.*) it causes an extreme suppression of mediator systems that normally have inhibitory effects on the activity of stress-implementing mechanisms. As a result, stress becomes excessive, causing damage to the body. In laboratory experiments on rats, emotional stress was used to help provoke such an additional effect. However, according to scientists, in the conditions of an oncological clinic, such an additional factor can have almost any effect on the patient's body or psyche, especially when it comes to powerful stress factors such as radiation or chemotherapy (Balitskiy K. P., Shmalko Y. P., 1987).

The psychological state in which the patient finds themselves following surgery is also very important. Increased stress levels, high anxiety, and an emotionally negative mood reduce the cellular immune response in cancer patients, including a decrease in the activity of natural killer and helper cells and a decrease in the synthesis of cytokines IL-2, IL-12, and gamma interferon (Andersen B. L. et al., 1998; Blomberg B. B. et al., 2009). They are necessary to enhance the immune response, for the purpose of effective anti-infective, anti-inflammatory and anti-metastatic postoperative protection of the body.

When commenting on the results of his research, Professor Ben-Eliyahu (2008) noted the exceptional importance of the period immediately after the operation. According to him, there is a short time window, about a week after the operation, when the immune system needs to function as well as possible in order to kill the remaining microscopic particles of tumor tissue that are spread throughout the body. To achieve this goal, scientists are developing drugs that can activate the immune system in the near-operative period.

26.2. Chemo– and Radiotherapy

Although, at present, chemotherapy is used to combat almost all the varieties of oncological diseases, the expediency of such a "universal" approach is increasingly doubted by specialists from different countries.

In 1992, Ulrich Abel of the University of Heidelberg (Germany) analyzed numerous clinical observations and studies of chemotherapy for tumors of epithelial origin, which account for 80% of all neoplasms. He came to an unequivocal conclusion: with the exception of the cases of small-cell lung cancer and ovarian cancer, chemotherapy is generally ineffective, as it does not increase the life expectancy of the vast majority of cancer patients and sharply worsens its quality.

In 2004, Graham Morgan and his colleagues from the Sydney Cancer Center (Australia) studied extensive statistical data on the effectiveness of chemotherapy for patients with cancer in various locations in Australia and the USA. It turned out that its impact on five-year patient survival was 2.3% in Australia and 2.1% in the United States. The authors found no significant progress in the effectiveness of cytotoxic chemotherapy over the past twenty years. They concluded that its main effect is palliative, that is, temporary relief of the symptoms of the disease, and the placebo effect cannot be excluded from the mechanism of its action.

In the last regard, Jeanne Achterberg (2002) argues: "Apparently, anything can work if you believe in it enough, including wheat grass, Navaho sand paintings, healing waters, and chemotherapy." She thinks that recovery of people after exposure to such a severe poison as chemotherapy can even be regarded as spontaneous remission because of their attitude—in spite of the treatment. Caryle Hirshberg and Marc Ian Barasch (1995) raise an even more radical question:

What percentage of medical cures may be instances of remarkable recovery mistakenly attributed solely to treatment? Since remission occurs with a yet unknown frequency, it can be convincingly argued that some of the apparent successes of conventional (as well as unconventional) therapies may be cases of remission that have little to do with medicines themselves. It is an overlooked challenge: Could a class of treatment be in reality a collaboration between medicine and the innate powers of the healing system?

Danish researchers arrived at the following conclusion in 2010 on the basis of a meta-analysis of available research: chemotherapy improves patient survival only in a short time frame—from six to twelve months, but not for two years; this improvement is observed only in men, not in women, and does not improve their quality of life (Ventegodt S. et al., 2010).

In the Ukrainian Research Institute of Oncology Problems in the 1980s, it was found that in response to the toxic effect of chemotherapy drugs, an excessive activation of stress-realizing mechanisms develops, which can have a stimulating effect on the process of metastasis (Balitskiy K. P., Shmalko Y. P., 1987). Recently Vladimir Mosienko (2014), a professor at the same institute, wrote:

> The use of standard antitumor therapy up to now has not significantly improved the treatment results of cancer patients. Surgical intervention, radiation and chemotherapy cure or prolong the lives of no more than 40% of cancer patients; the remaining 60% die in the first year of a malignant progression, which, according to many authors, can be stimulated by these treatment methods. Only 1 out of 4 radically operated patients in our country live for more than 5 years following the procedure. Chemotherapy cures no more than 7%–10% of patients with various forms of tumors, prolongs the lives of 25% of patients and improves the quality of life for 30% of people, but does not increase life duration. In other cases, the use of chemotherapy worsens the prognosis of a patient's life.

Russian oncologist and psychotherapist Nikolay Stepanov (2007) argues that the effectiveness of chemotherapy is still limited to malignant lymphomas, *seminomas*, and germ cell tumors of women. In most cases, the administration of polychemotherapy just prolongs the life of the patient for the duration of the intake of expensive drugs. "Research is funded by the pharmaceutical industry, and it claims that the new scheme is actually more easily tolerated by the patient and more effective than the old set of drugs. However, it does not say that, like the previous scheme, it only shifts the manifestation of the disease in time," the author notes.

If chemotherapy was simply not very effective, this could still be reconciled (if we do not take into account the financial side of the issue). However, it often happens that the negative impact of these drugs on human health exceeds their positive impact. Everyone knows the side effects of chemotherapy—damage to the digestive tract, bone marrow, hair follicles, the hematopoietic system. Long-term toxic damage to the cardiovascular and nervous systems, impaired cognitive functions of the brain—concentration, attention, memory, mental speed (known as "chemical brain" or "brain fog") are registered. Secondary leukemia often occurs, while young women experience problems with conception and sexual disorders (Azim H. A. et al., 2011; Meinardi M. T. et al., 2000).

The most important complication of chemotherapy is the damage it causes to the immune system. In particular, patients with breast cancer experience disorders of various immune parameters for nine to twelve months after the end of chemotherapy. This reduces the body's resistance to common infections, such as pneumonia or tetanus (Verma R. et al., 2016; Kang D. H. et al., 2009). Scientists from MD Anderson, one of the largest American cancer research centers, found that, following chemotherapy, the activity of natural immune killer cells is reduced by 95.7%, thereby increasing the risk of metastasis. And if surgical intervention occurs after that, then killer cell activity is reduced by even more (Beitsch P. et al., 1994).

Another problem with chemotherapy is the resistance of tumors to its effects. After the initial suspense of growth under the influence of drugs, the tumor resumes its growth and progresses without responding to the treatment. Researchers from the Seattle Cancer Center discovered the mechanism of this phenomenon in the tissues of the prostate, breast, and ovarian tumors: under the influence of a chemotherapy drug, the specific WNT16B protein is being synthesized in healthy cells surrounding the tumor. It is absorbed by tumor cells and in this way activates their growth, and also protects them against the effects of chemotherapy (Sun Y. et al., 2012). Thus, tumor growth is stimulated, instead of inhibited.

Alan Nixon, former president of the American Chemical Society, said: "As a chemist trained to interpret data, it is incomprehensible to me why physicians can ignore the clear evidence that chemotherapy does much, much more harm than good" (Bermel M. B., 2011).

Similar problems are noted when using radiotherapy: stress associated with the danger and complications of exposure, anxiety, worries, nausea, loss of appetite, fatigue, depression, impairment of physical and emotional well-being, and social relationships (Sehlen S. et al., 2000; Guzińska K. et al., 2014), deteriorated cognitive function due to inhibition of neurogenesis in the hippocampus, and damage to the subcortical white matter of the brain during irradiation to the central nervous system (Monje M., Dietrich J., 2012), long-lasting impaired immune function due to DNA damage (Pinar B. et al., 2007). If radiotherapy is used in combination with chemotherapy, the toxic side effects increase by 44% (Hickey B. E. et al., 2006).

* * *

The data discussed in this chapter may cause some patients to have hard thoughts about the appropriateness of standard medical therapy. Legally, only the attending physician can advise you on the choice of treatment. However, as they say, "who is forewarned is forearmed." Knowledge is also a weapon, and the reader of this book is much better armed than other patients. This knowledge suggests that patients need to ask the attending oncologist for a rationale as to whether their early-stage tumor really requires immediate surgical removal or if it is possible for it to be carefully observed for a certain period of time (especially in combination with psychotherapy). It is also necessary to demand the statistical data on the effectiveness of chemotherapy and radiotherapy, suggested by the doctor, for the specific diagnosis and stage of the disease. Remember, oncology appointments should be individualized for each patient and shouldn't be carried out merely on the basis of general protocols.

This way you will be able to take part in the decision on the appropriateness of the suggested therapy and consider alternatives to it, thereby increasing personal responsibility for your health and fate.

Chapter 27

Psychological Factors that Affect the Effectiveness of Medical Treatment

The prevalence of psychological distress in cancer patients varies depending on the type of cancer, the time that has passed since the diagnosis, the degree of physical impairment, the intensity of experienced pain, the survival prognosis, among other factors. Upon examining almost 4,500 patients aged nineteen years and older, American researchers found significant psychological distress in the range of 29% to 43% of patients with fourteen of the most common types of cancer (Zabora J. et al., 2001). However, even those patients who do not exhibit clear clinical syndromes of distress can experience hidden feelings of guilt, loss of control, anger, sadness, confusion, and fear (Charmaz K., 2000), as well as difficulties in their relationships with family members (Kornblith A. B., 1998).

Physical limitations that arise as a result of surgery or chemotherapy often make patients unable to perform simple daily tasks and procedures, since during this period these tasks require more physical strength and energy than they have. Accepting the fact that they should allow others to help themselves, and in some cases even allow others to perform certain functions for them, can be very difficult for previously active people, and can also create a significant sense of helplessness and even negatively influence their self-esteem. When they discover that they are not able to function in the same way as before the disease, patients are forced to abandon their goals and habitual behavior, despite previously having taken it for granted when it was crucial for their sense of comfort and self-confidence. Because of this, they may feel worthless and unnecessary. Psychological pain caused by such experiences can significantly exacerbate physical pain and often leads to deep depression and passivity (Yang W. et al., 2012).

When patients experience psychosocial stress, they have fewer white blood cells, decreased activity of their cytotoxic T-cells and natural killer cells, high levels of cortisol, and elevated concentrations of inflammatory cytokines, angiogenic factors, and protease enzymes, stronger inflammatory reactions, and DNA damage (Gidron Y., Ronson A., 2008). All of this promotes the activity of the tumor process.

The mood of a person in the process of treatment is no less important than their immunity indicators. Difficulties in adapting to the disease, insufficient social support, severe fatigue, and depression reduce the activity of immune killer cells, which affects the number of metastases in the axillary lymph nodes three months after the removal of the mammary gland (Levy S. M. et al., 1987, 1991). The habitual suppression of emotions (especially anger) during the course of chemotherapy leads to the appearance of a greater number of symptoms indicating disturbances in the immune and cardiovascular systems (Schlatter M. C., Cameron L. D., 2010).

Social support from relatives, friends, co-workers, and health workers provides tremendous assistance to patients in overcoming the stress of illness. A meta-analysis of eighty-seven studies conducted on over ten million patients demonstrated that high levels of social support, a wide circle of communication, and the presence of a spouse or partner reduce the mortality of cancer patients by 25%, 20%, and 12%, respectively (Pinquart M., Duberstein P. R., 2010). In contrast, according to long-term studies carried out at the University of Iowa, low social support and, consequently, higher levels of stress, particularly in patients with ovarian cancer, are reflected in greater anxiety and depression in patients, a decrease in their immune defense, an increased level of cortisol, and impaired function of its regulation, as well as increased pro-inflammatory activity. It also leads to a higher concentration of the vascular growth factor and metallopeptidase enzyme both in the blood and in the tissue of the tumor itself, which contributes to its further development (Lutgendorf S. K. et al., 2002; 2008a; 2012).

One of the significant sources of stress for the patient is the lack of sincere and open communication with their family concerning their illness, the possibility of healing, and death. The fake assurance of recovery, especially when the relatives themselves do not believe in it, is acutely felt by the sick person and causes them additional suffering (LeShan L., 1977).

Poor social support for women with early breast cancer is associated with impaired killer immune cell function both during surgery and three months later (Levy S. M. et al., 1985, 1987). Researchers observed 2,800 patients with the same diagnosis for six years and concluded that women who were socially isolated before being diagnosed had a 100% higher risk of death from the underlying disease and 66% from other causes during the observation period, compared with socially integrated women (Kroenke C. H. et al., 2006). A similar situation was found in newly diagnosed patients with rectal cancer: loneliness, which is the main symptom of poor social support, is correlated with a higher content of the

VEGF vascular growth factor in blood serum, which accelerates tumor development (Nausheen B. et al., 2010).

Interesting experimental observations were made by researchers at Carleton University in Ottawa. Mice were subjected to the stress of social isolation and during this period they were "grafted" with cancer cells. This resulted in more active tumor growth than what was observed in rodents under normal keeping conditions. However, when these isolated mice were exposed to additional stress following the injection of cancer cells, the result depended on the type of stress: the impact of limiting mobility (a situation of hopelessness) activated the development of cancer, whereas the stress of social conflict, when animals had to constantly fight, inhibited the development of tumors (Sklar L. S., Anisman H., 1980). This data emphasizes the need to maintain an active life position in the fight against the disease, that we repeatedly observe in humans.

What also plays an important role is how well the patient understands the mechanisms of their disease: insufficient knowledge on the topic in patients with ovarian cancer, in particular, is reflected in higher levels of depression, anxiety, and the indicator of the tumor marker CA-125 (Parker P. A. et al., 2006). In addition, patients with ovarian cancer, who were in deep depression and had low levels of social support, had an over-activity of about 200 genes responsible for the mechanisms of tumor growth and progression. The leading role in this gene activity is played by the intracellular response to stress hormones epinephrine and norepinephrine (Lutgendorf S. K. et al., 2009).

Depression, which develops as a result of a diagnosis, worsens the prognosis of the disease, as it further depresses the immune system. This has been proven during the observation of patients with breast cancer (Sephton S. E. et al., 2009), liver (Steel J. L. et al., 2007) and digestive tract cancer (Nan K. J. et al., 2004). All those molecular mechanisms that are common to stress and depression, which we considered in Chapter 19, continue to work. It is the patient's prolonged stay in a negative emotional state, which is manifested through depression and hopelessness, that influences the progression of the disease, and this is even more important than additional stresses currently ongoing in the patient's life (Moreno-Smith M. et al., 2010). One of the mechanisms of such activation of the disease is that during depression, tumor, when under the influence of an increased content of catecholamines, is capable of more easily releasing cancer cells, which in turn migrate throughout the body and become the causes of metastases (Sood A. K., Lutgendorf S. K., 2011).

Another problem is the increase in cytokine–endocrine imbalance during depression (Raison C. L., Miller A. H., 2003), leading to further progress of inflammation. This is confirmed by the fact on the increase in the activity of genes responsible for the synthesis of pro-inflammatory substances and agents of metastasis in depressive cancer patients (Cohen L. et al., 2012). Moreover, the tumor itself activates the synthesis of pro-inflammatory cytokines directly in its tissue (interleukin IL-1β) and in the hippocampus (interleukins IL-1β, IL-6, TNF, and IL-10), which stimulates the development of depression (Pyter L. M. et al., 2009).

The negative impact of stress on the treatment process is confirmed in animal experiments. One of the hormonal drugs (bicalutamide), which inhibited the growth of both the spontaneous and "grafted" tumors of the prostate in mice in non-stressful keeping, was ineffective when such mice were stressed by means of restriction of their mobility. However, this stress effect was stopped with a beta-adrenergic blocker (Hassan S. et al., 2013). A similar stress effect was observed while using the chemotherapy drug cyclophosphamide for the treatment of "grafted" lung cancer in mice (Zorzet S. et al., 1998).

Conclusion

The US National Comprehensive Cancer Network (NCCN, 2007) defines the distress felt by cancer patients as

> a multifactorial unpleasant experience of a psychological (i.e., cognitive, behavioral, emotional), social, spiritual, and/or physical nature that may interfere with the ability to cope effectively with cancer, its physical symptoms, and its treatment. Distress extends along a continuum, ranging from common normal feelings of vulnerability, sadness, and fears to problems that can become disabling, such as depression, anxiety, panic, social isolation, and existential and spiritual crisis.

As we have seen, distress of this kind begins during the diagnostic process and accompanies the patient throughout the entire treatment period. Moreover, the accumulation of distress has a significant impact: the initial (pre-diagnosis) chronic stress is aggravated by the distress of the diagnosis and is amplified by the distress of the treatment (operation, chemotherapy, and radiotherapy) and their consequences, as well as by the stress of impaired physical and social status and uncertainty about the future. This fact is also noted by Russian psychologists who have studied patients with breast cancer. In their opinion, a feature of chronic stress in this disease, is its cumulative nature: there is a combination of negative emotional experiences of psycho-traumatic events that occurred in the patient's life prior to the onset of the disease, acute stress that is caused by the diagnosis, and existential experiences the patient has when they know that their life is at risk (Tarabrina N. V. et al., 2008).

Another illustration is the study of the role of psychological factors over the course of oncohematological diseases. When compared with a group of recovered patients, patients who died within three years of the onset of the disease experienced twice as much burden, which was caused by psychosocial stress. According to the authors, patients who experience many stresses, including the distress of life-threatening situations, are not able to organize adaptive protection against new stress, such as leukemia (Umanskiy S. V., Semke V. Y., 2008).

The huge issue with post-Soviet practical oncology at all its levels—starting with the oncologist at the polyclinic and ending with specialized clinics—lies in the lack of knowledge and the misunderstanding of the enormous influence that the combined distress has on the effectiveness of treatment, the number of possible complications, and the potential for a relapse of the disease. Meanwhile, oncologists from many developed countries have already acknowledged the need to introduce standardized methods for identifying patients experiencing distress who need additional psychological assistance. Such an assessment aims to recognize the stressful condition of patients in a timely manner so that these problems can be solved as soon as possible.

This concept of Screening for Distress was, in particular, approved in 2004 by the Canadian Strategy for Cancer Control and is currently included in the oncology program accreditation system (Rebalance Focus, 2005). In 2007, the US National Comprehensive Cancer Network established the following as a standard: "All patients should be screened for distress at their initial visit, at appropriate intervals, and as clinically indicated especially with changes in disease status (i.e., remission, recurrence, progression)" (NCCN, 2007).

Based on the above-considered data on the stimulating effect of the distress resulting from the diagnosis and the distress at treatment on the mechanisms of tumor growth, from my point of view, it is necessary that preventive measures be taken as soon as possible in order to protect all patients, without exception, from distress—even at the stage of primary examination. Testing can reveal the severity of distress experienced by each patient in order to understand the amount of help each individual requires. There are no people who would not experience distress at all during this period. Therefore, anti-stress care can and should be started even before examination.

In such an anti-stress therapy, both pharmacological and psychotherapeutic actions should be taken.

A. Pharmacotherapy of Cancer Patients' Distress

We have repeatedly examined research results that demonstrated the effectiveness of drugs from the group of beta-adrenergic blockers (which eliminate the effects of the catecholamine stress hormones) to inhibit the growth of experimental tumors. At their core, beta-blockers have been long-known and widely used in clinical practice drugs for the treatment of hypertension and other cardiovascular diseases. After their effect of inhibiting the development of tumors was experimentally discovered, researchers analyzed the medical databases regarding the incidence of cancer in various patients who had been taking similar drugs for a long time, and noticed a decrease in their cancer incidence rates.

One such meta-analysis reviewed the twelve studies performed from 1993 to 2013, where beta-blockers were used to treat 20,898 patients with non-oncological diseases. It was discovered that those patients who subsequently became ill with cancer had a higher survival rate and fewer relapses of the disease. The strongest effect of beta-blockers was manifested in the early stages of the disease and in patients undergoing surgery (compared with other forms of treatment) (Choi C. H. et al., 2014). It was also found that breast cancer patients, who had previously taken beta-blockers to treat hypertension for ten years, had a significantly reduced frequency of metastases and the recurrence of the disease after treatment was significantly reduced, and mortality was 71% lower (Powe D. G. et al., 2010). In men, the risk of developing prostate cancer was decreased by 18% (Perron L. et al., 2004), and among those who still developed this type of cancer, mortality and the number of metastases were reduced as a result of the beta-blockers taken (Grytli H. H. et al., 2014).

MD Anderson's cancer research center analyzed the statistical data of 1,425 women who took various beta-blockers and were treated for ovarian cancer at various medical centers from 2000 to 2010. It turned out that not all beta-blockers work equally effectively on the cancer process. The most effective were the so-called non-selective beta-blockers,[1] which interact with both types of beta-adrenergic receptors, and they increased the average survival time of patients to up to 94.9 months. The average survival time for patients who did not receive beta-blockers at all was 42 months, and for those who took any selective beta-blocker the survival time was 47.8 months (Watkins J. L. et al., 2015).

The accumulation of such data on the influence of beta-blockers on patients' survival times allowed scientists to recognize the feasibility of targeted research on the use of beta-blockers in the course of antitumor therapy. The goal is to reduce psycho-emotional stress, angiogenesis, tumor growth and metastasis, and to improve immunity. The perspective of prescribing beta-blockers jointly with chemotherapy and radiation, as well as in combination with anti-inflammatory drugs such as aspirin and prostaglandin blockers is currently being studied, as well as the possibility of prescribing them during the postoperative period to improve wound healing (Nagaraja A. S. et al., 2013; Watkins J. L. et al., 2015; Benish M. et al., 2008). Clinical testing is already being done in this direction (Feasibility Study, 2012) and is recommended by the American Food and Drug Administration, as well as by the relevant EU body, as appropriate for clinical use (Watkins J. L. et al., 2015).

---

[1] The most common of these drugs is propranolol.

Recent studies show that the use of beta-adrenoblockers can reduce the speed of the proliferation of esophageal cancer cells (Liu X. et al., 2008), decrease the incidence of early breast cancer and lymph node metastasis (Barron T. I. et al., 2011), and reduce the probability of progression in melanoma (Lemeshow S. et al., 2011).

The use of beta-blockers to reduce the impact of psycho-emotional stress is also actively being explored outside of oncology, since prolonged activation of adrenergic mechanisms after an acute stressful event can increase the risk of developing post-traumatic stress disorder (PTSD) (Orr S. P. et al., 2000). By blocking these mechanisms, propranolol is able to reduce the intensity of emotionally "loaded" memories (Cahill L. et al., 1994), and therefore began to be used for the treatment of PTSD (Brunet A. et al., 2011). In particular, prescribing propranolol in the early stages after a traumatic event has occurred reduces generalized anxiety and reduces the incidence of PTSD in the long term (Pitman R. K. et al., 2002; Vaiva G. et al., 2003). However, some authors did not confirm this effect, which may be explained by differences in the dosages used and other factors (Amos T. et al., 2014).

Psycho-oncologists have become interested in beta-blockers for the same reason. At the University of Ohio researchers studied recently diagnosed rectum and breast cancer patients that were constantly taking beta-blockers to treat hypertension. It turned out that they developed less psychological distress after one to three months after the diagnosis was announced. This was reflected in the amount of disturbing obsessive thoughts, which was 32% lower. In this regard, doctors consider it expedient to assign beta-blockers immediately after the diagnosis is announced, when a peak in distress is observed (Lindgren M. E. et al., 2013).

There is no doubt that the most important studies in this area of psycho-oncology are still to come, especially if we consider that beta-blockers can cause serious side effects in some patients. This can prevent their widespread use in cancer patients (Watkins J. L. et al., 2015). However, taking into account the positive effect of these drugs on the patient's psyche and on the dynamics of the cancer development, we can hope that the study of beta-blockers will help scientists take a step forward in the treatment of cancer patients.

In addition, back in the 1970s and 1980s scientists at the Research Institute of Oncology Problems in Ukraine carried out experimental and clinical studies of phentolamine, a representative of another group of adrenoblockers—alpha-blockers (named according to another type of receptor for catecholamines). Phentolamine has proven to be effective in inhibiting the development of gastric tumors in rats and reducing the recurrence of gastric polyps (a precancerous condition) after their surgical removal in humans. Also, the Institute conducted studies of various psychotropic drugs (in particular, the psychic stimulant sidnofen and the antidepressant pirazidol), drugs modulating the activity of the

Vladislav Matrenitsky

adrenal cortex and the thyroid (chlorpromazine, metamizol, thyroliberin, liothyronine), and other pharmacological agents (lithium carbonate, Delta Sleep Inducing Peptide, Na-gamma-hydroxybutyrate, L-DOPA, leu-enkephalin). Their effects include the prevention of exhaustion and disruption of the mediator systems of the brain, antistress, immunostimulating, and adaptogenic effects on the neuroendocrine systems, increase in the effectiveness of the treatment prescribed to cancer patients and the inhibition of the metastasis process (Balitskiy K. P. et al., 1983; Balitskiy K. P., Shmalko Y. P., 1987).

Sadly, Ukraine has lost priority in this promising direction and such studies are no longer conducted at this Institute, which is currently called the Institute of Experimental Pathology, Oncology and Radiobiology after Kavetskiy. Meanwhile, foreign scientists continue to study various drugs designed to reduce the activating effects of psycho-physiological and operational stress on the mechanisms of tumor growth. Examples of such drugs are the anticoagulant heparin, which prevents the spread of cancer cells after surgery (Seth R. et al., 2013), anti-inflammatory substances (Kehlet H., 1997; Harris R. E. et al., 1999), an opiate of internal origin, beta-endorphin (Zhang C., Sarkar D. K., 2012), the adaptogen ginseng (Jia L., Qian K., 2011), and melatonin (Dziegiel P. et al., 2008), among others.

Significant results were obtained in the 1970s and 1980s in the course of research conducted by the team led by Prof. Liubov Garkavi at the Rostov Research Institute of Oncology (Russia). Scientists have learned how to translate the tumor-related stress, which has low levels of reactivity, into a reaction of training or activation of higher levels of reactivity. This makes it possible for the organism to overcome the stage of exhaustion caused by stress and once again restores the functional and organic reserves needed to fight the disease. The consequent elimination of central nervous system suppression enhances the functions of the endocrine and immune systems, which leads to the regression of some tumors in both experimental and clinical conditions. Such a translation of stress in the reaction of training and activation was achieved with the help of small and medium doses of neurotrophic substances, biostimulants, and a magnetic field (Garkavi L. H. et al., 1990). However, these developments are not presently included in the clinical practice of the Rostov's Institute—probably for the same reason as the studies of oncogenic stress are not done in the Kiev's Institute—they cannot be used to help produce expensive anti-cancer drugs...

Meanwhile, Professor Ben-Eliyahu (2008) from the University of Tel Aviv concluded:

By boosting the immune system and blocking its suppression by psychological and physiological stress, starting a day or two before surgery, during surgery and after surgery, we may be able to provide an intervention program that can extend people's lives and potentially increase their chances for long-term survival.

B. Distress Psychotherapy

The involvement of psychotherapy immediately after the announcement of the diagnosis is extremely important, since it helps the patient to cope with distress and prevents the development of PTSD (Helgeson V. S. et al., 2004; Koopman C. et al., 2002). Researchers at the University of West Virginia argue for the need for psychotherapeutic intervention at the first mention of the possibility of cancer. According to the authors, reducing the level of stress caused by the disease also contributes to a more rapid recovery and better quality of life in patients undergoing chemotherapy and radiotherapy (Montgomery M., McCrone S., 2010).

This is confirmed by studies conducted at the MD Anderson Cancer Center at the University of Texas. Before the prostate removal surgery, the patients were divided into three groups. Two sessions of anti-stress therapy were conducted for patients in the first group, which included methods of cognitive psychotherapy, deep breathing, and directed visualization to improve the results of the operation. Patients received guidance and audio records on stress management for self-preparation for surgery; had a brief activating session with a psychologist in the morning before the operation and a similar session forty-eight hours after the operation in order to improve their relaxation and stress management skills.

Patients that were assigned to the second group met twice with a psychologist one or two weeks before the operation. Their concerns were discussed in an empathizing and encouraging atmosphere, and they were taught some techniques of cognitive self-regulation. These patients also had a brief activating session with a psychologist in the morning before the operation and a second session forty-eight hours after it, during which their experience and emotions in connection with surgery and hospital stay were discussed. Patients belonging to the third group received standard medical care.

The study of the immune system of all patients conducted two days after the operation showed a significant increase in its activity in the first group, the absence of changes in the second and a decrease in the third one. The psychological state, determined by mood disorders, was also significantly better in the patients in the first group and did not differ in the second and third. The findings suggest the importance of psychological intervention to reduce preoperative stress and improve the results of the operation (Cohen L. et al., 2011).

Another program of early psychological care for cancer patients was proposed at the University of Los Angeles. It included teaching patients how to behave and overcome difficulties (learning the techniques of problem solving), informing them about the mechanisms of disease development and various aspects of treatment, and visiting psychosocial support groups. The program proved to be effective for patients who had recently been diagnosed with cancer and were in the initial stages of the disease. According to the authors, teaching the active forms of behavioral and cognitive psychological adaptation can weaken the distress caused by the disease, improve the quality of patients' lives in general, and increase their lifespan (Fawzy F. J., 1995).

In the surgical clinic at the University of Hamburg, patients with cancer of the gastrointestinal tract (experimental group), in addition to standard treatment, were given an average of seven psychotherapeutic sessions. The therapy was aimed at emotional and cognitive support in order to activate the "fighting spirit," decrease the feelings of helplessness and hopelessness, and to resolve emotional and existential problems. Patient survival time in the experimental group was twice as long as that of the control group that did not receive psychotherapy (Küchler T. et al., 2007).

The study performed in the University of Miami was focused on monitoring women in the early stages of breast cancer. Patients were offered a ten-week program of cognitive-behavioral stress management, with follow-up observation for a year. These patients had significantly decreased anxiety and serum cortisol, and in their leukocytes there was a lowered activity of genes responsible for inflammatory reactions and metastasis (Cruess D. G. et al., 2000; Antoni M. H. et al., 2012). The same group of scientists used a thirteen-week period of experimental existential group psychotherapy in another research study, as a result of which patients with a similar diagnosis were able to express their emotional needs more freely. This resulted in less impairment of immunity under stress (Van der Pompe G. et al., 2001).

The practice of mindfulness meditation, which psychotherapists presently often involve in therapy, also leads to a decrease in distress associated with a newly diagnosed cancer (we will look at this aspect in detail in Chapter 32). It helps to improve immunity, reduce cortisol levels in the blood, increase mental well-being, improve the quality of life, and decrease the incidence of PTSD (Bränström R. et al., 2010; Witek-Janusek L. et al., 2008). Creative art therapy, which reduces the level of negative emotions and increases the positive state, also proved to be effective (Puig A. et al., 2006).

Meta-analyses show that the positive effect of psychotherapy is also observed in subsequent stages of the disease. It reduces cancer-related stress and maladaptive behavior, emotional imbalance, fatigue, anxiety, depression, while the quality of life improves (Spiegel D. et al., 1989; Meyer T. J., Mark M. M., 1995; Duijts S. F. et al., 2011; Rehse B., Pukrop R., 2003). Increased psychological literacy of patients leads to similar results (Devine E. C., Westlake S. K., 1995).

Hypnotherapy has great potential for cancer patients. Hypnosis and self-hypnosis help them to effectively control the emotional distress and pain associated with the operation, improve and accelerate the process of subsequent recovery, reduce fatigue caused by chemotherapy, nausea and vomiting, to lower their levels of anxiety and depression, increase their self-esteem and motivate them to work on themselves, improve their physical well-being, quality of life, and indicators of immunity (Montgomery G. H. et al., 2002; Flory N., Lang E., 2008; Richardson J. et al., 2007; Walker L. G. et al., 1999; Levitan A. A., 1991; Devine E. C., Westlake S. K., 1995). A DNA study showed that hypnotherapy leads to changes in gene expression within 90–120 minutes from the beginning of the process (Rossi E. L., 2000).

Dr. Bernard Newton from California (1982) applied ten hours of hypnotherapy to a group of 105 oncological patients over a three-month period. After eight years, 54% of patients in this group were alive, whereas only 18% of patients that were in the control group and did not receive hypnotherapy survived. Russian scientists have not only confirmed the above data on the improvement of psychological parameters of patients with gastric cancer and melanoma under the influence of hypno-suggestive psychotherapy, but also found significant changes at the cellular-molecular level. For the first time, it has been demonstrated that the use of hypnosis can cause a long-term rise in the content of stem cells in peripheral blood and an increase in the length of lymphocytes' telomeres. This was reflected in the normalization of the immune status indicators of cancer patients. As a result, patients with melanoma were able to achieve an increase in five-year survival (Bukhtoyarov O. V., Arkhangelskiy A. E., 2008).

The growing number of such studies, showing the effect of psychotherapy on the physiological and biochemical processes in the body, encourages scientists to consider psychotherapy as an "epigenetic medicine," as a therapeutic agent that acts in an epigenetic way similar to pharmaceutical preparations. This data leads to a change in the paradigm of the use of psychotherapy: the effectiveness of the impact of various standardized, short-term, goal-oriented techniques can now be tested at the genome level, and it is possible to use them in cases where doctors previously relied solely on pharmacological agents (Stahl S. M., 2012).

C. Recommendations

All of the above indicates a significant potential benefit of early anti-stress therapy in preventing the stimulation of tumor growth caused by the announcement of the diagnosis and surgery, in the reduction of all types of complications of subsequent treatment and of the likelihood of recurrence of the disease.

In my opinion, the use of beta-blockers should begin from the moment when a person is referred for primary diagnostics and continue throughout the whole subsequent period of therapy (of course, this should take into account one's general health, individual contraindications, and aspects of interaction with other drugs).

Ideally, the announcement of the diagnosis should be carried out by a tandem of an oncologist and psychologist (or psychotherapist). Immediately after this, it is necessary to provide the patient with emergency psychotherapeutic aid, making use of techniques that aid in the removal of an acute affective stress state. In this situation, one can use the methods of short-term psychotherapy, such as EMDR (*Eye Movement Desensitization and Reprocessing*—Shapiro F., 2001), emotional-imaginative therapy (Linde N. D., 2006), "Key" methodic (Aliyev H., 2003), hypnosis, NLP, body-oriented, positive, and rational therapy (Vihristyuk O. V. et al., 2010; O'Hanlon B., Cade W. H., 1993), and so on. It is also advisable to use the recommendations and experience of army and emergency service psychologists (Shoygu Y. S., 2007; Kohanov V. P., Krasnov V. N., 2008). As with acute psychic trauma of any other origin, the application of sedative and tranquilizing drugs can be helpful (Kekelidze Z. I., 2001). All these activities should be carried out quite quickly—before the formation of post-traumatic stress disorder or other delayed neuropsychiatric disorders.

Started during a period of shock and crisis caused by the announcement of the diagnosis, psychotherapeutic observation and assistance should continue throughout the subsequent period, both before the start of medical procedures and during them. Having determined the level of the patient's distress, one can apply rational-informational psychotherapy, which consists of briefing the patient on the main mechanisms of stress disorders and their health risks, and teaching them methods of mental self-regulation, aimed to cope with anxiety and tension symptoms (in particular, autogenic training by Schultz, relaxation, visualization of a positive result of therapy, etc.).

Russian psycho-oncologists also believe that it is necessary to create special psychological programs for preparing patients for surgery in order to alleviate their fears and worries, to teach patients methods of self-regulation and of decreasing depression and anxiety (Rusina N. A., Moiseeva K. S., 2013).

The use of cognitive psychotherapy can help the patient ease the severity of maladaptive thoughts and alter negative beliefs. Person-centered therapy can influence the patient's attitude to the situation of the disease and help them take responsibility for their actions. Methods of positive therapy and gestalt therapy will help patients to realize that despite the problems associated with the disease, there are ways and possibilities to overcome them and these are available to everyone (Kohanov V. P., Krasnov V. N., 2008; Malkina-Pykh I., 2005). All of this contributes to an increase in the resources, capabilities, and skills of coping with the stress of the disease and treatment, and hence reduces the physiological distress, which is so dangerous to one's health and therapy results.

When the patient is in a more balanced and prepared state (this can be reached both in the process of and after the treatment, during the rehabilitation period), and the main complications of therapy (such as the "chemical brain") have been removed, it is necessary to begin the main part of psychotherapy. It is aimed at identifying and eliminating unresolved psychic traumas and conflicts, cancer dominant, self-destructiveness, hidden suicidality, and the loss of the meaning of life. We will discuss these aspects in the final section.

Part VII

The Outcome and
Consequences of Cancer

No one is ever defeated
until defeat has been accepted as a reality.
Napoleon Hill,
Think and Grow Rich

In my opinion, the depressing statistics on the survival of cancer patients that have been observed in modern oncology are directly related to the absence or insufficient quantity and quality of psychosocial services (especially in the ex-Soviet area). Even in places where a psycho-oncology service exists, it mainly performs the functions of palliative therapy, thus dealing with the psychological symptoms that have arisen as a result of the disease. Although it is much better than nothing, still the introduction of integrative multimodal programs, especially those focused on actively influencing the psychological sources of the disease, it is still at an early stage. Some of these programs have been described in the previous chapter, and we will take a look at some of the others in this chapter.

It is known that cancer patients can experience a high level of distress for up to fifteen months after diagnosis (Hinnen C. et al., 2008). As the reader already understands, this does not in any way contribute to recovery and remission. If, by the end of the first year after being diagnosed with the disease, the patient experiences significant hopelessness, then even if there is a positive medical prognosis, such a patient has poor survival chances (Filipp S. H., 1992).

Researchers at the Royal Marsden Clinic in the UK conducted a psychological examination of 578 women undergoing first-stage breast cancer treatment. Testing was conducted twice: during the period from one to three months after the diagnosis and then one year later. Over the next five years, the patients were under observation. At the end of this period, 133 women had died, 50 had a relapse of the disease, and the remaining 395 remained healthy. Analysis of the tests revealed that women in both the groups who died and got sick again experienced high levels of helplessness and hopelessness, and those who died additionally had higher rates of depression (Watson M. et al., 1999). This data once again emphasizes the importance of timely psychotherapy.

Under standard medical therapy, the outcome of the disease for different patients with the same diagnosis and treatment methods can be completely different, and from the point of view of the biomedical model of medicine, this is still a riddle for oncologists. From the standpoint of the biopsychosocial-spiritual model, there is no mystery, since the outcome is determined by the totality and severity of all those psychological factors that we have examined so far.

Unresolved psychic traumas and conflicts, distress caused by the diagnosis and treatment, loss of hope and will to live, as well as the absence of anti-stress and in-depth psychotherapeutic assistance lead to the rapid progression of the disease, despite ongoing antitumor therapy. In this case, as we will see later, the death of some patients may occur not even because of complications caused by the development of the disease, but because of the psychogenic imbalance of the main physiological systems of the body, reflecting the state of "surrendering."

Among the stronger personalities who have reached remission, many still suffer from a significant number of psychological disorders, including depression and post-traumatic stress disorder, to top off an entire accumulated "bunch" of distress, which we have talked about. These most often remain unattended and untreated, and owing to the fact that the patients often return to the same oncogenic lifestyle they led before the disease, these complications shorten the remission period and contribute to the relapse of the disease.

Nevertheless, a certain number of patients experience psychological and spiritual transformation, which becomes a powerful source of internal healing forces. This leads to sustained remission and often complete recovery. Moreover, in rare cases, such a personal transformation can heal a person even without the need for medical treatment—these cases are referred to as spontaneous remission.

In the next section, we will analyze why the same diagnosis can result in such different outcomes.

Chapter 28

Psychogenic Death

Being diagnosed with cancer can activate the deepest social "archetypical" attitudes about the inevitability of death due to cancer in the subconscious of an individual, which always has a catastrophic effect on their survival. Even with a relatively favorable prognosis, a number of patients condemn themselves to death, as if allowing themselves to die, and continue believing that cancer is incurable (Shutcenberger A. A., 1990).

Most of us either known or heard reports of an apparently healthy, vigorous person who died almost immediately after being diagnosed as having cancer, *write C. Simonton and co-authors (1978)*. Such patients are often so intimidated by the cancer diagnosis and have such a negative expectancy of their ability to survive, that they may never even leave the hospital following the diagnosis. The course of the disease goes downhill far more rapidly than the physicians anticipated. To explain such cases, doctors sometimes speak of the patient's 'giving up' or losing their "will to live".

As far back as in 1928 a similar phenomenon was described by the Kiev's Clinical Institute professor Georgiy Bykhovskiy. Before the operation to remove a breast tumor, the patient was very afraid and worried, claiming that she would not survive it. Despite the success of the operation, the patient died in the hours following the surgery. In the surgeon's opinion, the patient's death was due to mental depression or shock, which caused "a sudden drop in vital functions and heart failure."

Iatrogeny plays a major role in oncology; that is, mental or physical impairment or aggravation of the patient's symptoms caused by the health worker, because of their attitude toward the patient, their behavior, or the use of erroneous treatment methods. Iatrogeny is a particular case of the psychogenic death phenomenon, and its existence is recognized even in primitive cultures, where people sentenced to death by a shaman or sorcerer die in accordance with the pronounced sentence. The African tradition of "voodoo" (Cannon W. B., 1942) is best known for such cases. A psychiatrist from New Zealand, Professor Jennifer Barraclough (2001), who had had cancer in the past, said the following about herself: "Doctors have no right to play God by extinguishing hope. Had I passively accepted my doctor's death sentence I would have died years ago, another victim of sophisticated Western-style voodoo."

Dr. Andrey Gnezdilov (2002) provides a vivid example of iatrogeny:

At the Oncology Institute, upon bandaging a postoperative wound, a young doctor involuntarily pursed his lips and slightly rolled his eyes. The patient trusted the doctor very much and, during the dressing of the wound, watched the expression on his face, attempting to assess her condition by observing his reaction. When she returned to the ward, she began to cry and told her neighbors that when the doctor opened her wound, his face changed, he pursed his lips and rolled his eyes. This made her realize that her condition was hopeless. By evening, she developed a heart attack and died.

These observations of the Russian psycho-oncologist are confirmed by the above-mentioned study conducted by Swedish scientists: in the first week after being diagnosed with cancer, the cardiovascular mortality of patients increased by 5.6 times, in the first month, by 3.3 times, and during the year the rate quickly dropped to the usual level (Fang F. et al., 2012).

The prevalence and severity of iatrogeny are indicated by the fact that in 1990 the First World Congress of the International Society for the Prevention of Iatrogenic Complications (ISPIC) was held in Denmark, and adopted a special Statement on Safety in Health Protection. It considers iatrogeny as the final negative result of the functioning of the healthcare system as a whole (Shaposhnikov A., 1998).

A textbook example of how self-hypnosis influences the course of the disease is given in a story published in 1957 by Doctor Bruno Klopfer, from the University of Los Angeles. His patient, referred to as Mr. Wright, suffered from the most severe form of lymphosarcoma. The patient's body was covered with orange-sized tumors, no treatment had any effect, the spleen and liver were extremely enlarged, and he had to breathe with the help of an oxygen mask. According to the doctors, he had a few days to live. After hearing about a new drug called Krebiozen, which was being tested at the clinic he was at, Wright insistently asked Klopfer to administer it to him. Although he did not meet the criteria for this program, the doctor did decide to give the patient a single injection on Friday, believing that the patient would die by Monday.

However, to Klopfer's surprise, Wright's condition improved significantly on Monday, while the drug had no positive effect on other patients. Klopfer wrote that the masses of tumors dematerialized "like snow on a hot stove" and their number decreased by half in a few days. The treatment was continued, and after ten days almost all of the symptoms of the disease had disappeared. The patient then returned to his normal life.

Meanwhile, two months later, controversial news about Krebiozen appeared in the press, reporting that there were no positive results in any of the clinics that had tested Krebiozen. Because of this, Wright began to lose his faith in healing. A relapse began. After another two months his health returned to its original state, and he was gloomy and unhappy. We should give credit to Dr. Klopfer and his team, since they realized the psychogenic nature of the observed phenomenon, and told Wright that they were awaiting the arrival of a new, super-purified Krebiozen, a "double powered" drug. The patient was almost ecstatic, and his faith was strong. When the medicine arrived, Klopfer, with an air of great importance, gave the patient his first injection of this new, "twice as strong drug," which actually consisted of pure water. The result of this "course of treatment" was even more spectacular than the first time: the tumor masses disappeared, the patient returned to his normal life, and remained in a good state of health for the next two months.

But then, after analyzing the results of research in a large number of medical institutions, a respected medical journal published a report concluding that Krebiozen is useless in the treatment of cancer. Upon learning this, Wright lost his last hope: his belief in the drug disappeared, the disease flared up again, and after a few days he entered the hospital again in a hopeless state, where he died two days later (Klopfer B., 1957).

All these examples convincingly confirm the truth stated by the Buddhist master Zopa Rinpoche (2001), that illness is the mind indeed.

The most important influence on the course of the disease is the life expectancy predicted by doctors. Despite the fact that such a forecast reflects the average picture of the outcome of the disease and does not take into account the individual characteristics of the patient's personality, for many people the "set time" becomes a "self-fulfilling prophecy," triggering the mechanism of psychogenic death. The reason for this is that during the shocking psychic trauma of the diagnosis, the human consciousness goes into an altered state for protective purposes (Spivak L. I., 1988), which is characterized by hypersuggestibility (Bukhtoyarov O. V., Arkhangelskiy A. E., 2008). At this moment, information (forecast) emanating from an authoritative person (doctor), according to the principles of hypnotic suggestion, is fixed in the subconscious of a person, and thus triggers mechanisms for the realization of "prophecy".

According to D. S. Chernavskiy and his colleagues (2003), in this case the fear of death breaks out from the deep levels of consciousness and, without meeting the opposition of hope and faith, for they are lost, completely captures the hierarchical mental structures of the patient. As a result, there is a "narrowing" in all spheres of activity, including life activity. A person loses hope and submissively surrenders to the illness, almost counting the days until the specified time. The case stories are full of observations about how cancer patients dutifully die during the "appointed" period, but their autopsies do not reveal fatal complications caused by tumor growth. In particular, according to the Minsk city (Belarus) dissection bureau, in 22% of cases the cause of the deaths of cancer patients is from non-cancer reasons such as acute heart failure, regardless of the localization of the tumor process (Fridman M. V. et al., 2002).

The "good intentions" of the medical personnel, in particular, the advice "keep holding on, grit your teeth" can also become iatrogenic. Many patients (especially men) behave this way, to prevent their emotional tension from spilling out. As a result, some patients experience such a strong emotional overload that they have a cardiac arrest or cerebral hemorrhage even before the operation begins (Gnezdilov A. V., 2002).

A detailed analysis of the phenomenon of psychogenic death of cancer patients is undertaken by O. V. Bukhtoyarov and A. E. Arkhangelskiy (2006; 2008). They explain it as the psychological capitulation of patients as a result of the combination of the chronic psycho-emotional stress and its somatic consequences: anxiety, depression, feelings of social isolation, despair, hopelessness, as well as complications of chemo- and radiotherapy. All of these factors contribute to the rapid progression of the cancer process and cardiac abnormalities. The authors (2006) write that

> in cases of cancer diagnosis, psychogenic stress is inexhaustible, and the death sentence for an indefinite period turns into a chronic massive psychic trauma and a severe life crisis. In our opinion, in such situations, the cumulative effect of long-term psychogenic influences can be so powerful that it can cause organic changes or significantly aggravate the already existing organic pathology up to death.

Also, according to Japanese scientists, about 80% of oncological patients die owing to a psychological surrender to the disease (Fukunishi I., 1998).

In the opinion of O. V. Bukhtoyarov and A. E. Arkhangelskiy (2006), the mechanism of psychogenic death is based on the formation of the syndrome of the disintegration of brain structures under the influence of changes in the psyche of the patients. Its neurophysiological characteristics are consistent changes in the cortical-subcortical and hypothalamic-reticular connections, followed by prolonged, "stagnant" activation of the limbic-reticular complex and descending tonic effects on the sympathetic-adrenal and hypophyseal-adrenal apparatus. Such hyperactivation of the nervous system primarily affects the initial or acquired "weak places" in the body, which can be the myocardium and the neuro-conducting system of the heart, with the subsequent development of fatal arrhythmias. Also contributing to this outcome is the immune system, which is weakened by the cancer process and psychogenic disorders (and often chemotherapy). All of this leads to the cancer's progression and a general weakening of the body.

Psychogenic death can have both a rapid form, developing in a period of up to three to five days from the moment of the massive psychic trauma onset (often iatrogenic, as we saw above), and a slow form that occurs in the interval from five days to two months or more. The latter form is more common and is characterized by the occurrence of psychological surrender and clinical symptoms of depression up to the catatonic state, followed by death (Bukhtoyarov O. V., Arkhangelskiy A. E., 2006).

Undoubtedly, the loss of the will to live and the patient's avital experiences also play an important role in the mechanisms of psychogenic death. These can be significantly activated as a result of the cancer diagnosis, especially if the disease is subconsciously perceived as a way out of an unbearable life situation. Physician and homeopath Alla Osipova, who works with cancer patients, in her book *Cancer can be Beaten* (2014) shares her experience:

> ... some patients simply do not want to live. And no matter how hard I strived, no matter how hard I tried to help them believe in recovery, they had already sealed their fate and all the decisions about life and death had already been made. Eros and Thanatos, eternal struggle between the two beginnings. And the subconscious of many [patients] has already chosen death.

Chapter 29

Mental Disorders and the Survival of Patients

The "inexhaustible psychogenic stress" caused by cancer, even despite successful medical treatment and remission, without adequate psychotherapeutic help or spiritual transformation of the personality often has consequences in the form of psychological, somatic, or psychopathological disorders. The main ones are anxiety, fatigue, deep depression, and post-traumatic stress disorder (Stein K. D. et al., 2008; Schmidt M. E. et al., 2012; Marilova T. Y., Shestopalova I. M., 2008). As a rule, these negative conditions do not receive sufficient attention from medical staff, which reduces the physical and mental capabilities of patients, as well as their quality of life (Alfano C. M., Rowland J. H., 2006; Zebrack B. J. et al., 2008).

For example from one study, in 87% of patients with breast cancer who had undergone radical mastectomy, the initial fear and anxiety in the long-term period were transformed into severe neurotic disorders, depression of varying severity, anxiety for the future, and anxious expectation of the progression of the disease (Tkachenko G. A. et al., 2010).

Among other things, cancer patients often experience poor general well-being, vegetative-vascular and cardiovascular disorders, emotional lability, previously uncharacteristic aggressiveness, which is associated with anxiety over one's health and lack of confidence in recovery, asthenia, hypochondria, apathy, dysphoria, and negative feelings due to physical impairment caused by an operation (Gnezdilov A. V., 2002; Blinov N. N. et al., 1990; Marilova T. Y., 2002; Jacobsen P. B., Donovan K. A., 2011; Dudnichenko A. S. et al., 2003).

According to epidemiological studies, in general 50%–70% of oncological patients develop various mental disorders (Gnezdilov A. V., 2002; Pirl W. F., 2004; Grassi L. et al., 2005). Obviously, their causes are combined distress, as discussed. Besides, after treatment, almost all patients are faced with an additional powerful source of distress—the fear of relapse of the illness (Alfano C. M., Rowland J. H., 2006; Thewes B., et al., 2011; Deimling G. T. et al., 2006).

In fact, the fear of relapse is the fear of the unknown. Since the overwhelming majority of patients have no idea what role the psyche plays in the occurrence of the disease, the "enemy remains unknown," and patients do not have any of their own tools to monitor their state of health, except for general physician's recommendations to follow a "healthy lifestyle." Those rare patients who seek help from psychiatrists or psychotherapists mainly complain of severe anxiety or depression, and, as a rule, receive only symptomatic psychopharmacological treatment. Psychologists rarely explore the psychodynamics of the main oncogenic conflicts, and so do not make enough effort to correct the specific properties of the type "C" personality and to teach patients how to cope with stress in the future. Meanwhile, scientists insist on the need for psychotherapy in order to reduce the fear of relapse (Holmberg C., 2014).

Cyclist Lance Armstrong (with S. Jenkins, 2000) shares that while his treatment was ongoing, he actively fought the disease, but as soon as the therapy was over, he suddenly felt completely helpless:

> I was such an active, aggressive persone that I would have felt better if they'd given me chemo for a year. Dr. Nichols tried to reassure me: "Some people have more trouble after treatment than during. It's common. It's more difficult to wait for it to come back than it is to attack."

V. D. Mendelevich (2001) highlights the persistent deferred syndrome, characterized as "cancerophobia in patients with malignant neoplasms." This syndrome can be observed for ten years after the initial diagnosis and includes anxious-depressive disorders in the form of a slight, but permanently depressed mood, a decrease in or loss of the ability to enjoy life (anhedonia), pessimistic self-esteem (dysmorphophobia), loss of perspective on existence, overvalued fear of tumor recurrence.

Fear of relapse enhances the initial chronic stress, potentiates the development of PTSD (Tacon A., 2012), and actually creates conditions in the body for the reactivation of the tumor process.

29.1. Post-Traumatic Stress Disorder

PTSD is a complex of mental disorder symptoms that develops as a result of a powerful traumatic effect on the human psyche that has acquired a protracted course.

The most common symptoms of PTSD include the delayed experience of mental trauma in the form of intrusive memories (flashbacks) and nightmarish dreams, loss of interest in life with the development of depression, alienation from other people and emotional torpor. Overexcitement, excessive vigilance, increased reaction to fear, and insomnia may occur. In the absence of adequate therapy, PTSD can go into a chronic stage and can lead to sustained personality changes, as well as the development of severe somatic diseases, including bronchial asthma, hypertension, ulcers of the gastrointestinal tract, etc. (Davidson J. R. et al., 1991; Giaconia R. M. et al., 1995).

There is contradictory data on how frequently this disorder occurs. In the non-oncological population, PTSD after an acute stress disorder occurs in 25% to 80% of people, while overall it prevails in 5% to 8% of the population (Breslau N., Kessler R. C., 2001; Voloshin P. V. et al., 2004).

Owing to the serious psychotraumatic effect of the cancer diagnosis and treatment, many patients develop symptoms of PTSD over time. Everything that reminds the patient of their illness, including periodic medical examinations, supports the existence of this disorder (Tacon A., 2012). According to the observations made by Australian scientists, PTSD occurred in 53% of patients suffering from head, neck, or lung cancer within six months of the initial diagnosis, which was followed by an acute stress disorder, and only developed in 11% of those who did not experience an acute stress disorder (Kangas M. et al., 2005). A similar incidence of PTSD in clinical expression was found in patients with hemoblastosis (Korotneva E. V., Varshavskiy A. V., 2007). In more than 30% of patients, PTSD symptoms persisted or worsened during the next five years of remission (Smith S. K. et al., 2011).

According to the team of researchers at the Institute of Psychology of the Russian Academy of Sciences, PTSD is diagnosed in 65.3% of women with breast cancer during the remission period (Tarabrina N. V. et al., 2010). The main etiological factors leading to the development of the disorder in these patients include the chronic nature of the disease, the risk of loss of physical usefulness as a result of the operation, as well as the feeling of having one's life threatened, accompanied by intense negative emotions of fear, horror, and helplessness. These experiences are characteristic of patients who failed to integrate the traumatic experience of the disease and to reprocess the negative beliefs resulting from the impact of distress. The more intense the symptoms of post-traumatic stress that developed were, the more fully expressed were the psychopathological symptoms among them (Vorona O. A., 2005).

In such patients, approximately equally high levels of hostility, phobic anxiety, and paranoid symptoms were observed, along with high rates of somatization, *obsessiveness-compulsiveness*, depression, *psychoticism*, a more negative image of the "I," a belief in one's own failure, and inability to control events. These disorders were significantly more pronounced in patients with PTSD than in patients without signs of post-traumatic stress (Tarabrina N. V., 2014). The identified post-traumatic and psychopathological symptoms reflect the state of chronic stress experienced by patients with breast cancer and are associated with the suppression of cellular immunity (Tarabrina N. V. et al., 2008).

The likelihood of PTSD developing is closely related to the stress-reactivity of a person and their belonging to a specific phenotype, which is characterized by a reduced ability to cope with and recover from mental trauma. Therefore, it is not only the severity of the traumatic event that matters, but also personal characteristics, basic beliefs and ideas, cases of psychopathology and PTSD in the family, previous episodes of anxiety and depression, unfavorable childhood conditions, loss of affection, poor social support, low socio-economic status, and history of experienced stressful events (Yehuda R., LeDoux J., 2007; Vorona O. A., 2005; Auxemery Y., 2012), which generally correspond to the diathesis–stress concept of diseases.

Upon taking into account the factors preceding the development of PTSD, C. P. Korolenko and N. V. Dmitrieva (2010) argue that as a result of some single severe trauma, the isolated diagnosis of this disorder is insufficient and leads to inadequate therapy. This view is supported by studies done on women with breast cancer. Those who developed PTSD clearly revealed the phenomenon of cumulative stress: a high level of personal anxiety, a number of stressful events before the disease, a greater amount of stress in general, and the inability to cope with these events. As a result, depressive states arose while personal resources to combat the stress of the disease were exhausted (Tarabrina N. V., 2014). Newly emerging psychological tensions on top of previous ones led to the appearance of significantly more pronounced stress symptoms (Butler L. D. et al., 1999). A similar tendency to accumulation of traumatic experiences before PTSD is also determined in patients with hemoblastosis (Korotneva E. V., Varshavskiy A. V., 2007).

Such life-accumulating stresses create a predisposition to the development of PTSD by epigenetic mechanisms (Heinzelmann M., Gill J., 2013; Zovkic I. B. et al., 2013), similar to those we have discussed.

In particular, immunosuppression, which is characteristic of PTSD as a whole, is accompanied by epigenetic changes in the methylation of genes associated with the immune response (Uddin M. et al., 2010). Also in monocyte immune cells, the activity of genes responsible for the mechanisms of inflammation changes, leading to an increase in inflammation during PTSD (O'Donovan A. et al., 2011). What also contributes to such a disorder is the fact that when PTSD persists for a prolonged period of time, the level of cortisol in the blood decreases (Wingenfeld K. et al., 2015; Yehuda R., 2001). Such a reaction of the adrenal glands may indicate the onset of the third stage of the general adaptation syndrome—the depletion of stress-regulating resources.

During PTSD, as well as generally during chronic stress, the content of catecholamines in the blood increases (Southwick S. M. et al., 1999; Wingenfeld K. et al., 2015). This provides grounds to prescribe a two- or three-week course of the beta-blocker propranolol after a traumatic event to reduce the likelihood of developing this disorder (Auxemery Y., 2012), which often occurs in the early stages of cancer in response to the psychological trauma of diagnosis. Interestingly, in a study conducted at the University of Munich clinic, it was found that symptoms of impaired attention, memory, and cognitive functions, traditionally associated with the effects of chemotherapy, occur in many patients before this treatment begins as a result of the development of PTSD (Hermelink K. et al., 2015).

All this data confirms my statement that timely pharmaco- and psychotherapy for the acute stress disorder, which results from the diagnosis and treatment of cancer is vital for patients. Such therapy will help prevent the development of PTSD, which complicates the course of the disease and its treatment, as well as damaging the quality of life and survival of the patients. This opinion is shared by other scientists (Baum A., Posluszny D. M., 2001).

Depression caused by an oncological disease often aggravates the course of PTSD and makes it more protracted.

29.2. Deepening of Initial, or the Appearance of Secondary Depression

If the initial subconscious depression, which occurs as a result of unresolved intrapersonal conflicts, can be called primary, then experiences associated with cancer and the fear of relapse lead to the development of an aggravated depressive state, which can be regarded as secondary or reactive. According to authors from various countries, the prevalence of depression among cancer patients can vary from 12.5% to 72% (Wu S. M., Andersen B. L., 2011; Lloyd-Williams M., Friedman T., 2001; Ng C. G., Zainal N. Z., 2015; Massie M. J., 2004).

During advanced stages of cancer, an asthenic-depressive syndrome may develop and then progress to somatized depression. It is characterized by signs of "irritable weakness," vegetative lability, and a hypochondriac mood. When the clinical symptoms of disease progress, these disorders get transferred to their own depressive stage (Gindikin V. Y., 2000).

Earlier, I wrote that depression reduces the activity of the immune system and contributes to the occurrence of cancer. Studies show that patients with cancer of the liver, breast, rectum, and colon, esophagus, stomach, duodenum, gallbladder, and pancreas, who show symptoms of clinical depression, have a reduction in number of immune killer cells, a poorer quality of life, and less survival time than patients without the depressive syndrome (Steel J. L. et al., 2007; Sachs G. et al., 1995; Orsi A. J. et al., 1996; Zhou F. L. et al., 2005).

In particular, in almost all forms of cancer, the life expectancy of depressed patients is halved (Mols F. et al., 2013). In patients with cancer of the urinary bladder, the combination of depression with the shortening of chromosome telomeres in blood lymphocytes (which is a sign of the epigenetic alterations) reduces the survival of patients by three times (Lin J. et al., 2015). Conversely, reducing depressive symptoms in breast cancer patients contributes to their better survival rates (Giese-Davis J. et al., 2011).

Scientists believe that, similarly to PTSD, the risk of depression arising within five years after diagnosis is associated not so much with the disease or treatment itself, as with the personal qualities of patients. Periodically occurring cases of depression before an oncological illness or immediately after diagnosis, external locus of control, more stressful events, resignation to fate, inability to adapt to the cancer diagnosis, helplessness and hopelessness, anxiety about the future, intense feelings about disorders of bodily form and function (especially, in women, about their appearance and sexuality), poorer social support, and reduced work performance (Reich M. et al., 2008; Grassi L. et al., 1997; Stommel M. et al., 2002)—all of these are risk factors for the development of depression, and as we have seen above, these reflect the same personality traits that were the prerequisites for the formation of the precancerous state. Consequently, there is either an absence or insufficient effectiveness of psychotherapeutic and rehabilitation measures after the initial course of treatment. Neither the patient's personality nor their ability to cope with stress has changed. It is natural that this leads to an increase in depression, reduced survival, and relapse of the disease.

Moreover, the deepening of depression increases the risk of suicide among patients who are unable to make sense of their suffering. Between 30% and 50% of patients diagnosed with depression have suicidal readiness and are prone to attempt suicide, and about 15% complete suicide (Morev M. V. et al., 2010; Depression guideline panel, 1993).

Chapter 30

Relapse as a Result of Continuing Distress

I think that by this time the reader is already able to understand why many cancer patients experience a relapse of the disease. In short, the reason for this is that chronic distress in such patients does not only not decrease after treatment, but increases even more strongly. The initial unresolved psychological conflicts and psychic traumas, persisting states of helplessness and hopelessness, oncodominant and avital experiences are combined with distress caused by the diagnosis and treatment, as well as its complications (mostly manifested in psychopathology and disability), changes in social status, fear of the future, often deepened depression, and PTSD.

Although medical intervention eliminates the tumor, the patient's psychological state often remains unchanged, which is what leads them to a regressive defense reaction, without their realizing it themselves. It continues to support the disease, in this way solving some unconscious, deep, personal, or social problems (Pilipenko G. N. et al., 2009).

It is especially important to note that most often, the individual will attempt to return to their "normal life," which actually brought them to the disease, without changing their maladaptive personal qualities, lifestyle, "suffocating" relationships, or dreaded work.

Meanwhile, O. V. Bukhtoyarov and A. E. Arkhangelskiy (2008) note that

the psychogenic component of the oncodominant, which is usually untouched by a somatically oriented treatment, largely determines the fate of the entire oncodominant. As A. A. Ukhtomskiy repeatedly stressed, 'Even one of the elements of a complex of stimuli—an adequate stimulus—is capable of restoring the previous dominant in its cortical and somatic expression.' This means that in the case that the former psychogenic component of the oncodominant is preserved, or if there is an appearance of 'familiar' psycho-traumatic stimuli, a full reproduction of the oncodominant is possible, i.e. recurrence of tumor growth. This likelihood increases significantly if there are tumor cells remaining in the body after surgery.

On this basis, it is understandable why Tom Laughlin (1999) urges us:

Whenever you hear of someone who is being heralded as having 'licked the big "C," as they return to their previous job, profession, or lifestyle, watch out! Unless such people are being suffocated in some other area of their life other than the job, and are taking steps to change that suffocation, it is very likely that they will experience a recurrence.

Let's recall the story of Laughlin's patient Jerry. After a successful surgery to remove a brain tumor (which developed as a result of the inability to do what he loved), his father forced him to work in his company under the supervision of a less qualified employee and under worse conditions than those of that supervisor. "Jerry, who silently detested every minute of every day on this job since he began, took that as a brutal rejection, feeling that no matter what he did, he could never please his father, or live up to his extremely high standards—but until this session, Jerry had never even allowed himself to feel this hurt, let alone the anger he felt toward his father for humiliating him so", shares Laughlin. The result was a relapse of the disease.

The study conducted by Dutch scientists which was cited earlier testifies to the same causes of relapse. They found that the psychological characteristics of women with breast cancer, such as increased rationalization, emotional closedness, and emotional control, determined during the initial diagnosis of the disease, remained virtually unchanged upon re-examination a year and a half later (Bleiker E. M. et al., 1995). Even after leaving the hospital, such patients most often choose unconstructive life strategies and hardly take responsibility for their health. They still seek support mostly in external objects or roles (at work, at home, in the family), concentrate on caring for other family members, rather than on developing their own individuality and life competence. If such external support disappears for various reasons, then the risk of developing a depressive state and deterioration of health increases significantly (Rozhkova O. D., 2015).

As Carl Simonton and co-authors (1978) argue, disease gives a person a temporary right to be more open emotionally. But if they do not learn to maintain the same openness after being cured, then the old rules are followed again, and the individual finds themselves in a situation fraught with psychological and physical destruction, in a position that once led them to the disease. Authors believe that relapse does not mean that the person has been defeated in their fight against the disease, but is an important psychological signal of the body, and it can mean that the patient:

- was unable to cope with the new emotional problems and unconsciously did surrender;

- has not yet learned how to satisfy their emotional needs in ways other than with the help of a disease, so it is important to review the "benefits" of the disease and try to find new ways to help these needs get met;

- may be trying to change too many things in their life at the same time, which can become a source of strong stress. Then a symptom may give a signal to reduce the pace and their demands to themselves;

- has made some important changes, but then relaxed and fell into a state of complacency, finding it difficult to follow the path of change. To keep up with it, they need regular practice and self-discipline;

- by not listening to their emotional needs, they continued in their course of self-destruction, so the body reminds them of the need to pay attention primarily to their own emotional needs and health.

Therefore, as A. Y. Bergfeld (2011) showed, special attention should be paid to the emotional experience of a cancer patient as one of the factors that predict the likelihood of a relapse, and not just to evaluating the extent of changes in their current mental state.

In addition, according to the data scientists from the University of Vermont obtained on patients with cancers in different localizations, many patients not only lack the desire for change, but also actively avoid thoughts and feelings associated with the disease. However, the reluctance to remember, think, talk about the disease and everything connected with it is an ineffective survival strategy. Owing to persistent stress in the subconscious, in such patients, the progression of the disease occurs more often during the first year after the primary therapy. The authors attribute this to both the impaired function of the immune system and late requests for medical care (Epping-Jordan J. E. et al., 1994).

According to research done at the University of Antwerp, the level of chronic stress experienced by patients after breast cancer treatment is a convincing factor in relapse of the disease for three and a half years after surgery (De Brabander B., Gerits P., 1999). Similar results were obtained at Harvard and Copenhagen universities: a decrease in the survival rate of patients with the same diagnosis is associated with a high level of emotional distress, fatigue, and anxiety (Weisman A. D., Worden J. W., 1977; Groenvold M. et al., 2007).

Often, new stressful events in the patient's life become a source of relapse. In particular, such data was presented by N. V. Finagentova (2010), who studied patients with cancer in different localizations. I see the reason for this that most of these patients are in the dark about the role of stress in their illness. They do not take any actions to change the way they react to the difficulties life presents them with and are not trained in new behavioral strategies. In other words, they do not learn their lesson from their first encounter with the disease.

Dr. Don Colbert, author of *Deadly Emotions* (2006), cites the example of a patient from his practice whose wife left him soon after successful cancer therapy:

> Brokenhearted, Charlie was overcome by emotions he could not seem to vent. Less than three months after this experience, his cancer came out of remission with a raging fury, and he died within a year. Charlie's experience was one more vivid example to me of the link between emotion and disease.

Researchers at Guy's Hospital in London determined that severe life events that occurred during a period of about three years after the initial diagnosis (death of a loved one, divorce, etc.) increased the risk of breast cancer recurrence by 5.67 times, and serious life difficulties experienced for at least six months (caring for another patient, an alcoholic child, etc.) increased the recurrence of the disease by 4.75 times (Ramirez A. et al., 1989). According to a professor of oncology, Theodore Miller (1977), the occurrence of relapse in patients who are in long-term remission is associated with severe emotional trauma that occurred six to eighteen months earlier. Other scientists have found that high levels of depression, helplessness, and hopelessness significantly increase the risk of relapse by the fifth year after the initial diagnosis (Watson M. et al., 1999).

One of the biological causes of relapse is the result of previously experienced stress and the continued imbalance of the hypothalamic-pituitary-adrenal system. At three to five years after the initial diagnosis of breast cancer, the baseline cortisol level, which is measured in the saliva of women, remains elevated. However, their adrenal reactivity to additional stress (such as control mammography) is reduced—they produce less cortisol in response to stress than healthy women (Porter L. S. et al., 2003). This once again confirms the fact of exhaustion of stress-regulatory resources under chronic stress associated with cancer. It was also shown that the more the activity of immune killer cells decreased during the seven years after the initial diagnosis, the greater was the likelihood of the disease recurring (Levy S. M. et al., 1991).

According to psychologists in Perm (Russia), women with gynecological oncology who have a relapse of the disease are characterized by a low level of neuropsychic resistance to stressful effects. They have a high risk of maladaptation to stress, and when dealing with it, these patients use ineffective methods that are focused on avoiding problems. These women are characterized by being immersed in their experiences, which results in the appearance of internal tension, anxiety, and confusion (Sirotkina M. Y., Bergfeld A. Y., 2012). On the other hand, patients who do not have a recurrence of the disease after treatment of ovarian cancer for an average of seven years were identified by the following main health factors: reduction of stress, positive attitude to life, medical control, healthy lifestyle, prayers, diet, and physical exercise (Stewart D. E. et al., 2001).

As we can see, the peculiarities of the psyche and behavior of an individual are interrelated with both the causes of cancer and the occurrence of relapse in the future. The negative personality qualities include: a sense of their inability to influence the course of the disease as a whole, difficulty in finding meaning in it, responding to distress with passivity and stoic acceptance, a tendency to helplessness, hopelessness, suppression or non-expression of negative emotions, a type of psychological defense referred to as "denial", staying in a depressed, gloomy-irritable mood, hostility, feeling more isolated from others, low assessment of their communication skills and weak self-confidence, and a narrow repertoire of coping behavior (Tomich P. L., Helgeson V. S., 2006; Weisman A.

D., Worden J. W., 1977; Pettingale K. et al., 1985; Jensen M. R., 1987; Levy S. M. et al., 1988; Finagentova N. V., 2010).

M. F. De Boer and his colleagues (1998) investigated the psychosocial factors for the recurrence of head and neck tumors. They found three significant aspects in patients before the start of primary medical treatment:

a) a low level of physical activity,

b) substantial loss of autonomy (for example, "I am not or am only partly able to work or keep house," or "I become more dependent on others"),

c) fewer complaints that patients allowed themselves to voice (for example, "During the past three days I have suffered from worrying and from feeling tense."), i.e. low level of emotional openness.

Similar results were obtained in studies on patients with melanoma: a relapse of the disease was characteristic of those who did not adapt to the disease and treatment, refusing to recognize (or displacing the significance of) the effects of the disease on their lives (Rogentine N. G. et al., 1979), avoided thoughts and feelings associated with the disease, did not perceive their treatment as complete healing, paid less attention to their problems and more to their families (*preference for the interests of others—V. M.*) (Brown J. E. et al., 2000), had a greater level of anxiety and depression (Bergenmar M. et al., 2004).

Lama Zopa Rinpoche (2001) provides an example of one of his students who had a relapse of the disease:

> She told me that it happened because her life had become very messy and out of control. For a long time she had maintained discipline in her spiritual practice, but at that time she had stopped doing the practices, and her life had become very confused. Alice's experience shows that healing the mind is much more important than healing the body. Her cancer returned because she stopped doing her practices and stopped disciplining her mind; she did not protect her mind by practicing the meditations. Disciplining your life means disciplining your mind.

The history of previous stresses also contributes to the relapse of the disease: even one, and certainly several traumatic events, as well as less severe stressful events that do not meet the criteria of psychic trauma, that occurred before the onset of the primary disease, halved the remission period for breast cancer patients (Palesh O. et al., 2007).

At the same time, some scientists did not confirm the connection between the experienced stress or psychological peculiarities of a person and cancer recurrence (Graham J. E. et al., 2002; Saito-Nakaya K. et al., 2012; Cassileth B. R. et al., 1988). The reasons for this discrepancy are discussed in Chapters 9 and 12.

In my opinion, the correctness of the research that found such a relationship is confirmed by the results of psychosocial programs demonstrating that psychotherapy and the reduction of stress decrease the frequency of cancer recurrence. The need for such an approach was pointed out by Professor Theodore Miller in 1977: "Once the existing tumor has been treated, much more attention should be paid to the psycho-dynamic aspects to aid in the prevention of recurrence."

Psychiatrist F. I. Fawzy and his colleagues from the University of California at Los Angeles (1990, 1993) studied sixty-eight patients who had undergone surgery to remove a malignant melanoma. Half of these patients participated in the six-week group therapy program which included psychotherapy, group support, an explanation of the mechanisms of the onset of melanoma, and training in coping with stress (relaxation, etc.). At the end of the program, a lower level of stress was found in these patients, and six months later they had lower rates of depression, fatigue, and mood disorders, and increased immunity compared with those who did not attend group classes. After six years, the group that completed the additional program still maintained a lower level of basic distress and was able to cope with stress better. Relapse occurred in seven of them and three out of the thirty-four people died, whereas in the control group, relapse occurred in thirteen people and ten out of the thirty-four died.

For eleven years, 227 women suffering from breast cancer with metastases in the lymph nodes of the second and third stages have been monitored at the Oncology Center of the University of Ohio, under the guidance of psychology professor Barbara Andersen and her team (2008). All of them received standard cancer therapy, after which a part of the group participated in a one-year program for the formation of a new lifestyle, similar to that described above. As a result, those women who took part in the program had a significantly reduced frequency of relapses and mortality compared with other patients. Over the course of further research, it was found that being in a group program led to a steady improvement in immunity, and this is effected by an increase in the level of NK cells.

At least three studies of large groups of women who took beta-blockers for the treatment of hypertension for a long time, including during the period of illness and treatment of breast cancer, found a significantly lower incidence of disease recurrence (Powe D. G. et al., 2010; Melhem-Bertrandt A. et al., 2011; Ganz P. A. et al., 2011), which confirms the role of the stress hormones catecholamines in the relapse phenomenon.

Although the possibility of reducing the likelihood of recurrence with the help of beta-blockers looks attractive to patients, we should not forget that this drug has its own complications and side effects. And since the same effect can be achieved by learning to regulate one's reactions to stress, in this situation, patients have a choice: they can rely on medications for the rest of their lives or they have the option to start changing themselves. In my opinion, the use of beta-blockers is justified during the period of diagnosis and therapy, when the patient is demoralized and in a state of acute distress, but in the long term it is necessary for patients to rely more and more on their own resources.

The reappearance of the same type of cancer or the emergence of a new one for some patients becomes an even more stressful event than the first manifestation of the disease and often leads to PTSD. Other patients experience less distress, which probably indicates that they have acquired the skill of overcoming difficulties (Green B. L. et al., 1998; Cella D. et al., 1990; Andersen B. L. et al., 2005). Depression, anxiety, and a fear for life, loss of hope for a cure, complications associated with disability often appear or deepen (Andersen B. L. et al., 2005). In many patients, relapse is accompanied by a deepening of an existential crisis and requires courage in the further struggle for life. According to M. M. Rawnsley (1994), this period can become a "crisis of courage." For the psychological adaptation of patients at this time, they must accept responsibility for their lives and health, especially if they have not learned this before (Pestereva E. V., 2011).

The need for serious psychotherapeutic care in relapse, good social support, and the active actions of patients to change their psychological attitudes are beyond doubt.

Chapter 31

Post–Traumatic Growth as a Source of Remission

> If a significant part of the cause of cancer
> is trying to be who we are not,
> then healing cancer involves opening to who we are.
> Carl Simonton,
> *The Healing Journey*

Although we have seen that many cancer patients develop post-traumatic stress disorder due to the psychic trauma caused by the disease and the fear of death, there is also a significant amount of evidence suggesting that such a trauma and the crisis associated with it can provide an impetus for personal, social, and spiritual transformation (Sumalla E. C. et al., 2009; Shand L. K. et al., 2015; Jayawickreme E., Blackie L. E., 2016).

According to S. S. Uchadze (2008), the psychospiritual crisis can be defined as a special moment of human existence when two opposing tendencies are present at the same time—the destruction of the old, obsolete, and interfering, and the creation of the new, holistic, and harmonious—whether it is the death and revival of the cellular structures or a radical change in worldviews.

In various philosophical and religious systems, historical and literary works, there are ideas and observations suggesting that suffering can be beneficial for the individual. Vissarion Belinsky, a well-known Russian philosopher and writer of the nineteenth century, said: "Those, who do not know suffering, do not know bliss either" (quoted in Korolkov A. V., 2005). In his book *Creative Malady*, George Pickering (1974), an English physician and writer, describes the central role that the disease played in the fate of a number of prominent people—Charles Darwin, Sigmund Freud, Marcel Proust, and others. The suffering caused by the disease awakened a brilliant vital force in each of them.

Ivan Ilyin (2006), another Russian philosopher, writes:

Suffering testifies to a discrepancy, a discord between a suffering person and divinely created nature: it expresses this individual's falling away from nature, signifying the beginning of their return and healing. Suffering is the mysterious self-healing of man, his body and soul: it is he himself who is fighting for the renewal of the inner order and the harmony of his life, he is working on his transformation, he is looking for a 'return'.

According to the observations of modern transpersonal psychologists, more than a third of people who survived an unexpected encounter with death experienced a deep and unique spiritual revelation. C. and S. Grof (1989) argue that a critical illness, like cancer, can be seen as a "spiritual crisis" or a crisis of change, a radical personal transformation, and spiritual awakening. Such a crisis can lead to emotional and psychological healing and the evolution of consciousness.

31.1. Cancer as a Life "Reset Button"

A terrifying symptom is usually
your greatest dream trying to come true.
Arnold Mindell,
Working With the Dream Body

For an ordinary person, the idea that cancer can mean something positive and bring about anything other than pain, suffering, and death seems blasphemous. However, for many cancer patients, having an awareness of the meaning of the appearance of cancer made it possible for them to revise, or even discover for the first time, the meaning of their life. This is accompanied by personal and spiritual development known as post-traumatic growth (PTG). It is characterized by changes in the patient's life perspective in three main aspects: self-perception, relationships with other people, and life philosophy, or worldview (Tedeschi R. G., Calhoun L. G., 1995).

Post-traumatic growth does not mean that the person returns to their former way of life. Instead, they acquire a new one—the disease turns out to be a springboard for deep self-improvement. Various changes can occur: the emergence of new meanings, an increase in optimism and endurance, an awareness of the value of life, a transformation of life priorities, a feeling of increasing one's own strength, improving interpersonal relationships, and an increase in the spiritual and existential components of life (Tedeschi R. G., Calhoun L. G., 2004). Irvin Yalom (1980) wrote that death is an event of such immense importance that, with the right attitude, an encounter with it can lead to a change in one's life perspective and provide an incentive for the authentic immersion into life.

Over the course of an illness, a person can understand that the trials and sufferings they experience are not only negative, but also positive. They allow the individual to rise above their former, limited level of world perception, to sort out their problems, and to change their life for the better. The ongoing spontaneous self-actualization and spiritual revelation lead to the awakening and liberation of the Essence. As a rule, this is accompanied by a marked improvement in health. According to Lawrence LeShan (1989), the freedom and joy that are brought by self-realization become a powerful medicine that may inhibit or even reverse the cancer.

Alexander Solzhenitsyn, a famous Russian writer, said that in the days when he was dying of cancer, he was able to get to know himself, to know the laws of the universe. And then a miracle happened: the disease receded. The writer saw God's Providence in this: he was given a respite so that he could tell about the sufferings of the Russian people after 1917 on behalf of all the victims. This insight is embodied in his literary masterpieces (Danilenko L. V., 2008).

Psychologists at the University of Kentucky found that just 52% of patients who had breast cancer named their experience as traumatic only. Many others patients reported that post-traumatic stress disorder was accompanied by simultaneous intensive processes of post-traumatic growth (Cordova M. J. et al., 2007). Korean psychologists came to a similar conclusion, when they found PTG among 53.3% of patients who had stomach cancer (Sim B. Y. et al., 2015). After analyzing twenty-four scientific papers published between 1990 and 2010, Greek researchers concluded that the number of breast cancer patients who reached PTG was significantly higher than the number of patients with post-traumatic stress (Koutrouli N. et al., 2012). Having reviewed eighty-eight articles from 1985 to 2014, Australian scientists noted that PTSD often develops during the initial stage of the disease, while PTG tends to occur during the treatment process (Parikh D. et al., 2015).

Fifty-nine percent of patients with a similarly heavy AIDS illness told about significant changes that occurred in their lives after they were diagnosed with the disease. Their religiosity, self-control, and attention to their health increased, as well as their sense of community and involvement with other people. They have formed or strengthened the belief in life after death, developed focusing on the value of life "here and now" and the desire to perform altruistic actions (Milam J. E., 2004). Fifty-two percent of patients who are in remission for five or more years after being treated for malignant melanoma realized the cause of their disease, revised their outlook on life, and took responsibility for overcoming the disease (Dirksen S. R., 1995). An even greater proportion, 75%, was detected among patients who had ovarian cancer, representing those who found the disease had a positive effect on their lives (Kornblith A. B. et al., 2010).

According to the observations of C. O. Simonton and associates (1978), some patients experienced a feeling that they became "more than just healthy" as a result of treatment. Cancer gave them the opportunity to break those limiting social norms in which they were brought up and begin to develop and grow as a person. The disease taught them to express their feelings, to openly and explicitly state their needs. Otherwise, they would continue to lead a quiet life, "full of unspoken despair."

V. A. Sotnikov (2014) noted that it was the disease that made women with gynecological cancers ask themselves the question of the meaning of life, stimulated the reassessment of life values and priorities, and led to religious faith. There was a decrease in the desire for material well-being and demonstration of financial success, while the turn to spiritual values became the main direction. Many "survivors" patients believe that only the disease gave them the opportunity to understand how valuable life is, and therefore they stopped "worrying in vain." As one breast cancer patient in prolonged remission said to researchers, the Lord gave her the strength to endure cancer not in order to kill her, but to open her eyes (Allen D. J. et al., 2009).

I often observe a similar experience in my patients. For example, the following is the immense comprehension that was experienced by my patient S. during our seventh therapy session, after we had worked on her main conflicts in previous sessions:

I felt the Highest Divine Presence and turned to Him with the question of why I am here and why I suffer from illness. And at that very moment I realized that I had an answer to these questions from the very beginning—I felt that my life was stuck, that it was not going anywhere, but I did not want to admit it. However, the main answer I received told me to not worry about the future, that I was on my way, and that the main thing that matters now is to learn to keep my awareness inside me. I also experienced contact with an unusually white light, and was told that it is my Essence. It was like a light outside the light ... Extraterrestrial light! I still feel it now, but not that strong. I now have a feeling of greater presence in myself, a feeling that there is more space inside me. I also clearly see that everything that occurs during journeys (*sessions of transpersonal psychotherapy—V. M.*) can be transformed into something useful in everyday life.

That is why a certain number of cancer patients who have reached remission are grateful for the disease—otherwise they would not have changed, and their whole life would have passed in a "daze," inspired by a false personality. Reid Henson writes: "Most people find it shocking when I say that I now see cancer as a blessing because it was the key stimulus that moved me closer to God. I see cancer, as well as all other adversity in my life, as a precious gift from God helping me to better understand my role in life in relation to Him" (Simonton O. C., Henson R., 1992). Psycho-oncologist Tom Laughlin believes that there is a covert meaning hidden in cancer, a secret message that can reveal to the patient, and those they love, the sense of life—but only if it happens to be correctly interpreted (Laughlin T., 1999).

Here is how Lance Armstrong (2000, with S. Jenkins) assessed the role of his illness:

> The truth is that cancer was the best thing that ever happened to me. I don't know why I got the illness, but it did wonders for me, and I wouldn't want to walk away from it. Why would I want to change, even for a day, the most important and shaping event in my life? …So if there is a purpose to the suffering that is cancer, I think it must be this: it's meant to improve us. I am very firm in my belief that cancer is not a form of death. I choose to redefine it: it is a part of life.

"Although cancer often kills, it can also be the beginning of a new life," argues Lawrence LeShan. The search for one's own being, the discovery of the life that a person really needs to live, can be the strongest weapon against illness. That is why the psycho-oncologist titled his bestseller *Cancer as a turning point*. LeShan asserts that pain and suffering are "the divine reset button," since serious suffering sometimes becomes the only thing that can awaken a person, make them understand who they are, and stimulate deep changes (LeShan L., 1989). Prior to this, most people lack the motivation to truly get to know themselves. However, the emergence of a new meaning requires the destruction of the old; for growth to start, stagnation must first occur. As the Grofs (1989) emphasize, the crisis should be understood correctly and treated as a difficult stage in the natural development process. Then it is possible to achieve a spontaneous healing from various emotional and psychosomatic disorders, secure favorable personality changes, and resolve important life problems. This is the evolutionary movement toward what is called higher consciousness.

Caryle Hirshberg and Mark Ian Barasch (1995) noted that among the people who had a spontaneous remission of cancer, some had a certain quality that they called "congruence": an ability to discover a way to be deeply true to themselves in the midst of crisis and manifest a set of behaviors growing from the roots of their being.

> [Cancer] changed my life in an extraordinary way. The unparalleled stares I receive, the exceptional strength and confidence that I have and the moment I take each day to recognize the beauty in my blemish, together have all made me who I am today,

concluded Leslie Lambert (2014), who recovered from a medulloepithelioma, a rare form of eye cancer.

A keen sense of mortality can be paralyzing, but it can also be an important catalyst for change, asserts psycho-oncologist Linda Carlson from the University of Calgary and psychoneuroendocrinologist Michael Speca from the Tom Baker Cancer Center (2011). According to their observations, the diagnosis of cancer can be a springboard for self-inquiry, personal discovery, and growth for a person. It provides a valuable opportunity to start living differently, consciously, more richly and naturally than before. A cancer diagnosis is the most sobering wake-up call that can be heard during a life crisis. "We have seen many people who have used the turning point that cancer provides (time off work, willingness to try new things, appreciation for the preciousness of every moment) as a chance to learn how to be more present at each moment of their lives," scientists write.

Psychologists at the University of Nijmegen in the Netherlands studied what happens to cancer patients as a result of passing through an existential crisis caused by the disease. If patients could abandon their long-cultivated image of "I," they would undergo significant changes in their perception of themselves and others. The most important of these changes was the acceptance of oneself ("Now I allow myself to be what I am," said one patient). This acceptance of oneself includes the acceptance of one's emotions and experiences, especially the negative ones, and this was of great importance in strengthening patients' self-esteem. Now they wanted to make their own decisions, to choose the direction of their life. Shifts in self-perception also caused important changes in the relationships the patients had with other people—their emotional dependence on others diminished significantly. This transformation allowed patients to reach a new level of awareness of themselves and the universe, which led to radical changes in their views on life and death. The shifts were not limited to a certain segment of life or a specific aspect of awareness of their identity, but permeated all aspects of self-perception. This allowed scientists to call these changes "fundamental" (Yang W. et al., 2012).

Post-traumatic growth occurs even in children. Although "even" is not very appropriate in this case, since the Essence is not yet so suppressed by the false personality in children, and the transformation process can take place more easily and faster. Upon interviewing 784 young people about thirty years of age who had cancer in their teens, researchers from the University of Ulm (Germany) found that 94.3% of them encountered at least one very important positive consequence as a result of their illness (Gunst D. C. et al., 2016). When interviewing adults who had suffered from cancer before twenty years of age, American psychologists revealed the following positive effects of the disease: personal strength (psychological confidence and emotional maturity), improved relationships with other people (family intimacy, empathy for others), the emergence of new possibilities (having a passion to contend with cancer), appreciation for life (new priorities), and spiritual development (strengthened spiritual beliefs, participating in religious rituals and activities) (Zamora E. R. et al., 2017).

Take, for example, Anya's story from Renata Ravitch's (2013) book, *The Hymn of Life. Life stories of children who conquered cancer.* Anya shares:

> Six years after the end of the treatment I realized that although my illness was both an unpleasant and painful experience, it led me to a wonderful moment in my life: to the feeling of benefit and meaningfulness of my life. There were (*in the rehabilitation center—V. M.*) Irish children, and when they were interviewed, they said almost the same thing that I understood myself: they felt that their illness was 'correct', that it helped put everything into its place, gave them strength for the

future. I remember that before the illness I was in a stressful situation, I wanted to be like everyone else but I did not succeed. Now, I am glad that I went through this test, through this disease, through cancer, through the understanding that I am me, and everything fell into its proper place.

One of my first cancer patients, Anna Z., said during the psychotherapy process: "Now I realized the gift and lesson that cancer brought to my life."

Thus, although losing the meaning of life sometimes leads to cancer, passing through this disease can be a way to find that meaning. Holger Kalweit (1999), a clinical psychologist and anthropologist, says that those who were able to understand illness and suffering as processes of physical and mental transformation achieved a deeper and less biased look at psychosomatic and psychospiritual processes and would begin to realize the diversity of possibilities that is contained in suffering and the death of the ego. For them, disease becomes a cleansing process that washes away everything that was bad, miserable, and weak, it floods one like a fierce river and clears one of all that is dull and limited. In this way the disease becomes the gateway to life.

Kalweit is supported by the psychiatrist R. D. Laing (1999):

> True sanity entails in one way or another the dissolution of the normal ego, that false self competently adjusted to our alienated social reality: the emergence of the "inner" archetypal mediators of divine power, and through this death a rebirth, and the eventual reestablishment of a new kind of ego-functioning, the ego now being the servant of the Divine, no longer its betrayer.

Many cancer patients of Stanislav Grof have passed through such a death of the ego and the subsequent transpersonal experiences of rebirth and cosmic unity during psychedelic therapy. This often led to radical and lasting changes in their fundamental views on human nature and relationships with the world. There were striking changes in the hierarchy of their life values—an understanding of the absurdity and futility of exorbitant ambitions, of attachment to money, social standing, fame, power, or the race for transient values. The experiences of emotional and psychodynamic discomfort were significantly reduced (in particular, the traumatic events of childhood were recalled and therapeutically processed). Depression, anxiety, tension, and feelings of guilt declined, while self-perception and self-esteem increased significantly. Patients had new spiritual feelings of a cosmic or pantheistic nature, developed a great interest in philosophy, religion, and mysticism. According to the patients who experienced death and rebirth during the sessions, they began to feel cleansed and reborn. Their inner life was filled with deep clarity and joy, a feeling of physical health and good physiological functioning appeared (Grof S., Halifax J., 1978).

Such changes are reminiscent of ancient legends, which talk about the rebirth after burning in the fire of death. After all, every cancer patient who reached post-traumatic growth and was healed can be truly called a phoenix! In the mythology of various ancient and modern cultures, stories can be found telling about heroes who, after visiting the world of the dead and having endured hardships, came back and acquired new abilities (Grof S., Halifax J., 1978). This is told, for example, in the ancient Babylonian and Assyrian tales of Tammuz and Ishtar, in the legend of the Thracian singer Orpheus, who descended into the darkness of the underworld in search of his beloved Eurydice, in the Dionysian legends of Bacchus, killed by the Titans and resurrected by Afina Pallada, Scandinavian tales of the resurrected Baldr, son of the god Odin, Inanna in the Sumerian legend who returned from Underworld, and, of course, the life of Jesus Christ.

K. V. Yatskevich (2007) writes that the self-transformation that is necessary for cancer patients is to some extent similar to death and the crucifixion of Christ, but this is the crucifixion of oneself. And only after passing through the symbolic death of the former system of thinking and attitude to life, "having been on the cross of the crucifix, can one feel the resurrection, renewing and inspiring Power of higher Love." The possibility of such a transformation, or "rebirth," as a stage on the inner path of a person, was expressed by the Russian philosopher Valerian Muravyev (1992) back in 1922:

This state can be called the second birth, just as the previous state of complete despair and death can be considered to be a passage through death ... Resurrection consists of degrees: the more we revive, the more we live. But, you can die in one life aspect and rise again in another. This is the secret of 'if you don't die, you will not rise.' Death is thus associated with resurrection.

The Soviet singer Aida Vedischeva, who defeated cancer, had a similar experience (Rak, 2014):

... such a resurrection is a real miracle: [I] died and was resurrected! And resurrected not only in the direct, but also in the spiritual sense. ... But if I dare relax, the misfortune will come back. Many of my former comrades in disease, who did not want to understand that it was necessary to change in everything, had already died down.

In this regard, Carl Simonton emphasizes that healing from cancer requires significant and long-term efforts to change. In the deepest sense, it implies the healing of one's life, and this is not something that one can do overnight. Simonton found that patients who explore their core beliefs and consider, again and again, such issues as the purpose of their life and their ideas about God, often experience profound changes leading to a new physical, mental, and spiritual balance that promotes health (Simonton C. O., Henson R., 1992).

31.2. Post–Traumatic Stress or Post–Traumatic Growth?

But why do some cancer patients experience personal growth, while others do not or even more, become prone to post-traumatic stress disorder and a greater loss of the meaning of life? Probably, it is a degree of the manifestation of all factors considered in previous chapters that define an outcome. Among them, the most important role is played by a mental resistance to stress, embedded in a person by their parents, as well as the peculiarities of the psychosomatic personality, formed as a result of violations of children's attachment. This is confirmed by the data obtained stating that cancer patients with safe attachment can better cope with the stress of the disease and more often experience post-traumatic growth (Hamama-Raz Y., Solomon Z., 2006; Schmidt S. D. et al., 2012). On the other hand, people with the avoiding coping style more often suffer from PTSD, in contrast to those who are able to feel happiness, to be realistic, and acknowledge the need for social support—such individuals are more likely to have PTG (Kamali M. et al., 2015). Basic beliefs are also important: people who have negative ideas about their own "I" and are convinced of the hostility of the external world suffer much more from symptoms of distress than those whose picture of the world and their own "I" are more positive (Padun M. A., Zagryazhskaya E. A., 2006).

According to O. A. Vorona (2005), the individual response of cancer patients to stress is not so much due to the effectiveness of treatment (all patients in the author's study completed the treatment successfully), but rather to the cognitive-personal characteristics of patients, their basic beliefs and ideas; it is these that determine success in overcoming the trauma of disease. Patients who failed to integrate the traumatic experience and reprocess negative beliefs formed as a result of exposure to stress pass into the stage of chronic distress with aggravation of the negative psychological consequences of the disease. This, as we saw in the previous chapter, is fraught with the relapse of the disease.

The mode of response to the stress currently experienced is also significantly influenced by previous life stresses or mental trauma (McKenna M. C. et al., 1999). For example, the higher the number of traumatic situations experienced by breast cancer patients throughout their lives, and the more significant they assessed their impact to be, the more pronounced became the psychopathological symptoms of post-traumatic stress in response to the disease (Tarabrina N. V., 2014). In other studies of patients with the same diagnosis, it was found that a higher incidence of PTSD is associated with stronger previous psycho-traumatic experience, less social support, and a shorter period since the end of medical treatment (Andrykowski M. A., Cordova M. J., 1998), as well as with less confidence of women in their strength and abilities to cope with difficult situations (Koopman C. et al., 2002).

Annick Shaw and his colleagues from the University of Warwick, UK (2005) analyzed eleven scientific papers that determined a connection between religion, spirituality, and post-traumatic growth. According to these studies, as a rule, religion and spirituality are useful for people in dealing with the effects of psychic trauma. On the other hand, the traumatic experiences themselves can lead to a deepening of religious consciousness or spirituality. In addition, spirituality as a way to overcome psychic trauma, openness, willingness to consider existential issues, and inner religiosity are usually associated with post-traumatic growth.

However, it is especially important, according to the psychotherapist Ruediger Dahlke (1999), that any crisis can be consciously accepted or, conversely, ignored and fought off. In accordance with this, a crisis will be either a danger or a chance for an individual, which will determine the picture of the disease. Taking a disease as a message, a person turns it into a chance. Fighting a disease, he acquires a dangerous enemy.

A similar view is expressed by psychologists from the Institute of Oncology in St. Petersburg (Russia), who revealed two basic ways for patients to experience a situation of disease. Some patients evaluate it as extreme, highly difficult, and tragic. They believe that they need to "endure it until something changes," strain all internal forces in order to "keep this life," although with an unknown result. At the same time, they are trying to live in the same way as before, to hold on to the "old," in spite of the changed life situation. This leads to an increase in tension, which people cannot always withstand. As a result, a "breakdown," disadaptation, fixation on painful experiences, depression, and even suicide ensue.

Other patients perceive their cancer as a crisis. Although they also feel the complexity and tragedy of the situation, their mental state is concentrated on the feeling of the "turning point" of the moment, on the difficult realization that they can no longer live as they had before, and they cannot be who they were before the illness. These thoughts force patients to reconsider their ideas about themselves, to acutely recognize their own "I," to think about the course of their lives and understand that they are the ones that play the main role in it, and the situation will change only when they themselves can change. Patients begin the search for a new vision and ways to establish their reincarnated "I," which requires a painful parting with the old life, a courageous opening of themselves to a new life, and accepting it as it is (Chulkova A., Moiseenko M., 2009).

While studying the methods of overcoming critical life situations employed by patients with different diseases (including cancer), A. A. Bakanova (2000) similarly discovered two main methods that depend on the attitude of the individual to the crisis: they experience a critical situation either as an opportunity for spiritual growth or as endless suffering. In the first variation, a person is aware of the possibility of a deeper, authentic being, which is accompanied by the acceptance of fate, a sense of ontological security and meaningfulness of life, responsibility, striving for inner growth, acceptance of the spiritual and physical aspects of one's personality, tolerance for the variability of life, acceptance of one's feelings in relation to death, and faith in the immortality of the soul. In the second case, the critical situation is experienced as punishment or redemption and manifests in the form of a concentration of a person on their sufferings— illness, old age, fear, evil, helplessness, and loneliness, which results from the notion of death as an absolute end and, accordingly, causes fear of it.

According to Vladislav Sotnikov, the choice of a specific type of patient response to a situation of cancer is associated with those sense-bearing formations that are embedded in the foundation of their personality. When only basic life meanings and values serve as this foundation, a collision with a fatal disease can lead to a mismatch of sense between being and reality. This is accompanied by a feeling of deadlock and tension, the destruction of the individual's usual activities, beliefs, and attitudes. A person finds themselves in a situation of impossibility to realize their needs, so as a result an identity crisis develops (Sotnikov V. A., 2014). Such a situation may contribute to a shift toward PTSD.

Upon comparing two groups of women suffering from breast cancer, one with post-traumatic stress and one without it, N. V. Tarabrina (2014) determined that patients without signs of PTSD have a significantly higher level of education. They, as a rule, work or are involved in some significant field of activity, which allows them to switch from thoughts about the disease and have a noticeably more positive image of their own "I." In contrast, patients with advanced PTSD have high levels of hostility, anxiety, depression, and other psychopathological manifestations. They have a negative image of their "I," a belief in their own failure and inability to control the events happening to them. They consider the world and the people around them as unfriendly, dangerous, and unworthy of trust, and over the course of their lives a chain of accumulating stressful events can be traced prior to the disease.

The author of the study concluded that a lower level of intellectual development is very important in the appearance of PTSD in these cancer patients. Education, possession of professional skills in any field of activity helps to find meaning in what is happening and has a positive effect on the personal resources for successfully overcoming the traumatic stress of the disease (Tarabrina N. V., 2014). A low level of intellectual development as a predisposing factor for PTSD has been confirmed by other scientists (Van der Kolk B. A., 1987). On the other hand, N. Koutrouli and his colleagues (2012) found that education, economic status, age, subjective assessment of the threat of disease, medical treatment, support of relatives and friends, as well as possession of positive coping strategies, are the main factors leading to PTG in patients with the same diagnosis.

It should be realized that the currently dominant bio-pharmacological model of medicine plays an important role in inhibiting the development of PTG in cancer patients. By focusing all its activities on suppressing the symptoms of diseases, orthodox medicine actually programs people to only believe in this possibility of treatment, to depend on physicians, and not to rely on their own capabilities. I fully agree with my colleague, psychotherapist Vyacheslav Gusev (2014):

> What medicine can do thanks to many of its interventions allows us to not learn anything. Medicine provides us with numerous cheatsheets. It makes it possible to expand the bronchi instead of [feeling] the real anger, to expand the vessels of the heart instead of experiencing sadness, to excite and stimulate instead of genuine adherence to one's interests, etc. Now that person has become a puppet! ... I have a sad aphorism on this topic: modern medicine inhibits the development of mankind.

Indeed, how can a person think that the appearance of pain in the body is a sign of trouble in their psychological state, if they are convinced from childhood that pain is an enemy that needs to be fought with an analgesic?

In the above observations we can see a clear parallel with the previously discussed topic of psychological infantilism, dependence, self-centeredness, and existential vacuum in many cancer patients. In all likelihood, the more pronounced these personality traits are, the higher the probability of experiencing the disease as a life crash, with the subsequent development of PTSD. Also, the chances for the emergence of post-traumatic growth are reduced owing to the intensity of the experienced stress, low levels of general development and spirituality, as well as a high dependence on the material side of life. Such patients, as opposed to "self-seeking" patients, during the course of the disease may even more rapidly lose the meaning of life. The threat of death leads them into a state of demoralization and despair (Kissane D. W. et al., 2001). As death approaches, existential themes become particularly relevant for such materialistic patients (Greisinger A. J. et al., 1997).

At the same time, even those people who have reached the end of their lives are able to achieve post-traumatic growth. Irvin Yalom (1980) notes the amazing shifts occurring with end-stage cancer patients. For them, the significance of life's relative trivialities decreases, the experience of life in the present sharpens, deeper contact is established with loved ones, a feeling of liberation and other positive changes arise. This transformation is indeed the personal growth. Viktor Frankl (1984) explains this in that when a person is faced with a hopeless and inevitable situation, meets a fate that cannot be changed (as happens during an incurable disease or a natural disaster), this gives them a chance to actualize the highest values and to realize the deepest meaning—the meaning of suffering.

And if a person even fails to heal the body, the attainment and liberation of their Essence, their true nature, can become an event that is more significant than physical recovery. There is a wonderful example given in a book by the remarkable psychologist Stephen Levine (1989), who developed a program of harmonious dying for terminal patients. He writes about two people of about the same age and cultural level who got the same disease. One of them was fighting against the disease, resisted it, and saw disease as something unnatural and himself as a victim. He became tense and scared, was clinging to life with all his might. When he had some relief from his symptoms, he felt cheerful and wonderful, but when the disease activated again he became discouraged and upset, his opinion of himself worsened, and then the aggression that was hidden inside him turned into self-loathing and guilt. In this way, his self-esteem depended on whether he could help himself.

Another patient considered the illness as a message to understand and work with, an opportunity to regain his harmony and balance the heart and mind. He sought to improve the quality of his life and change what seemed to be erratic, not just clinging to prolonging life by any means but plunging into the inner wealth that gives him the meaning of life.

When the first man felt that he could not be cured, he decided that everything was lost. The second one, instead, had a place both for life and for death, so he explored his life, and did not resist it. He was open to healing, but accepted that conscious death could also make sense. This made his life deeper, filled it up with a new understanding, and this living truth could be felt in communication with him. He did not fight or curse the disease but investigated the questions, "What is a disease?" and "Who is sick?" As a result, this patient came to the conclusion that spiritual healing does not exclude the possibility of death.

31.3. Post–Traumatic Growth Leads to Comprehending the Meaning of Life and Improving Health

> Life will give you whatever experience is most helpful
> for the evolution of your consciousness.
> How do you know this is the experience you need?
> Because this is the experience you are having at the moment.
> Eckhart Tolle,
> *A New Earth: Awakening to Your Life's Purpose*

Upon getting rid of the false "I," a person transforms their personality and allows it to grow, thereby reviving their authentic Essence, and this is extremely important for gaining physical and mental health.

The possibility of such changes was shown by N. V. Finagentova (2010) when studying in her dissertation the psychological resources of cancer patients in the prevention of disease recurrence. She demonstrated that the desire for self-improvement as opposed to the motivation to achieve material well-being, as well as the ability to take responsibility and desire to do good things, are directly related to the degree of life satisfaction and mental health of a person. The aspiration for spiritual development, developed skills in managing emotions, resistance to stressful and uncertain situations, a high level of self-acceptance and self-confidence can be identified as the main factors contributing to the best quality adaptation to the situation of disease for all patients examined.

S. A. Moskvitina (2012) observed the transformations that occurred with patients who had breast cancer. The researcher has determined that in the minds of these women the profound changes and re-estimation of values occur, which significantly distinguish them from healthy women who have never encountered a serious illness. If healthy women are more characterized by an orientation to material values, such as a "secure life," "entertainment," and to a lesser extent, altruistic impulses ("to do something for the sake of others"), then for women who have had cancer, spiritual values come in first place: "productive life," "active life," "development," "self-confidence," "love," "the presence of true friends." Interestingly enough, in the process of therapy the desire for spiritual development in patients significantly increased compared with how it was the time of admission to treatment.

I would not like the reader to get the wrong idea, on the basis of the data shared above, that material welfare is not significant. Of course, there is nothing bad in material well-being; when it is in the list of other values, it contributes to the satisfaction of our needs and brings comfort to our lives. However, when money-grubbing completely absorbs a person's mind and becomes the dominant of their life goal, suppressing other needs and talents, then the result can be a protest of Essence and the development of an existential crisis, which leads to various diseases. That is why a change in the value system is so necessary to achieve healing.

According to N. A. Rusina (2012), the actualization of the process of "meaning-building," i.e. the discovery of new life meanings, turns out to be an effective coping resource for cancer patients, significantly contributing to the improvement of their adaptation to the disease and increasing the quality of their life.

Several research teams independently monitored the mental state of women with breast and ovarian cancer and arrived at a similar conclusion (Vickberg S. M. et al., 2000, MacKinnon D. P. et al., 2002; Gall T. L., Cornblat M. W., 2002; Meraviglia M., 2006; Ferrell B. R. et al., 2003). The presence of a meaning of life, especially spiritual meaning, reduces the number of obsessive, restless thoughts about the disease, diminish distress, and significantly improves the psychological well-being of patients. At the biochemical level, this was reflected in a decreased content of the stress hormone cortisol in the blood (Cruess D. G. et al., 2000). It is self-actualization, the comprehension of the meaning of one's life, according to Iranian psycho-oncologists, that underlies the PTG in cancer patients (Fazel M. et al., 2016).

Dr. Bernie Siegel (1989), based on his own clinical experience, writes that a disease often reveals the spiritual reality hidden before the disease. One of his "exceptional patients" said that the disease was given to her as a challenge and a gift. It prompted her to study the thoughts, desires, and beliefs hidden in the very depths of her consciousness, allowing her to experience what the unity of spirit and flesh is and thus rebuild her life. As result, the destructive process in her body ceased and the process opposite to the chaos that the disease caused, began.

More than five hundred cancer patients were examined at universities in South Florida and Ohio to determine the effect of their psychological state on the course of the disease. It has been found that the existence of a life meaning is the most important factor that decreases the severity of distress resulting from impaired physical and social activity of patients (Jim H. S., Andersen B. L, 2007). According to an analysis of forty-three studies conducted in fourteen countries, cancer patients of various profiles who have attained higher psycho-spiritual well-being (self-awareness, effective coping with stress, feelings of faith, increased opportunities and self-confidence, living with meaning and hope, favorable relations with other people), are able to more effectively cope with a serious illness and find meaning in what is happening (Lin H. R., Bauer-Wu S. M., 2003).

Scientists from the Russian Cancer Research Center came to the conclusion that only as a result of the patient's activity that is significant for him, with the support of the nearest social environment, it is possible to change his self-consciousness and restructure the motivational and sense-bearing sphere. As a result of this activity, a very special type of personality aspirations is formed in the human at advanced stages of the disease, and the very concept of a "cancer patient" is transformed. It is no longer associated by the person with a life threat. Nothing else, the researchers believe, contributes to the real motivation of cancer patients to achieve an active life (Martova T. Y., Malygin E. N., 2002).

Such a strategy corresponds to the principle of the dominant of Alexey Ukhtomskiy (2000): "In order to not be a victim of the dominant, one must be its commander," he wrote. R. M. Granovskaya (1988) adds that in order to help a person go through a severe loss, it is necessary to contribute to the formation of the new dominant, which can suppress or at least weaken the focus of arousal that is associated with mental trauma.

Even experiments on mice have shown that individuals leading an active life more successfully resist the development of cancer. Biologists from the

University of Ohio and Cornell University, NY, divided the young rodents into two groups: the control group lived in standard laboratory cell conditions, while the test group was provided with larger cells with "entertainment": a labyrinth, "squirrel wheels" and various toys. Then melanoma cells, one of the most deadly forms of cancer, were injected under the skin of mice. Three weeks later, it turned out that in the control group the size of the developed tumors was approximately two times larger than in the experimental group, and in another three weeks this difference increased to 77%. Moreover, in 17% of the mice from the experimental group, tumors did not appear at all (Cao L. et al., 2010).

Similar results were observed by the same researchers in experiments with the "inoculation" of colon cancer cells in rodents. The authors of the study believe that the reason for the protective effect of "entertainment" is not just in the increased physical activity of the mice, but also in the stimulating effect of mild stress (*"eustress" according to Selye—V. M.*), which was confirmed by a slightly elevated level of the corticosterone hormone. At the same time, there was a significant reduction in these mice of the hormone leptin, which is responsible for energy metabolism and affects obesity and cancer development, and in the hypothalamus, the expression level of the gene encoding the synthesis of the nerve tissue growth factor BDNF increased (Cao L. et al., 2010). This suggests a sufficiently active body resistance.

Considering the positive impact of acquiring the lost meaning of life on the favorable outcome of cancer, Tom Laughlin (1999) argues:

> Nothing is more thrilling then for a cancer patients to discover that the most important thing they must do in their recovery program along with their medical regimen, is to consciously develop some exciting new talent or ability they never knew existed. ... Ending the suffocation and discovering a new talent in the cancer patient immediately relieve the unconscious depression and transform the patient's life. ... [If you start] to build upon these new values and insights and discover all the unknown abilities and talents that are buried in your unconscious, then your cancer can become a starting point for the real life you were meant to live from the beginning.

Lawrence LeShan (1977) shares the same opinion: the main thing for the patient is to find a way to return to life, to start developing that part of it that was previously rejected by him, to realize desires and impulses that previously seemed impracticable, and to understand what he really wants to do with them.

Similar thoughts were expressed by Steve Jobs (2005), who also was a cancer patient:

> You've got to find what you love. And that is as true for your work as it is for your lovers. Your work is going to fill a large part of your life, and the only way to be truly satisfied is to do what you believe is great work. And the only way to do great work is to love what you do. If you haven't found it yet, keep looking. Don't settle. As with all matters of the heart, you'll know when you find it. And, like any great relationship, it just gets better and better as the years roll on. So keep looking until you find it. Don't settle.

In Jobs' case, definitely, the main oncogenic conflict was of another origin.

Psycho-oncologist Tieng-Sheng Hsu (2010) believes that cancer leads patients to the discovery of their inner strength. When they are diagnosed with cancer, most people do not pay attention to the fact that they have blocked creative vital energy. In order to cure the disease, they use all kinds of medical technology to attack the result of this distorted vital energy. However, according to Dr. Hsu, the key to effective cancer treatment is to understand how this creative energy is blocked. When it is normalized, it can significantly revitalize the functions of the body, render the life full of creativity, and make the soul overflow with life.

The research performed at the Cancer Institute and the University of Sao Paulo, Brazil, found that introduction of spiritual practices in the program of psychological rehabilitation of cancer patients contributes to their realization of the power of their own life to fight the disease, and makes it possible for them to recognize and use their own resources and energy to build a better, wholer life. The ongoing transformation of the personality is accompanied by the restoration of a healthy libido in patients and dissociation from the craving for death, creates favorable conditions for the emergence of thoughts about the need for self-care. Positive self-esteem, self-confidence, feeling worthy of protection by Divine Love is growing. All these transformations naturally lead to the onset of new opportunities for the external expression of the individual's potential (Elias A. C. A. et al., 2015).

During the period of such a personality transformation, a patient may experience a state similar to that described by my patient S., who for the first time had contact with her Essence and repressed interests:

> What I have found for myself as most important at the present moment directs me to the future. I feel joy and inspiration in what is happening to me, in what the new personality that I am becoming is. I know that this "new I" will be able to realize all those plans and goals in life that I stopped hoping to realize about ten years ago.

Upon analyzing twenty-seven scientific works, A. Visser and his colleagues (2010) came to the conclusion that spirituality has a positive effect on the well-being of cancer patients. Sixteen scientific papers reviewed by H. G. Koenig (2012) showed that spiritual and/or religious people have a lower risk of developing cancer, and those who fall ill have a better prognosis for therapy. Working in the same direction, scientists from the San Gerardo Hospital in Milan found that patients with deep spiritual faith showed significantly better results with chemotherapy. The activity of their immune system after treatment (determined by the number of lymphocytes) was significantly higher than in the control "weak-believing" group, and their survival after a course of therapy during three years of observation was better (Lissoni P. et al., 2008).

At the same time, researchers from the Rochester Cancer Center noted that it is not so much religiousness, but the spiritual meaning discovered by breast cancer patients during the disease that helps them to reduce the traumatic stress and increase their well-being (Purnell J. Q. et al., 2009). Moreover, fatalistic religious beliefs (cancer as God's punishment for sins) can even negatively influence the overcoming of stress caused by an oncological disease (Baider L., Sarell M., 1983).

In connection with the above, A. A. Gostev's (2007) view on the metaphysics of sin seems legitimate. The philosopher regards a sin as the incompatibility of man with his true nature and purpose:

> The characteristics and measure of this inconsistency determine the pathological bodily, mental, and spiritual life. In psychological terms, the fall is a violation in the hierarchy of structures in man, leading to a change in his psychological nature. At the top there must be the Spirit, which gives clarity and harmony to the psychic life, centering the life of man on God.

According to S. A. Kulakov's biopsychosocial-spiritual cancer model (2009a), "the accumulation of sins and the long existence of [uncontrolled] passions weaken the spirit and increase the body's entropy, which leads to a decrease in immunity and the emergence of various diseases."

With this approach, religiosity can become a positive factor, significantly contributing to the overcoming of the disease. This is confirmed by the studies conducted by S. Feher and R. C. Maly (1999) from the University of California: 64% of women with newly diagnosed breast tumors were able to understand the meaning of the disease in their lives by relying on their religious faith. Psychologists at the University of Health Sciences in Bethesda found that cancer patients with religious belief suffer less pain, anxiety, hostility, and social isolation, and feel more satisfied with life than unbelieving patients (Jenkins R. A., Pargament K. I., 1995).

Italian expert Dr. P. M. Biava (2009) writes that cancer will be healed only when we realize that healing must occur on all levels of life, to which we are all connected:

> Healing cancer also means finding meaning in our existence. In these difficult times, I think the only path pursuable is within ourselves, in our profound self. We must tap into our inner strength to fight our egoistic instincts and have faith that something has meaning, regardless of the results achieved.

Returning to the topic of the hidden propensity to suicide as a factor of the initiation of cancer, as well as the common origin of avital experiences in precancerous and pre-suicidal periods, it is appropriate to cite the observation of Stanislav Grof: "The best remedy for self-destructive tendencies and the suicidal urge is, then, the experience of ego death and rebirth and ensuing sense of cosmic unity" (Grof S., 2000). Several of his patients who experienced the death-rebirth process independently stated that their past suicidal tendencies were in fact an incomprehensible desire to overcome the ego. Since they did not have such an understanding at that time, they chose in physical reality a situation very similar to the death of the ego, which was the bodily self-destruction. "Following the ego death individuals saw human existence in a much broader spiritual framework; no matter how difficult their life situations and circumstances were from an objective point of view, suicide somehow no longer appeared to be a solution." (Grof S., Halifax J., 1978).

In his book *Ultimate Healing* (2001), the Buddhist teacher Lama Zopa Rinpoche draws our attention to how important it is to have complete clarity regarding the highest goal of our life. If getting rid of one particular disease is the most important goal that the patient set for themselves, then they did not understand anything, because even if they get rid of this disease, nothing will change in a bigger sense. Their attitude to life will remain the same and they will continue, as before, to do all the same bad deeds and create causes for future problems, particularly the cause of the disease. Changing one's view of things, according to this spiritual teacher, is much more important than a cure for a physical disease.

This opinion is supported by Antonina Derzhavina (2008), who healed herself from cancer. She urges:

> Think about the meaning of life. Is there something worth living for? If, when ill with cancer, you have not found the goal, but just want to live out your remaining days, then you will not be able to recover. But if your "I" rebelled against the aimlessness of existence, then you have a chance.

Thus, it is the change in worldview and spiritual development in the course of post-traumatic growth that can serve to restore the patient's psychological and energy resources, necessary to defeat the disease.

Chapter 32

Ways to Achieve Post–Traumatic Growth

> If we treat people as if they were
> what they ought to be,
> we help them become
> what they are capable of becoming.
> Johann Wolfgang von Goethe,
> *Wilhelm Meister's Apprenticeship*

Post-traumatic growth can be either spontaneous, arising in a patient without any help as a result of their personal transformation and spiritual awakening, or induced, that is, directed by specialists. PTG can be initiated by means of psychotherapeutic techniques, especially those developed in existential-humanistic psychology: logotherapy (Frankl V., 2016), supportive-expressive (Spiegel D., Yalom I. D., 1978) and cognitive-existential group therapy (Kissane D. W. et al., 2004), as well as meaning-centered therapy (Breitbart W., 2002; Lee V. et al., 2006), therapy of dignity (Chochinov H. M. et al., 2005), transpersonal psychotherapy (Grof S., 1985, Clarkson P., 2002), combined methods of therapy (Ramos C. et al., 2018). Special programs of personal and spiritual growth created by teams of psycho-oncologists in different countries, such as psychospiritual integrative therapy (Fauver R., 2011) and the "Healing Journey" (Cunningham A. J., Edmonds C. V., 1996) are also effective.

32.1. The Help of Specialists in Attaining Post–Traumatic Growth

Undoubtedly, during the main stage of working with the patient, psychologists and psychotherapists should identify and resolve the main intrapersonal conflicts and psychic traumas, since these are the source of the individual's current chronic stress. At the same time, the patient needs to begin exploring their personality, while the specialist should correct their individual maladaptive properties, attitudes, and behavioral patterns, as discussed in Part II: alexithymia, suppression or repression of negative emotions, psychological infantilism, negative self-image, preference of other people's interests, dependence and subordination, the suppression of creative potential in favor of material well-being, lack of understanding of their life goals. These personality traits impede the achievement of PTG and lead the patient in the direction of post-traumatic disorders.

One of the main tasks of the psycho-oncologist or psychotherapist is to help the patient overcome the existential crisis and the avital experiences that contributed to the formation of the oncodominant. To do this, it is necessary to, together with the patient, find a new meaning in their life, which will become their reason to fight for life. When an understanding of the meaning and purpose of the struggle appears, the hope for healing begins to rise in the patient, and thus triggers active recovery processes in the body. One such mechanism is establishing a healthier diurnal cortisol rhythm, which is associated with enhanced positive emotions that result from finding benefit in one's experience with cancer (Wang A. W., Hoyt M. A., 2018).

According to Nietzsche (2009), "He, who has a why to live, can bear almost any how." Resolving existential problems becomes a powerful internal resource for overcoming a crisis situation, choosing effective coping strategies, and successfully managing to deal with life difficulties (Bakanova A. A., 2001). Therefore, turning to spirituality can play an important role in resolving an existential crisis.

To reach these goals, at least the following requirements must be met:

- training of health workers in the principles of spirituality and awareness;

- study of and support for the spiritual needs of patients to achieve mental stability and successfully endure the stress of the disease, especially during periods of diagnosis, hospitalization, relapse, and worsening of the course of the disease. Since patients have different spiritual needs, it is important to understand and respect the place of the spiritual component in each of their lives (Webster A., 2008; Puchalski C. M., McSkimming S., 2006; Motenko J. S., 2012);

- the inclusion of the development of spirituality in the integrative programs of treatment and rehabilitation.

This helps to improve the quality of patients' lives, increase their self-esteem and self-confidence, enhance their emotional state, realize their potential (Elias A. C. A. et al., 2015), and also leads to the activation of immunity and greater effectiveness of medical therapy (Lissoni P. et al., 2008).

In the framework of the biopsychosocial-spiritual model, when conducting the case interview, an authorized medical professional or clinical psychologist should clarify both the social (including family) aspects of the patient's life and their spiritual and religious position. Based on this data, a diagnosis of mental pain or distress is made, specific spiritual questions, needs, or goals are identified, and the ways to implement relevant spiritual assistance are determined (Puchalski C. M., 2013). It is very important for healthcare workers to be able to support patients in the search for new spiritual meanings and help to re-evaluate their life values (Motenko J. S., 2012). Spiritual and psychological assistance to patients is recommended to be directed to the:

- attraction of faith in spiritual reality,
- involvement of faith in God or Higher Forces,
- understanding of the differences between the different forms of religion,
- recognition of spirituality as the core element of human experience,
- recognition of an innate human need for the search for meaning and spirituality,
- recognition of the possibilities of religion in dealing with extreme situations,
- consideration of issues relating to the ultimate goal and meaning of life,
- involvement of certain spiritual exercises,
- use of a complex of religious beliefs and rituals,
- bringing of the patient to experience holiness, reverence, and unity,
- development of transcendental connections,
- integration of religion and spirituality into everyday life,
- recognition of the limitations and conventions of religiosity in dealing with stress,
- assistance in the search for spiritual guidance and education.
(Pargament K. I., 2002; Wong P. T., 1998)

Even general psychotherapeutic care, as shown in the group of patients with gastrointestinal cancer, significantly increases the ten-year patient survival (Kuchler T. et al., 2007). Analysis of fifteen randomized controlled trials published between 1989 and 2009 showed that thirty and more hours of psychosocial treatment yielded a significant survival benefit in the first two years following intervention (Xia Y. et al., 2014). The involvement of the spiritual, existential dimension in therapy increases its effectiveness.

The studies conducted by Prof. David Spiegel and his colleagues from Stanford University (1989) that have become well-known provide a good illustration. After organizing a therapeutically supporting group for women who had been treated for breast cancer, the researchers did everything possible so that these women began to actively work on their development. The patients were taught self-hypnosis and assisted in solving the existential questions—what they can do to improve their lives, what their needs are, and how to satisfy them. As a result of this development, the quality of life of these women has noticeably improved and their life term almost doubled compared with the control group.

A two-month course of psycho-spiritual integrative therapy developed by the American Institute of Transpersonal Therapy showed a significant improvement in overall spiritual well-being, an increase in the feeling of meaningfulness of life, peace and faith, and a decrease in mood disorders (Fauver R., 2011). Another two-month course called "Steps Toward Spiritual Healing," which is part of the "Healing Journey" program developed at the Cancer Institute in Ontario, helped patients resolve many existential issues, problems of condemnation, guilt, and forgiveness, self-worth, meanings of love and life. Patients learned to accept everyday life and engage in fewer conflicts with other people (Cunningham A. J., 2005; Cunningham A. J., Edmonds C. V., 1996). The three-month holistic healing program, created at the University of Texas, focused on developing a balance between the mental, emotional, spiritual, and physical health of cancer patients. At its end, patients showed a decrease in distress, an improvement in the quality of life, a deeper awareness of the purpose and meaning of existence, and an increase in the sense of general well-being (Kinney C. K. et al., 2003).

Another example is research conducted at the Baptist University of Houston, which showed that with the help of religious beliefs, positive *reframing*, and acceptance of the disease situation, 46% of breast cancer patients developed PTG (Bussell V. A., Naus M. J., 2010). Other authors came to the conclusion that timely and active psychological intervention after a person is diagnosed with cancer can reduce distress and potentiate PTG (Knobf M. T., 2007).

F. B. Levenson and colleagues (2009) analyzed the results of their more-than-thirty-year practice in psycho-oncology involving the use of clinical holistic psychotherapy (psychodynamic psychotherapy that involves therapeutic touches). Of the seventy-five patients with metastatic cancer treated during this period, at the time of the publication of the article, 44% were alive, 80% lived more than five years and 45% lived more than ten years. Researchers have identified the following common factors that characterize the surviving patients:

1. Their life has changed—most often in the aspects of home, job, partner.

2. They got married or formed close relationships with a partner, including full-fledged sexual relationships.

3. They developed close relationships with friends and family members. In these relations, bodily contact (hugs) takes up an important place.

4. They developed a positive life philosophy, expressed the will to live and responsibility for their lives. This was manifested in the behavior of the patients.

5. Their quality of life has improved markedly, regardless of the presence of the disease.

6. Goals appeared in their lives (life mission).

7. They got rid of the habit of becoming irritated.

8. They developed a sense of harmony (coherence).

9. They began to view the disease as a lesson for the soul.

Using the therapy, which is centered on meaning, William Breitbart and his colleagues from the Department of Psychiatry at the Memorial Sloan-Kettering Cancer Center in New York (2010) achieved a significant increase in spiritual well-being and sense of meaningfulness, as well as a decrease in anxiety, hopelessness, and desire for early death in patients with advanced forms of cancer. As a result of the psychotherapeutic and musical therapy program conducted at the St. Gallen Hospital (Switzerland), cancer patients reported spiritual and transcendental experiences that led to significant changes. At the physical level, this was expressed though the reduction of pain and (sometimes) shortness of breath, at the psychological level—less anxiety, better endurance of the disease, acceptance of life and death, and at the spiritual level—a change in spiritual identity (Renz M. et al., 2013).

"The main purpose in the treatment of cancer is to set some kind of objective," writes Russian psycho-oncologist Alexander Danilin (2011). "... I have often seen how people who found a goal and strength to fight against the feeling of total uselessness, grew well." Such a task, in my opinion, should be a challenge for the patient; it should go beyond the everyday goals of material well-being. As Joseph Murphy (2008) writes, we live in order to unleash the splendor imprisoned in our dungeon, to express our talents. If we think that we live only to earn the right to exist, then this is all that we will do for all our days.

That is why, in Lawrence LeShan's opinion (1977), the idea of "settling for material sufficiency foremost" has little impetus for the cancer patient; for this, he will not work hard, endure pain, fight for his life. Paul Rosch (1996), director of the American Institute of Stress, tells the life story of the famous Hungarian composer Bela Bartok. He was at the terminal stage of leukemia, when the conductor of the Boston Symphony Orchestra, Sergey Kusevitsky, suggested that he write a new composition. While working, Bartok experienced an inexplicable (by medicine) remission, which lasted until the composer finished his work. After that, the disease broke out with a new force, soon resulting in his death. While this story does not have a "happy ending," nevertheless it demonstrates the great potential of our mind when it is aware of the meaning of existence.

Although the cited data on the occurrence of remission or full healing of cancer by a change effected in patients' outlook and lifestyle today appears to us as the cutting edge of science, this approach has been known to humanity for several thousand years. Historians have discovered that, in order to cure his patients, the famous ancient Greek physician Hippocrates (460–377 BC) helped them to gain a new character, find direction in life, and use their talents for the benefit of the outside world (Jones W. H. S., 1923).

When planning post-traumatic growth programs for patients, it is very important that the significant person, especially the spouse, participate together with the patient. Otherwise, a situation may arise when the patient, owing to the ongoing personal and spiritual development, can no longer lead the former "normal" way of life, while his family or relatives, who remain at the initial level, expect him to return to his former existence (which is often the source of oncogenic distress). Such dissonance leads to misunderstanding, stress in relationships, and the emergence of social isolation in the life of a patient, which is extremely harmful to the recovery process.

Science is still far from understanding all the mechanisms by which PTG promotes the improvement of health or even the remission. However, there is already evidence of a marked increase in immunity among those who have found meaning in the experienced grief (Bower J. E. et al., 2003), have gone through spontaneous PTG in cancer (Dunigan J. T. et al., 2007), went through a program of cognitive-behavioral stress management that helped them find meaning in the disease (McGregor B. A. et al., 2004), went through an integrative therapy program aimed at increasing the spiritual level of cancer patients (Nakau M. et al., 2013). Since PTG is accompanied by an increase in a person's satisfaction with life, that is, an increase in positive emotions, this also certainly should be accompanied by an increase in the content of the hormone dopamine in the brain, which, as I reported in Chapter 19.2, reduces depression and is able to suppress tumor growth. Another interesting fact was discovered by scientists from the University of Toronto: experiencing positive emotions, such as amusement, compassion, contentment, joy, love, pride, and especially awe, helps to reduce the content of the pro-inflammatory cytokine IL-6 (Stellar J. E. et al., 2015).

32.2. Self-Knowledge—the Path to Spontaneous Post-Traumatic Growth

> I am not what happened to me;
> I am what I choose to become.
> Karl Gustav Jung,
> *Collected Works*

But what actions can the patient him/herself take, he or she, who before the disease was in the grip of a false personality, not knowing about its limitations, not caring about self-improvement? What path can lead him/her from an existential vacuum to self-actualization, post-traumatic growth, and further to self-transcendence and remission? How can one heal oneself from the noogenic neurosis and activate the healing powers of the body?

I once again emphasize that first of all the patient needs to work with the psychotherapist to process his main psychological problems. However, it is necessary to understand that working with a therapist is only the initial stage on the path of healing. Together with it, active actions taken by the patient himself, self-change and self-development, transformation of his personality and the discovery of the Essence are necessary. Martin Buber (2003) wrote that every crisis not only leads a person to a situation of loneliness, hopelessness, and loss, but also to the need to overcome them. Therefore one is faced with the main task of life—self-knowledge, and as a result, it becomes possible to overcome the crisis and get out of it.

The importance of self-knowledge and self-development has been known to mankind for many millennia. Aristotle (2006) wrote that "Get to know thyself" was written above the doorway of the Delphic sanctuary in ancient Greece. And the first step in this direction is the knowledge of the difference between one's Essence, one's true self, and a false personality. The problem of the modern man is that he thinks that his physical body with his personality are all that he is. And as long as he does not have the direct experience of comprehending the existence of his Essence, his true nature, he will continue to make mistakes and spend his life in vain.

"When our consciousness ceases to identify with our personality, unprecedented perspectives will unfold in front of us," writes Mario Alonso Puig (2012), a physician and psychologist at Harvard University. Knowing one's Essence and striving to "nourish, love and cherish it, as the most enlightened and caring parent would have done" leads to the situation when it begins to grow gradually and use those opportunities, knowledge, and power that were previously automatically used by a false personality. Then, instead of a miserable two percent of the Essence and ninety-eight percent of a false personality, as is observed in most people, a person who has stepped onto the path of self-knowledge begins a gradual shift to an increasing manifestation of the Essence, and with it to an ever-increasing vitality and natural joy of being. And since the false personality will continue to fade in such a person, he will develop a higher type of consciousness. This state is called awakening (Tart C., 1987).

Awakening leads to self-realization—"a state of consciousness characterized by joy, serenity, inner security, a sense of calm power, clear understanding, and radiant love. In its highest aspects it is the realization of essential Being, of communion and identification with the Universal Life" (Assagioli R., 1999). Jack Kornfield (1999), a psychologist and a dedicated Buddhist monk, writes that systematic spiritual practice is one of the most profound, exciting, intense, wonderful and difficult adventures that we, as human beings, can undertake. This is a journey where a person can explore the deepest, inner regions of consciousness, waking up to observe countless parts of himself, while leading his mind and heart to the very boundaries of their penetration into our deep connection with the whole universe.

All seeking individuals followed a similar path. For example, the Russian philosopher Nikolai Berdyaev wrote about himself in his book, *Self-knowledge* (2009):

My personality is not a ready-made reality; I create my personality; I create it also when I perceive myself; I am first and foremost an act.

George Gurdjieff taught that a person is not complete—from birth he is only able to develop to a certain level. He must achieve further development himself, making his own efforts, and for this he needs to know himself. However, while being under the influence of a false personality, a person does not get to truly know herself and only uses a small part of her potential. The true birth has yet to happen and it occurs if a person becomes the creator of herself and her soul. This birth is a product of inner creativity, of inward movement helping one to find their unique source of vital energy (Ouspensky P. D., 1959).

According to Abraham Maslow (1967), the best way to a good life for a patient can be only one thing: to be even more authentic. He has to learn how to release the suppressed, to get to know his own Self, listen to the "voice of the impulse," reveal his majestic nature, reach understanding, penetration, and comprehend the truth.

The development of the ability to hear the "voice of the impulse," or "the voice of the subconscious" is especially important for a sick person, because it allows him to control his own health condition. Studies show that every individual possesses such abilities, but few are capable of developing them. Meanwhile, if they were developed, a person could feel the approach of a disease in time and take the necessary measures. For example, R. Schwartz and S. Geyer (1984) found that 74% of those who underwent a biopsy for diagnosis had a premonition of having cancer. Upon using the Han symbol test (patient's interpretation of the meaning of various figures and models) conducted on women before a breast biopsy, psychologists from the University of California confirmed that the subconsciousness of the patients reported on the presence of a tumor through the characters, and it was even possible to distinguish benign and malignant tumors (Engelman S. R., Craddick R., 1984).

In addition, an individual's subconscious manifests information about the disease through dreams: 94% of the women who were tested for breast cancer reported specific dreams that they had before being diagnosed with the disease—bright, realistic, creating a sense of importance, certainty, threat, often associated with the breast or even specifically cancer (Burk L., 2015). My patient A. from Kazakhstan told me that several months before being diagnosed with rectal cancer he had a dream where something dark was trying to catch him and he was running away to escape. Then right before the operation a similar dream appeared: the dark entity caught and gripped him while some people were trying to free him from its grip. When he awoke, he felt free, as if they had succeeded in releasing him. The operation went quite well, so finishing the story he told me, "Now I know that it is my surgeons and you who wrestled me out of darkness!"

That is why C. Simonton and colleagues (1978), after having been exposed to similar facts in their practice, began to successfully use the technique of interaction with the subconscious in the form of a dialogue with the "inner mentor" in their famous rehabilitation program. Carl Simonton writes that over time he stopped puzzling over the question of why one kind of therapy works for one patient and does not work for another, and what to recommend to them. In his opinion, the main way to help patients is to teach them to listen to their own inner source, which will tell them what kind of therapy they need. Then they will cease to grasp at each new method of treatment only because it has helped some other patient. It takes time and patience to develop this ability to contact one's own inner wisdom, and this is not always possible, but the result is worth the effort (Simonton O. C., Henson R. M., 1992).

Anita Moorjani's (2012) experience has taught her that the best way to cultivate faith and feel the connection with the life energy of the universe is to look inside herself:

> I understand that cancer in itself was neither my enemy, nor even a disease. I know exactly what it wanted to tell me, and in my case it turned out to be really only the way my own body tried to cure me. Now I realize that an attempt to present cancer as an external enemy, which must be destroyed, would never lead to getting rid of the main problem that became the original cause of its appearance. ... Cancer is just my own power and energy, which did not find a way out to the outside world, and had to somehow express itself inside of me, attacking my defenseless body.

The same experience got Japanese survivor Shin Terayama (Weil A., 2000):

> Gradually, I began to realize that I had created my own cancer. I had created it by my behavior. And as I came to that realization, I saw that I had to love my cancer, not attack it as an enemy. It was part of me, and I had to love my whole self.

The most important questions for a cancer patient, according to Tom Laughlin (1999), are exactly what ability, what emotion, what talent, what need, or what unknown part of his personality is suppressed and cannot begin to develop. It is impossible to achieve complete liberation from the paralyzing seizure of subconscious depression until this question is sorted out, and that is why the success of medical therapy remains extremely small.

Reginald Ray (2002) writes that the experience of closeness of death generated by a cancer diagnosis brings with it a sense of spontaneity and even freedom. Since a person understands that his future is indeed uncertain, the moment that is existing now becomes more important—in fact, this is all he or she has or can ever have, and the rest is just an empty guess. Realizing that everything that one is and what he does will one day become nothing, a person is free to be anyone and do what lives in his heart. The same is true about the spiritual path—one has to live more and more in the present, become fully and completely who one is, the person one truly is, the one already recorded in the depths of her own soul. In this way the understanding of death powerfully leads one to spiritual practice and therefore, to the discovery of our true Essence.

Buddhist Lama Zopa Rinpoche (2001) calls us to learn to use the disease to help us see our needs, not as something we seek to get rid of, not an obstacle but the tool for the development of love, compassion, and wisdom. In the same way as a poison can be used to prepare a medicine, the disease can be used as a path to happiness. Our experiences in the process of illness can bring a deep meaning should we transform our mind and develop the precious human qualities of love and compassion. Thus we will get the ability to bring peace and happiness to every living being we come into contact with.

The main goal of self-exploration is to find ways to health, abandoning the views that lead a person to self-destruction. If one could contribute to the onset of the disease, one can also participate in one's own recovery (Simonton C. et al., 1978). Brandon Bays (2012) confirms that such an understanding came from her inner knowledge:

> I realized that the same part of me that had been responsible for creating the tumor would also be responsible for un-creating it, ... that, in fact, this tumor was a gift, that it had something important to teach me, and that somehow I would be guided to heal myself.

A similar transformation of consciousness often occurs in my patients. Their attitude to the tumor changes: it is no longer perceived as a separate, alien enemy that needs to be destroyed. There comes an understanding that there is only a diseased organ with a deformation that has arisen in it, that it needs help, love, and sympathetic attention—just as a sick child does. And the more a person expresses such love and attention for a sick organ and him/herself as a whole, the more actively his or her general harmony will increase, and hence his or her own healing potential increases.

Starting from a basic study of oneself, a diligent practitioner can achieve self-actualization first, revealing his natural talents, and then the self-transcendence by choosing one or more spiritual traditions. By changing his life philosophy and priorities, he can reach a state where stresses lose their power over him. "Very often people have such a profound experience of Source (*transcendental experience—V. M.*) that they find many old habits and limiting beliefs drop away spontaneously without them consciously working at it," says Brandon Bays (2012). "The more they get in touch with their true Self, the more the old, destructive patterns become obsolete and unnatural."

Tibetan Lama Yongey Mingyur Rinpoche (with E. Swanson, 2008) explains that when one dedicates oneself to developing one's Buddhahood awareness, one inevitably begins to notice changes in everyday experiences: what once bothered one, gradually loses the ability to get one out of the state of mental equilibrium. This develops intuitive wisdom, helps a person to be more relaxed and more open, to see the obstacles as opportunities for further growth. Then the illusory feeling of limitation and vulnerability gradually disappears, and one discovers the true greatness of one's own nature deep within.

32.3. Self-awareness and Meditation as a Way of Transforming One's Personality and Activating Internal Resources

One of the most important ways of knowing our real "I" is the development of the self-awareness skill, which is the feeling of the presence of the "inner observer" in everything that happens in our life. The initial actions on this path can be, for example, the development of the ability to correctly perceive ("listen to") your body and understand its signals, in the form of sensations in organs and systems, before a disorder occurs. It is necessary to learn relaxation skills, properly evaluate and manifest your emotions, understand the mechanisms of the psyche, manage your own energy, and perceive the information that is coming from the subconscious. Upon observing our desires and aversions, attachments and fears, we gradually realize that at the core of our behavior there are social patterns, which, like computer programs, determine and limit the work of our mind. In this kind of self-observation, we can learn to track and recognize manifestations of a false personality and its maladaptive actions. We begin to consciously control ourselves and our behavior, become aware of our needs, intelligently analyze and regulate our emotions and activities.

As a practical method, I recommend learning the technique of mindfulness meditation. Coming from Indian yoga and Buddhist spiritual traditions, this method is currently actively conquering the Western world because of its simplicity and efficiency. Moreover, it is intensively studied by scientists, who find that it has remarkable positive influence on mental and physical health. Since 1983, scientists have been meeting with the leader of the Tibetan Buddhists—the Dalai Lama XIV, Tenzin Gyatso. During these meetings, various issues of nature and consciousness were discussed. It turned out that the views of Buddhism on many aspects of human mental life not only do not contradict, but coincide with the latest scientific discoveries in the field of neurophysiology and quantum physics.

Subsequently, the Mind and Life Dialogues Institute was established, where scientists had the opportunity to conduct various studies on the brains of meditating monks. It turned out that the latter, both in a state outside of meditation, and especially during it, had a significantly increased activity of gamma waves in the brain, reflecting the processes of attention, memory mechanisms, learning, and conscious perception. This suggests the ability of the meditative state to create long-lasting positive changes in the brain. An increased activity in the areas of the brain that are associated with positive emotions, in particular, experiences of happiness, was also detected (Lutz A. et al., 2004). The number of such studies is increasing every year (see the review by Boccia M. et al., 2015).

During the mindfulness meditation, a focused and clear state arises, leading to the transformation of consciousness and subsequent behavioral, mental, and bodily changes. It allows one to go beyond the limits of a false personality and to come into contact with one's Essence, which always remains whole and is not subject to any suffering experienced by a false personality. It is the reunion with one's own Essence, in my opinion, that becomes the source of post-traumatic growth for patients.

The first step to mastering the art of meditation is to learn how to relax a tensed body.

In the late 1960s, Dr. Herbert Benson, now a professor of medicine at Harvard University, was studying Buddhist practices. He proposed the concept of a "relaxation response" to describe the physiological changes that occur in the body during meditation. However, it took many more years before the concept of "mind-body" was adopted by the general scientific community. Benson recalled that for a long period he felt like a "persona non grata" and incurred the condemnation of his colleagues' after the publication of his book on the relaxation response in 1975 (with M. Z. Klipper). However, the book later became a bestseller, while in 1994 Benson founded the Institute for Mind Body Medicine at Harvard University. Modern studies show that the practice of relaxation activates the expression of genes associated with energy metabolism, mitochondrial functions, insulin secretion, and maintenance of telomeres, and inhibits the activity of genes that are responsible for inflammatory and stress-implementing reactions (Bhasin M. K. et al., 2013).

In 1979, John Kabat-Zinn, at that time a young scientist and now an honorary professor at the Medical School of the University of Massachusetts, was trained by the famous Vietnamese Buddhist teacher Thich Nhat Hanh. Using this knowledge, Kabat-Zinn founded the first US clinic aimed at reducing stress. The Mindfulness-Based Stress Reduction (MBSR) program he developed has been widely recognized as an effective adjuvant method for treating a large number of diseases. At the core of this program is the same concept of self-awareness, or mindfulness, regarding the processes taking place in the mind and body. The processes of perception, physical sensations, emotional reactions, thoughts, imagination—all this is realized and observed during every moment, without evaluations, impartially, which makes it possible to learn to recognize and prevent the damaging effects of stress (Kabat-Zinn J., 2005). Now more than 250 hospitals and clinics around the world offer MBSR programs to their patients, and their number is increasing every year. The method developed by

Professor Kabat-Zinn is taught at the medical faculties of Stanford and Harvard Universities.

Studies of the mechanisms by which meditation helps to improve health have shown its profound impact at all levels of the body. In addition to the previously noted activation of brain regions associated with positive moods (Davidson R. J. et al., 2003; Lutz A. et al., 2004), meditation directly changes the structure of the brain owing to the thickening of the cortex in the somatosensory area, which is responsible for perceiving body signals, and in the right insula—an islet that is part of the hemispheres. The right insula is involved in the regulation of emotions, perception, cognition, self-awareness, and, as I reported above, does not develop enough in children with negative feelings of guilt and depression. This thickening of the cortex areas strengthens the body's physiological resistance to anxiety, depression, and alexithymia (Santarnecchi E. et al., 2014).

Mindful meditation can increase the level of daily attention and self-compassion, which leads to a growth in positive mental attitudes toward oneself and others (Rodríguez-Carvajal R. et al., 2016). It is worth mentioning the research data which found that the spiritual, Divine-oriented context of meditation practiced for twenty minutes a day for two weeks leads to a greater decrease in testee anxiety, a more positive mood, an increase in spiritual health and spiritual experience compared to "secular" meditation that did not involve Divine context (Wachholtz A. B., Pargament K. I., 2005).

In response to meditative practices, anxiety and blood pressure are reduced (Ospina M. B. et al., 2007), the content of stress hormones epinephrine, norepinephrine (Infante J. R. et al., 2001), and cortisol (Jevning R. et al., 1978) decreases. The level of cell lipid oxidation caused by free radicals drops (Schneider R. H. et al., 1998), including in the lymphocytes that are involved in immune protection. This is due to changes in the activity of genes responsible for the synthesis of the antioxidant enzyme glutathione peroxidase (Sharma H. et al., 2008). At the same time, salivary IgA level increases, as an indicator of an improved immune response (Bellosta-Batalla M. et al., 2018).

In fact, meditation is a factor in the epigenetic regulation of the genome. Scientists from Navarra Institute for Health Research (Spain) found that in meditators the methylation level of forty-three genes changes, compared to those in the control group. Almost half of these genes are linked to common human diseases, such as neurological and psychiatric disorders, cardiovascular diseases, and cancer (García-Campayo J. et al., 2018). Meditation also changes the acetylation of chromosomal histone proteins, followed by a decrease in the activity of a number of pro-inflammatory genes. This correlates with rapid physical recovery from a stressful situation (Kaliman P. et al., 2014). The stress-induced growth of the pro-inflammatory cytokine interleukin-6 and the concentration of the inflammatory marker C-reactive protein are also reduced (Pace T. W. et al., 2009; Fang C. Y. et al., 2010).

An intensive three-month course of meditation aimed at the development of self-awareness helped to increase realization of the meaning of life and reduce the stress experienced by practitioners. At the same time, the activity of the telomerase enzyme, which is responsible for the length of chromosomal telomeres in immune cells, increased, which led to the activation of immune protection (Jacobs T. L. et al., 2011). Improvement in the functions of the immune system and reduction of the body's inflammatory response as a result of mindfulness meditation have been confirmed by scientists from the University of Wisconsin (Davidson R. J. et al., 2003; Rosenkranz M. A. et al., 2013).

As we have seen in previous chapters, a decrease in immunity, an increase in the level of catecholamines, cortisol, inflammation, and oxidation of lipids are closely related to the development of the tumor process. Therefore, all the above data undoubtedly indicates the profound influence of the mindful state on the functions of the genome. The result is the increased anticancer protection of the body.

It is natural that meditation in various forms, particularly based on the MBSR, has been actively used in therapeutic and rehabilitation programs for cancer patients, positively affecting the quality of life and patient survival (Meares A., 1978; Manzaneque J. M. et al., 2011; Smith J. E. et al., 2005; Carlson L. E. et al., 2004; Shennan C. et al., 2011). Awareness acts as a buffer, which softens the physiological effects of chronic psychosocial stress associated with a cancer diagnosis. The practice also leads to a decrease in the activating effect of stress on low-level chronic inflammation and immunosuppression. This contributes to a more effective course of traditional medical treatment. In addition, mindfulness meditation helps patients cope with the many side effects of therapy (Joyce P. D., 2015).

Back in 1978, the Australian psychiatrist Ainsley Meares, using daily two-hour meditation in seventy-three patients with advanced forms of cancer, was able to help five patients achieve complete remission. One of them is already familiar to us and quoted in this book, Dr. Ian Gawler, who later founded The Gawler Cancer Foundation, dedicated to helping other cancer patients combat the disease. Dr. Meares explains Gawler's success in the following manner (Hirshberg C., Barasch M. I., 1995):

> He has developed a degree of calm about him which I have rarely observed in anyone, even in Oriental mystics with whom I have had some considerable experience. When asked to what he attributes the regression of metastases, he answers: "I really think it is the way we experience our life." In other words, it would seem that the patient has let the effects of the intense and prolonged meditation enter into his whole experience of life. His extraordinarily low level of anxiety is obvious to the most casual observer. It is suggested this has enhanced the activity of his immune system by reducing his level of cortisone.

In the other five patients, tumor growth slowed significantly. For most of the group, the quality of life has improved significantly and suffering has decreased

(Meares A., 1978). A meta-analysis of sixteen studies using similar meditation practices showed a significant improvement in immune functions in cancer patients. They also exhibited decreased levels of anxiety, depression, stress, sexual dysfunction, and physiological arousal (Shennan C. et al., 2011). Other meta-analyses of fourteen, ten, and nineteen scientific papers revealed a steady improvement in psychological functioning, a reduction in stress symptoms, and an increase in the ability to combat stress, as well as an improvement in the quality of life of cancer patients (Ott M. J. et al., 2006; Ledesma D., Kumano H., 2009; Musial F. et al., 2011). A Mindfulness-Based Cancer Recovery program was also developed for patients (Carlson L. E., Speca M., 2011), in addition to a therapeutic technique for psycho-oncologists: a Mindfulness-Based Cognitive Therapy for Cancer (Bartley T., Teasdale J., 2011).

The above data on the molecular mechanisms of the action of meditation in healthy people is confirmed by studies conducted on cancer patients. Meditative practices cause a decrease of cortisol in their blood and saliva, and also the activity of cytokines and immune killer cells return to normal levels (Witek-Janusek L. et al., 2008; Carlson L. E. et al., 2003). According to a study done by the University of Calgary (Canada), following a three-month course of meditation based on MBSR, which was applied after standard medical therapy in cancer patients, the length of telomeres of their chromosomes remained stable, whereas in patients who did not participate in this program, the length of telomeres decreased (Carlson L. E. et al., 2015). An increase in telomerase enzyme activity corresponding to these results was also observed at the end of the six-week program organized at the University of South Florida. Based on the MBSR, this program was designed to reduce stress in women undergoing surgery and treatment for breast cancer (Lengacher C. A. et al., 2014).

Curious data was obtained by scientists from the University of Taiwan. They studied the effect of bioenergy emitted from the hands of an experienced Buddhist meditation master toward the culture of prostate tumor cells for one minute. The impact resulted in a significant inhibition of cell growth in the next forty-eight hours of observation and caused an increase in the content of the specific antigen PAcP in the cells, which indicates that the cells lost their state of tumor un-differentiation (Yu T. et al., 2003). These results indirectly suggest the change in activity of the corresponding genes.

Buddhism holds that it is through meditation that even the most ordinary and un-gifted person can make contact with the awakened state (Ray R. A., 2002), which in other words, is his Essence. According to Buddhism, it is only by transforming our mind that we can destroy the causes of suffering and create the causes of happiness. Lama Zopa Rinpoche (2001) calls meditation an inner medicine used by our own mind to create an inner positive attitude for self-healing. Since both happiness and suffering arise from our mind, Lama Zopa claims that meditation is the main tool in healing. In his book, he cites the stories of several of his students who were able to get rid of cancer and AIDS with the help of Buddhist meditative practices.

However, it is important to understand that meditation is a tool to work with the psyche, and if it is used incorrectly, it can do more harm than good. With the growth of popularity, as in any other field of human activity, many unskilled "teachers" appear claiming to teach meditation, when all they seek is to earn money at the peak of demand. They discredit this practice among those students who could not achieve the promised results. Therefore, I urge readers to carefully approach the choice of a teacher or instructor, preferring direct carriers of the tradition—for example, Buddhist lamas, or at least practitioners with long experience. It is worth considering this: do they have students that you would like to be similar to?

32.4. The Importance of an Integrative, Multimodal Approach to Therapy

At the same time, it is necessary to realize that the practice of meditation in psycho-oncology is an important, necessary, but not self-sufficient method of therapy and rehabilitation. A comprehensive, integrative approach is needed, which includes various combinations of relaxation, self-hypnosis, autogenic training, art therapy, biofeedback, body-oriented therapy, and guided visualization. Methods that are also effective include music therapy, psychophysical practices of yoga, Chinese energy arts Tai Chi and Qigong, physical exercises, special diets, etc. Participation in these programs can stimulate post-traumatic growth in cancer patients, improve the quality of their life, reduce stress and depression, activate the immune system, and reduce inflammatory reactions (Lee M. S. et al., 2001; Shpak V. S. et al., 2016; Dobos G. J. et al., 2012; Culos-Reed S. N. et al., 2006; Kiecolt-Glaser J. K. et al., 2010; Zeng Y. et al., 2014). As we have seen, this contributes to a significant increase in the time of remission and can even result in complete healing.

In fact, thanks to the achievements of epigenetics and psychoneuroimmunology, the general public has finally had the opportunity to see that these practices are not just a "pleasant pastime" that distracts patients from thoughts about the disease. These methods are real health improvement tools that act at the genome level, and the patient's mind and his motivation for recovery play a crucial role in treatment. For most of these practices, the epigenetic effects underlying their positive health effects have already been proven, both separately and in combination. I have mentioned above the epigenetic effects of meditation; similarly, in patients with breast cancer, after a three-month course of yoga (Bower J. E. et al., 2014) and a three-month course of the Tai Chi (Irwin M. R. et al., 2014), the activity of the genes responsible for the synthesis of pro-inflammatory agents decreases. Positive epigenetic changes were also found in cancer patients as a result of changes in diet and the use of bioactive foods (Ross S. A. et al., 2008).

In the Department of Oncology at the University of California, it was found that a course of psychological counseling for women who have been treated for cervical cancer results in a significant reduction in their state of stress. In parallel, telomere length in chromosomes of their macrophage immune cells increases (Biegler K. A. et al., 2012). In patients with early-stage breast cancer, following a ten-week program of cognitive-behavioral stress management, reduction of serum cortisol level and anxiety, higher progress in the ability to relax, and inhibition of the activity of genes responsible for inflammatory reactions were observed (Phillips K. M. et al., 2008; Antoni M. H. et al., 2012).

Another group of patients with breast cancer underwent a six-month course of physical exercises. At the end of the course, patients experienced a change in the methylation of forty-three genes in blood leukocytes, and the activity of three of these genes correlated with an increase in the survival rate of patients. One of the genes, L3MBTL1, is believed to be the source of the inhibition of tumor growth, and its increased expression in this study corresponded to a lower probability of disease recurrence and death (Zeng H. et al., 2012).

As for other cancer rehabilitation programs, including combined ones, their number increases every year. An interested reader can familiarize themselves with these programs in reviews and meta-analyses (Meyer T. J., Mark M. M., 1995; Rehse B., Pukrop R., 2003; Elkins G. et al., 2010; Subnis U. B. et al., 2014). A good example is the one-year program of physical and mental health, developed in 2005 at the University of San Francisco under the guidance of Professor of Medicine Dean Ornish. The peculiarity of this experiment was that, for the duration of this program, ninety-three early-stage prostate cancer patients abandoned classical oncological treatment, choosing an active surveillance strategy. During the year, they adhered to a vegetarian diet enhanced with bio-supplements (antioxidants–vitamins E and C, selenium, and omega-3 polyunsaturated fatty acids), exercised, used stress management techniques (yoga, breathing techniques, visualizations, and progressive relaxation), and once a week met with other patients for communication in a support group. In fact, the program led to a radical change in the lifestyle of patients who had previously lived in a state of chronic stress.

The results of research have become unprecedented for oncology. In forty-one patients who carefully followed the program, there was a significant improvement in health, and the content of tumor markers in their blood decreased. The ability of the blood of these patients to inhibit the growth of typical prostate cancer cells was seven times higher than the ability of the blood of patients who did not change their lifestyle. However, the main thing was that these patients did not have the need for traditional treatment! In his further experiments, Dr. Ornish found that even three months after the end of the program, in these people an increased activity of genes that protect against cancer and a decrease in the activity of genes that promote tumor growth in these people an increased activity of genes maintained. In general, as a result of the program, patients have changed the activity of more than 500 genes (Ornish D. et al., 2008, 2008a).

I have also cited data on programs that promote post-traumatic growth, spiritual awakening, and the search for meaning in the disease. I will write about these programs in more detail in my next book. One such integrative program – "Anticancer" - was created by me and successfully tested at our Expio psycho-oncology center in Kiev (see the appendix). It is important to understand that the task of such a programs is not to "cure the patient," as is commonly understood in orthodox medicine, but to help patients understand the personal and behavioral problems that created a predisposition to cancer. The aim is to eliminate the oncodominant, change the patient's attitude toward himself and his life, to get to know his own capabilities and learn how to use them, to find a new goal in life, in order to awaken and activate his own healing resources. This process of self-knowledge and self-transformation requires a significant amount of effort and involvement of the patient himself.

Chapter 33

Spontaneous Healing: The Result of a Spiritual Transformation?

> Cancer is a blocked spiritual flow.
> Reid Henson,
> *The Healing Journey*

In Chapter 22 we were already introduced to the data on the self-destruction of tumors at early stage. In addition to that observation, more and more data is beginning to appear indicating the existence of spontaneous regression not only of precancerous cells and initial tumors, but also tumors in advanced stages, including those with metastases. Already in 1940, Dr. Ewing noted cases of spontaneous healing of certain tumors in special conditions.

In 1966, T. C. Everson and W. H. Cole published a monograph describing 176 well-documented cases of spontaneous regression (or remission) of cancer. All these cases were published in medical periodicals from 1900 to 1964. The criteria for the diagnosis of spontaneous regression were: a documented histological study of metastases biopsies; x-ray examination; regression of such a metastatic tumor, where therapy is generally considered ineffective.

In 1990 G. B. Challis and H. J. Stam analyzed 564 cases of cancer regression published between 1966 and 1987. Among these cases were most of the known forms of cancer.

In 1993, the Institute of Noetic Sciences (USA) issued an annotated bibliography of spontaneous remission of cancer. This collection of worldwide cases of the disease stopping or its complete cure registered more than 3,500 references from 800 journals in 20 different languages. The data from this study suggests that the phenomenon of spontaneous remission may not be as rare as was previously thought. The impression of its rarity could arise, at least in part, owing to the lack of public disclosure of such cases. (The online version of this book is freely available on the institute's website—see Hirschberg C., O'Regan B., 1993).

33.1. Psychospiritual Mechanisms of Spontaneous Cancer Regression

Most hypotheses about possible mechanisms of spontaneous regression explain this phenomenon through the activation of the immune system due to the influence of some external factors, for example, surgical trauma or parallel infection (Sindelar W. F., Ketcham A. S., 1976; Thomas J. A., Badini M., 2011). However, there is growing evidence that the psyche can be the mysterious link that leads to spontaneous remissions. As early as 1954, Dr. Louise Rose wrote: "Accumulating evidence of body-mind relationship constantly reveals new psycho-physiological rationale in 'cures' hitherto inexplicable." At about the same time Carl Jung (2015) claimed: "Just as carcinoma can develop for psychic reasons, it can also disappear for psychic reasons. Such cases are well authenticated."

Today, this is confirmed by clinical observations on positive psychological changes in patients shortly before remission, as well as by results of psychotherapy, hypnosis, meditation, visualization methods that are increasingly used in psycho-oncological practice (Meares A., 1978, 1980; Simonton C. et al., 1995; Weinstock C., 1983; Schwarz R., Heim M., 2000; Schilder J. N. et al., 2004; Kent J. et al., 1989).

The role of central nervous system in spontaneous healing is confirmed by some animal experiments already described. Here is another example: scientists caused an initial skin cancer in mice by using high doses of ultraviolet radiation. If the exposure was stopped, 50% of cases, on average, resulted in the spontaneous regression of tumors. But if irradiation was carried out under chronic stress, then no regression occurred (Saul A. N. et al., 2005).

C. Hirshberg and M. I. Barasch (1995) note that behind the dry medical reports of spontaneous remission cases, describing such details as age, physical condition, diagnosis, and treatment, it is impossible to see the person him/herself, to understand his or her character and those personality features that may in fact play a vital role in his or her healing.

Researchers from the Helen Dowling Institute of Psycho-Oncology (Denmark) studied the psychological mechanisms that could contribute to the occurrence of spontaneous regression of histologically confirmed tumors of various origins in eleven patients. To do this, the authors retrospectively studied what happened to these patients before the first signs of their clinical improvement. As it turned out, shortly before the regression of the tumor a situation arose in each patient's life associated with negative experiences or unsatisfactory activity. In order to counteract the unbearable, abusive behavior of other people or another unusual negative event, a nonstandard adaptation reaction developed in patients. As a result, they had significantly activated syntonic reactions (built on values, ideas, and feelings that are perceived as meaningful and acceptable to the consciousness) (Schilder J. N. et al. 2004).

It is possible that these patients were able to, for the first time, fully respond to repressed negative emotions associated with "suffocating" experiences in terms of Tom Laughlin, and to initiate personal changes. An example of such healing is the clinical case described by Ceril Hirshberg and Mark Ian Barasch (1995). A fifty-two-year-old woman had carcinoma of the uterus (originating near or in the cervix). It spread to the intestine and her death was expected within weeks; however, before this happened, her much-hated husband suddenly died. She entered unexpected remission and a year and a half later was still entirely well.

Scientists from California and Denmark have come to the conclusion that surviving metastatic cancer and its spontaneous remission are likely to result from the process of personality development. This allows patients to receive a degree of proximity, intimacy, and free sexuality in relationships that they have always dreamed of, but never had before. Closeness and intimate attachment to a partner, according to researchers, is the most important factor in improving the quality of patients' lives, along with the emergence of a positive attitude toward oneself, to other people, and to life in general (Levenson F. B. et al., 2009).

When such changes are the result of the work of psycho-oncologists, we can call it an ultimate post-traumatic growth, or directed cancer regression. An example is the case of Alice Epstein (1989), who suffered from a hypernephroma that had metastasized to both lungs. She was receiving psychotherapy on a daily basis and manifested a major personality transformation, so her cancer-prone personality attributes ameliorated. During a few months of therapy, her tumors began to shrink, and she was completely free of the disease in less than a year.

Dr. Søren Ventegodt, along with his colleagues (2004c, 2005), argues: it is the restoration of a person's life goal and character that is able to activate health reserves and lead to this kind of cure for cancer, which is commonly called "spontaneous." This can be called existential healing—not the local treatment of some tissue, but the healing of the individual as a whole, giving him or her far more resources, love, and knowledge of his or her own needs and desires. By releasing negative attitudes and beliefs, a person returns to a more responsible position in life and achieves a significant improvement in their quality of life. Such a holistic approach has already proven its effectiveness: the author helped two patients to fully recover from cancer without medical therapy.

However, even more significant in the phenomenon of spontaneous regression can be spiritual awakening. A person's ability to heal from bodily ailments in the process of spiritual transformation caused by an existential or personal crisis was first described by psychoanalysts who were developing a psychosomatic medicine in the middle of the last century. This phenomenon was given the name "kairos," which in Greek means the exact or critical time, or an opportunity (it is also the name of the God of Chance). In existential psychology, kairos is a critical moment for an individual to take a life-changing decision regarding her own life, when her values, meanings, and personality as a whole change in the most radical, fateful way (Verbitskiy A. A., 2013).

Paul Tillich (1964), a well-known theologian and existentialist philosopher, considers kairos as a moment of fullness of time, a flash, when the Eternal breaks into the temporary. Such an intervention is usually called a miracle or a revelation, something that falls out of the chain of cause and effect. The philosopher emphasizes that these moments need to be heeded, for God turns to us in them. When applied to medicine, kairos is a turning point in illness, a person's awareness of his problems, and a decision to change his life (Booth G., 1969; Kelman H., 1969). It is kairos, which has analogs in many spiritual traditions, that leads, as G. R. Slater (1982) believes, to spontaneous remission in cancer.

Carl Simonton writes that contact with our spiritual essence provides us with a resource that cannot be obtained using the traditional psychological approach. It enables us to access healing powers that exceed our imaginary limits by far. And it is possible to learn how to bring these forces into our lives. Simonton's patient and coauthor Reid Henson confirms:

> Once I invited the spiritual aspect of me into the [cancer] problem, I found that Spirit can transform the human mind. It was only then that I realized I did not have to figure out all aspects of my illness in order to get well. At this point, my approach shifted from mental analysis toward developing trust in the spiritual dimension (Simonton O. C., Henson R. M., 1992).

C. Hirshberg and M. Barasch (1995), who studied cases of spontaneous cancer regression, have seen that the healing system may be activated by a strong emotional charge, by the power of ceremony, or by the stimulus of expectant faith. They also found that spectacular healing can be internally generated by powerful beliefs, and many of these people told about an experience of a divine presence.

In his bestseller *Spontaneous healing* (2000), Dr. Andrew Weil attributes a great role to mental and spiritual transformation. He cites the experience of Japanese survivor Shin Terayama that preceded his recovery: "I was just so happy to be alive. I saw the sun as God. When I came back down to my apartment, I saw auras around all my family members. I thought everyone was God."

Danish scientist Ulrik Dige, in the book *Cancer Miracles* (2000), published more than forty cases of spontaneous healing. According to him, two thirds of these patients experienced a spiritual awakening before healing. C. Weinstock (1983) describes eighteen cases of spontaneous regression of cancer in which patients experienced significant psychosocial changes one to eight weeks before the manifestation of the phenomenon: they came out of depression and found meaning in life.

An excellent illustration of the role of spiritual awakening in spontaneous healing is the story of Anita Moorjani (2012), which I have already mentioned several times. She lived an ordinary life in Hong Kong, had a happy family and a successful career in business, until one day she was diagnosed with lymphoma. After four years of struggling for life and testing different ways of healing, her illness reached stage four, and Anita was admitted into the hospital. While in a coma, she had an amazing experience of consciousness leaving the body and visiting her loved ones, as well as being present during the conversations of physicians in other rooms. The details of these conversations were confirmed after she awoke from the coma. But the most important thing is that she visited the "other world," the spiritual dimension, where the truth about the causes of her illness and the laws of the universe were revealed to her.

Anita was given the possibility to return to her body, almost destroyed by cancer, and then in an incredible way to be healed within a week with the help of a force which she called "infinite love." Here is what she writes about her healing:

> I understood that my body is only a reflection of my internal state. If my inner self were aware of its greatness and connection with all-that-is, my body would soon reflect that and heal rapidly.... My healing wasn't so much born from a shift in my state of mind or beliefs as it was from finally allowing my true spirit to shine through.

Anita described her experience of comprehending inner strength, as well as knowledge gained beyond the earthly life, in her books. She believes that it was only through illness that she was able to wake up from the dream she had been in during her entire life:

> My soul was finally realizing its true magnificence. And in doing so, it was expanding beyond my body and this physical world. ... All I ever had to do was to be myself, without judgment or feeling that I was flawed. At the same time I understood that at the core, our essence is made of pure love.

In fact, the near-death experience enabled Anita to fully unlock the potential of her Essence, which became the most effective means of healing.

Researchers at Erasmus University in Rotterdam studied seven cases of spontaneous cancer regression. They found that prior to recovery these patients made a transition from dependence and helplessness to full or increased autonomy, and also experienced a more or less radical existential shift in their worldviews. The authors of the study, as well as scientists from the Institute of Noetic Sciences and Norwegian researchers, came to the following conclusion: the phenomenon of spontaneous cancer regression is more common than it is considered to be officially (Van Baalen D. C. et al., 1987). Dr. Paul Roud (1989) conducted interviews with nine patients who had survived cancer despite the fact that the official medical forecast gave them no more than a 25% survival probability. For four of them, the chances were less than 0.1%. Dr. Roud determined that all these patients had common features: assuming responsibility for the occurrence and outcome of the disease and the quality of their life, letting go of fears and worries, changes in communication style, recognition of the importance of close relationships and support, more independent behavior, and a strong desire to live.

People who had a spontaneous remission,

> accept the diagnosis but reject the prognosis, they make decisions according to their own particular belief systems and understandings; there is at least one special healing relationship with a loved one, a health professional, a friend, a support group, or a therapist; they get in touch with unexpressed emotions, they rediscover creativity, a purpose in life, a sense of worth, a reason to be on this planet, a feeling of fulfillment; they transform their lives, careers, cities, marriages (Hirshberg C., Barasch M. I., 1995).

Scientists from the Fukuoka University School of Medicine (Japan) analyzed five cases of spontaneous remission in cancer patients from the psychosomatic point of view. They found that the reason behind the full activation of their innate self-recuperative potentials was that they were able to get rid of anxious and depressive reactions and underwent a dramatic change in their life views. Their religious faith, a positive change in their environment, and possibly a nature of Oriental thought provided them with significant support and encouragement. In three of these people an unchanged or elevated immunity was observed, while usually this is lowered in cancer patients (Ikemi Y. et al., 1975).

The story of Sir Francis Chichester (2012), an English yachtsman, is a vivid example of spontaneous healing that followed the acceptance of full responsibility for his life and the transition to full autonomy. Before the disease, he made several single round-the-world voyages. When he was diagnosed with lung cancer, Chichester refused the proposed lung removal surgery and went on another single round-the-world trip on a yacht, although the doctors gave him a maximum of one month's life. Perhaps, he initially simply wanted to die on his beloved sea, but in the end Francis returned after his journey without any signs of illness, believing that health is determined mainly by the mental state of a person.

A survey of forty-five people who experienced spontaneous remission of cancer revealed the following factors that were of primary importance in their healing (in decreasing order of frequency of mention): faith in recovery, fighting spirit, acceptance of the disease, seeing the disease as a challenge, reviving the will to live, taking responsibility for illness and its outcome, positive emotions, religious faith, a sense of new meaning, a change in habits and behavior, a sense of control over what is happening, a change in lifestyle, self-care, social support. The main activities used by these people for recovery were: prayer, meditation, physical exercises, guided visualization, walking, music and singing, stress reduction techniques. The authors (Hirshberg C., Barasch M. I., 1995) tell the story of one of the respondents:

"I thought, well, if I only have months to live, I would be completely crazy to just do what society or my parents want from me. It's no longer necessary do things I hate; it is necessary I do things I love." What followed was an overnight transformation. She had been miserable; now "I felt very happy within me, laughing a lot." She had been afraid of meeting people. Suddenly, she says, "I felt connected to people for the first time in my life, like a dream coming true." Whereas she had been silent, now she "was talking very much, telling my girlfriends and my boyfriend I was convinced I didn't have to die. And they told me, 'Whatever your decision is, we will stay behind you'. They believed in me. And we developed a deep trust. Everything I sent to them, they sent back to me, and that made me stronger.

These observations are confirmed by Belarusian psycho-oncologist K. V. Yatskevich (2007): "Spiritual evolution is the basis for an effective cancer cure," and the main factor of healing is "the unbending intent of a person to heal. ... Without the patient him/herself participating in the treatment, without his dedication and hard work, no method of treatment, nor any healer, will help to cope with this ailment." A similar opinion is expressed by Dr. A. Osipova (2014): "No one can cure anyone—neither the best doctor, nor the most wonderful medicine. The decision about recovery must be made by the patient themselves."

In the book cited above, T. C. Everson and W. H. Cole (1966) give an example of a patient with pancreatic cancer in an inoperable stage (the tumor was three times the size of the gland itself). Being a deeply religious believer and following the instructions of her spiritual mentors, the patient began intensive prayers for the intercession of higher powers. Within a month, her condition improved so much that the patient was able to go to work. After her death in seven years from another cause (pulmonary embolism), it was revealed that there were no traces of cancer in her pancreas.

Psychological and spiritual development can reverse the course of the disease, Dr. Bernie Siegel (1998) is convinced:

It's as though cancer's energy is channeled into self-discovery, and the tumor is attacked by the immune system. The tumor is not an estranged and unnecessary part. It's almost as though the individual is reborn and rejects the old self, and its disease, thereby becoming able to identify the tumor as something distinct and separate from the new self.

According to Dr. J. Kent and his colleagues (1989), who have investigated spontaneous healing cases, faith, coping style, and emotions, through the modulation of immune functions, may play a role in the mechanisms of this phenomenon.

In addition to the activation of the immune system, another biological mechanism of tumor regression can be the activation of apoptosis—the genetic mechanism of cell death, which we discussed in Chapter 23.2. According to Søren Ventegodt and colleagues (2004, 2004a), the ability of tissues to engage in "metamorphosis" remains accessible in humans even after the end of the period of embryonic development, but resides in an inactive state. However, under certain conditions, especially spiritual awakening and the restoration of the meaning of life, the psyche is able to activate this process again. The authors describes how, in the process of holistic therapy (short-term psychodynamic therapy, supplemented by body-oriented therapy), the tumor size in the breast of the patient decreased by half within a few hours.

Other scientists suggest that spiritual experience can activate an organism's "sleeping" healing potential (*i.e., actually, cause kairos—V. M.*) according to mechanisms similar to the placebo effect (we were introduced to this in Chapter 28, where the outstanding example of Mr. Wright's remission and relapse was described). "Placebo" can be defined as anything that causes the meaning response, i.e. as the physiological or psychological effects of subjective meaning in the origins or treatment (Moerman D. E., Jonas W. B., 2002). N. B. Kohls and his coauthors (2011) expand this understanding by involving the concept of spirituality and defining the placebo as the "existential meaning response." Thus, any phenomenon or event that can result in significant spiritual experiences can activate specific neuro-psycho-physiological reactions in the body that affect the immune and endocrine systems. Such a mechanism has even received a special name—"neurosprituality" (D'Aquili E., Newberg A., 2002).

As for the placebo, it is important to note that this effect of the mind manifests not only with the use of placebo drugs, but also with various other medical manipulations. Henry Beecher (1961) describes an experiment when a number of patients suffering from heart failure, instead of a real coronary artery bypass surgery,[1] got a sham operation, which was a similar skin incision near the sternum, followed by suturing. After "surgery," these patients experienced the same significant reduction in the intensity of heart pain and improvement in the function of the heart muscle as the patients that were actually operated on. A similar result was obtained by Dr. Bruce Moseley and his colleagues (2002) in simulating a surgery for osteoarthritis (inflammation of the knee joint): the improvement in the condition of the knees of the group of such patients was almost the same as in those who actually had the surgery.

Ian Gawler (1984) tells the story of an illiterate country guy who had throat cancer. Upon referring the patient to one of the largest cancer clinics in the USA, the local doctor said that there he would be prescribed a new, very effective course of radiation therapy that could cure him immediately. When the patient arrived at the clinic, during the general examination a thermometer was placed in his mouth. At that moment, the "reverent" expression on the patient's face showed the doctor that the guy took the thermometer for a new wonderful method of radiotherapy. The doctor probably decided to conduct a placebo

---

[1] Coronary bypass surgery is an operation that allows the restoration of blood flow in the arteries of the heart by connecting a shunt—a link from the another blood vessel.

experiment and therefore arranged for the patient to have several sessions of such "treatment." As a result, the patient was completely healed.

This is how one of the functions of our powerful mind manifests—the state of faith, in particular, faith in the power of medicine. And faith, whatever it is, is already a spiritual phenomenon, even if a person does not understand this.

33.2. Psychic Traumas and Inner Conflicts Block Spiritual Growth and the Healing Process

Despite the obvious connection between spiritual awakening and spontaneous remission, it should be noted that one's previous spiritual experience is not always capable of protecting one from cancer. There are many cases when this disease has arisen, both in famous spiritual and religious teachers and in ordinary practitioners. In my psychotherapeutic practice, I repeatedly encountered cases when cancer or another serious disease developed in people who led a healthy and seemingly spiritual lifestyle, practiced yoga, Qigong or other developmental systems, or even conducted teaching seminars themselves. For such people, a serious illness, especially cancer, becomes doubly distressing, because they cannot find an answer to the question "out of all people, why is it happening to me?"

Of course, it matters whether such a person is actually a serious practitioner, or is just playing at spirituality in conformance with the "new-age" fashion, to fit in with friends, or to maintain a positive self-image.

These considerations are supported by data from research that studies the influence of the type of religiosity on the sense of well-being of cancer patients. Those who experienced religion as an integral part of the inner world coped with the stress of illness much better, had a more conscious sense of life and a sense of general well-being than those whose faith had an outward orientation—who were following religion as a way of obtaining social and/or emotional support or status (Acklin M. W. et al., 1983).

Reginald Ray (2002), a college teacher, Buddhist researcher and practitioner, describes his encounter with a cancer diagnosis:

> I realized how I had wasted so much of my life. I became aware that I had spent far too much of my time doing things that were reflections of how I and others thought I should act but were not expressions of who I really was. ... And though I followed a spiritual path, I did so to often by rote and acted as if I had all the time in the world.

At the same time, my practical experience shows that the more important causes of illness in people that are engaged in spiritual practices are the same unprocessed psychic traumas or intrapersonal conflicts, especially those that arose during childhood. Even in the absence of an existential crisis in these people, the accumulated strength of the pathogenic effects of these problems can create oncogenic distress, almost never acknowledged. Also, according to Frederick Levenson (1985),

> the puzzling questions for researchers in this field can be answered by looking at the intangible (emotional and life event) carcinogens. These intangibles are intangible only because we choose to ignore what we cannot observe and understand simply and directly. The major carcinogen for all of us is an aberrant processing of all irritants.

Jan Bastiaans (1982) writes that the difficulty of eliminating the psychosomatic symptom is attributed to both the severity of the narcissistic defense processes and the deeply imprinted personal traumatic experiences. Extremely unpleasant feelings and affects associated with such psychic trauma are repressed or split off with such intensity that it is possible to achieve the disappearance of symptoms only through the complete liberation of the "trapped" experiences.

For many people spiritual practices become merely a way of avoiding the difficulties life presents them with, soothing emotional tensions, and finding ways to satisfy their material needs. John Welwood (2000) calls such behavior a "spiritual bypass." Such avoidance of reality leads to the situation where behind the "spiritual facade" there are hidden psychological problems that have not been processed, and are repressed into "the Shadow," causing internal conflicts with all their dysfunctional consequences (Cashwell C. S. et al., 2004).

Tom Laughlin (1999) argues that when the conflict is hidden in a person's subconscious, where the conscious part of his mind cannot reach, the situation becomes extremely dangerous. It leads to the deadly variant of subconscious depression and creates a predisposition to cancer. "The pain, agony, fear, resentment, anger and rage work their deadly poison on the body by festering unnoticed day after day, year after year in this invisible part of the patient's personality," the author writes. As a result, whatever alternative therapies are used by a cancer patient, in whatever support or development groups he would participate—if he does not go through an effective psychotherapeutic study of the hidden psychological factors underlying his illness, the chances of healing are extremely small. Psycho-oncologists Linda Carlson and Michael Speca (2011) point out that healing from emotional pain is central to our growth as human beings. Without the reconciliation with these "dark" emotions in our life, healing is not possible.

Let me recall the conclusion that was reached by German scientists stating that future cancer patients often do not realize the social pressure they are experiencing, which leads to "subdued depression" (Grossarth-Maticek R. et al., 1982), and the observations of Dr. Gabor Maté (2003) revealing that in most cases of breast cancer, stress is hidden and flows chronically. Such stresses are associated with childhood experiences, early emotional programming, and unconscious psychological styles of coping with adversity. Also, Lydia

Temoshok (1987), the author of the "C" type personality concept, as well as Russian researchers (Bukhtoyarov O. V., Arkhangelskiy A. E., 2008), note that the chronic hopelessness and helplessness of people prone to cancer may not be realized by them.

A prominent Soviet and Russian psychiatrist and psychotherapist, Professor B. D. Karvasarskiy (1990; 2008), wrote that the pathogenicity of intrapersonal conflict under psychosomatic diseases is that it occurs at an unconscious level. The conflict is not realized, and therefore not controlled. A similar opinion is expressed by Søren Ventegodt and colleagues (2005): old traumas, such as, for example, rape during childhood, are often deeply repressed. Therefore, they cannot rise to the surface of consciousness without the help and serious support of a caring and attentive psychotherapist, who has established a close and trusting relationship with the patient. Research conducted by psychologists at the University of Seville (Spain) showed that in the hypnotic state, the patients recounted 9.8 times more traumatic life events than in the waking state (Almeida-Marques F. X. D. et al., 2018).

A telling example is that of psychotherapist Gerald Harris (2005), who becomes ill with bladder cancer after the death (also from cancer) of a very close friend of his. Upon analyzing the psychological causes that led to the disease in his own case, Harris writes that the death of a friend reactivated in him the emotional trauma of rejection from very early childhood and "opened up a door which had been firmly shut" since that time. The illness has revealed a significant amount of emotion that he has suppressed since childhood, and the psychotherapist had to work a lot on himself to correct some very early unconscious beliefs. They existed in his subconscious mind and, despite being completely contrary to his conscious notions, they had become a part of his personality.

The reason for such a deep repression of the conflict may be associated with the type of attachment disorder that has arisen in childhood. According to the research done by M. Mikulincer and I. Orbakh (1995), individuals with an avoidant type demonstrate stronger defense and anxiety when trying to process the negative experiences from childhood in therapy. They are also less able to recall these experiences than people with other types of attachment.

Therefore, I retain a calm understanding of the emotional objections of some of my cancer patients at the beginning of their therapy. Being unable to personally remember some repressed stresses or even psychic traumas, especially from childhood, many were convinced that these events never happened, until they encountered them during a trance treatment session.

For example, we investigated the cause of the failures of one of my patients who was trying, but without much success, to develop self-love. The following is what she realized:

This session showed me that I can't build a heavenly castle of self-love at the top of a volcano filled with emotions of anger, anxiety, and discontent. And then I remembered a dream I had a few weeks ago. In it, I was going to move to live in a wonderful warm place near the sea, but a few meters from my future home there was a volcano with a big jam on the top, ready to explode at any moment. It turns out that my subconscious sent me signals, but I did not hear them!

A good illustration of the above are also the stories of some well-known New Age leaders and best-selling authors—Barbel Mohr, Louise Hay, and Brandon Bays. All of these women were active and well-known spiritual "seekers" before the onset of cancer. For about fifteen years, Barbel Mohr conducted seminars on the topic of joy of life and positive thinking, has published many books on self-help and healing, including a bestseller translated into fourteen languages (Mohr B., 2001). Louise Hay has been practicing meditation and therapy with affirmations for almost a decade. She has been a popular seminar leader on how positive thinking can change the body. At the onset of her disease, Brandon Bays was an expert in spiritual and bodily health, an NLP practitioner for twelve years.

Mohr was diagnosed with breast cancer, Hay and Bays with uterine cancer. Barbel Mohr believed that a person's responsibility for his illness was limited to his lifestyle (and she herself was an example of a healthy lifestyle), while in truth, ancestral traumas play a major role in the disease. Maybe that's why she did not deeply investigate her own traumas? In addition, as she admitted herself in one of her books—*The Miracle of Self-Love* (Mohr B., Mohr M., 2012)—it was difficult for her to find time to meet her needs, which makes me doubt in her real love for herself. As a result, Barbel died within a year after being diagnosed with the disease, disappointing thousands of her readers. In a conversation with me, one of my foreign patients commented on her death: "I came to the conclusion that no matter how many positive thoughts were in my head, the soul has its own intentions when something oppresses it."

Louise Hay (1984), in search of a healing path, found the cause of her disease in the negative experiences of her childhood, which were cruel treatment and rape. Brandon Bays (2012), upon exploring her subconscious, also came face to face with her psychic trauma from childhood—the death of her sister and how the way her parents treated her was negatively impacted following this tragedy:

> Unexpected emotions that I had buried and long since forgotten seemed to be arising, and the true expression of how I felt at the time seemed to be surfacing. I hadn't realized how intensely I had felt at the time. I'd been too successful, even then, at masking my true emotions by putting on a brave face.

Both of these women realized the need for forgiveness and letting go of their old grievances to make room for liberation from long-standing internal conflict and for healing. Having freed themselves from the traumas of the past, rejecting surgery, and actively using alternative treatment, healthy eating, meditation, and purification, Louise Hay claimed to be healed within six months; Brandon Bays—within two months. As a result, both former patients not only experienced post-traumatic growth, but also achieved significant personal and spiritual progress, wrote books that became international bestsellers, and created healing systems that help thousands of people around the world.

In her book (2012) Brandon shares:

> It occurred to me that all along I had thought this tumor was clinging to me, when in fact I had been clinging to it—protecting myself from the memory and painful feelings stored there. ... It seemed as if I had literally put the painful memory into a package, and put a lid on it. Then the cells had grown and grown to keep the old memory encapsulated, protecting me from having to face it over the years.

Thus, although the previous experience of self-development and self-actualization did not protect all these women from cancer, for two of them their previous experience enabled a deeper and more effective understanding of the causes of the disease and healing from past traumas, which became the basis for launching the process of spontaneous tumor regression.

C. Simonton and colleagues (1978) confirm that when the basic attitudes that have been blocking the normal course of life are discovered and destroyed, life once again begins to flow quietly and without hindrance. Then the vital energy that restores the healthy functioning of the human natural defense mechanism comes back.

It can be concluded that in the phenomenon of spontaneous cancer regression the leading role is played by kairos—awakening from the sleep of a false personality. It contributes to the liberation from the main psychic traumas and intrapersonal conflicts ("suffocating factors"), with subsequent post-traumatic growth, fundamental personality changes, and spiritual transformation, referred to as the discovery of Essence.

Conclusion

Based on the studies and observations considered in this part, it clearly follows that the outcome of cancer, just like its occurrence, mostly depends on the patient's mental state, ability to manage stress, and level of spiritual development.

We have seen that the numerous negative consequences of diagnosis and treatment of oncological diseases, from psychological disorders to relapses and psychogenic death, are due to the underestimation of the enormous harm to health that is the result of the patient's distress during this period.

The physical and chemical treatment of a tumor affects merely the tip of that iceberg which is the cancer. Therefore, the passage through the standard medical treatment is only the first step in the struggle with disease and return to health. Upon leaving the hospital, most patients are left alone with their fear of cancer, not knowing what to do, not receiving specialized psychological help, being in a state of tension in waiting for the return of the disease. It is not surprising that such stress complicates post-treatment rehabilitation, causes pain, fatigue, sleep disorders, anxiety, depression, and thus lowers these patients' quality of life.

Even in such a developed country as the UK, 60% of surviving patients have unmet physical or psychological needs, more than 33% experience problems with personal relationships or job, or have difficulty in performing household duties, and more than 90% experience financial losses (Burton C., 2010). And what is there to say about the post-Soviet countries, where even psycho-oncology is a new thing?

Such a powerful negative impact of stress on a sick person is primarily a social problem. Nobody teaches us how to behave during a period of illness, especially a life-threatening one. We do not know what to do when we face a death, either our own or that of someone close, because we don't want to even think about it during periods of well-being. Coping with the disease and with the situation of death (as well as with the difficulties of life) is not taught in our schools, although these are the main issues of human life. In this way we are implicitly implanting into the minds of children the idea that death cannot happen to them, that illness and death are not important, since there is no place for them in education. Because of this, generation after generation find themselves in situations where fear and confusion during illness, as well as ignorance of their internal reserves, create an unnecessary distress that significantly complicates treatment or even blocks it.

As a result, a sick person experiences a deep existential crisis, where he or she is forced to look for a way out almost alone, weakly understanding the direction of movement. And although a certain number of patients, as we saw above, overcome the crisis, heal, and transform their lives, the majority of patients (and not only oncological) who are not as strong in their spirit cannot find a way out of the situation and therefore die, in fact, because of their own ignorance and the insolvency of society.

What is equally surprising and regrettable is the lack of extensive study and introduction into preventive medicine of the invaluable experience of those who have overcome the crisis, experienced kairos, and recovered, for cases of remarkable recovery are

> inspiring human sagas, priceless raw material, sources of information and hope, and new clues to the healing process. But they are also an impetus and, in some way, a blueprint for the remarkable recovery of the medical system itself (Hirshberg C., Barasch M. I., 1995).

As Vladimir Kozlov (2015) writes, the value of people who have lived through a deep crisis is extremely great not only for the spiritual, but also for the social and material life of society. The experience of a personal crisis often has such a quality, which can become an invaluable gift of insight for hundreds of thousands of people.

According to the scientist, the crisis is an evolutionary challenge, the last mechanism of natural selection of the most powerful and strong personalities in the struggle for social survival. Although it comes as an unwelcome guest, its experience leads to the utmost efficiency of a person as a carrier of human qualities, and is able to uncover the potential for development hidden in the human psyche. This crisis can lead to such a reconstruction of the psyche, personality, and consciousness, which is necessary for the evolution of this person and mankind as a whole.

Bernie Siegel (1998) explains that people who managed to get ahead of their ailment and live as full a life as possible, give this invaluable gift to those close to them—to relatives, friends, physicians. We can learn from them not only how to defeat a disease, but also how to live in the broad sense of the word, thus understand what healing really means.

Such people who have healed themselves share their experiences with other patients, showing them the path to healing through the transformation of their lives. The following are titles of some of the books they wrote: *Cancer Was My Lifecoach: A 10 Step Survivor's Handbook* (Beaufort J. L., 2015), *Cancer My Personal Story: Pulling the positives out of the negatives* (Nelson J. D., 2015), *Cancer: The Best Gift of My Life* (Rudoy Y., 2016), *Cancer is My Teacher* (O'Donnell L., 2014), *The Cancer Whisperer: How to let cancer heal your life* (Sabbage S., 2016), and others.

From these positions, cancer is not only an instrument of evolutionary "screening out" of those who could not cope with it, as I mentioned above, but also an instrument of the evolutionary development of humanity. After all, as Tom Laughlin insightfully writes, what turns out to be "suffocated" in a cancer patient is his or her Essence, and the Essence is the embodiment of God, of the Creator. Therefore, when we help patients to realize the fact that they have a unique role in the transformation of God within themselves, a role that no one else can play better, then they will finally "understand that the answer to the question 'Why me?' is Because you were called. ... In having been called by their cancer, they now choose to make the transformation of this Greater Personality (*the Essence—V. M.*) within their life work, they will understand the psychology behind the words, 'Many are called, and few are chosen'" (Laughlin, 1999).

"And then—long live the crisis," proclaims Vladimir Kozlov (2015), because it is the crisis that gives birth to a new person that is less conflicted, free from the past, less attached to his conditions and herd mentality, to a person that is more healthy and holistic; "It is the crisis that creates all that is best in the human."

We see this result in those cancer patients who have experienced post-traumatic growth and achieved sustained remission or complete healing. The crisis of the deadly disease transforms their life and leads to personal evolution, which is usually impossible without spiritual growth and involvement in helping other people, that is, without the evolution of society. The disease removes a person from an existential vacuum and helps him answer the question about the meaning of life, finding it in spiritual development and unfolding the hidden potential.

In light of the above, a logical question arises: why do so many people have to suffer and go through serious illnesses in order to reach their potential and develop, when this can be achieved by changing social standards and the educational system?

Upon reflecting in this same direction, Professor V. D. Troshin rightly argues that the main goal of spiritual and moral upbringing, education, and rehabilitation is a systematic and purposeful impact on human consciousness and behavior through the introduction of concepts, principles, hygienic attitudes, personality values, the formation of a healthy lifestyle, i.e. promotion of behavior that contributes to the preservation and strengthening of health.

Without effective spiritual and moral education as a preventative measure against disease, it is impossible to achieve significant success in the improving of national health. Spiritual aspects of a healthy lifestyle (spiritual hygiene) should be developed by representatives of various disciplines, and in the medicine of the future these aspects should be central to human activities and in the organization of healing and health systems (Troshin V. D., 2009).

Summing Up

It turns out that there are no incurable diseases or unsolvable problems
but a lack of knowledge, a lack of
understanding of the reasons for their occurrence,
lack of knowledge of remedies and of methods of eliminating
the causes of these problems and diseases.
Vladimir Vernadskiy,
Prominent scientist, first president
of the Academy of Sciences of Ukraine

The materials on the causes of cancer that have been reviewed in this book, from an interdisciplinary position that covers psychology, oncology, physiology, stressology, spirituality, and molecular biology, lead to an unequivocal conclusion that this pathology has a psychosomatic nature, and therefore that the central role in cancer is played by the mind—hence the book's title: *Carcinogenic Mind*.

In 1962, an eminent Ukrainian oncologist and academician, Rostislav Kavetskiy, clear-sightedly wrote:

... there is no doubt that the tumor [-provoking] factor can realize its action, just as the tumor cell that has emerged is able to manifest its properties, only under certain conditions—conditions of the whole organism.

The totality of the data analyzed in this book suggests that these "certain conditions" are chronic psychophysiological distress generated by an imbalance of mind. Moreover, the conclusion itself suggests that oncological diseases develop in general on the same universal diathesis–stress mechanisms as any other pathology, be it somatic or mental.

Summarizing, we can briefly describe the process of cancer development as follows.

Cancer in humans is a multi-step time process that is formed sequentially at the levels of the mind, brain, and body (end organ or system). This process begins in the early stages of ontogenesis with the formation of a nonspecific psychosomatic predisposition (diathesis) due to a different combination of the five main factors:

1. Epigenetic and genetic heredity that increases one's vulnerability to stress;

2. Dysfunctions of a fetus' nervous, endocrine, and immune systems due to stress experienced by the mother during pregnancy, and/or her negative attitude to the fetus and thoughts about abortion;

3. The psycho-traumatic experiences of the child during childbirth when delivery is complicated;

4. The psycho-traumatic experiences and disorders of the child's attachment to the parents in a dysfunctional family in the postpartum period (with the ongoing imbalance of the psycho-physiological systems);

5. The formation of a specific psychosomatic type of "C" personality, where the main features (in various proportions) are: avoidance of expressing negative emotions, psychological infantilism, avoidance of conflicts, dependence and subordination, orientation to the interests of other people and not their own ("psychological masochism").

The number of these factors and the way that they are combined in a child, along with their intensity, defines the age at which cancer will occur: the greater the strength of these factors, the earlier the disease will manifest.

If one even safely overcame the stresses of childhood, that is, the number and intensity of the predisposing factors did not exceed the reserve of one's psychophysiological "strength," then in adulthood it will be subjected to testing by provocation factors. By this time, the type "C" personality is usually formed and this creates difficulties in overcoming a new stress. Often, this personality is burdened by a merely vague understanding of the meaning of life (existential vacuum), obsession with the material aspects of life, and excessive attachment to an overvalued subject or object.

Later in life, powerful psycho-traumatic situations, usually based on loss, or on unresolved intrapersonal conflicts that emerged owing to the inability of the person to satisfy his or her own important needs (especially the need for love and free expression of the individuality), act as provoking factors. The result in both cases is the development of chronic psycho-physiological stress, gradually weakening the body's protective reserves, in particular the immune system (on top of the fact that the reserves are already weakened by diathesis factors). This forms the metabolic syndrome and increases the body's sensitivity to the carcinogenic agents of the external environment.

Such a situation can continue sluggishly into old age, when the gradual accumulation of the psychobiological consequences of life stresses leads to a further weakening of protective resources, increased reactivity to new stresses, and high sensitivity to carcinogens. Therefore, it becomes very easy for provoking factors to trigger the cancer process during this period.

At a younger or a mature age, a situation may arise when it is not possible for a person to resolve the psychic trauma(s) and/or satisfy significant needs, especially if the person is in a state of being "suffocated" by relationships in the family or at work (subordinate suppression of individuality). One begins to develop a state of helplessness and hopelessness, leading to depression—mostly unconscious, sometimes clinical. Increased chronic psychophysiological distress, as well as metabolic syndrome, form a precancerous condition.

The persistence over a long period of the situation described gradually leads the individual to experience a psychospiritual crisis, when both the hope for a positive change in life and the desire to continue the former way of life are lost. Thus an avital experience arises. This crisis and avital feelings are often not identified by a person owing to the presence of alexithymia. Therefore, these experiences take place in the subconscious and, as a rule, one is unable to comprehend them as they appear on the external level only as a markedly depressed mood. The systems of immunity, DNA repair, and apoptosis are significantly violated, and inflammation is growing. The loss of the will to live and the unconscious desire to die bring about the appearance of an oncodominant—first in the psyche, and then in the brain as a focus of chronic neurophysiological arousal. It affects the associated organ or system—the target—and initiates in it the transition of precancerous disorders to early-stage cancer.

If, at this moment, a person manages to realize the crisis and/or seek the help of a psychotherapist, resolve a basic conflict, and/or heal a psychic trauma, discover a new meaning for his or her life, and especially achieve spiritual awakening, then the cancer dominant loses its power. The activity of the body's defense systems increases, and the initial tumor can self-degrade or stop in its development. In this case, the individual usually does not even suspect that he or she had cancer.

However, if a way out of the crisis is not found, and the chronic stress continues to develop, then the tumor or systemic oncological disease progresses and manifests at the clinical level. The same happens with the "dormant" primary tumor: if the crisis is not fully resolved, or, if after some time a new crisis or acute distress occurs, then the tumor "awakens" and resumes its growth.

In rare cases during the clinical stage of the disease, the diagnosis of cancer becomes a source of a deep spiritual awakening for the individual and comprehension of the causes of his or her psychological problems. This brings about kairos—spontaneous psycho-spiritual transformation leading to a powerful restoration of the body's defenses and spontaneous healing without medical care, or by using alternative healing methods.

But more often, the psychic traumas of diagnosis and surgery, and of standard medical treatment, result in additional distress, depleting the already weak protective resources of the body. Chemotherapy depresses the immune system. Metastases occur. The psychospiritual crisis is manifesting and deepening, often leading to the rapid progression of the disease and/or psychogenic death. The chances of survival in the absence of specialized psychological assistance are very small.

In the post-clinical period, if the psychospiritual state of the person has not changed (usually the case in the absence of professional help) or has even deteriorated, then hopelessness and depression increase, post-traumatic stress disorder occurs, various psychopathologies develop. Following treatment, the patient usually returns to the same life conditions that often were the source of his or her psychological conflicts or traumas, and, as a rule, resumes the same lifestyle. Chronic stress continues, the body's defense systems are not restored. This results in a relapse.

If a patient requests psychotherapeutic help in time, becomes aware of the psychological causes of his illness, gets rid of psychic traumas and conflicts, begins to engage in self-knowledge, and decisively changes his life, then he has a high chance of achieving the post-traumatic growth and psychospiritual transformation that activate natural healing resources of his body and restore the immune system. This leads to a state of prolonged remission or even complete healing.

Based on the information presented above, it is obvious that the speed of development and progression of cancer depends on the patient's mental state. The more anxious, emotionally closed, and prone to helplessness and depression her character is (that is, the more pronounced the psychosomatic type "C" personality is), the more difficult it is for her to cope with stresses. Hence, the person will suffer more from psychic traumas and conflicts, the state of chronic psycho-physiological stress will be deeper, and the body's defense systems will weaken more. The same factors determine the effectiveness of treatment.

1. A "Roadmap" of the Development and Course of Cancer

Based on the data presented in this book, and also using the concept of the biopsychosocial-spiritual origin of human pathology and its diathesis–stress mechanisms, the models of the multifactorial structure of development of psychosomatic diseases by M. V. Korkina, V. V. Marilov (1998) and D. N. Isaev (2000), synergistic concepts of the formation of psychosomatic and oncological diseases by P. I. Sidorov, I. A. Novikova (2007), P. I. Sidorov, E. P. Sovershaeva (2015), and S. A. Kulakov (2009a), I propose as a hypothesis the following detailed scheme of six successive stages in the development of cancer. Conditionally, each stage is divided into the psychological, social, spiritual, and biological levels of human existence:

Levels of human existence/ Stages of disease	Psychological	Social	Spiritual	Biological

Predisposition	Fetal psychic trauma during unwanted pregnancy, *or/and* The psychic trauma of the newborn child due to complicated childbirth, *or/and* Child's attachment disorders and psychic traumas. Imprinting of maladaptive behavior of parents. Formation of the psychosomatic type of personality with oncogenic accentuation ("type C"). Ineffective coping with the stresses of life. The weakening of the first level of the barrier of mental adaptation.	Psychosoma-togenic family. Family dysfunction.	Violation of the existential safety of the child. Weak or absent spiritual education.	Epigenetic and genetic heredity. Fetal developmental disorders due to maternal stress. Disorders of somatic development. Defects of neuroimmune-endocrinolo-gical interactions, distortion of the hypothalamic-pituitary-adrenal system. Psychosomatic diathesis.

| Provocation | Acute psychic trauma that becomes chronic.

Long time unresolved intrapersonal conflict.

Reactivation of childhood psychic trauma(s).

The effect of stresses accumulation.

Disorder of the second level of the barrier of mental adaptation. | Disharmonious interpersonal relationships.

Lack of self-actualization. | Noogenic neurosis. | State of chronic psycho-physiological distress.

Reduced activity of body's antitumor protection mechanisms, particularly immune and DNA repair systems.

Somatization of affect related to psychic trauma or intrapersonal conflict.

Increased sensitization to carcinogenic agents of the environment. |

Precancerous condition	Clinical or subliminal (unconscious) depression with traits of helplessness and hopelessness. The destruction of the second level of the barrier of mental adaptation.	"Suffocating" relationships. Lack of social support.	Existential vacuum.	Activation of proto-oncogenes and deactivation of suppressor genes. Blocked apoptosis. Inflammatory process. Psychosomatic and precancerous diseases. High sensitization to carcinogenic agents of the environment.
Initialization	Loss of the life goal dominant. Formation of the cancer dominant. Pronounced degree of helplessness and hopelessness. Avital experiences, hidden suicidality.	Disharmony of one's socialization. Reduced quality of life.	Existential crisis. Loss of will to live.	Exceeding the individual's threshold of chronic stress tolerance. Disintegration of the hypothalamic-pituitary-adrenal axis. Transformation of cells into cancerous.

	The destruction of the third level of the barrier of mental adaptation.			
Promotion and progression (Clinical manifestation)	Psychic trauma of diagnosis. Clinical depression. High degree of helplessness and hopelessness.	Loss of social status and relationships ("social inferiority").	Loss of the meaning of life. Suicidal ideas.	Tumor growth ("progressi-on"). Metastases. Disorders of the structure and function of organs and systems. Additional suppression of immunity by tumor.
Outcome and consequences of the disease	Post-traumatic stress disorder. Other psychological disorders. Psychopatholo gy. *or* Post-traumatic growth.	"Social hypochondria". Disability. *or* Social progress.	Deep existential crisis. Suicide. *or* Kairos. Spiritual and personal growth.	Complicati-ons of medical therapy. Relapse. Death (including psychogenic death). *or* Mobilization of immunity. Remission. Spontaneous tumor regression.

This scheme allows psycho-oncologists to analyze in detail the patient's life and development of the illness, determine the role of each of the etiological factors in the overall structure of the disease, their contribution and "proportion" in the corresponding phase of the disease.

2. Clinical Example: Movie Star Audrey Hepburn

As an illustration, let us consider the life and illness story of the famous Hollywood actress, Oscar winner Audrey Hepburn. The idol of hundreds of thousands of fans, a beautiful woman, millionaire, beloved by all her friends for her wonderful character … how could such a woman have lost the joy of life to the point of getting cancer? However, the information contained in a number of biographical books and articles about her life (Paris B., 2001; Hepburn Ferrer S. H., 2003; Spoto D., 2007; River C. E., 2013; Holborn K., 2018), is enough to provide at least a close understanding of the reasons that led her to develop intestinal cancer at the age of 64.

The analysis performed on the base of the scheme above allows us to see a typical picture of the formation of the psychosomatic type "C" personality.

Factors of predisposition

Audrey grew up during World War II, experiencing the stresses associated with it, with fear for her life and the life of her mother, who participated in the work of the Resistance. Her uncle and other relatives were shot for acts of disobedience. She endured the famine of 1944 and as a result developed a number of health problems.

As a child she suffered psychic traumas associated with the conflicts, scandals, and finally the divorce of her parents after her mother left her father. It was aggravated by her believing that it happened because her father was not happy with her. There was also the lack of a feeling of love and recognition from an emotionally cold mother, along with her strictness and domination. Her mother taught her to hold back emotions and think first about others and then about herself, be benevolent even when she wanted to howl, not to allow tears in public or show her grief to others. This resulted in a trait of suppression of emotions and the first signs of depression.

Audrey's desire for her mother's approval and praise taught her to behave in an amiable and tolerable way. As a consequence, Audrey developed psychological infantilism and low self-esteem. Her dominant goal in life was "a reliable marriage," in which the husband was subconsciously expected to be the compensation for the love and reliability that she did not receive from her father and mother. Even when she was a recognized actress, she thought that she acted less well than others, that she was talentless, and absolutely did not deserve people's love and adoration. According to Audrey's son, Sean, "she was a star who could not see her own light."

Factors of provocation

Despite Audrey's success in cinema, she still could not gain her mother's approval, sensing instead her critical and politely cold attitude, even when she was rewarded with an Oscar. This, of course, only increased her inner conflict around not being good enough.

Upon having found her father as an adult, after having dreamt of him for many years, Audrey discovered that he was indifferent to her, her work, and his grandson. What occurred once again was the re-traumatization of the childhood trauma of neglect and abandonment.

Financial stress: despite her successful projects, she was severely short of money. The actress, who caused such delight, lived in an extremely constrained manner.

Audrey felt dependence and subordination in family life. She tried to meet her husband's requirements, as she did during childhood when she strove to satisfy her mother's ideals. This brought about a state of "suffocation" by her obligation to be a public person and make money, by the suppression of the need to be just a wife and housewife, to raise children. This suggests that the profession of an actress was not her true desire, despite all the success that she achieved in this field.

A miscarriage caused the heavy mental trauma, depression, and avital feelings, but finally she was able to give birth.

Despite her dissatisfaction with her first husband, Audrey stayed married long enough in order to make a father available for her son (psychological masochism). When she left the husband, she felt guilty because of her son and experienced heavy depression because of the divorce. We can assume here that an overvaluing of the importance of marriage followed the childhood trauma of her parents' divorce.

In her second marriage, Audrey repeated the same pattern, getting into dependence and subordination again. Her husband's betrayals "confirmed" her perception of herself as "not good enough," not deserving happiness. The powerful psychic trauma of the second divorce aggravated the depression. Also in this period she felt contempt from her film co-star, actor Humphrey Bogart. Audrey resented him, but never expressed her emotions. Chronic stress increased. She discharged it with the help of heavy tobacco smoking (factor of physical provocation). Audrey was deeply disappointed in herself and even hated herself at certain times (development of self-aggression).

Pre-cancer state

According to a her friend, actress Marian Seldes, Audrey was "chronically unhappy," felt constant dissatisfaction with life. Because of the "star disease," an emptiness formed around her, and she felt extremely lonely. In his book, Audrey's son, Sean, writes that his mother often experienced deep sadness, melancholy, which he associated with her negative childhood experiences. Her depression intensified.

Initialization of disease

Avital experiences appeared again, reaching the stage of suicide attempts. It can be assumed that, at this moment, the actress's life goals were dominated by her children, so her suicide attempts were subconsciously not serious enough. But after the children matured and left home, a non-dominant state was probably established, inner emptiness, and it is possible that the cancer dominant was initiated at that moment as a way out of "chronic unhappiness," despite the appearance of a third (civil) marriage in her life.

The emergence of a new life dominant—being an ambassador for UNICEF—filled her non-dominant emptiness for five years. However, frequent meetings with abandoned children who were dying from hunger and thirst undoubtedly reactivated Audrey's own childhood psychic traumas and served as a source of additional distress, which happened to be stronger than the dominant of social activity. Or perhaps this dominant has weakened over time owing to her inability to provide help to all those suffering children she saw.

As a result, the general strength of the accumulated conflicts and psychic traumas resulted in chronic distress, destroyed the third barrier of the actress's mental adaptation, brought her to the stage of depletion of the general adaptation syndrome, significantly weakened the anticancer protection of the body, and activated the oncodominant. Upon reading her biographical sources, I did not find any mention of her requesting psychological help, except for the period when her second husband, a psychiatrist, prescribed her some pharmaceuticals during her depression.

Manifested clinical state

The first abdominal pains appeared in September 1992 during a difficult trip on behalf of UNICEF to Somalia and Kenya. On this trip, Audrey said that she went to hell and back. Following her relatives' insistence in October, diagnostic laporoscopy was performed, which revealed appendix cancer. In early November, surgery was performed to remove the tumor.

Outcome of the disease

Despite the surgery, the cancer cells remaining at the site of the operation continued their rapid growth, spreading to the large intestine and neighboring tissues. This can be attributed to the psychic trauma of the diagnosis, her hopelessness, and loss of the will to live. On January 20, 1993, Audrey died.

As for the target organ of her cancer, the intestine, it could be somatically a "weak link" following the famine she suffered during childhood. On the other hand, symbolically, Audrey probably could "not digest" or "not let out" all those negative emotions that she accumulated as a result of her distresses but could not release.

Was it possible to prevent cancer in Audrey Hepburn using psychotherapy? I am sure that yes, it was—if she had sought help at least a year before the manifestation of the disease. Could it have been possible to prolong her life with psycho-oncological methods after the cancer diagnosing? Undoubtedly, yes, but it is impossible to answer to what extent without having direct contact with the patient. Given the speed of the progression of her disease, it is obvious that her oncodominant was very strong.

As we can see, by using the proposed roadmap, psycho-oncologists and psychotherapists can effectively make a diagnosis and define the extent of psychosocial care for the patient at each stage of the disease from the point of view of integrative medicine, thereby ensuring the maximum possible effectiveness of therapy.

3. Are There Specific Psychological Predisposing Factors for Cancer?

In the process of studying the materials presented in the book, we discovered that cancer arises according to the same general laws as other chronic diseases. In almost every somatic or mental illness, we can find predisposing factors in the form of disorders of children's attachment and/or psychic traumas. They are reflected in personalities and behavioral disorders, the most pathogenic of which is the suppression or repression of negative emotions, particularly anger, anxiety, and fear. Provocation factors in adulthood are also widespread in the form of psychic traumas and/or chronic unresolved conflicts. Often there are premorbid factors in the form of depression, hopelessness, and helplessness, which can cause avital experiences.

This leads us to the fundamental question: are there any unique factors in the psychological mechanisms of cancer that direct psychosomatic imbalances toward cancer? To date, I believe that there are no unique factors, but there is a specific constellation, or combination, of psychosomatic properties of character and ways of responding to stress which together lead to the emergence of an oncodominant:

A. Suppression or repression of negative emotions;

B. Psychological masochistic sacrificing;

C. The overvalue of the lost subject or object of attachment (that was the life goal dominant) and/or the inability to realize one's talents and abilities, to live one's desired life, "to be what I really am" (described as the factors of "suffocation" by Tom Laughlin (1999), "submissive despondency" by R. Grossarth-Maticek et al. (1982) and "unsung song of life" by Lawrence LeShan (1989));

D. Subliminal (unconscious) depressive hopelessness;

E. Avital experiences (hidden suicidality).

However, even the combination of these factors causes a carcinogenic effect only in the presence of non-specific predisposing factors, discussed in the second part of the book. Hence, there is a combined, cumulative effect of all factors, according to the above scheme and the diathesis–stress model of pathology.

4. Perspectives of Psycho-oncology

Despite the persuasiveness of the scientific data presented in this book, orthodox medicine still considers it merely from the standpoint of potential pharmacotherapy of the "broken link." Meanwhile, it is time to realize that it is impossible to invent a "pill for cancer," since no medicine is capable of altering the contents (rather than the state) of our mind. Drugs can only slow down the progression of the disease, which, in the absence of fundamental personal and spiritual changes, will most often recur.

If we look at the reviewed facts from a biopsychosocial-spiritual point of view, it becomes obvious that the accumulated knowledge is already enough to change the approach to oncological (and, in fact, to any other) diseases. Dividing diseases into "psycho" and "somatic" has become completely meaningless in today's world. The diathesis–stress model of pathology is confirmed by a multitude of studies that finally allow us to recognize that any human disease is primarily a psychosocial problem. Therefore, pharmacologically oriented medicine should, in fairness, be referred to as symptomatic medicine, focused only on leveling bodily signals of psychological problems.

Even in epigenetics, the science that proves the role of the mind in the regulation of the genome, many scientists still can not get rid of pharmacological blinders, trying to find means of chemical influence on the epigenome. In this way, in the consumer's consciousness, a vicious understanding of progress is cultivated, a kind of "we will do everything for you, do not strain yourself." It is with regret that we have to admit that such a policy of medical science is in line with the wishes of many people—to solve health problems quickly by using a "magic pill" and return to their old way of life. Few people understand the need for active and continuous work on themselves, for taking responsibility for their health. Orthodox medicine also corresponds to the interests of corporations—to earn money from the illiteracy of people. Fortunately, sensible scientists understand that epigenetic therapy is devoid of specificity and attempts to induce, for example, global hypomethylation of the genome (which can be achieved by using substances that suppress the activity of the DNA methyltransferase enzyme) can be very dangerous for health (Romani M. et al., 2015).

The studies presented in the book prove the need for the widespread introduction of anti-stress and psychotherapeutic care to cancer patients, starting from the moment of suspected diagnosis. We have seen that a massive psychic trauma of diagnosis activates the malignant process and increases the risk of metastasis. The traditional treatment process and its complications increase the distress even more. Mental imbalance that develops on top of that, and especially post-traumatic stress disorder, block the body's natural ability to heal itself and often cause a recurrence of the disease.

After the treatment of the psychic trauma of the diagnosis, the systemic work of the psychotherapist, focusing on the correction of maladaptive traits of the type "C" personality, is necessary. For this purpose, a diagnostic approach for psychosomatic patients proposed by L. P. Velikanova and Y. S. Shevchenko (2005) is expedient. It allows us to find out:

- why stress in the life of a person turned into distress;
- why the conflict that caused the distress is insoluble for him or her;
- why distress is expressed as a psychosomatic pathology, and not as neurotic or pathopsychological;
- why the psychosomatic "channel" of the psychological problem led to the pathology of this particular organ or system;
- why external and internal sanogenic factors, such as the compensatory forces of the body, life experience, family microclimate, and others, did not ensure the recovery of a person from the initially functional psychogenic disorders.

The solution of these problems is assisted by a careful analysis and correction of the factors of predisposition—disorders of attachment and psychic childhood traumas—and distortions of perception of oneself and the external world that have arisen on their basis. According to the observations of Søren Ventegodt (2004a, 2005), psychotherapeutic work aimed to eliminate the suppression of character, which has become fixed in childhood as a strategy for adapting to family circumstances, helps to improve the quality of life of the psychosomatic patient, his mental and physical health, and to define the purpose of life.

It is necessary to diagnose and deactivate the pathogenic effect of provocation factors—unresolved conflicts and psychic traumas of the past and present, that acts as a source of chronic stress. Achieving these goals alone makes it possible to reduce the severity of such premorbid factors as depression, helplessness, and hopelessness. Additional therapy for these mental distortions will help the patient to gain access to previously blocked energy resources necessary for restoring his health. Dr. David Servan-Schreiber (2009), a scientist and a cancer patient himself, believed that in order to cultivate the will to live in a patient, the first step should be the diagnosis and therapy of past traumas, since poorly healed wounds continue to deplete vitality and block the body's ability to protect itself.

The attention of psychologists should also be directed to help patients to improve the quality of their lives. This is achieved by involving patients in social support groups, teaching them how to express emotions and resolve conflicts, and developing their psychological adaptation skills. The main objective when acting in this direction, as has been repeatedly emphasized, is to help the patient realize that, when experiencing stress, he or she usually reacts not to the fact itself, but to the meaning attributed to it. Having learned how to change the meaning of the stress, he or she can change his or her reaction to what is happening. Changing the non-adaptive patterns of behavior will help the patient in improving communication skills, getting rid of dependence and "suffocation," and optimizing his or her interpersonal and intra-family relationships. It is also important to educate patients about pain management, openly consider the possibility of death, and get rid of the stigma of cancer.

At the same time, in my opinion, the time has come for the role of psychotherapy in oncology to be expanded. We must move on from focusing mainly on the treatment of personality and psychopathological disorders that arise *as a result* of the disease, to active involvement of the patient's mind and resources for eliminating *the causes* of the disease and activating the body's natural healing resources.

As one of the recognized experts, Stanford University professor David Spiegel, writes (2012), the branch of psycho-oncology is currently hung up on the hyphen between psycho and onco, and its further movement depends on our recognition of the connection between mind and body. "Is that hyphen merely an arrow to the left, indicating that cancer in the body affects the mind?" The scientist asks,—"Can it be an arrow to the right as well, mind affecting the course of cancer?" And with the help of his own research, he is able to prove: the second direction in psycho-oncology is certainly effective (Spiegel D. et al., 1989).

S. V. Umanskiy and V. Y. Semke (2008) consider psychotherapeutic influence on certain cognitive, emotional, or behavioral disorders of cancer patients as a tactical-symptomatic approach. The main, strategic, psychotherapeutic approach consists not only of improving the quality of the patient's life and his rehabilitation after successful therapy, but also in the direct therapeutic effect on cancer. The main point is the formation and maintenance of a patient's positive attitude to life in all its manifestations (job, family, children, creativity, etc.).

Belarusian psycho-oncologists also believe that in the process of psychotherapy and rehabilitation of cancer patients, both symptomatic and pathogenetic measures should be applied. The former contributes to the reduction of anxious-depressive manifestations and distraction of attention from painful experiences; while the latter provides access to the internal resources of the individual, processes the psycho-traumatic experience, and changes the rigid, inadequate cognitive structure, which forms distorted ideas about the disease and prospects for its cure (Igumnov S. A., Grigorieva I. V., 2014).

O. V. Bukhtoyarov and A. E. Arkhangelskiy (2008), who demonstrated the positive effect of hypnotherapy on the survival of cancer patients and the epigenetic mechanisms underlying this effect, state:

> The significant involvement of the psychogenic component at all stages of cancer requires a revision of views on the role of psychotherapy in the practice of oncology. The use of psychotherapy should not be based on a symptomatic approach aimed only at "improving the quality of life of a dying patient," which is justified in the palliative care of terminal patients, for example, in the hospice. In all other cases, in the absence of signs of generalization of the tumor process and cachexia, pathogenetically oriented psychotherapy is needed to correct psychological problems and treat mental disorders of cancer patients, aimed at the destruction of the psychogenic component of the cancer dominant after the elimination of the somatogenic factor.

To achieve this goal, these scientists substantiate the need to form a lasting recovery-oriented internal suggestion in patients in the process of postoperative rehabilitation, in order to completely replace the cancer dominant with the health dominant. Otherwise, if the patient remains pessimistic about his recovery and does not restore the dominant of life goal, the powerful psychogenic component of the cancer dominant will significantly impede the attainment of remission. Professor V. S. Mosienko (2014) agrees with this opinion. Noting that the tumor dominant prevails in the cerebral cortex and inhibits the function of the central nervous system, he points out the importance of dispersing this dominant to prevent the progression of the malignant process.

However, as we already know, the health dominant is only one of the constituent parts of the life goal dominant. Therefore, it is vital to aid cancer patients in acquiring the meaning of life, paying special attention to spirituality. Dr. Bernie Siegel (1998) came to the conclusion that the resolution of conflicts, an awareness of the true self, spiritual insight, and affection release unbelievable energy that contributes to the biochemistry of treatment.

Psycho-oncologist N. A. Rusina (2009) takes a similar stance: if psychological, psychotherapeutic, and medical care does not affect the spiritual sphere of the personality and cannot bring it to a higher level of spiritual development, it does not bring relief and provides a superficial explanation of what is happening. Finally, as psychotherapist Vyacheslav Gusev (2014) writes,

> I dare to assert that the basis of all the sufferings and illnesses of mankind is that their light is not manifested. Hence, the only real way of healing is the manifestation of this light, the disclosure of the potential of the soul. All other treatment methods cannot be called healing.

It seems to me that the advice from John Kabat-Zinn (2005) for those who study meditation fully corresponds to the goals that a cancer patient should strive to achieve with the help of a psychotherapist:

> TRY: Seeing your own life this very day as a journey and as an adventure. Where are you going? What are you seeking? Where are you now? What stage of the journey have you come to? If your life were a book, what would you call it today? What would you entitle the chapter you are in right now? Are you stuck here in certain ways? Can you be fully open to all of the energies at your disposal at this point? Note that this journey is uniquely yours, no one else's. So the path has to be your own. You cannot imitate somebody else's journey and still be true to yourself. Are you prepared to honor your uniqueness in this way?

In such manner, we help the patient to find and develop those depressed, unrealized aspects of his or her personality that manifested through a spiritual-existential crisis and avital experiences. The release of these resources can be the basis for personal and spiritual development, or, in the words of Lawrence LeShan, for helping the patient to find his "song of life." Getting awareness in the course of therapy on how her false personality was formed and what impact it had on the occurrence of the disease, and understanding of the possibility of changing it, allow the patient to embark on the path of post-traumatic growth. As a result, a person can achieve the kairos, a deep transformation of life, comprehension of her Essence, and transcendental perception of reality. This, apparently, is a prerequisite for sustained remission and even complete healing.

Such a result is possible because the possibilities of our mind are endless. The restrictions that block these possibilities manifest mainly in self-disbelief and social programming such as "this cannot be." Elimination of these restrictions allows a person to learn of his amazing abilities, that open up in so-called "altered states of consciousness." For example, under hypnosis, a burn may appear when a coin at room temperature is placed on one's skin if one is told that it is red-hot. In states of hypnosis or trance, one can gain access to the memory of a distant past—well-forgotten or repressed by the defense mechanisms of the psyche. In such states, which are often used in regression therapy, access can also be opened up to powerful creative abilities, the existence of which one does not even suspect in an ordinary state.

Many of us have heard about the extraordinary psychic reserves manifested in people in the state of affect—for example, when a fragile woman lifts with her bare hands a truck that her child is pinned under, or an unfit person easily jumps over a two-meter fence, fleeing from a pursuer. Science has extensively studied the placebo effect, which we discussed above (remember Mr. Wright?). Cases of duality of consciousness (dual personalities) in the same person are of great interest— when the personality in which the disease develops seems to disappear, and another appears in its place, the disease also disappear. For decades research has been ongoing on the amazing abilities of some yoga practitioners to change the physiological functions of their bodies.

In my opinion, it is this state of consciousness in which one can consciously have access to these abilities that should be considered the true one, natural to the human who has awakened his or her Essence. The overwhelming majority of people, unfortunately, live just in the "altered state of consciousness" created by the false personality. And only a life crisis created by a severe illness or other adversity is able to, through the process of kairos and post-traumatic growth, push such a person out of this "altered state" of mind and give him or her access to dormant abilities. One of their manifestations is healing from cancer, which we still define as mysteriously "spontaneous."

However, if the most important way to help a cancer patient is to direct him to post-traumatic growth, to reveal the potential of his soul, to manifest his inner light, to find his "song of life," then this makes the highest demands on the psycho-oncologist or psychotherapist. Such work cannot be done mechanically. It is not enough to be just a highly qualified specialist: you need to have a sufficiently high level of spirituality yourself. It is necessary for an opened potential of the therapist's soul to be present in order for the patient to discover his own inner light. You cannot bring a traveler to where you have never been yourself. There is a need for the therapist to invest in constant work on himself, constant self-knowledge, increasing his own harmony, reaching a level where psychotherapy becomes the flow of creativity, not work. Only the therapist's own powerful dominant of the life goal can "pull out" the faded life dominant of the patient.

In this regard, the practice of the psycho-oncologist is akin to the practice of a shaman who sends her soul to the "lower worlds" to search for and return the "lost soul" of the client. These "lower worlds" of suffering and depression are controlled by the "evil spirits" of helplessness, hopelessness, and despair. Therapists need an extraordinary power of their own will to live in order not to "burn out" by working with those who have lost theirs. Otherwise, the therapist's own soul may not be able to rise from the "lower world" of negative emotions. And if the psychotherapist acts not from her false personality, not from pride, but from the Essence, if she stays in the stream of spiritual creativity during therapy, then both she and her client go to the transcendental level. They find themselves during a session in the "upper world" where the patient can touch her Essence and see its inner light. And so her post-traumatic growth begins... I call this approach transpersonal psycho-onco-therapy.

That is why such work cannot be "put on stream." In fact, this is the art, and every creator is individual. And it is only when the psychotherapist uses not the "protocols" but his creativity that he can help the client co-create himself and his health.

5. Ways to Prevent Cancer and Other Serious Diseases

All of the above also applies to preventive medicine and early diagnostic. Instead of eliminating the psychosocial problems of an individual with a family history of cancer, deactivating the maladaptive behaviors inherited by him or her, helping to resolve an existential crisis and its consequences, avital activity, orthodox medicine, while remaining disconnected from psychology, tries to remove the organ where a tumor may occur.

For example, Professor E. N. Imyanitov, the head of the department of biology of tumor growth of the leading Russian Research Institute of Oncology, in his article (2010) recognizes that the effectiveness of early detection of breast and ovarian cancer is far from desirable. Therefore, women over the age of thirty to forty with a genetic predisposition are "strongly recommended" to have preventive mastectomy and oophorectomy, leading to an "inevitable loss of the quality of life." Moreover, he admits that there is still a risk of cancer from the residual cells of the removed breast.

One of the factors of this predisposition is the carriage of BRCA genes, which, as we learned in Chapter 19.5.2, are activated by the stress hormone cortisol. However, have you ever heard of these women being advised to learn about stress management instead of having an operation?

As for the prevention of hereditary cancer, the most advanced solution that medicine can offer today to families planning to have children, where a close relative has cancer, is assisted reproductive technology. Under it, embryos are diagnosed for the presence of mutations, and then a "healthy" embryo is transferred to the uterus of the woman. Unfortunately, we are still far from using psychosocial interventions to change the epigenetic regulation of the parent's genome. This would give us a chance to get rid of dangerous "records" in their reproductive cells without passing them on to the children (I presented data on such experiments in the second part of the book). Meanwhile, the US National

536   Vladislav Matrenitsky

Institute of Health has already recognized that cancer prevention is impossible without the complex relationship between genetic changes and the influence on genes caused by behavioral factors and the external environment (both physical and social) being taken into account (Mabry P. L. et al., 2008).

Based on the material discussed in the second part of the book, it is obvious that the prevention of cancer and other diseases should begin with an analysis of prenatal (if the parents are available) and postnatal periods of the person's development, since childhood adversities change the epigenetic regulation of the genome and increase the risk of health impairment. The social environment in the early stages of development determines how a person will react to stress in the future. Therefore, children whose early social environment is unfavorable should be automatically enrolled by social services into a group of people at risk of developing somatic or mental pathology and advised to take a course of preventive psychotherapy. This approach will help any state to save significant funds on the treatment of these people in the future.

With the same purpose, it is absolutely necessary for secondary schools to introduce a subject dealing with the basis of self-regulation, self-analysis, emotional literacy. This book is full of studies demonstrating the pathogenic potential of alexithymia, suppression and repression of emotions, psychological infantilism. By teaching children to understand and express their emotions and needs properly, we can significantly reduce their likelihood of developing psychosomatic diseases. Children should know that whatever their emotions are, they should not feel ashamed of them or avoid them, but on the contrary, they should be aware of, understand, and adequately express—and particularly, speak openly about—them.

It is just as worthwhile to teach children about body literacy, explain how the body gives signals in a state of imbalance or overstrain. They need to know how the symptoms of disorders of various organs can manifest and how they can help themselves at primary psychosomatic imbalance, how to understand pain and spasms, not taking these body signals solely as a reason for taking pills.

An important way to achieve these goals is to introduce daily meditation practice in school. It would be ideal for both pupils and teachers to begin and end each class with a five-to-seven-minute meditation. In some schools in different countries where this practice has already been implemented, the positive effects of meditation on pupils' health and their academic performance have been repeatedly confirmed (Nidich S. et al., 2011; Joyce A. et al., 2010; Campion J., Rocco S., 2009). A meta-analysis of such studies demonstrates that learning awareness methods afford the most optimal way for children at an early age to effectively cope with stress and anxiety, as well as to develop focused attention (Nieminen S. H., Sajaniemi N., 2016).

In the United States, for example, several foundations such as InnerKids, Impact Foundation, Lineage Project, developed programs to teach children awareness. What is especially important is their initiative to educate adolescents who are in the at-risk group—in particular, those living in poor and dangerous areas or in prison. Something else that is worth mentioning is the "Learn to learn" course of self-regulation, developed by teachers and pediatricians in Irkutsk (Russia) for first- to fourth-grade pupils. It is aimed at teaching children the skills of psycho-emotional self-management, proper cognitive activity, healthy psychosocial interactions, working rationally with information, in order to preserve their health and optimize development processes (Belozertseva I. N., 2001). Waldorf schools, which are based on the spiritual teaching of anthroposophy, are becoming increasingly popular. Their goal is the development of the child's creativity, subtle feelings, and intuition for an objective experience of spiritual reality.

With such approaches, inherited or acquired adverse epigenetic changes can be eliminated. The child receives knowledge and skills for overcoming stressful situations and the negative emotions they cause. It is also necessary for high schools to introduce a psychological educational course about genders and family relationships, how to deal with losses and disappointments in life. It is especially important to be literate in how to endure the stresses of disease and the deaths of loved ones, how to help ourselves psychologically during serious illnesses, and how to understand our own death. If this is done, then those psycho-traumatic factors that provoke cancer and other chronic diseases will not have enough power in the future to have a destructive effect on the body. A good example is the experimental program conducted at the University of California for women who suffered the death of a loved one: they found new life orientations, and achieved personal growth and awareness of new meaning in life. This helped women to go through a difficult period of life more confidently and improve the protective functions of the immune system (Bower J. E. et al., 2003). Imagine how many people would be able to save their health and life if such programs were offered in schools!

Ronit Peled and his colleagues from Ben-Gurion University of Israel (2008), upon examining 255 women with breast cancer, came to the conclusion that young women who have been exposed to a number of negative life events should be considered a "risk group" for cancer of the mammary gland, and they should be given appropriate psychological help.

In general, the materials reviewed in the book indicate that, in accordance with the biopsychosocial-spiritual paradigm of medicine, it is time to gradually shift the emphasis from researching diseases to studying what health is and how to achieve and maintain it. In other words, the time has come for the transition from pathology to sanology and *valeology*.

The basis of modern medicine is pathogenesis (from the Greek "pathos (παθος),"—suffering and "genesis (γενεσις)," —origin). Accordingly, the main objective of medicine is considered to be searching for the causes of diseases and fighting them. On the contrary, sanology (from the Latin "sanitas," health and "logos,'" words, reason) seeks to achieve public health, protect and strengthen it. In turn, valeology (from the Latin "'valere," to be strong or healthy and "logos," the study of how to be healthy) explores the essence, mechanisms, and manifestations of individual health, the methods of its detection, prediction, and optimization with the aim of improving the quality of life and increasing the social adaptation of humans.

In other words, these two sciences are looking for the answer to the question "Where does health come from and how can it be strengthened?" and not to the question "Where does the disease come from and how can it be cured?" These ideas, of course, are not new. According to legend, in ancient China, the doctor was paid only for the time when the person he helped was healthy, and not during the illness. In the Soviet Union, I. I. Brekhman (1982) came up with the idea of the need to change the entire healthcare strategy, studying the origin, quality, and level of an individual's health, and formulated methodological foundations for the preservation and promotion of health in healthy people.

The concept of salutogenesis (from the Latin "salus," well-being, health, and Greek "genesis," origin), which was developed by Israeli sociologist Aaron Antonovsky, is also becoming increasingly popular. He investigated the issue of why a person is able to stay healthy and happy, despite the effects of pathogenic stress. The scientist discovered a stress tolerance factor, which he called a sense of connectedness (coherence). This feeling reflects the extent to which life challenges are comprehensible, manageable, and meaningful for a person, and determines the individual's experience of the psychological well-being that underlies health. As characteristics of such well-being the author considers the presence of conscious strategies of coping instead of unconscious defense mechanisms, a feeling of joy instead of a feeling of suffering, the ability for constant creative adaptation and growth, the productive use of emotional energy instead of its waste, dedication instead of narcissism, interaction instead of exploiting other people, and so on. In this case, stress can be not only pathogenic, but also, under certain conditions, a salutogenic factor, since successfully overcoming a critical situation can be a positive life experience (Antonovsky A., 1979, 1987).

For this to happen, it is necessary for both schools and universities to run special educational programs with the support of mass media. The goal is to inform young people that an existential crisis may occur in life, with subsequent avital experiences, and this can lead to serious diseases, including cancer. Knowing the symptoms of such a crisis and being able to recognize it in oneself is no less important, in my opinion, than knowing the basic physical symptoms of various diseases, although even the last is not given the attention it deserves in our society owing to the underdevelopment of educational programs.

Such an integrated approach to education can also help young people who have created a family to acquire the right ideas and skills to adequately educate and raise their children. Unfortunately, today we are witnessing the blatant ignorance of young parents, followed by attachment disorders and psychic traumatization of their children. The result is the transmission of pathogenic patterns of behavior from generation to generation.

In order for a child's proper salutogenic psychosomatic development to be achieved, in other words, for him to grow up healthy in both spirit and body, we need to start with good physical and psychic health in the mother. It is necessary for her own traumas to be healed before pregnancy, and for the pregnancy itself to come consciously and be desired. If, after birth, the child has a positive and harmonious relationship with his parents, with himself, and with the world, then he will develop adequately in each period of ontogenesis. Then a positive attitude toward his own body, the ability to properly sense and use it will be formed, getting joy and pleasure from it and from bodily contact with parents (Kravtsova N., 2009). This way the child will have a positive self-attitude, self-esteem, and self-image, proper motor functions, and emotional competence, and not psychological infantilism, subordination, dependence, and self-centeredness.

I warmly support Sandor Ferenczi (1908), a renowned Austro-Hungarian psychiatrist and psychoanalyst, who, as early as the beginning of the last century, first declared that deep psychology should become the basis of modern pedagogy. Such an approach to education, in his opinion, will serve to prevent neurosis, and will be a much stronger influence on the formation of a person's character than the factors of heredity. Ferenczi believed that the introduction the analytical principles of mental hygiene into one's life by means of pedagogy could be one of the greatest revolutions in the history of mankind.

That is why I will keep repeating that the health of the nation is the responsibility of the educational system to a greater extent than of the healthcare system. If school would teach a person self-analysis and self-regulation, ways of calming the mind and relaxing the body, then this person will develop not only cognitive but also emotional intelligence that makes him or her capable of coping with stress. He or she will certainly run a much lower risk of getting sick and will have every opportunity to achieve active and creative longevity. In addition, such a person has a much lower chance of becoming a criminal since he knows from childhood how to control (not suppress!) his aggression and frustration. And again, he knows how to bring up healthy, free, developed, and independent children of his own.

However, at this point another question arises—is the government, that is in its current form most often ruled by monopolies and corporations, ready for such changes in its citizens?

Since psychological health and awareness cannot be patented and run on a conveyor belt, neither corporations nor state institutions are really interested in people getting sick less often. A thinking, informed, and independent citizen is not needed by the state or the hospital—he asks too many questions and requires too much attention and too many answers. It is much better for the state to have to deal with a simple "cog" in the system. When such a loyal citizen is told to defend a religious faith or "brothers by nationality" in other countries, he believes what is suggested and dutifully goes to the slaughter. Since the existential vacuum often prevails in these people, the suggestion by political technologists of such ideas brings meaning to their lives, allows them to feel their "significance," being part of the "great idea of a fighter for ...," creates the dominant of life goal. When such a person becomes ill, he also believes that there is no choice except for the pharmacy, and will use his last money to buy an expensive drug.

There are very few patients like the cyclist Lance Armstrong (2000, with S. Jenkins), who described his treatment in the following way:

I was not a compliant cancer patient. I was salty, aggressive, and pestering... When LaTrice (*the nurse—V. M.*) said, "Drink five glasses of water in a day," I drank fifteen, draining them one after the other until the water ran down my chin.

... I insisted on behaving as if I was a full participant in the cure. I followed the blood work and the X rays closely, and badgered LaTrice as if I were the Grand Inquisitor.

... This was a typical day for her:

"What dose am I getting, LaTrice?" I'd ask.

"What's that based on?

"Am I getting the same thing as yesterday?

"Why am I getting a different one?'

"What time do we start, LaTrice?'

"When do I finish, LaTrice?'

Undoubtedly, for the average patient, especially one who is accustomed to dependence or the suppression of individuality, it is incredibly difficult to behave in this way. That is why psychotherapeutic care is important from the first days of treatment: it is necessary to change ineffective patterns of patient behavior, to teach him or her independence and responsibility for his or her health. According to Dr. Vyacheslav Gusev (2015), "The main task of psychotherapy in psychosomatic diseases is to return to the patient the opportunity to choose whether to remain ill or become healthy. In other words—to return to the patient responsibility for what happens to him. And that's all. This is enough. When there is a choice, people prefer to recover." The main psychotherapeutic processes in achieving this task considered by the author are helping the patient to become aware of his or her needs, to understand the mechanisms that block the realization of his or her needs, and assist in the search for optimal ways of meeting the needs. Taking into account the data on the central role of unmet needs in the origin of cancer considered in Part III, this approach seems to me to be absolutely correct.

The outstanding Soviet researcher into oncogenic stress, Professor L. H. Garkavi (et al., 1998), wrote:

All of us who stand for the whole organism and not just against the symptoms of the disease, are just awakening its natural defenses, raising the vitality of the human body, increasing the level of health by bringing it in harmony with itself and with the environment. This means that we promote self-organization and further human evolution, which, as we know, is not yet complete. The health and harmonious development of ourselves and of future generations is in our hands and depends on the level of our consciousness.

6. Both Ancient and Modern Knowledge Asserts: It is our Mind that Creates our World and our Health!

However, as they say, "Nothing is new under the Moon." All this knowledge of the problems and abilities of the mind that is being rediscovered and recognized by mankind today with the help of the latest scientific research, has been known for more than one millennium. Ancient Indian, Chinese, Greek, and Tibetan thinkers were studying the properties of the mind with the same care and attention with which modern scientists study the phenomena of the material world. The ancient researchers have achieved greater success on this path than modern psychology. In fact, the basic commandments of all world philosophies and religions are aimed at teaching a person to be in the most harmonious state of mind and bring this harmony to the world around him.

For example, there are interesting parallels with Buddhist philosophy. The term "suffering," which is the traditional translation of the Pali term "dukkha," has a broader interpretation—unsatisfactoriness, disturbance, irritation, dejection, worry, despair, anxiety, inferiority, frustration, suppression, hopelessness, and even "stress" these days (Dukkha, 2013). Therefore, the central position of Buddhism, the so-called "four noble truths," may also sound as follows:

1. There is dissatisfaction (with unmet needs) in life.

2. Dissatisfaction has a cause— ignorance, that causes disturbing emotions.

3. Dissatisfaction can be stopped by removing ignorance.

4. There is a definite way to stop dissatisfaction—the realization of one's true nature (the Essence).

From this we see that humankind has been able to understand that dissatisfaction lies at the root of conflicts and suffering for a long time. The main emotions that create it, according to Buddhism, are affection (desire) and hostility (disgust). Affection arises when a person does not possess something and wants it (whether it is material objects, relationships, or a position in society), when he has achieved this something and tries to retain or maintain it with all his might, and then when he has lost this something. From another angle, toward everything that prevents him from possessing these objects of affection, such a person feels hostility, anger, and fear.

Over the millennia of civilization's development, significant changes have occurred mainly at the level of technology and social organization, while the personal qualities of humans have changed little—we continue to experience all the same problems and emotions as humans did many centuries ago. Therefore, Buddhism actually describes the same intrapersonal conflicts due to unmet needs that modern psychology explores so intensively (probably that is why the techniques of meditation developed in Buddhism to manage our suffering are of such interest to science). The negative emotions that arise under the suffering of dissatisfaction are indeed what creates that chronic stress that leads to various diseases, including cancer.

The most important source of dissatisfaction, as has been repeatedly explored in this book, is loss. In a sense, all the negative events occurring in the life of a cancer patient can be referred to as experiences of loss. Consider this yourself:

- In childhood: the loss of a parent or close relative; loss of parental warmth, attachment, attention, love, security; loss of freedom of expression, including the freedom to express one's emotions;

- In adulthood: the loss of a significant object or subject (partner, social status, business); loss of love, freedom of expression, faith in oneself and in one's future;

- Before the disease: loss of hope for a better life, for an exit from a "suffocating" situation or relationship; loss of social support, the joy of life, the purpose and meaning of life, the desire to live;

- During or after illness: loss of an organ or part of the body; loss of hope for a full life after treatment, loss of hope to be healed, of hope for survival.

As an "antidote" to suffering caused by loss, Buddhism offers a teaching on impermanence. It is based on the fact that everything in the universe is transitory. Everything around us exists in the process of continuous change—nothing remains the same. It would seem that there is nothing that is difficult to understand. Whatever we look at around us—nothing remains in a static state. Day and night, seasons, life and death ... Everything appears, exists for a limited amount of time, and disappears. But if we look at our lives impartially, we have to admit that despite the incontestability of the impermanence of all things, we basically behave as if we don't want to see and accept this inevitability. We do not want to see ourselves as part of the universe. We strive for something unchanging, stable, often considering such constancy as "happiness." And if we achieve the desired permanence, then we hold on to it with all our strength, as if it depends on us to keep it from changing. As a result, problems appear, such as affection and hostility, clinging to material things and to other people, and suffering because of their loss. In this way, life for many people becomes an endless experience of loss, because what we want to possess and try to save will inevitably change or disappear. To struggle with the laws of the universe is meaningless—everything has its time limit.

Therefore, at each moment of time we also change, and our feelings, thoughts, and ideas, no matter how beautiful or unpleasant they are, also change. The concept of impermanence implies that there cannot be any kind of finite or unchanging truth—and this is another reason that motivates us to reflect on our beliefs and worldview. We can only talk about a certain level of understanding that corresponds to a specific time and place. As conditions change, what seems to be true at one moment in time becomes inevitably false or worthless at other times. In fact, it is the acceptance of impermanence that is the basis for creativity and non-stagnation, for the absence of existential emptiness and depression.

Accepting changes is a necessary factor in getting rid of a significant part of the suffering that we cause ourselves. For example, we often force ourselves to suffer when refusing to part with the past. If we evaluate and perceive ourselves only on the basis of what we have achieved, accumulated, and maintained, then with each loss we will increase the level of internal strain and create the basis for the development of diseases. Conversely, by consciously observing and accepting the changes brought by life, we can stay in maximum harmony with the universe, like a windsurfer who has mastered the formidable waves of an ocean that changes every second. Buddhism calls such a mind, which is "pure and perfect," the "All-Almighty King."

Unfortunately, most people are too clouded by their false personality to turn to this knowledge, and therefore continue to suffer and get ill. That is why all the causes of suffering in Buddhism ultimately boil down to ignorance—the inability of the undeveloped mind to realize itself and the true nature of the universe. As a result, we stay in the thrall of delusions. By the way, Buddhists often compare dissatisfaction, or suffering, with illness. In this case, the external and internal conditions that cause the disease are the causes of suffering. When these conditions and causes are eliminated, recovery from the disease begins—that is, suffering is stopped.

I hope that modern people will finally listen, if not to ancient philosophy or religion, then at least to science, which has become a kind of religion for most of us these days. Epigenetics, psychoneuroimmunology, and psychoneuroendocrinology, placebo and hypnosis effects have proved that our mind is capable of changing the state and functions of the body at both physiological and genetic levels. This convincingly demonstrates the priority of consciousness over matter.

Numerous studies reviewed in this book confirm that it is our subjective perception of what is happening—what we think about it and how our emotions reflect our thoughts—that affects the regulation of various genes and our health (Chen E. E. et al., 2009; Irwin M. R., Cole S. W., 2011). Let me remind you of some of these studies:

- the more threatening a social situation seems to us (as opposed to its objective characteristics), the more CTRA stress-activating transcription factors of the genome are activated. In contrast, psychological and meditative practices that reduce the significance of perceived threats inhibit the activity of these factors (Antoni M. H. et al., 2016; Creswell J. D. et al., 2012);

- schoolchildren who subjectively experience a higher level of stress caused by life troubles, physical violence, or loss, are more severely depressed (Rakhimkulova A. V., Rozanov V. A., 2015);

- students who have a higher subjective level of stress during exams have a higher level of DNA damage, which is normalized after the holidays (Cohen L. et al., 2000);

- in women who believe that their daily stress level is high (subjective assessment), the length of chromosomal telomeres decreases in the same way as in women who are actually in chronic stress caring for sick children (Epel E. S. et al., 2004);

- the more old women who care for their demented husbands doubt their ability to cope with the expected difficulties, the more their telomeres are reduced (O'Donovan A. et al., 2012);

- the presence of suicidal thoughts, rather than the number of actual negative life events, is associated with an increase in the methylation of the gene responsible for the synthesis of the nerve tissue growth factor BDNF (Kang H. J. et al., 2013).

We have also seen that mental practices such as meditation, hypnosis, visualization, and even restructuring the way of thinking under the influence of psychotherapy, lead to positive and healing epigenetic and physiological changes. Moreover, scientists from the HeartMath Institute in the United States demonstrated that the meditative state called "cardiac coherence" can affect even the physical structure of DNA, unwinding its helix (McCraty R. et al., 2003).

That is why if a patient thinks that cancer is death and believes in it, then his body will follow these thoughts, while if he thinks he can be healed and believes in it, then this will happen. Why? Because his mind is the "All-Almighty King."

Quantum physics has also come to the conclusion about the priority of consciousness. Max Planck (1931), the Nobel Prize winner and the creator of this branch of physics, stated: "I regard consciousness as a fundamental. I regard matter as derivative from consciousness. We cannot get behind consciousness.

Everything that we talk about, everything that we regard as existing, postulates consciousness." The "Copenhagen interpretation" of quantum physics, developed by another Nobel laureate, Niels Bohr, says that the results of the experiment depend on the expectations of the experimenter. If the task of the experiment is to detect the electron as a particle, then it behaves like a particle. If the experimenter expects the electron to be a wave, then he will find the wave; that is, the mind controls matter. Finally, the famous physicist Albert Einstein (et al., 1930) believes that

> ... people have grown tired of materialism, in the popular sense of the term; it shows that they find life empty and that they are looking toward something beyond mere personal interests. This popular interest in scientific theory brings into play the higher spiritual faculties, and anything that does so must be of high importance in the moral betterment of humanity.

Thus, if both the ancient and modern sciences, including all the data in this book, testify in favor of the fact that it is our mind that creates our reality—which means also our body and health—then this message is of great importance for cancer patients. This is the good news that each ill person has inside himself a perfect tool for changing the physical reality of his body. However this tool, the mind, has been incorrectly tuned since childhood and, under the influence of life adversities, has increasingly deviated from the effective mode of operation. But this tool is not broken! It is only necessary to understand the principles of its functioning, adjust it with the help of specialists, and learn how to use it correctly. The harmonized mind, in turn, will harmonize the brain, our "central processor," which will now be able to activate the body's self-regulation mechanisms.

This message can be a source of hope for many cancer patients in the sense that they have the potential to master the power of their mind, so it will make self-healing possible. And as the patient goes deeper into self-knowledge, develops his capabilities, invests in his health, his disbelief in himself will be transformed into a Desire to examine his capabilities. The first positive results will bring the Trust, and then, with further progress, the Confidence that overcoming the disease is possible. And when the disease begins to recede, an invincible Faith in oneself will arise, which will create the main medicine for each patient—Love for oneself and for the world. The Love that grants us comprehension that each of us is an equivalent part of the universe and that the meaning of our life is to co-create the evolution of the universe.

Glossary

Adrenoreceptors—a family of binding proteins located on the surface of cells that transmit signals from the stress hormones epinephrine (adrenaline) and norepinephrine (noradrenaline) inside the cell. Depending on the effects they cause, their location, and their affinity for different substances, they refer to two main types—alpha and beta, and their subspecies: α1-, α2-, β1-, β2, β3.

Affect—a short-term, violently flowing, positively or negatively colored psychogenic emotional reaction to a highly irritating factor.

Alexithymia—the difficulty or inability of a person to realize and express his own feelings and understand the feelings of other people, with a display of excessive attention to external events in detriment to internal processes, and difficulties in finding differences between feelings and bodily sensations.

Amygdala—the part of the limbic system of the brain responsible for experiencing threats, fear, pleasure, and for memories associated with these feelings.

Anergy—the loss of energy, the inability to be active, and the body's loss of resistance to the pathogenic effects of the environment.

Angiogenesis—the formation of new blood vessels in the embryo, the affected organ or tissue.

Anhedonia—the feeling of joylessness, the monotony of life, pessimism, not previously characteristic indecision, remorse.

Anoikis—the precursor of apoptosis (natural cell death), when a damaged or mutated cell detaches from other cells of any tissue.

Basal cell *carcinoma*—a malignant tumor of the skin that develops from the lower layer of the epidermis.

Beta(β)-blockers—a class of pharmacological drugs that prevent epinephrine from connecting to its receptors (*adrenoreceptors*) and thereby block its effects on organs and tissues.

Cancer dominant or oncodominant—a dominating psycho-physiological formation with a function of host self-destruction that determines development of pathology in the form of an oncological disease.

Carcinoma—a tumor of a class that are in the initial stage, formed from skin cells or tissues that cover the surface of internal organs and ducts of the glands.

Catatonia—a psychopathological syndrome, which has the main clinical manifestations of various motor disorders such as stupor, muscle rigidity, agitation, or impulsive behavior. It occurs in schizophrenia, affective and other mental disorders, somatic and neurological diseases, as well as during poisoning.

CEID—see cognitive-emotional imbalance or deficiency.

Celiac disease, or gluten enteropathy—an autoimmune disease, caused by persistent gluten intolerance, that disrupts the digestive process.

Cell culture—a population of cells of a certain type of microorganism, plant, animal, or human tissue, which is artificially grown in controlled laboratory conditions.

Chromatin—a substance that forms the basis of *chromosomes*. Formed of DNA, *RNA* and *histones*.

Chromosomes—the structure of the cell nucleus consisting of *chromatin* and containing the hereditary information of the body.

Circadian cycle, or rhythm—daily fluctuations in the level of corticosteroid hormones in the blood.

COEX—see *system of condensed experience*.

Cognitive-emotional imbalance or deficiency (CEID)—1. lack of either cognitive abilities (including processes of attention, memory, logical thinking, imagination), or abilities to realize and express emotions; 2. an imbalance between these two functions of the psyche.

Constitution—the functional and morphological features of an organism, formed on the basis of hereditary and acquired properties and determining the organism's reactivity to various influences.

Culture of cells—see *cell culture*.

Cycloidal trait—periodic mood changes when a decline in mood is replaced by its improvement. Some clinicians consider it to be a mild form of bipolar disorder.

Cytokines—peptides (short forms of proteins) that transmit information inside the body. They regulate the intercellular and intersystem interactions, control the growth, activity and destruction (apoptosis) of cells and the inflammation process, and also coordinate interaction of the nervous, immune, and endocrine systems.

Diathesis—*constitutional* (biological) predisposition of an organism to certain diseases due to inherited, congenital, or acquired properties and physiological features. As a result, the functions of the organism are in a state of unstable equilibrium for a prolonged period of time.

DLG—the dominant of the life goal, the main dominant of the individual that defines their mental state and life in general.

DNA methylation—the addition of a special chemical label—a methyl group (formed from one carbon atom and three hydrogen atoms)—to the cytosine bases of a specific gene. As a result, this gene becomes less active in *transcription*, since access to it becomes limited.

DNA repair—restoration of lesions in the structure of DNA that have emerged as a result of *mutations*.

Dysphoria—the predominance of a gloomy-angry mood, frequent sensations of tension, melancholic irritability, aggressiveness.

Dystrophy—disorders of cellular metabolism leading to pathological structural and functional changes in the organ or tissue.

Ego—a psychological concept proposed by Sigmund Freud to denote one of the structures of the human psyche that provides a link between the external and internal world. This is a complex of ideas and views, perceived by the individual as the center of consciousness.

Endothelium—a monolayer of endothelial cells that constitutes the inner cellular lining of the blood vessels and the lymphatic system, an interface between the blood stream and the vessel wall.

Eniology—the study of objective phenomena, processes and patterns of subtle energy, and interaction of information, as well as the circulation of physical matter, in nature and society.

Enneatype—according to Claudio Naranjo (1994), this is a personality classification in accordance with the enneagram—the psychological model developed by George Gurdjieff—which describes nine deep-seated motives driving us on a subconscious level.

Enzyme—a specific protein that acts as a catalyst in living organisms. Enzymes accelerate the utilization of substances both entering the body and formed during metabolism, as well as regulating biochemical and genetic processes in response to changing conditions.

Epigenetic—the branch of genetic that study a changes in gene activity under the influence of environmental signals, where the structure of DNA, unlike what occurs during *mutation*s, remains unchanged.

Existential vacuum—the absence of meanings and values of existence which are crucial for the individual.

Existentialism—a branch of philosophy dedicated to the analysis of existence and exploring the unique way that humans experience their existence in the world.

Expression of a gene—the process by which information encoded in genes is converted into products—*RNA* or proteins—that are necessary for the structure or function of a cell.

Frustration—a kind of negative psychological state that arises owing to regular problems with the satisfaction of desires and human needs. It manifests in the inadequate experience of failures or inconsistencies in the desired and the real, including the real and ideal images of "I."

Gene transcription—synthesis of *RNA* molecules on the corresponding DNA segments, the first stage of the reproduction of genetic information in the cell.

Genome—a set of genes contained in the *chromosomes* of a given organism.

Genotype—a set of genes of a given organism, localized in its chromosomes and forming the organism's hereditary basis.

Glia—auxiliary nerve tissue that takes up to 40% of the total volume of the brain and spinal cord. It performs the functions of supporting neurons, their nutrition, metabolism, growth, and regulation of their activity.

Hippocampus—an area of the human brain that is mainly responsible for memory. As a part of the *limbic system*, it is associated with the regulation of emotional responses. It also provides spatial orientation.

Histones— special proteins that compose the *chromosomes*. They ensure the assembly and packaging of DNA into a structure of the optimal density for the current chromosome task.

Holistic approach, or holism—(from ancient Greek ὅλος—whole, integral) is a "philosophy of integrality," implying that the whole is always something more than a simple sum of its parts. As the annex to medicine, it reflects the vision of "the person as a whole," and not just an arbitrary carrier of specific disease.

Hypochondria—an excessive concern for one's health in the absence of objective reasons for this, a fairly consistent unfounded conviction of the presence of a serious disease.

Hypophysis (pituitary gland)—a neuroendocrine organ located at the base of the brain, the center of the endocrine system, closely associated with the *hypothalamus*. It controls the function of other endocrine glands, growth, maturation, and the function of various organs by producing the signal hormones.

Hypothalamic-pituitary-adrenal system (axis)—a set of specific parts of the body that ensure the maintenance of homeostasis and the body's resistance to the stressors in the external environment.

Hypothalamus—the structure of the intermediate section of the brain, the highest center of regulation of the *vegetative* and reproductive functions of the body, the location of interaction of the nervous and endocrine systems.

Interleukins—a type of *cytokines* produced predominantly by leukocytes; they are mediators of inflammation and immunity.

Intra-personal conflict—psychological state of a person in which there is a confrontation between opposing (up to mutually exclusive) needs, values, and goals, resulting in an inability to choose behavioral priorities.

Intropunitive reactions—a type of autoaggressive response in a state of *frustration*, characterized by an internal orientation ("turning into oneself"), self-blame, and depression.

Kairos—in existential psychology, the critical moment for an individual to make a pivotal decision regarding his or her own life, when his or her values, meanings, and personality in general change in the most radical and fateful of ways.

Libido—according to Sigmund Freud, libido is sexual desire or sexual instinct (energy) that determines the normal and pathological development of a person. By redirecting it in any activity, for example, in creativity, a person discharges this energy.

Limbic system—several anatomically and functionally connected parts of the brain that include the hypothalamus, hippocampus, amygdala, reticular formation, and others. It participates in the control of emotional and instinctive behavior.

Locus of external control—psychological mechanism of attributing the responsibility for the events in one's life to external environmental factors, fate, surrounding people, i.e. to solely external objects and circumstances seemingly independent of the person himself.

Lymphocytes—a type of white blood cells, the main cells of the immune system responsible for the production of antibodies, involved in the destruction of alien and "sick" cells and regulating the activity of other types of cells.

Lymphogranulomatosis (Hodgkin's disease or Hodgkin's lymphoma, or malignant granuloma)—an oncological disease of the lymphatic system, characterized by the abnormal growth of the lymphoid tissue and the formation in it of specific giant cells of Berezovsky-Sternberg, which are the structural elements of granulomas.

Lymphoma—a group of blood cancers that start in the *lymphocytes*. Hodgkin's lymphoma—see *Lymphogranulomatosis*.

Macrophages—*monocytes* that have migrated from the bloodstream into tissues and grown into them in full. They accumulate in large quantities at the foci of inflammation, actively destroying bacteria.

Mammography—X-ray examination of the mammary glands.

Messenger RNA—a type of *RNA* that transmits information from DNA to the ribosomes, the intracellular protein "factories."

Meta-analysis—a scientific methodology combining statistical data from a number of research studies to test scientific hypotheses.

Metabolic syndrome—a complex of metabolic, hormonal, and clinical disorders, most often manifested in the deterioration of carbohydrate and lipid metabolism and arterial hypertension. It is a risk factor for diabetes, cardiovascular, oncological, and other diseases.

Metabolism—chemical reactions taking place in a living organism to sustain life.

Micro-RNA—a type of *RNA* that regulates the *expression* of genes by blocking the function of *messenger RNA*.

Myeloid cells—differentiated blood cells that arise from a common progenitor derived from hematopoietic stem cells in the bone marrow.

Myoma (uterine fibroid)—the most common benign solid pelvic tumor occurring in females of reproductive age.

Monocytes—large blood leukocytes (a class of phagocytes), which are responsible for antitumor, antiviral, antimicrobial, contraceptive, and antiparasitic immunity. They produce cytotoxins, interleukin-1, tumor necrosis factor, and interferon, and participate in the regulation of blood formation.

Mononuclear blood cells—a specific class of white blood cells involved in the immune response.

Mutations—sudden changes in genes that occur under the influence of an external or internal environment. They cause changes in functions and properties of the organism and are inherited.

Narcissism—a manifestation of a person's increased interest in him/herself, ranging from healthy to pathological aspects.

Nerve tissue growth factors (neurotrophic factors)—protein compounds that are synthesized by neurons and *glial* cells. They are involved in regulating the processes of growth, differentiation, plasticity, and maintenance of the vitality of the tissues of the central and peripheral nervous system.

Neurasthenia (asthenic neurosis or exhaustion neurosis)—a mental disorder that is characterized by increased excitability and irritability, emotional instability, and *vegetative* disorders, fatigue, loss of ability for prolonged physical and mental work, and sleep disorders.

Neuroblastoma—a malignant tumor of the sympathetic nervous system, most often arising during early childhood.

Neuropil—a neural network in the gray matter of the brain, formed primarily by the outgrowth of neurons (axons and dendrites) and their junctions—synapses.

Neurosis—a consequence of an intrapersonal conflict, a functional (reversible) disturbance of the nervous system, when sensitivity to signals from the external and internal environment significantly increases. This leads to impaired psychological adaptation, which is often manifested in increased irritability, anxiety, and fatigue, and results in the depletion of the nervous system and *vegetative* disorders.

Neuroticism—a personality trait characterized by emotional instability, anxiety, and low self-esteem.

Neurotransmitters—a group of body chemicals, biologically active messengers released by nerve cells to transmit impulses to other nerve, muscle, or endocrine cells.

NLP (neuro-linguistic programming)— a kind of suggestive psychotherapy intended for the correction of human behavior through the formation of predetermined programs in a "masked" verbal form. Uses different communicative/learning styles for different characteristic sensory modes.

Noogenesis—the emergence and evolution of the mind.

Obsessive-compulsive syndrome (disorder)—constantly arising, unwanted ideas, fears, thoughts, images, or motivations (obsessions) and stereotypically repeated actions or rituals (compulsions) that interfere with normal life. Obsessions usually create anxiety, and compulsive actions aid in reducing this anxiety.

Oncodominant—see *cancer dominant.*

Ontogenesis—the process of individual development of the organism.

Ontology—the doctrine of being (existence) as such, the direction of philosophy which studies the fundamental principles of being.

Papillomaviruses—more than 600 types of viruses that infect the body's epithelial tissues and can cause the formation of warts, genital pointed condylomas, as well as benign or malignant tumors.

Parasympathetic nervous system—part of the autonomic (peripheral, vegetative) nervous system of vertebrate animals and humans. Its stimulation leads to inhibition of the functions of a number of internal organs and to muscle relaxation.

Phenotype—a set of biological properties and characteristics of the organism, that were formed in the process of its individual development and are based on the interaction of the *genotype* and the external environment.

Post-traumatic growth (PTG)—personal and spiritual development and changes in the meaning of life as a result of traumatic experiences and/or serious illness.

Post-traumatic stress disorder (PTSD)— a complex of symptoms of a mental disorder that developed as a result of a powerful traumatic effect and persist for a prolonged time. Its main symptoms are a delayed experience of mental trauma in the form of intrusive memories and nightmares and loss of interest in life, followed by the appearance of depression, alienation from other people, and emotional bluntness.

Prefrontal cortex—an area of brain's gray matter that is involved in cognitive and behavioral functions, emotions, and abstract thinking.

Pro-inflammatory agents—various biological substances that activate the processes of inflammation in tissues.

Propranolol—a pharmacological drug from the group of *beta-adrenergic blockers*, one of the most common in the market.

Prospective study—a scientific approach in which a group of people selected on certain grounds is observed for a certain period of time following an experiment or survey.

Prostaglandins—bioactive lipid derivatives that both sustain homeostatic functions and mediate a number of pathogenic mechanisms.

Proto-oncogene—a gene that is responsible, as a rule, for the synthesis of proteins that regulate cell growth, reproduction, and differentiation (the acquisition of specific functions by the cell in the process of maturation).

Psychedelic therapy—psychotherapy with the use of psychoactive substances that alter the perception, affecting the emotional state and most of the mental processes. It is used to obtain *transpersonal experiences* and to achieve personal and spiritual changes.

Psychodynamics—a direction of psychology that studies the patterns of the activity of an individual's mental forces—their movement, unfolding, growth and attenuation, interaction, and struggle.

Psychological defense—an adaptive mental process directed against negative emotional overload.

Psychosis—is a mental condition that causes one to lose touch with reality and results in strange or bizarre thinking, perceptions, behaviors, and emotions.

Psychoticism—a personality trait which, according to Hans Eysenck, is characterized by a tendency to solitude and insensitivity to others, wild imagination, inflexibility, lack of realism, self-centeredness, difficulty in contacting others, strong internal tension, inadequate emotional responses, increased predisposition to *psychosis*, and other features.

Receptor—a protein or glycoprotein molecule that binds a hormone or other chemical substance on the cell membrane (or inside it) and transmits a regulatory signal reflecting this contact further into the cell, including the genome. This triggers a response from appropriate organs and tissues.

Reframing—a technique used in *NLP* to achieve a restructuring of the mechanisms of perception, thinking, and behavior of the client in order to allow him to rid himself of unsuccessful mental patterns and change his point of view on something, even as far as to an opposite point of view.

Regressive therapy—a therapeutic process where the person experiences a return to an earlier age, earlier events, states, and emotions through trance, hypnosis, or other methods.

Reticuloendothelial system (RES or a system of *macrophages*)—reticular connective tissue, spread throughout different parts of the body, performing barrier, protective, and metabolic functions. It is mostly concentrated in the spleen, lymph nodes, and bone marrow.

RNA (ribonucleic acid)—a long-chain macromolecule used by the cell to program protein synthesis. It is synthesized on the DNA template during the *transcription* process.

Self—according to Karl Jung, this is the center of the integrity of the conscious and unconscious mental existence of man, the principle of their integration.

Self-actualization—desire to achieve the fullest possible identification and development of one's personal capabilities, as well as the transition from a state of possibility to a state of reality.

Self-transcendence—the stage of development that leads to the comprehension of one's spiritual nature, the meaning of life, the creative power of the universe, and the unity of the universe; and to the aspiration to contribute to the evolution of the universe.

Seminoma—the most common testicular tumor, accounting for ~45% of all primary testicular tumors.

Shadow—according to C. G. Jung, an unconscious complex containing the repressed, suppressed, or alienated features of the conscious part of the personality.

Somatization—"embodiment" of emotions, when the psychological stress is experienced at the body level. It ranges from discomfort to disorders of the structure and function of internal organs.

Subconscious— a symbolic part of the mind, responsible for psychic activity (needs, emotions, desires, etc.) that is not available to conscious awareness but affects one's feelings and behavior.

Superego—one of the components of the personality structure according to S. Freud. It is a system of moral attitudes and requirements for the behavior, actions, and decisions of the *Ego* ("I") of the subject, established in early childhood under the influence of education.

Symbiotic relationships—mutually beneficial and useful connections between organisms with different needs, resulting in their successful complementation of each other. In psychology, a relationship where one or, more rarely, both partners desire to be together constantly, as if to "merge" physically and spiritually, even to think and feel in the same way.

Sympathetic nervous system—part of the autonomic (peripheral, vegetative) nervous system of vertebrate animals and humans. Its stimulation leads to the activation of the functions of a number of internal organs and muscles, including the stimulation of cardiac activity.

Synergetics—an interdisciplinary area of science; the study of the general laws of phenomena and processes of self-organization and spontaneous disorganization in complex non-equilibrated systems of diverse natures (physical, biological, social).

System of condensed experience (COEX)—memories related to different periods of life but that have similar factors of origin, especially with similar emotional content. They are concentrated in closely related conglomerates in the subconscious.

Teleology—the doctrine of the expediency of being as it is. It claims that in any development process there is a pre-established goal.

Telomeres—end regions of *chromosomes*, that ensure the safety of the *genome* and give the cell a possibility of beginning preparation for the next division.

Trance—a special resource state of consciousness linking and mediating conscious and unconscious mental functioning. In this state, attention is directed to the inner, imaginative world but not to the outer, as it happens in the usual state of consciousness. Trance is a healing state in which a person gets access to the repressed content of the psyche and its potential.

Transcendence—going beyond one's personal limits; a state that is supernatural, beyond the rational framework. This state is accessible to human knowledge, although not as a result of subjective experience. In Christian theology, transcendence is the spiritual principle that unites the soul of man and God.

Transcription factors—specific protein complexes. By translocating to the cell nucleus, they activate certain genes and result in their *expression*.

Transpersonal experience— a state of the psyche when a sense of self-identity passes the limits of an individual or personal self, embracing humanity as a whole, life, spirit, and the cosmos. According to C. and S. Grof (2000), it refers to *transcendence* and includes many experiences, usually known as spiritual, mystical, or religious.

Transpersonal psychology—a direction in psychology involving the study of religious and *transpersonal experiences* and altered states of consciousness. It combines modern psychological concepts, theories, and methods with traditional spiritual practices of the East and West.

Tumor microenvironment—various cells and structures that surround the tumor: simple chemicals and complex macromolecules, in particular, blood vessels, connective tissue elements, intercellular fluid, hormones, enzymes, immune cells, *metabolic* products, etc.

Valeology— study of the essence, mechanisms, and manifestations of individual health, the methods of its determination, prediction, and optimization with the aim of improving the quality of human life and social adaptation.

Vegetative functions—the main physiological functions of the body responsible for digestion, blood circulation, respiration, and metabolism.

Bibliography[1]

Aardal-Eriksson E., Eriksson T. E., Thorell L. H. (2001). Salivary cortisol, posttraumatic stress symptoms, and general health in the acute phase and during 9-month follow-up. *Biological Psychiatry*, 15, 986–993.

Abel U. (1992). Chemotherapy of advanced epithelial cancer-a critical review. *Biomedicine & Pharmacotherapy*, 46(10), 439–452.

Abitov I. R., Mendelevich V. D. (2008). Osobennosti sovladayushchego povedeniya pri psikhosomaticheskikh i nevroticheskikh rasstroystvakh. *Vestnik Psikhiatrii i Psikhologii Chuvashii*, 4, 35–49.

Abrams R. D., Finesinger J. E. (1953). Guilt reactions in patients with cancer. *Cancer*, 6(3), 474–482.

Abramson L. Y., Metalsky G. I., Alloy L. B. (1989). Hopelessness depression: A theory-based subtype of depression. *Psychological Review*, 96, 358–372.

Achterberg J. (2002). *Imagery in Healing*. Boulder, CO: Shambhala Publications.

Achterberg J., Collerain I., Craig P. (1978). A possible relationship between cancer, mental retardation and mental disorders. *Social Science & Medicine. Part A: Medical Psychology & Medical Sociology*, 12, 135–139.

Acklin M. W., Brown E. C., Mauger P. A. (1983). The Role of Religious Values in Coping with Cancer. *Journal of Religion & Health*, 22(4), 322–333.

Adachi S., Kawamura K., Takemoto K. (1993). Oxidative Damage of Nuclear DNA in Liver of Rats Exposed to Psychological Stress. *Cancer Res*, 53, 4153–4155.

Adamson J. D., Schmale A. H. Jr (1965). Object loss, giving up, and the onset of psychiatric disease. *Psychosom Med*, 27(6), 557–576.

Ader R., Felton D. L., Cohen N. (eds) (2000). *Psychoneuroimmunology*. Cambridge, MA: Academic Press Inc; 3rd rev. edn.

Ader R., Cohen N. (1975). Behaviorally Conditioned Immunosuppression. *Psychosomatic Medicine*, 37(4), 333–340.

Adimoolam S., Ford J. M. (2003). p53 and regulation of DNA damage recognition during nucleotide excision repair. *DNA repair*, 2(9), 947–954.

Adler A. (1907). *Studie über Minderwertigkeit von Organen*. Munich: Urban & Schwarzenberg.

Adler A. (1932). *What Life Could Mean to You*. Sydney: Allen & Unwin.

Adler N. E., Page A. E. (2008). *Cancer Care for the Whole Patient: Meeting Psychosocial Health Needs* Washington, DC: The National Academies Press.

Ahadi B., Ariapooran S. (2009). Role of self and other forgiveness in predicting depression and suicide ideation of divorcees. *Journal of Applied Sciences*, 9(19), 3598–3601.

Akhmerov R. A. (1994). *Biograficheskie krizisyi lichnosti*. Avtoref. dis. kand. psihol. nauk. Moscow: MGU.

---

[1] The sources in Cyrillic are transliterated.

Akhmerov R. A. (2013). Kartina zhiznennogo puti u onkologicheskih bolnyih. *Psihologiya v zdravoohranenii. Materialyi nauchnoy konferentsii "Ananevskie chteniya-2013".* Saint Petersburg: Skifiya-print, 381–382.

Ainsworth M. D. S., Bowlby J. (1991). An ethological approach to personality development. *American Psychologist.* 46, 333–441.

Ainsworth M. D. S., Blehar M., Warers E., Wall E. (1987). *Patterns of Attachment. A psychological study of the strange situation.* Hillsdale, NY: Erlbaum Associates.

Aizawa T., Ishizaka N., Usui S. et al. (2002). Angiotensin II and catecholamines increase plasma levels of 8-epi-prostaglandin F(2alpha) with different pressor dependencies in rats. *Hypertension*, 39, 149–154.

Akil H., Haskett R. F., Young E. A. et al. (1993). Multiple HPA profiles in endogenous depression: effect of age and sex on cortisol and beta-endorphin. *Biological Psychiatry*, 33(2), 73–85.

Akulenko L. V. (2004). O nasledstvennom rake molochnoy zhelezy, yaichnikov i endometriya (klinicheskaya lektsiya). *Probl. reprod*, 10, 20–27.

Albo D., Akay C. L., Marshall C. L. et al. (2011). Neurogenesis in colorectal cancer is a marker of aggressive tumor behavior and poor outcomes. *Cancer*, 117(21), 4834–4845.

Alcala H. E., Tomiyama A. J., von Ehrenstein O. S. (2017). Gender Differences in the Association between Adverse Childhood Experiences and Cancer. *Women's Health Issues*, 27(6), 625–631.

Aleksandrovskiy Y. A. (1976). *Sostoyaniya psihicheskoy dezadaptatsii i ih kompensatsiya.* Moscow: Nauka.

Aleksandrovskiy Y. A. (2005). Posttravmaticheskoe stressovoe rasstroystvo i obschie voprosy razvitiya psihogennyih zabolevaniy. *Rossiyskiy Psihiatricheskiy Zhurnal*, (1), 4–12.

Aleksandrovskiy Y. A. (2008). Sotsialnyie kataklizmy i psihicheskoe zdorove. *Sotsiologicheskiye Issledovaniya,* (4), 99-104.

Alekseeva A. S. (2010). *Kliniko-morfologicheskie proyavleniya hronicheskih gepatitov i tsirrozov pecheni razlichnoy etiologii vo vzaimosvyazi s psihologicheskim profilem i kachestvom zhizni patsientov.* Avtoref. dis. d-ra med. nauk. Tomsk: SGMU.

Alexander F. (1939). Psychological aspects of medicine. *Psychosomatic Medicine*, 1(1), 7–18.

Alfano C. M., Rowland J. H. (2006). Recovery issues in cancer survivorship: a new challenge for supportive care. *Cancer J*, 12(5), 432-443.

Aliyev H. (2003). *Metod Klyuch v borbe so stressom.* Rostov-na-Donu: Feniks.

Allen D. J., Savadatti S., Gurmankin Levy A. (2009). The transition from breast cancer "patient" to "survivor". *Psycho-Oncology*, 18, 71–78.

Almeida-Marques F. X. D., Sánchez-Blanco J., Cano-García F. J. (2018). Hypnosis is More Effective than Clinical Interviews: Occurrence of Trauma in Fibromyalgia. *International Journal of Clinical and Experimental Hypnosis*, 66(1), 3–18.

Almgren M., Schlinzig T., Gomez-Cabrero D. et al. (2014). Cesarean delivery and hematopoietic stem cell epigenetics in the newborn infant: implications for future health? *American Journal of Obstetrics and Gynecology*, 211(5), 502, e1.

Altieri A., Hemminki K. (2007). Number of siblings and the risk of solid tumours: a nation-wide study. *British Journal of Cancer*, 96(11), 1755–1759.

Al-Wadei H. A., Ullah M. F., Al-Wadei M. H. (2012). Intercepting neoplastic progression in lung malignancies via the beta adrenergic (β-AR) pathway: implications for anti-cancer drug targets. *Pharmacological Research*, 66(1), 33–40.

Amaral A. P., Vaz Serra A. (2009). Traumatic childhood events and potential consequences in adult health. *Eur Psychiatry*, 24(Suppl. 1), S1233.

Ammon G. (1972). *Dynamische psychiatrie (dynamic psychiatry): internationale zeitschrift fur psychiatrie und psychoanalyse.* Berlin: Pinel-publikationen.

Amos T., Stein D. J., Ipser, J. C. (2014). Pharmacological interventions for preventing post-traumatic stress disorder (PTSD). *Cochrane Database Syst Rev*, 7.

Amritanshuram R., Nagendra H. R., Shastry A. S. et al. (2013). A psycho-oncological model of cancer according to ancient texts of yoga. *Journal of Yoga & Physical Therapy*, 3(1), 129.

Amussat J. (1854). *Quelques Reflexions sur la Curabilité du Cancer.* Paris: E. Thunot et Cie.

Andersen B. L., Farrar W. B., Golden-Kreutz D. et al. (1998). Stress and immune responses after surgical treatment for regional breast cancer. *J Natl Cancer Inst*, 90, 30–36.

Andersen B. L., Shapiro C. L., Farrar W. B. et al. (2005). Psychological responses to cancer recurrence. *Cancer*, 104(7), 1540–1547.

Andersen B. L., Yang H. C., Farrar W. B. et al. (2008). Psychologic intervention improves survival for breast cancer patients: a randomized clinical trial. *Cancer*, 113(12), 3450–3458.

Anderson G. (1990). *The Cancer Conqueror: An Incredible Journey to Wellness.* Kansas, MO: Andrews Mcmeel Pub.

Anderson R. M., Birnie A. K., Koblesky N. K. (2014). Adrenocortical status predicts the degree of age-related deficits in prefrontal structural plasticity and working memory. *The Journal of Neuroscience*, 34(25), 8387–8397.

Ando N., Iwamitsu Y., Kuranami M. et al. (2009). Psychological characteristics and subjective symptoms as determinants of psychological distress in patients prior to breast cancer diagnosis. *Support Care Cancer*, 17(11), 1361–1370.

Andrykowski M. A., Cordova M. J. (1998). Factors associated with PTSD symptoms following treatment for breast cancer: test of the Andersen model. *J Trauma Stress*, 11, 189–203.

Anisimov V. N. (2008). *Molekulyarnyie i fiziologicheskie mehanizmyi stareniya.* Saint Petersburg: Nauka.

Anisman H., Hayley S., Turrin N., Merali Z. (2002). Cytokines as a stressor: implications for depressive illness. *Int J Neuropsychopharmacol*, 5(4), 357–373.

Anokhin P. K. (1980). *Uzlovyye voprosy teorii funktsional'noy sistemy.* Moscow: Nauka.

Anokhina I. P., Yumatov E. A., Ivanova T. M., Skotselyas Y. G. (1985). Soderzhanie biogennyih aminov v raznyih strukturah mozga u kryis, adaptirovavshihsya k hronicheskomu emotsionalnomu stressu. *Zhurn Vyissh Nervn Deyat*, 2, 348–353.

Antokhin E., Budza V., Gorbunova M. et al. (2008). Koping-povedenie u bolnyih shizofreniey s pervyim psihoticheskim epizodom i ego dinamika v protsesse psihoobrazovaniya. *Sotsialnaya i Klinicheskaya Psihiatriya*, 18(3), 5–12.

Antoni M. H. (2013). Psychosocial intervention effects on adaptation, disease course and biobehavioral processes in cancer. *Brain, Behavior, and Immunity*, 30, S88–S98.

Antoni M. H., Bouchard L. C., Jacobs J. M. et al. (2016). Stress management, leukocyte transcriptional changes and breast cancer recurrence in a randomized trial: an exploratory analysis. *Psychoneuroendocrinology*, 74, 269–277.

Antoni M. H., Lutgendorf S. K., Blomberg B. et al. (2012). Cognitive-behavioral stress management reverses anxiety-related leukocyte transcriptional dynamics. *Biol Psychiatry*, 71(4), 366–372.

Antoni M. H., Lutgendorf S. K., Cole S. W. et al. (2006). The influence of bio-behavioural factors on tumour biology: pathways and mechanisms. *Nat Rev Cancer*, 6, 240–248.

Antonova L., Mueller C. R. (2008). Hydrocortisone down-regulates the tumor suppressor gene BRCA1 in mammary cells: A possible molecular link between stress and breast cancer. *Genes, Chromosomes and Cancer*, 47(4), 341–352.

Antonovsky A. (1979). *Health, Stress and Coping.* San Francisco, CA: Jossey-Bass.

Antonovsky A. (1987). *Unraveling The Mystery of Health—How People Manage Stress and Stay Well.* San Francisco, CA: Jossey-Bass.

Antonyan Y. M. (1997). *Psihologiya ubiystva.* Moscow: Yurist.

Antropov Y. F. (1997). *Psihosomaticheskie rasstroystva u detey i podrostkov (klinika, atogenez, sistematika i differentsirovannaya terapiya)*. Moscow: NGMA.

Antsupov A. Y., Shipilov A. I. (2002). *Konfliktologiya*. Moscow: Yuniti-Dana.

Anufriev A. K. (1985). Psihopatologicheskaya struktura i forma nevroticheskogo sostoyaniya. *Trudyi 5-go Vseros. s'ezda nevropatologov i psihiatrov*. Moscow, 184–186.

Apanel E. N. (2012). K obosnovaniyu strukturno-funktsionalnogo zaschitnogo kompleksa normalnogo krovosnabzheniya mozga. *Meditsinskiy Zhurnal*, 2, 136–139.

Aphrodisiensis A. (1841). Problematurn physicorum et medicorum eclogae. In: J. L. Ideler, *Physici et Medici Graeci Minores*, Vol. I, Berlin: Reimer, 3–81.

Archakova T. O. (2009). Zhiznestoykost protiv faktorov riska. V: *Elektronnyiy sbornik statey portala psihologicheskih izdaniy PsyJournals.ru*. Retrieved 06.01.2015 from: http://psyjournals.ru/pj/2009-1/22860.shtml.

Archer S., Brathwaite F., Fraser H. (2005). Centenarians in Barbados: The importance of religiosity in adaptation and coping and life satisfaction in the case of extreme longevity. *Journal of Religion, Spirituality & Aging*, 18(1), 3–19.

Argaman M., Gidron Y., Ariad S. (2005). Interleukin-1 May Link Helplessness—Hopelessness with Cancer Progression: A Proposed Model. *International Journal of Behavioral Medicine*, 12(3), 161–170.

Arkhipov G. N. (1971). Vliyanie nevroticheskih izmeneniy na funktsionalnoe sostoyanie zheludka i kantserogenez. *Voprosyi Onkologii*, 17(2), 14–21.

Aristotle (2006). *On Rhetoric: A Theory of Civic Discourse*, Book 2. Oxford: Oxford University Press.

Armaiz-Pena G. N, Allen J. K., Cruz A. et al. (2013). Src activation by β-adrenoreceptors is a key switch for tumor metastasis. *Nat Commun*, 4, 1403-1423.

Armaiz-Pena G. N., Lutgendorf S. K., Cole S. W., Sood A. K. (2009). Neuroendocrine modulation of cancer progression. *Brain Behav Immun*, 23, 10–15.

Armstrong L., Jenkins S. (2000). *It's Not about the Bike: My Journey Back to Life*. New York: Putnam Adult.

Arshavskiy V. V., Rotenberg V. S. (1984). *Poiskovaya aktivnost i adaptatsiya*. Moscow: Nauka.

Aschbacher K., O'Donovan A., Wolkowitz O. M. et al. (2013). Good stress, bad stress and oxidative stress: insights from anticipatory cortisol reactivity. *Psychoneuroendocrinology*, 38(9), 1698–1708.

Aseev A. V. (1993). Psihologicheskie problemyi, svyazannyie s rakom molochnoy zhelezyi: obzor. *Klinicheskaya Meditsina*, 3, 30–34.

Aseev A. V. (1998). *Kachestvo zhizni zhenshchin, bolnyih rakom molochnoy zhelezyi i melanomoy kozhi*. Avtoref. dis. d-ra med. nauk. S-Pb: TMA.

Assagioli R. (1999). Self-realization and psychological disturbances. In: S. Grof, C. Grof (eds), *Spiritual Emergency: When Personal Transformation Becomes a Crisis*. New York: Tarcher/Putnam US, 27–49.

Astin J. A., Reilly C., Perkins C., Child W. L. (2006). Breast cancer patients' perspectives on and use of complementary and alternative medicine: A study by the Susan G, Komen Breast Cancer Foundation. *J Soc Integr Oncol*, 4(4), 157–169.

Astvatsaturov M. I. (1935). Sovremennyie nevrologicheskie dannyie o suschnosti emotsiy. *Sovetskaya Nevropatologiya, Psihiatriya i Psihogigiena*, 4, 9–10.

Atamanov A. A., Buykov V. A. (2000). Osobennosti trevozhnyih sindromov pri psihosomaticheskih zabolevaniyah: o pravomochnosti ponyatiya «psihosomaticheskaya trevoga». *Sots i Klinich Psihiatriya*, 4, 16–20.

Auxemery Y. (2006). [Posttraumatic stress disorder (PTSD) as a consequence of the interaction between an individual genetic susceptibility, a traumatogenic event and a social context]. *Encephale*, 38(5), 373–380 (in French).

Avery C. M. (2008). *The relationship between self-forgiveness and health: Mediating variables and implications for well-being.* Ann Arbor, MI: ProQuest.

Averyanova S. V. (2012). Psihologicheskie osobennosti zhenschin, bolnyih kolorektalnyim rakom. *Rossiyskiy Meditsinskiy Zhurnal*, 3, 27–29.

Azim H. A., De Azambuja E., Colozza M. et al. (2011). Long-term toxic effects of adjuvant chemotherapy in breast cancer. *Annals of Oncology*, 22(9), 1939–1947.

Bacon C. L., Rennecker R., Cutler M. A. (1952). Psychosomatic Survey of Cancer of the Breast. *Psychosomatic Med*, 14, 453–460.

Bahnson C. B. (1969). Psychophysiological complementarity in malignancies: past work and future vistas. *Ann N Y Acad Sci*, 164, 319–334.

Bahnson C. B. (1980). Stress and Cancer: The State of the Art. Part 1. *Psychosomatics*, 21(12), 975-981.

Bahnson C. B. (1981). Stress and Cancer: The State of the Art. Part 2. *Psychosomatics*, 22(3), 207-220.

Bahnson C. B. (1996). Families as producers of and sufferers from malignant disease: Therapeutic goals. *Giornale Italiano Di Oncologia, 16, 145-148.*

Bahnson C. B., Bahnson M. B. (1964). *Cancer as an alternative to psychosis: A theoretical model of somatic and psychologic regression. Psychosomatic aspects of neoplastic disease.* London: Pitman Medical Publishing Co., Ltd.

Baider L., Sarell M. (1983). Perceptions and causal attributions of Israeli women with breast cancer concerning their illness: the effects of ethnicity and religiosity. *Psychotherapy and Psychosomatics*, 39(3), 136–143.

Baider L., Peretz T., Hadani P. et al. (2014). Transmission of response to trauma? Second-generation Holocaust survivors' reaction to cancer. *Am J Psychiatry*, 157, 904–910.

Bakanova A. A. (2000). *Otnoshenie k zhizni i smerti v kriticheskih zhiznennyih situatsiyah.* Avtoref. diss. kand. psihol. nauk. Saint Petersburg: RGPU.

Bakanova A. A. (2001). Ekzistentsialnyiy kontekst preodoleniya krizisnyih situatsiy v zrelom vozraste. V: *Aktualnyie problemyi stanovleniya lichnosti v sovremennom mire.* Materialyi Vserossiyskoy nauchno-prakticheskoy konferentsii 30–31 maya 2001 g. Magnitogorsk.: MaGU, 44–46.

Baldessarini R. J., Hennen J. (2004). Genetics of suicide: an overview. *Harvard Review of Psychiatry*, 12, 1–13.

Balint M. (1970). *Therapeutische Aspekte der Regression.* Stuttgart: Klett.

Balitskiy K. P., Shmalko Y. P. (1987). *Stress i metastazirovanie zlokachestvennyih opuholey.* Kiev: Naukova dumka.

Balitskiy K. P., Veksler I. G. (1975). *Reaktivnost organizma i himioterapiya opuholey.* Kiev: Naukova dumka.

Balitskiy K. P., Veksler I. G., Vinnitskiy V. B. et al. (1983). *Nervnaya sistema i protivoopuholevaya zaschita.* Kiev: Naukova dumka.

Balliet R. M., Capparelli C., Guido C. et al. (2011). Mitochondrial oxidative stress in cancer-associated fibroblasts drives lactate production, promoting breast cancer tumor growth: understanding the aging and cancer connection. *Cell Cycle*, 10(23), 4065–4073.

Baltrusch H. J. F., Santagostino P. (1989). The Type C behavior pattern: New concepts. *International Journal of Psychophysiology*, 7(2), 126–128.

Baltrusch H. J. F., Waltz M. (1985). Cancer from a biobehavioural and social epidemiological perspective. *Social Science & Medicine*, 20(8), 789–794.

Baltrusch H. J. F., Waltz M. (1987). Stress and cancer: A sociobiological approach to aging, neuroimmunomodulation and the host-tumor relationship. In: J. Humphrey (ed.), *Human Stress: Current Selected Research.* New York: AMS Press, Inc., 2, 153–200.

Baltrusch H. J. F., Stangel W., Titze I. (1991). Stress, cancer and immunity: New developments in biopsychosocial and psychoneuroimmunologic research. *Acta Neurologica*, 13(4), 315–327.

Banerjee T., Chakravarti D. (2011). A peek into the complex realm of histone phosphorylation. *Mol Cell Biol*, 31(24), 4858–4873.

Baranovskiy A. Y. (ed.). (2011). *Gastroenterologiya: Spravochnik*. Saint Petersburg: Piter.

Baranskaya L. T., Polyanskiy M. A. (2001). Depressivnaya lichnost kak faktor riska k razvitiyu abdominalnoy zlokachestvennoy patologii. *Psihologicheskiy Vestnik Uralskogo Gosudarstvennogo Universiteta*, 2, 118–122.

Barber L., Maltby J., Macaskill A. (2005). Angry memories and thoughts of revenge: The relationship between forgiveness and anger rumination. *Personality and Individual Differences*, 39(2), 253–262.

Bardini G., Dicembrini I., Cresci B., Rotella C. M. (2010). Inflammation markers and metabolic characteristics of subjects with 1-h plasma glucose levels. *Diabetes Care*, 33(2), 411–413.

Barger S. W., Moerman A. M., Mao X. (2005). Molecular mechanisms of cytokine-induced neuroprotection: NFκB and neuroplasticity. *Current Pharmaceutical Design*, 11(8), 985–998.

Barker D. J. P. (1998). In utero programming of chronic disease. *Clin Science*, 95, 115–128.

Barnes D. E., Lindahl T. (2004). Repair and genetic consequences of endogenous DNA base damage in mammalian cells. *Annu Rev Genet*, 38, 445–476.

Barnum B. S. (1996). *Spirituality in Nursing: From Traditional to New Age*. New York: Springer.

Barraclough B., Bunch J., Nelson B., Sainsbury P. (1974). A hundred cases of suicide: clinical aspects. *Br J Psychiatry*, 125, 355–373.

Barraclough J. (2001). *Integrated cancer care: holistic, complementary and creative approaches*. Oxford: Oxford University Press.

Barrett H. (2003). *Parenting programmes for families at risk: A source book*. London: National Family and Parenting Institute.

Barrios A. (2012). *Breaking Free With SPC - The Road to Self Actualization*. Mumbai: Nextgen Interactivity Publishing Inc.

Barron T. I., Connolly R. M., Sharp L. et al. (2011). Beta blockers and breast cancer mortality: a population-based study. *J Clin Oncol*, 29(19), 2635–2644.

Barry M. (2010). *The Forgiveness Project: The Startling Discovery of How to Overcome Cancer, Find Health, and Achieve Peace*. Grand Rapids, MI: Kregel Publication.

Barsky A. J., Klerman J. L. (1983). Overview: Hypohondriasis, Bodili Complains and Somatic Style. *American J of Psychiatry*, 3, 273–283.

Bartley T., Teasdale J. (2011). *Mindfulness-Based Cognitive Therapy for Cancer*. Hoboken: Wiley-Blackwell.

Bartrop R. W., Lazarus L., Luckhurst E. et al. (1977). Depressed lymphocyte function after bereavement. *The Lancet*, 309, 8016, 834–836.

Baruk H. (1964). *Psychoses et névroses*. Coll. "Que sais-je?" Paris: PUF.

Baruk H. (1972). *L'hypnose et les méthodes dérivées*. Coll. "Que sais-je?" Paris: PUF.

Basowitz H., Persky H., Korchin S., Grinker R. (1955). *Anxiety and Stress: An Interdisciplinary Study of a Life Situation*. New York: McGraw-Hill.

Bastiaans J. (1982). Der Beitrag der Psychoanalyse zur psychosomatischen Medizin. In: *Tiefenpsychologie, Band 2: Neue Wege der Psychoanalyse – Psychoanalyse der Gesellschaft. Die psychoanalytische Bewegung*. Weinheim: Beltz, 225–261.

Bastiaans J., Groen J. (1954). Psychogenesis and psychotherapy of bronchial asthma. In: D. O'Neill (ed.), *Modern Trends in Psychosomatic Medicine*, 242.

Basu S., Dasgupta P. S., Chowdhury J. R. (1995). Enhanced tumor growth in brain dopamine-depleted mice following 1-methyl-4-phenyl-1,2,3,6-tetrahydropyridine (MPTP) treatment. *J Neuroimmunol*, 60(1–2), 1-8.

Basu S., Nagy J. A., Pal S. et al. (2001). The neurotransmitter dopamine inhibits angiogenesis induced by vascular permeability factor/vascular endothelial growth factor. *Nat Med*, 7(5), 569–574.

Bateson G. (1960). The Group Dynamics of Schizophrenia. In: L. Appleby, J. M. Scher and J. Cummings (eds), *Chronic Schizophrenia: Explorations in Theory and Treatment*. Illinois: The Free Press, 90-105.

Batty G. D., Russ T. C., Stamatakis E., Kivimäki M. (2017). Psychological distress in relation to site specific cancer mortality: pooling of unpublished data from 16 prospective cohort studies. *BMJ*, 356, j108.

Bauer K. H. (1928). *Die Mutationstheorie der Geschwulstentstehung: Ubergang von Korperzellen in Geschwulstzellen durch Genanderung*. Berlin: J. Springer.

Bauer-Wu S. M. (2002). Psychoneuroimmunology. Part 1: Physiology. *Clinical Journal of Oncology Nursing*, 6, 167–170.

Baum A., Posluszny D. M. (2001). Traumatic stress as a target for intervention with cancer patients. In: A. Baum, B. L. Andersen (eds) *Psychosocial interventions for cancer*. Washington, DC: APA, xix, 143–173.

Baumeister R. F., Vohs K. D., Aaker J. L., Garbinsky E. N. (2013). Some key differences between a happy life and a meaningful life. *The Journal of Positive Psychology*, 8(6), 505–516.

Baykova I. A. (1999). *Psihosomaticheskie rasstroystva (klassifikatsiya, klinika, diagnostika i lechenie). Metod. rekomendatsii*. Minsk: Belorusskiy GIUV.

Bays B. (2012). *The Journey: A Practical Guide to Healing Your Life and Setting Yourself*. New York: Atria Book.

Beadle B. (2014). Psychosis risk associated with the loss of a parent or sibling in early childhood. *Nursing Standard*, 28(24), 17.

Beard C. J., Chen M. H., Cote K. et al. (2004). Perineural invasion is associated with increased relapse after external beam radiotherapy for men with low-risk prostate cancer and may be a marker for occult, high-grade cancer. *Int J Radiat Oncol Biol Phys*, 58(1), 19–24.

Beaufort J. L. (2015). *Cancer Was My Lifecoach: A 10 Step Survivor's Handbook*. E-book, Amazon Media.

Beck A. T. (1999). *Hostility: Cognitive basis of anger*. New York: Harper Collins Publishers.

Beck A. T. (ed.) (1979). *Cognitive therapy of depression*. New York: Guilford Press.

Beck A. X, Kovacs M., Weissman A. (1975). Hopelessness and suicidal behavior: An overview. *Journal of the American Medical Association*, 234, 1146–1149.

Beck S. J. (2011). *Cognitive Behavior Therapy, Second Edition: Basics and Beyond*. New York: Guilford Press.

Becker H. (1979). Psychodynamic aspects of breast cancer. *Psychotherapy and psychosomatics*, 32(1–4), 287–296.

Becker-Stoll F. (1997). *Interaktionsverhalten Zwischen Jugendlichen und Müttern im Kontext längsschnittlicher Bindungsentwicklung*. Doctoral dissertation, University of Regensburg.

Bedi R. P. (1999). Depression: an inability to adapt to one's perceived life distress? *J Affect Disord*, 54(1–2), 225–234.

Beecher H. K. (1961). Surgery as placebo: A Quantitative Study of Bias. *JAMA*, 176(13), 1102–1107.

Bekhtereva N. P., Kambarova D. K., Pozdeev V. K. (1978). *Ustoychivoe patologicheskoe sostoyanie pri boleznyah mozga*. Leningrad: Meditsina.

Beitsch P., Lotzova E., Hortobagyi G., Pollock R. (1994). Natural immunity in breast cancer patients during neoadjuvant chemotherapy and after surgery. *Surgical Oncology*, 3(4), 211–219.

Belden A. C., Barch D. M., Oakberg T. J. et al. (2015). Anterior insula volume and guilt: neurobehavioral markers of recurrence after early childhood major depressive disorder. *JAMA Psychiatry*, 72(1), 40–48.

Belik I. A. (2006). *Chuvstvo vinyi v svyazi s osobennostyami razvitiya lichnosti.* Avtoreferat kand. psihol. nauk. Saint Petersburg: SPGU.

Belinskaya E. V. *Vliyanie vinyi na zdorove cheloveka.* Psihologicheskiy tsentr "Gelios". Retrieved 15.03.2015 from: http://rasstanovki-rostov.ru.

Belitskiy G. A. (2006). Himicheskiy kantserogenez. *Problemyi klinicheskoy meditsinyi,* 1, 10–15.

Bellosta-Batalla M., Ruiz-Robledillo N., Sarinana-Gonzalez P. et al. (2018). Increased Salivary IgA Response as an Indicator of Immunocompetence After a Mindfulness and Self-Compassion-Based Intervention. *Mindfulness,* 9(3), 905–913.

Belozertseva I. N. (2001). *Obuchayem rebenka samoregulyatsii (uchebnaya programma po kursu "Uchis' uchit'sya").* Irkutsk: Serviko.

Belyalova N. S., Belyalov F. I. (2005). Faktoryi riska i profilaktika raka. Chast1. *Klinicheskaya Meditsina,* 11, 17–21.

Ben-Arye E., Bar-Sela G., Frenkel M. et al. (2006). Is a biopsychosocial-spiritual approach relevant to cancer treatment? A study of patients and oncology staff members on issues of complementary medicine and spirituality. *Supportive Care in Cancer,* 14(2), 147–152.

Ben-Dat Fisher D., Serbin L. A., Stack D. M. et al. (2007). Intergenerational predictors of diurnal cortisol secretion in early childhood. *Infant and Child Development,* 16(2), 151–170.

Ben-Eliyahu S. (2003). The promotion of tumor metastasis by surgery and stress: immunological basis and implications for psychoneuroimmunology. *Brain, Behavior, and Immunity,* 17(1), 27–36.

Ben-Eliyahu S., Page G. G., Schleifer, S. J. (2007). Stress, NK cells, and cancer: Still a promissory note. *Brain, Behavior, and Immunity,* 21(7), 881–887.

Ben-Eliyahu S., Page G. G., Yirmiya R., Shakhar G. (1999). Evidence that stress and surgical interventions promote tumor development by suppressing natural killer cell activity. *Int J Cancer,* 80, 880–888.

Ben-Eliyahu S., Yirmiya R., Liebeskind J. C. et al. (1991). Stress increases metastatic spread of a mammary tumor in rats: evidence for mediation by the immune system. *Brain Behav Immun,* 193–205.

Ben-Eliyahu S. et al. (2008). Stress And Fear Can Affect Cancer's Recurrence. Tel Aviv University. Retrieved 05.05.2015 from: www.sciencedaily.com/releases/2008/02/080227142656.htm.

Beniashvili D. S., Benjamin S., Baturin D. A., Anisimov V. N. (2001). Effect of light/dark regimen on N-nitrosoethylurea-induced transplacental carcinogenesis in rats. *Cancer Lett,* 10, 163(1), 51–57.

Benish M., Bartal I., Goldfarb Y. et al. (2008). Perioperative use of β-blockers and COX-2 inhibitors may improve immune competence and reduce the risk of tumor metastasis. *Annals of Surgical Oncology,* 15(7), 2042–2052.

Benjamin H. (1989). *Basic Self-Knowledge.* Newburyport, MA: Red Wheel.

Bennett J. M., Fagundes C. P., Kiecolt-Glaser J. K. (2013). The chronic stress of caregiving accelerates the natural aging of the immune system. In: J. A. Bosch et al. (eds), *Immunosenescence.* New York: Springer, 35–46.

Bennett K. K., Compas B. E., Beckjord E., Glinder J. G. (2005). Self-blame and distress among women with newly diagnosed breast cancer. *J Behav Med,* 28, 313–323.

Benson H., Klipper M. Z. (1975). *The relaxation response.* New York: Morrow.

Berard R. M. (2001). Depression and anxiety in oncology: the psychiatrist's perspective. *J Clin Psychiatry,* 62, Suppl 8, 58–61, discussion 62–63.

Berdyaev N. A. (1996). Tragediya i obyidennost. V: *Lev Shestov.* Soch. v 2 tomah. Moscow: Vodoley, 2, 465–491.

Berdyaev N. A. (2009). *Self-Knowledge: An Essay in Autobiography.* New York: Semantron Press. Reprint edn.

Berenbaum H., James T. (1994). Correlates and retrospectively reported antecedents of alexithymia. *Psychosom Med*, 56, 353–359.

Berezin F. B., Barlas T. B. (1994). Sotsialno-psihologi-cheskaya adaptatsiya pri nevroticheskih i psihosomaticheskih rasstroystvah. *Zhurn Nevropat i Psihiatrii im. S. S. Korsakova*, 94(6), 38–43.

Berezin F. B., Beznosyuk E. V., Sokolova E. D. (1998). Psihologicheskie mehanizmyi psihosomaticheskih zabolevaniy. *Rossiyskiy Meditsinskiy Zhurnal*, 2, 43–49.

Berezina T. N. (2013). Faktoryi sredyi i ih vliyanie na individualnuyu prodolzhitelnost zhizni. *Mir Psihologii*, 4(76), 165–178.

Berg M. T., Simons R. L., Barr A. et al. (2017). Childhood/Adolescent stressors and allostatic load in adulthood: Support for a calibration model. *Social Science & Medicine*, 193, 130–139.

Bergelt C., Prescott E., Grønbaek M. et al. (2006). Stressful life events and cancer risk. *British Journal of Cancer*, 95(11), 1579–1581.

Bergen A. W., Mallick A., Nishita A. et al. (2012). Chronic psychosocial stressors and salivary biomarkers in emerging adults. *Psychoneuroendocrinology*, 37, 1158–1170.

Bergenmar M., Nilsso B., Hansson J., Brandberg Y. (2004). Anxiety and depressive symptoms measured by the Hospital Anxiety and Depression Scale as predictors of time to recurrence in localized cutaneous melanoma. *Acta Oncol*, 43, 161–168.

Bergfeld A. Y. (2011). Emotsionalnyiy opyit kak prediktor retsidiva onkologicheskih zabolevaniy. *Vestnik Permskogo universiteta. Filosofiya. Psihologiya. Sotsiologiya*, (3), 60–72.

Berglas A. (1957). *Cancer: Nature, Cause and Cure*. Paris: Institute Pasteur.

Bergler E. (1992). *Principles of Self-Damage*. Madison, CT: International Universities Press.

Berman H., Zhang J., Crawford Y. G. et al. (2005). Genetic and epigenetic changes in mammary epithelial cells identify a subpopulation of cells involved in early carcinogenesis. *Cold Spring Harbor symposia on quantitative biology*, 70, 317–327.

Bermejo J. L., Sundquist J., Hemminki K. (2007). Risk of cancer among the offspring of women who experienced parental death during pregnancy. *Cancer Epidemiology Biomarkers & Prevention*, 16(11), 2204–2206.

Bermel M. B. (2011). *The Cancer Odyssey: Discovering Truth and Inspiration on the Way to Wellness*. Bloomington: Xlibris.

Bernal A. J., Jirtle R. L. (2010). Epigenomic disruption: the effects of early developmental exposures. *Birth defects research Part A: Clinical and molecular teratology*, 88(10), 938–944.

Bernay-Roman A., Hubbard-Brown J. (2011). *Deep Feeling, Deep Healing: The Heart, Mind, and Soul of Getting Well*. Jupiter, FL: Spectrum Healing Press.

Berry D. S., Pennebaker J. W. (1993). Nonverbal and verbal emotional expression and health. *Psychother Psychosom*, 59(1), 11–19.

Berry J. W., Worthington E. L. Jr (2001). Forgiveness, relationship quality, stress while imagining relationship events, and physical and mental health. *Journal of Counseling Psychology*, 48, 447–455.

Berry J. W., Worthington E. L. Jr, Parrott L. III et al. (2001). Dispositional forgivingness: development and construct validity of the Transgression Narrative Test of Forgivingness (TNTF). *Personality and Social Psychology Bulletin*, 27, 1277–1290.

Bershteyn L. M. (2000). *Gormonalnyiy kantserogenez*. Saint Petersburg: Nauka.

Berthelot N., Ensink K., Bernazzani O. et al. (2015). Intergenerational transmission of attachment in abused and neglected mothers: the role of trauma-specific reflective functioning. *Infant Ment Health J*, 36(2), 200–212.

Besedovsky H. O., del Rey A. (2007). Physiology of psychoneuroimmunology: a personal view. *Brain, Behavior, and Immunity*, 21(1), 34–44.

Beslija S. E., Bonneterre J., Burstein H. J. et al. (2003). For the Central European Cooperative Group. Consensus on the medical treatment of metastatic breast cancer. *Breast Cancer Res*, 81, 1–7.

Bessey P. Q. (1995). Metabolic response to critical illness. In: D. W. Wilmore et al. (eds), *Scientific American Surgery*. New York: Scientific American Inc, 1–31.

Bhasin M. K., Dusek J. A., Chang B. H. et al. (2013). Relaxation response induces temporal transcriptome changes in energy metabolism, insulin secretion and inflammatory pathways. *PLoS One*, 8(5), e62817.

Biaggio M. K., Godwin W. H. (1987). Relation of depression to anger and hostility. *Psychological Reports*, 61, 87–90.

Biava P. M. (2009). *Cancer and the Search for Lost Meaning: The Discovery of a Revolutionary New Cancer Treatment*. Berkeley: North Atlantic Books.

Bibring E. (1953). The mechanism of depression. In P. Greenacre (ed.), *Affective Disorders*. New York: International Universities Press.

Biegler K. A., Anderson A. K., Wenzel L. B. et al. (2012). Longitudinal change in telomere length and the chronic stress response in a randomized pilot biobehavioral clinical study: implications for cancer prevention. *Cancer Prevention Research*, 5(10), 1173–1182.

Bieliauskas L. A., Shekelle R. B., Garron D. et al. (1979). *Prospective studies of psychological depression and cancer*. Read before the 87th Annual American Psychological Association Convention, New York, Sept 1.

Bierhaus A., Wolf J., Andrassy M. et al. (2003). A mechanism converting psychosocial stress into mononuclear cell activation. *Proc Natl Acad Sci USA*, 100(4), 1920–1925.

Biondi M., Picardi A. (1996). Clinical and biological aspects of bereavement and loss-induced depression: a reappraisal. *Psychotherapy and Psychosomatics*, 65(5), 229–245.

Biryukova I. V. (2005). Primenenie tantsevalno-dvigatelnoy terapii v reabilitatsii onkologicheskih patsientov. *Zhurnal prakticheskoy psihologii i psihoanaliza*, 1. Retrieved 14.07.2014 from: http://psyjournal.ru.

Black D. S., Cole S. W., Irwin M. R. et al. (2013). Yogic meditation reverses NF-κB and IRF-related transcriptome dynamics in leukocytes of family dementia caregivers in a randomized controlled trial. *Psychoneuroendocrinology*, 38(3), 348–355.

Black P. H. (2002). Stress and the inflammatory response: a review of neurogenic inflammation. *Brain Behav Immun*, 16(6), 622–653.

Black P. H. (2006). The inflammatory consequences of psychologic stress: relationship to insulin resistance, obesity, atherosclerosis and diabetes mellitus, type II. *Med Hypotheses*, 67, 879–891.

Bleichmar H. (1996). Some subtypes of depression and their implications for psychoanalytic treatment. *Int J Psycho-Anal*, 77, 935–961.

Bleiker E. M., van der Ploeg H. M. (1997). The role of (non) expression of emotions in the development of cancer. In: A. Vingerhoets, F. van Bussel, J. Boelhouwer (eds), *The (non)expression of emotions in health and disease*. Tilburg: Tilburg University Press, 221–236.

Bleiker E. M., van der Ploeg H. M., Adèr H. J. et al. (1995). Personality traits of women with breast cancer: before and after diagnosis. *Psychol Rep*, 76(3 Pt 2), 1139–1146.

Bleyer A., Welch H. G. (2012). Effect of Three Decades of Screening Mammography on Breast-Cancer Incidence. *N Engl J Med*, 367, 1998–2005.

Blinov N. N., Homyakov I. P., Shipovnikov N. V. (1990). Ob otnoshenii onkologicheskih bolnyih k svoemu diagnozu. *Voprosyi Onkologii*, 8, 966–969.

Blomberg B. B., Alvarez J. P., Diaz A. et al. (2009). Psychosocial adaptation and cellular immunity in breast cancer patients in the weeks after surgery: An exploratory study. *J Psychosom Res*, 67(5), 369–376.

Bloom F. E., Lazerson A. (2000). *Brain, Mind, and Behavior* (3rd edn). New York: Worth.

Blumberg E., West P., Ellis A. A. (1954). Possible Relationship Between Psychological Factors and Human Cancer. *Psychosomatic Med*, 16, 277–286.

Boccia M., Piccardi L., Guariglia P. (2015). The Meditative Mind: A Comprehensive Meta-Analysis of MRI Studies. *Biomed Res Int*, 419808.

Bock J., Wainstock T., Braun K., Segal M. (2015). Stress in utero: Prenatal programming of brain plasticity and cognition. *Biological Psychiatry*, 78(5), 315–326.

Bogdanova M. V. (2005). *Osobennosti psihologicheskih zaschit pri psihomaticheskih rasstroystvah: na primere chasto i dlitelno boleyuschih*. Diss. kand. psihol. nauk. Tomsk: Tyumen.

Bogomolets A. A. (1926). *V vedeniye v uchenie o konstitutsiyakh i diatezakh*. Moscow: izd-vo Sabashnikovykh.

Bogoyavlenskiy N. A. (1955). K istorii proishozhdeniya i razvitiya vzglyadov u russkogo naroda na opuholevyie bolezni. *Vopr Onkologii*, 1, 106–111.

Bolen J. (2016). A Virtual Interview with Jean Shinoda Bolen, MD. Retrieved 15.05.2016 from https://www.oncolink.org.

Boor de, C. (1965). Strukturunterschiede unbewußter Phantasien bei Neurosen und psychosomatischen Krankheiten. *Psyche*, 18(11), 664–673.

Booth G. (1969). The auspicious moment in somatic medicine. *The American Journal of Psychoanalysis*, 29(1), 84–88.

Booth G. (1973). Psychobiological aspects of "spontaneous" regressions of cancer. *J of Am Acad of Psychoanalysis*, 1(3), 303–17.

Booth G. (1979). *The Cancer Epidemic: Shadow of the Conquest of Nature*. Lewiston, ME; New York: Edwin Mellen Press.

Borges G., Benjet C., Medina-Mora M. E. et al. (2008). Traumatic events and suicide-related outcomes among Mexico City adolescents. *J Child Psychol Psychiatry*, 49(6), 654–666.

Borghol N., Suderman M., McArdle W. et al. (2012). Associations with early-life socio-economic position in adult DNA methylation. *International Journal of Epidemiology*, 41(1), 62–74.

Bos J. L. (2006). Epac proteins: multi-purpose cAMP targets. *Trends Biochem Sci*, 1(12), 680–686.

Boscaglia N., Clarke D. M., Jobling T. W., Quinn M. A. (2005). The contribution of spirituality and spiritual coping to anxiety and depression in women with a recent diagnosis of gynecological cancer. *Int J Gynecol Cancer*, 15(5), 755–761.

Bottomley A., Jones L. (1997). Social support and the cancer patient—a need for clarity. *European Journal of Cancer Care*, 6(1), 72–77.

Bovbjerg D. H., Valdimarsdottir H. (1993). Familial cancer, emotional distress, and low natural cytotoxic activity in healthy women. *Annals of Oncology*, 4(9), 745–752.

Bovbjerg D. H., Redd W. H., Maier L. A. et al. (1990). Anticipatory immune suppression and nausea in women receiving cyclic chemotherapy for ovarian cancer. *J Consult Clin Psychol*, 58, 153–157.

Bower J. E., Ganz P. A., Aziz N. et al. (2007). Inflammatory responses to psychological stress in fatigued breast cancer survivors: relationship to glucocorticoids. *Brain, Behavior, and Immunity*, 21(3), 251–258.

Bower J. E., Greendale G., Crosswell A. D. et al. (2014). Yoga reduces inflammatory signaling in fatigued breast cancer survivors: A randomized controlled trial. *Psychoneuroendocrinology*, 43, 20–29.

Bower J. E., Kemeny M. E., Taylor S. E., Fahey J. L. (2003). Finding positive meaning and its association with natural killer cell cytotoxicity among participants in a bereavement-related disclosure intervention. *Annals of Behavioral Medicine*, 25(2), 146–155.

Bowlby J. (1984). *Attachment and Loss*. London: Penguin UK.

Bowman R. E., Ferguson D., Luine V. N. (2002). Effects of chronic restraint stress and estradiol on open field activity, spatial memory, and monoaminergic neurotransmitters in ovariectomized rats. *Neuroscience*, 113(2), 401–410.

Boyd A. L., Salleh A., Humber B. et al. (2010). Neonatal Experiences Differentially Influence Mammary Gland Morphology, Estrogen Receptor α Protein Levels, and Carcinogenesis in BALB/c Mice. *Cancer Prev Res (Phila)*, 3(11), 1398–1408.

Bränström R., Kvillemo P., Brandberg Y., Moskowitz J. T. (2010). Self-report mindfulness as a mediator of psychological well-being in a stress reduction intervention for cancer patients—a randomized study. *Annals of Behavioral Medicine*, 39(2), 151–161.

Brassai L., Piko B. F., Steger M. F. (2011). Meaning in life: Is it a protective factor for adolescents' psychological health? *International Journal of Behavioral Medicine*, 18(1), 44–51.

Bräutigam W., Paul C., von Rad M. (1997). *Psychosomatische Medizin: Ein kurzgefaßtes Lehrbuch.* Taschenbuch. Stuttgart: Thieme.

Brekhman G. I. (2011). Emotsionalnaya zhizn ploda: ot smutnyih dogadok k nauchnyim issledovaniyam. *Zhinochiy Likar*, 2, 10–15.

Brekhman I. I. (1982). Filosofsko-metodologicheskie aspektyi problemyi zdorovya cheloveka. *Voprosyi filosofii*, 2, 48–53.

Breitbart W. (2002). Spirituality and meaning in supportive care: spirituality-and meaning-centered group psychotherapy interventions in advanced cancer. *Supportive Care in Cancer*, 10(4), 272–280.

Breitbart W., Rosenfeld B., Gibson C. et al. (2010). Meaning-centered group psychotherapy for patients with advanced cancer: a pilot randomized controlled trial. *Psycho-Oncology*, 19(1), 21–28.

Brémond A., Kune G. A., Bahnson C. B. (1986). Psychosomatic factors in breast cancer patients. Results of a case control study. *Journal of Psychosomatic Obstetrics & Gynecology*, 5(2), 127–136.

Brent D. A., Melhem N. (2008). Familial transmission of suicidal behavior. *Psychiatric Clinics of North America*, 31, 157–177.

Breslau N., Kessler R. C. (2001). The stressor criterion in DSM-IV posttraumatic stress disorder: an empirical investigation. *Biol Psychiatry*, 50(9), 699–704.

Brezo J., Klempan T., Turecki G. (2008). The genetics of suicide: a critical review of molecular studies. *Psychiatric Clinics of North America*, 31, 179–203.

Briggs M. K., Shoffner M. F. (2006). Spiritual wellness and depression: Testing a theoretical model with older adolescents and midlife adults. *Counseling and Values*, 51(1), 5–22.

Bright M. A., Hinojosa M. S., Knapp C. et al. (2014). Adverse childhood experiences and health outcomes in childhood/adolescence: co - morbidity of physical, mental, and learning disorders. Abstracts of 72nd Annual Scientific Meeting of American Psychosomatic Society: *Stretching the Boundaries: From Mechanisms of Disease to Models of Health.* San Francisco, CA.

Brisch K. H. (2009). *Bindungsstorungen. Von der Bindungstheorie zur Therapie.* Klett-Cotta: Nachfolger GmbH.

Brodie D. (2015). The cancer personality: its importance in healing. In: *Cancer Report: The Latest Research - How Thousands are Achieving Permanent Recoveries.* Retrieved 10.11.2015 from: http://www.healingcancer.info/ebook/douglas-brodie.

Bronk K. C., Hill P., Lapsley D. K. et al. (2009). Purpose, hope, and life satisfaction in three age groups. *Journal of Positive Psychology*, 4(6), 500–510.

Brooker R. J., Davidson R. J., Goldsmith H. H. (2015). Maternal negative affect during infancy is linked to disrupted patterns of diurnal cortisol and alpha asymmetry across contexts during childhood. *Journal of Experimental Child Psychology*, 142, 274–290.

Brown D. W., Anda R. F., Felitti V. J. et al. (2010). Adverse childhood experiences are associated with the risk of lung cancer: a prospective cohort study. *BMC Public Health*, 10(1), 20.

Brown J. E., Butow P. N., Culjak G. et al. (2000). Psychosocial predictors of outcome: time to relapse and survival in patients with early stage melanoma. *British Journal of Cancer*, 83(11), 1448–1453.

Brown P., Finkelhor D. (1986). Impact of child sexual abuse: A review of research. *Psychol Bull*, 99(1), 66–77.

Brunet A., Poundja J., Tremblay J. et al. (2011). Trauma reactivation under the influence of propranolol decreases posttraumatic stress symptoms and disorder: 3 open-label trials. *J Clin Psychopharmacol*, 31(4), 547–550.

Buber M. (2003). *Two Types of Faith*. Syracuse, New York: Syracuse University Press.

Buccheri G. (1998). Depressive reactions to lung cancer are common and often followed by a poor outcome. *European Respiratory Journal*, 11(1), 173–178.

Buettner D. (2008). *The blue zones: lessons for living longer from the people who've lived the longest*. Washington, D.C.: National Geographic.

Bufalino C., Hepgul N., Aguglia E., Pariante C. M. (2013). The role of immune genes in the association between depression and inflammation: a review of recent clinical studies. *Brain, Behavior, and Immunity*, 31, 31–47.

Bukhtoyarov O. V., Arkhangelskiy A. E. (2006). Psihogennaya smert v onkologii: obosnovanie ponyatiya, patogenez, formyi razvitiya, vozmozhnosti profilaktiki. *Voprosyi Onkologii*, 52(6), 708–715.

Bukhtoyarov O. V., Arkhangelskiy A. E. (2008). *Psihogennyiy kofaktor kantserogeneza. Vozmozhnosti primeneniya gipnoterapii*. Saint Petersburg: Aleteyya.

Bukhtoyarov O. V., Samarin D. M. (2010). Edinstvo psihiki i tela: kontseptsiya dominantyi zhiznennoy tseli. *Mir psihologii*, 3, 210–220.

Bulgakova O. S. (2010). Psihofiziologicheskie disfunktsii: mehanizmyi, diagnostika. *Mezhdunarodnyiy Zhurnal Prikladnyih i Fundamentalnyih Issledovaniy*, 7, 45–51.

Burchfield S. R. (1979). The stress response: a new perspective. *Psychosomatic Medicine*, 8, 661–672.

Burdick K. E., DeRosse P., Kane J. M. et al. (2010). Association of genetic variation in the MET proto-oncogene with schizophrenia and general cognitive ability. *American J of Psychiatry*, 167(4), 436–443.

Burg M. M., Lampert R., Joska T. et al. (2004). Psychological traits and emotion-triggering of ICD schock-terminated arrhythmias. *Psychosom Med*, 66, 898–902.

Burk L. (2015). Warning dreams preceding the diagnosis of breast cancer: a survey of the most important characteristics. *Explore*, 11(3), 193–198.

Burlachuk L. F., Grabskaya I. A., Kocharyan A. S. (1999). *Osnovyi psihoterapii*. K.: Nika-Tsentr.

Burns M. O., Seligman M. E. (1989). Explanatory style across the life span: evidence for stability over 52 years. *Journal of Personality and Social Psychology*, 56(3), 471–477.

Burrows J. (1783). *A new practical essay on cancers*. London: printed for the author.

Burton C. (2010). The effects of surviving cancer. GP newspaper, 14 May.

Burtovaya E. V. (2002). *Konfliktologiya. Uchebnoe posobie*. Moscow: Yuniti.

Bussell V. A., Naus M. J. (2010). A longitudinal investigation of coping and posttraumatic growth in breast cancer survivors. *J Psychosoc Oncol*, 28, 61–78.

Butler L. D., Koopman C., Classen C. et al. (1999). Traumatic stress, life events, and emotional support in women with metastatic breast cancer: cancer-related traumatic stress symptoms associated with past and current stressors. *Health Psychol*, 18, 555–560.

Buzunov A. F. (2010). *Formirovaniye somaticheskikh posledstviy adaptatsionnogo sindroma. Tsena tsivilizatsii*. Moscow: Prakticheskaya meditsina.

Bykhovskiy G. B. (1928). K voprosu o znachenii psihicheskogo momenta v hirurgii. *Vestnik Hirurgii i Pogranichnyih Oblastey*, 37–8, 1–15.

Bykov K. M., Kurtsin I. T. (1960). *Kortiko-vistseralnaya patologiya*. Leningrad: Medgiz.

Byilkina N. D. (1997). Razvitie zarubezhnyih psihosomaticheskih teoriy (analiticheskiy obzor). *Psihologicheskiy Zhurnal*, 18(2), 149–160.

Byuleten Natsionalnogo Kantser-reestru No 16. *Rak v Ukrayini*, 2013-2014. Retrieved 19.10.2015 from: http://www.ncru.inf.ua/publications/BULL_16/index.htm.

Cacioppo J. T., Kiecolt-Glaser J. K., Malarkey W. B., Laskowski B. F. (2002). Autonomic and glucocorticoid associations with the steady-state expression of latent Epstein-Barr virus. *Horm Behav*, 42(1), 32–41.

Cahill L., Prins B., Weber M., McGaugh J. L. (1994). Beta-adrenergic activation and memory for emotional events. *Nature*, 371, 702–704.

Calado R. T., Young N. S. (2009). Telomere diseases. *N Engl J Med*, 361(24), 2353–23265.

Campbell J. P., Karolak M. R., Ma Y. et al. (2012). Stimulation of host bone marrow stromal cells by sympathetic nerves promotes breast cancer bone metastasis in mice. *PLoS biology*, 10(7), e1001363.

Campion J., Rocco S. (2009). Minding the mind: the effects and potential of a school-based meditation programme for mental health promotion. *Advances in School Mental Health Promotion*, 2(1), 47–55.

Camus A. (1990). *The Myth of Sisyphus*. London: Penguin.

Cannon W. B. (1916). *Bodily changes in pain, hunger, fear, and rage: An account of recent researches into the function of emotional excitement*. New York: D. Appleton & Company.

Cannon W. B. (1942). "Voodoo" death. *American Anthropologist*, 44 (new series),169–181.

Cao L., Liu X., Lin E. J. et al. (2010). Environmental and genetic activation of a brain-adipocyte BDNF/leptin axis causes cancer remission and inhibition. *Cell*, 142(1), 52–64.

Caplan G. (1963). Emotional crises. In: W. A. Deutsch, H. Fishman (eds), *Encyclopedia of Mental Health*, 2, 521–532.

Cardenal V., Cerezo M. V., Marti'nez J. et al. (2012). Personality, Emotions and Coping Styles: Predictive Value for the Evolution of Cancer Patients. *The Spanish Journal of Psychology*, 15(2), 756–767.

Cardenal V., Ortiz-Tallo M., Frias I. M., Lozano J. M. (2008). Life stressors, emotional avoidance and breast cancer. *The Spanish Journal of Psychology*, 11(02), 522–530.

Carlson L. E., Speca M. (2011). *Mindfulness-based cancer recovery: A step-by-step MBSR approach to help you cope with treatment and reclaim your life*. Oakland: New Harbinger Publications.

Carlson L. E., Beattie T. L., Giese-Davis J. et al. (2015). Mindfulness-based cancer recovery and supportive-expressive therapy maintain telomere length relative to controls in distressed breast cancer survivors. *Cancer*, 121(3), 476–484.

Carlson L. E., Speca M., Patel K. D., Goodey E. (2004). Mindfulness-based stress reduction in relation to quality of life, mood, symptoms of stress and levels of cortisol, dehydroepiandrosterone sulfate (DHEAS) and melatonin in breast and prostate cancer outpatients. *Psychoneuroendocrinology*, 29(4), 448–474.

Carlson L. E., Speca M., Patel K. D. et al. (2003). Mindfulness-based stress reduction in relation to quality of life, mood, symptoms of stress, and immune parameters in breast and prostate cancer outpatients. *Psychosom Med*, 65, 571–581.

Carlsson E., Frostell A., Ludvigsson J., Faresjo M. (2014). Psychological Stress in Children May Alter the Immune Response. *The Journal of Immunology*, 192(5), 2071–2081.

Carpenter J. S., Brockopp D. Y., Andrykowski M. A. (1999). Self-transformation as a factor in the self-esteem and well-being of breast cancer survivors. *J Adv Nurs*, 29(6), 1402–1411.

Carpenter L. L., Gawuga C., Tyrka A. et al. (2010). Association between Plasma IL-6 Response to Acute Stress and Early-Life Adversity in Healthy Adults. *Neuropsychopharmacology*, 35, 2617–2623.

Carvalho F., Beblo T., Schlosser N. et al. (2012). Associations of childhood trauma with hypothalamic-pituitary-adrenal function in borderline personality disorder and major depression. *Psychoneuroendocrinology*, 37(10), 1659–1668.

Cashwell C. S., Myers J. E., Shurts W. M. (2004). Using the developmental counseling and therapy model to work with a client in spiritual bypass: Some preliminary considerations. *Journal of Counseling & Development*, 82, 403–409.

Caspi A., Sugden K., Moffitt T. E. (2003). Influence of life stress on depression: moderation by a polymorphism in the 5-HTT gene. *Science*, 301, 386–389.

Cassileth B. R. (1995). History of psychotherapeutic intervention in cancer patients. *Supportive Care in Cancer*, 3(4), 264–266.

Cassileth B. R., Walsh W. P., Lusk E. J. (1988). Psychosocial correlates of cancer survival: a subsequent report 3 to 8 years after cancer diagnosis. *J Clin Oncol*, 6(11), 1753–1759.

Cassoni P., Marrocco T., Deaglio S. et al. (2001). Biological relevance of oxytocin and oxytocin receptors in cancer cells and primary tumors. *Ann Oncol*, 12(Suppl 2), S37–39.

Catts V. S., Catts S. V., McGrath J. J. et al. (2006). Apoptosis and schizophrenia: a pilot study based on dermal fibroblast cell lines. *Schizophrenia Research*, 84(1), 20–8.

Cavigelli S. A., Yee J. R., McClintock M. K. (2006). Infant temperament predicts life span in female rats that develop spontaneous tumors. *Horm Behav*, 50(3), 454–462.

Cella D., Mahon S., Donovan M. (1990). Cancer recurrence as a traumatic event. *Behav Med*, 16, 15–22.

Chakroborty D., Sarkar C., Basu B. et al. (2009). Catecholamines regulate tumor angiogenesis. *Cancer research*, 69(9), 3727–3730.

Challis G. B., Stam H. J. (1990). The spontaneous regression of cancer. A review of cases from 1900 to 1987. *Acta Oncol*, 29, 545–549.

Chan K. T., Cortesio C. L., Huttenlocher A. (2009). FAK alters invadopodia and focal adhesion composition and dynamics to regulate breast cancer invasion. *The Journal of Cell Biology*, 185(2), 357–370.

Chandola T., Brunner E., Marmot M. (2006). Chronic stress at work and the metabolic syndrome: prospective study. *BMJ*, 332(7540), 521–525.

Chapman B. P., Fiscella K., Kawachi I. et al. (2013). Emotion suppression and mortality risk over a 12-year follow-up. *J Psychosom Res*, 75(4), 381–385.

Chapuys C. (1607). *Traité des cancers tant occultes qu'ulcérés, auquel il est enseigné leur curation certaine, comme aussi des fistules.* Lyon.

Chardin de P. T. (2008). *The Phenomenon of Man*. New York: Harper Perennial Modern Classics.

Charmaz K. (2000). Experiencing chronic illness. In: G. L. Albrecht, R. Fitzpatrick, and S. C. Scrimshaw (eds), *Handbook of social studies in health and medicine*. Thousand Oaks, CA: Sage Publications, 277–292.

Chatfield C. (2015). *A Formula for Healing Cancer: The Latest Research in Mind-Body Medicine.* Retrieved 02.09.2015 from: http://www.healingcancer.info/ebook.

Chekhun V. F. (2013). Vzaimodejstvie opuholi i organizma kak aktualnoe napravlenie nauchnyh issledovanij. *Zdorov'ya Ukrayini*, 1(26), 12–13.

Chen C. C., David A. S., Nunnerley H. et al. (1995). Adverse life events and breast cancer: case-control study. *BMJ*, 311(7019), 1527–1530.

Chen E. E., Miller G. E., Walker H. A. et al. (2009). Genome-wide transcriptional profiling linked to social class in asthma. *Thorax*, 64(1), 38–43.

Chen E. E., Miller G. E., Kobor M. S., Cole S. W. (2011). Maternal warmth buffers the effects of low early-life socioeconomic status on pro-inflammatory signaling in adulthood. *Mol Psychiatry*, 16, 729–737.

Chen Y. C., Shen Y. C., Hung Y. J. et al. (2007). Comparisons of glucose–insulin homeostasis following maprotiline and fluoxetine treatment in depressed males. *Journal of Affective Disorders*, 103(1–3), 257–261.

Chen Y. H., Lin H. C. (2011). Increased risk of cancer subsequent to severe depression—a nationwide population-based study. *Journal of Affective Disorders*, 131(1), 200–206.

Cherkas L. F., Aviv A., Valdes A. M. et al. (2006). The effects of social status on biological aging as measured by white-blood-cell telomere length. *Aging Cell*, 5(5), 361–365.

Chernavskiy D. S., Voronov M. V., Grimblat S. O., Rodshtat I. V. (2003). Psihoterapiya v kompleksnom lechenii onkologicheskoj patologii. *Mezhdunarodnyj Medicinskiy Zhurnal*, 4, 27–32.

Chichester F. (2012). *The Lonely Sea and the Sky*. Chichester: Summersdale. Reprint edn.

Chida Y., Hamer M., Wardle J., Steptoe A. (2008). Do stress-related psychosocial factors contribute to cancer incidence and survival? *Nat Clin Pract Oncol*, 5(8), 466–475.

Chochinov H. M. (2001). Depression in cancer patients. *Lancet Oncol*, 2(8), 499–505.

Chochinov H. M., Hack T., Hassard T. et al: (2005). Dignity therapy: a novel psychotherapeutic interventions for patients near the end of life. *J Clin Oncol*, 23, 5520–5525.

Chodak G. W., Thisted R. A., Gerber G. S. et al. (1994). Results of conservative management of clinically localized prostate cancer. *N Engl J Med*, 330, 242–248.

Chogyal Namkhai Norbu. (2003). *Dzogchen: The Self-Perfected State*. Boulder, CO: Snow Lion.

Choi C. H., Song T., Kim T. H. et al. (2014). Meta-analysis of the effects of beta blocker on survival time in cancer patients. *Journal of cancer research and clinical oncology*, 140(7), 1179–1188.

Choy C., Raytis J. L., Smith D. D. et al. (2016). Inhibition of β2-adrenergic receptor reduces triple-negative breast cancer brain metastases: The potential benefit of perioperative β-blockade. *Oncol Rep*, 35, 3135–3142.

Choi J., Fauce S. R., Effros R. B. (2008). Reduced telomerase activity in human T lymphocytes exposed to cortisol. *Brain Behav Immun*, 22(4), 600–605.

Christian L. M., Glaser R., Porter K. et al. (2011). Poorer self-rated health is associated with elevated inflammatory markers among older adults. *Psychoneuroendocrinology*, 36, 1495–1504.

Chukhrova M. G., Openko T. G., Korepanov S. V. (2010). Psihoemocionalnye sostoyaniya i lichnostnye harakteristiki pri rake. *Mir Nauki, Kultury, Obrazovaniya*, 1, 236–238.

Chulkova A., Moiseenko M. (2009). Psihologicheskie problemy v onkologii. *Rossijskiy Onkologicheskiy Zhurnal*, 10(3), 151–157.

Chung Y. C., Chang, Y. F. (2003). Serum interleukin-6 levels reflect the disease status of colorectal cancer. *J. Surg. Oncol*, 83, 222–226.

Ciccia A., Elledge S. J. (2010). The DNA Damage Response: Making It Safe to Play with Knives. *Molecular Cell*, 40(2-22), 179–204

Ciechanowski P. S., Walker E. A., Katon W. J., Russo J. E. (2002). Attachment theory: A model for health care utilization and somatization. *Psychosomatic Medicine*, 64(4), 660-667.

Cimprich B. (1999). Pretreatment symptom distress in women newly diagnosed with breast cancer. *Cancer Nursing*, 22(3), 185–194.

Ciring D. A. (2009). Semya kak faktor formirovaniya lichnostnoj bespomoshnosti u detej. *Voprosy Psihologii*, (1), 22–31.

Clarkson P. (2002). *The Transpersonal Relationship in Psychotherapy*. London: Whurr Publishers.

Clifford T. (1996). *Tibetan Buddhist Medicine and Psychiatry: The Diamond Healing*. Delhi: Motilal Banarsidass.

Clougherty J. E., Levy J. I. (2018). Psychosocial and Chemical Stressors. In: Rider C., Simmons J. E. (eds), *Chemical Mixtures and Combined Chemical and Nonchemical Stressors*. Berlin: Springer, 493–514.

Cobb A. B. (1952). *A Socio-psychological Study of the Cancer Patient*. Doc. Thesis. Austin, TX: University of Texas.

Coe C. L., Rusenberg L. T., Levine S. (1985). Immunological consequences of maternal separation in infant primates. In: H. Spector (ed.), *Neuroimmunomodulation. Proceedings of the First International Workshop of Neuroimmunomodulation*. Bethesda: IWGN, 213–216.

Coe C. L., Lubach G. R., Karaszewski J. W., Ershler W. B. (1996). Prenatal endocrine activation alters postnatal cellular immunity in infant monkeys. *Brain Behav Immun*, 10(3), 221–234.

Cohen L., Cole S. W., Sood A. K. et al. (2012). Depressive symptoms and cortisol rhythmicity predict survival in patients with renal cell carcinoma: role of inflammatory signaling. *PLoS One*, 7, e42324.

Cohen L., Marshall G. D. Jr, Cheng L. et al. (2000). DNA repair capacity in healthy medical students during and after exam stress. *J Behav Med*, 23(6), 531–544.

Cohen L., Parker P. A., Vence L. et al. (2011). Presurgical stress management improves postoperative immune function in men with prostate cancer undergoing radical prostatectomy. *Psychosomatic Medicine*, 73(3), 218–225.

Cohen R., Bavishi C., Rozanski A. (2015). Purpose in Life and its Relationship to All-Cause Mortality and Cardiovascular Events: A Meta-Analysis. *Circulation,* 131(Suppl 1), A52–A52.

Cohen S., Rabin B. S. (1998). Psychologic stress, immunity, and cancer. *J Natl Cancer Inst*, 90, 3–4.

Cohen S., Miller G. E., Rabin B. S. (2001). Psychological stress and antibody response to immunization: a critical review of the human literature. *Psychosom Med*, 63(1), 7–18.

Cohen S., Tyrrell D. A., Smith A. P. (1991). Psychological stress and susceptibility to the common cold. *N Engl J Med*, 325(9), 606–612.

Cohen T., Nahari D., Cerem L. W. et al. (1996). Interleukin 6 induces the expression of vascular endothelial growth factor. *J Biol Chem*, 271(2), 736–741.

Cohen-Woods S., Fisher H. L., Ahmetspahic D. et al. (2017). Interaction between childhood maltreatment on immunogenetic risk in depression: discovery and replication in clinical case-control samples. *Brain, behavior, and immunity*, 67, 203–210.

Coker A. L., Bond S., Madeleine M. M. et al. (2003). Psychosocial stress and cervical neoplasia risk. *Psychosom Med*, 65, 644–645.

Colbert D. (2006). *Deadly Emotions: Understand the Mind-Body-Spirit Connection That Can Heal or Destroy You.* Nashville: Thomas Nelson.

Cole B. (2005). Spiritually-focused psychotherapy for people diagnosed with cancer: A pilot outcome study. *Mental Health, Religion & Culture*, 3(3), 217–226.

Cole S. W. (2012). Social regulation of gene expression in the immune system. In: Segerstrom S. (ed.). *The Oxford Handbook of Psychoneuroimmunology.* New York: Oxford University Press, 254–273.

Cole S. W. (2009). Social regulation of human gene expression. *Curr Dir Psychol Sci*, 18(3), 132–137.

Cole S. W. (2013). Nervous system regulation of the cancer genome. *Brain, Behavior, and Immunity*, 30, S10–S18.

Cole S. W. (2014). Human social genomics. *PLoS Genet*, 10(8), e1004601.

Cole S. W., Arevalo, J., Takahashi, R. et al. (2010b). Computational identification of gene-social environment interaction at the human IL6 locus. *Proc Natl Acad Sci USA,* 107, 5681–5686.

Cole S. W., Conti, G., Arevalo, J. M. et al. (2012). Transcriptional modulation of the developing immune system by early life social adversity. *Proc Natl Acad Sci USA*, 109(50), 20578–20583.

Cole S. W., Naliboff B. D., Kemeny M. E. et al. (2001). Impaired response to HAART in HIV-infected individuals with high autonomic nervous system activity. *Proc Natl Acad Sci USA*, 98, 12695–12700.

Cole S. W., Korin Y. D., Fahey J. L., Zack J. A. (1998). Norepinephrine accelerates HIV replication via protein kinase A-dependent effects on cytokine production. *J Immunol*, 161, 610–616.

Conger R. D., Neppl, T., Kim, K. J., Scaramella, L. (2003). Angry and aggressive behavior across three generations: A prospective, longitudinal study of parents and children. *Journal of Abnormal Child Psychology*, 31(2), 143–160.

Contractor A. A., Brown L. A., Weiss N. H. (2018). Relation between Lifespan Polytrauma Typologies and Post-Trauma Mental Health. *Comprehensive Psychiatry*, 80, 202–213.

Cook S. C., Wellman C. L. (2004). Chronic stress alters dendritic morphology in rat medial prefrontal cortex. *J Neurobiol*, 60(2), 236–248.

Cooper C. L., Faragher E. B. (1993). Psychosocial stress and breast cancer: the inter-relationship between stress events, coping strategies and personality. *Psychological Medicine* (London), 23, 653–653.

Cooper C. L., Cooper R., Faragher E. B. (1989). Incidence and perception of psychosocial stress: the relationship with breast cancer. *Psychol Med*, 19, 415–422.

Cordova M. J., Davis J. G., Golant M. et al. (2007). Breast cancer as trauma: Posttraumatic stress and posttraumatic growth. *Journal of Clinical Psychology in Medical Settings*, 14, 308–319.

Costanzo E. S., Sood A. K., Lutgendorf S. K. (2011). Biobehavioral influences on cancer progression. *Immunol Allergy Clin North Am*, 31, 109.

Costanzo E. S., Lutgendorf S. K., Sood A. K. et al. (2005). Psychosocial factors and interleukin-6 among women with advanced ovarian cancer. *Cancer*, 104, 305–313.

Costello P. C. (2013). *Attachment-based psychotherapy: Helping patients develop adaptive capacities*. Washington, DC: American Psychological Association.

Cotrufo P., Galiani R. (2014). The Body of Libido and The Imploded Organ-Some Reflections on the Economy (and on the Topography) of Libido on People Affected by Cancer. *J Psychol Psychother*, 4(148), 2161–0487.

Courtney J. G., Longnecker M. P., Theorell T., de Verdier M. G. (1993). Stressful life events and the risk of colorectal cancer. *Epidemiology*, 4(5), 407–414.

Cousijn H., Rijpkema M., Qin S. et al. (2010). Acute stress modulates genotype effects on amygdala processing in humans. *Proc Natl Acad Sci USA*, 107(21), 9867–9872.

Cowdry E. V. (1955). *Cancer cells*. Philadelphia and London: W. B. Saunders.

Cowles M. K. (2009). Stress, Cytokines and Depressive Illness. In: Larry R. S. (ed.), *Encyclopedia of Neuroscience*. 3th. Oxford: Academic Press, 519–527.

Cox M. E., Deeble P. D., Lakhani S., Parsons S. J. (1999). Acquisition of neuroendocrine characteristics by prostate tumor cells is reversible: implications for prostate cancer progression. *Cancer Res*, 59, 3821–3830

Cox T., Mackay C. (1982). Psychosocial factors and psychophysiological mechanisms in the aetiology and development of cancers. *Soc Sci Med*, 16(4), 381–396.

Coyne J. C., Palmer S. C., Shapiro P. J. et al. (2004). Distress, psychiatric morbidity, and prescriptions for psychotropic medication in a breast cancer waiting room sample. *Gen Hosp Psychiatry*, 26, 121–128.

Crawford J. S. (1981). The role of rehabilitative medicine. In: D. A. Gordon (ed.), *Rheumathoid Arthritis*. New York: Medical Examination Publishing.

Creswell J. D., Irwin M. R., Burklund L. J. et al. (2012). Mindfulness-based stress reduction training reduces loneliness and pro-inflammatory gene expression in older adults: a small randomized controlled trial. *Brain Behav Immun*, 26, 1095–1101.

Crispen P. L., Viterbo R., Fox E. B et al. (2008). Delayed intervention of sporadic renal masses undergoing active surveillance. *Cancer*, 112(5), 1051–1057.

Crittenden P. M., Landini A. (2011). *Assessing Adult Attachment: A Dynamic-Maturational Approach to Discourse Analysis*. New York: W. W. Norton & Company.

Crosswell A. D., Bower J. E., Ganz P. A. (2014). Childhood adversity and inflammation in breast cancer survivors. *Psychosomatic Medicine*, 76(3), 208–214.

Cruess D. G., Antoni M. H., McGregor B. A. et al. (2000). Cognitive-behavioral stress management reduces serum cortisol by enhancing benefit finding among women being treated for early stage breast cancer. *Psychosomatic Medicine*, 62, 304–308.

Culos-Reed S. N., Carlson L. E., Daroux L. M., Hately-Aldous S. (2006). A Pilot Study of Yoga for Breast Cancer Survivors: Physical and Psychological Benefits. *Psycho-Oncology*, 15, 891–897.

Cunningham A. J. (2005). Integrating spirituality into a group psychological therapy program for cancer patients. *Integrative Cancer Therapies*, 4(2), 178-186.

Cunningham A. J., Edmonds C. V. (1996). Group psychological therapy for cancer patients: a point of view, and discussion of the hierarchy of options. *International Journal of Psychiatry in Medicine*, 26, 51–82.

Curry J. M., Hanke M. L., Piper M. G. et al. (2010). Social disruption induces lung inflammation. *Brain, Behavior, and Immunity*, 24(3), 394–402.

Curtin S. C., Minino A. M., Anderson R. N. (2016). Declines in Cancer Death Rates Among Children and Adolescents in the United States, 1999–2014. *NCHS data brief*, (257), 1-8.

Curtis M. A., Kam M., Faull R. L. (2011). Neurogenesis in humans. *European Journal of Neuroscience*, 33(6), 1170–1174.

Cutler M. (1954). The nature of the cancer process in relation to a possible psychosomatic influence. *The Psychological Variables in Human Cancer*. A symposium presented at the Veterans Administration Hospital, Long Beach, Calif., October 23, 1953. Berkeley: University of California Press, 1–16.

Cutter E. (1887). Diet on Cancer. *Albany Med J*, 8, 218–251.

Cwikel J. G., Gidron Y., Quastel M. (2010). Low-dose environmental radiation, DNA damage, and cancer: the possible contribution of psychological factors. *Psychology, Health & Medicine*, 15(1), 1–16.

Czéh B., Welt T., Fischer A. K. et al. (2002). Chronic psychosocial stress and concomitant repetitive transcranial magnetic stimulation: effects on stress hormone levels and adult hippocampal neurogenesis. *Biological Psychiatry*, 52(11), 1057–1065.

Dada R., Kumar S. B., Tolahunase M. et al. (2015). Yoga and Meditation as a Therapeutic Intervention in Oxidative Stress and Oxidative DNA Damage to Paternal Genome. *J Yoga Phys Ther*, 5(4), 217.

Dagan O., Asok A., Steele H. et al. (2017). Attachment security moderates the link between adverse childhood experiences and cellular aging. *Development and Psychopathology*, 1–13.

Dahlen H. G., Kennedy H. P., Anderson C. M. et al. (2013). The EPIIC hypothesis: intrapartum effects on the neonatal epigenome and consequent health outcomes. *Med Hypotheses*, 80, 656–662.

Dahlke R. (1997). *Krankheit als Sprache der Seele*. Munchen: Goldmann Wilhelm Verlag.

Dahlke R. (1999). *Lebenskrisen als Entwicklungschancen: Zeiten des Umbruchs und ihre Krankheitsbilder*. Munchen: Goldmann Wilhelm Verlag.

Damjanovic A. K., Yang Y., Glaser R. et al. (2007). Accelerated telomere erosion is associated with a declining immune function of caregivers of Alzheimer's disease patients. *J Immunol*, 179, 4249–4254.

Danese A., Pariante C. M., Caspie A. et al. (2007). Childhood maltreatment predicts adult inflammation in a life-course study. *Proc Natl Acad Sci USA*, 104(4), 1319–1324.

Danilenko L. V. (2008). Urok Aleksandra Solzhenicyna: razmyshlenie o ego povesti "Rakovyj korpus". *Literaturnaya ucheba*, 6.

Danilin A. G. (2011). *Tabletka ot smerti*. Moscow: Isolg.

Dantzer R., O'Connor J. C., Freund G. G. et al. (2008). From inflammation to sickness and depression: when the immune system subjugates the brain. *Nat Rev Neurosci*, 9(1), 46–56.

D'Aquili E., Newberg A. (2002). *The mystical mind*. Minneapolis: Fortress Press.

Dattore P. J., Shontz F. C., Coyne L. (1980). Premorbid personality differentiation of cancer and noncancer groups: A test of the hypothesis of cancer proneness. *Journal of Consulting and Clinical Psychology*, 48, 388–394.

Daura-Oller E., Cabre V., Montero M. A. et al. (2009). Specific gene hypomethylation and cancer: New insights into coding region feature trends. *Bioinformation*, 3(8), 340–343.

Davidson J. R., Hughes D., Blazer D. G., George L. K. (1991). Post-traumatic stress disorder in the community: an epidemiological study. *Psychol Med*, 21(3), 713–721.

Davidson R. J., Kabat-Zinn J., Schumacher J. et al. (2003). Alterations in Brain and immune Function produced by mindfulness meditation. *Psychosomatic Medicine*, 65, 564–570.

Davies P. C., Lineweaver C. H. (2011). Cancer tumors as Metazoa 1.0: tapping genes of ancient ancestors. *Phys Biol*, 8(1), 015001.

Davis C. G., Nolen-Hoeksema S., Larson J. (1998). Making sense of loss and benefiting from the experience: Two construals of meaning. *J Pers Soc Psychol*, 75, 561–574.

Davis D. E., Ho M. Y., Griffin B. J. et al. (2015). Forgiving the self and physical and mental health correlates: A meta-analytic review. *Journal of Counseling Psychology*, 62(2), 329–335.

Davis L. Z., Slavich G. M., Thaker P. H. et al. (2015). Eudaimonic well-being and tumor norepinephrine in patients with epithelial ovarian cancer. *Cancer*, 121(19), 3543–3550.

Davydov M. I., (ed.) (2005). *Profilaktika, rannyaya diagnostika i lechenie zlokachestvennyh novoobrazovanij.* Moscow: Izdatelskaya gruppa RONC.

Davydovskiy I. V. (1962). *Problema prichinnosti v medicine (etiologiya).* Moscow: Medicina.

De Bellis M. D., Baum A. S., Birmaher B. et al. (1999). Bennett Research Award. Developmental traumatology. Part I: Biological stress systems. *Biological Psychiatry*, 45(10), 1259–1270.

De Boer M. F., Van den Borne B., Pruyn J. F. et al. (1998). Psychosocial and physical correlates of survival and recurrence in patients with head and neck carcinoma. *Cancer,* 83(12), 2567–2579.

De Brabander B., Gerits P. (1999). Chronic and acute stress as predictors of relapse in primary breast cancer patients. *Patient Education and Counseling*, 37(3), 265–272.

Deci E. L., Ryan R. M. (1985). *Intrinsic motivation and self-determination in human behavior.* New York: Plenum.

DeCicco T. (2007). Finding Your «Self» in Psychology, Spirituality and Religion. *Psychology. Journal of Higher School of Economics*, 4(4), 46–52.

Dedov I. I., Melnichenko G. A. (ed.) (2004). *Ozhirenie: etiologiya, patogenez, klinicheskie aspekty.* Moscow: MIA.

Deimling G. T., Bowman K. F., Sterns S. et al. (2006). Cancer-related health worries and psychological distress among older adult, long-term cancer survivors. *Psycho-Oncology*, 15(4), 306–320.

De Jong M. L. (1992). Attachment, individuation, and risk of suicide in late adolescence. *Journal of Youth and Adolescence*, 21(3), 357–373.

Delahanty D. L., Raimonde A. J., Spoonster E., Cullado M. (2003). Injury severity, prior trauma history, urinary cortisol levels, and acute PTSD in motor vehicle accident victims. *Journal of Anxiety Disorders*, 17, 149–164.

Delgado-Guay M. O., Hui D., Parsons H. A. et al. (2011). Spirituality, religiosity, and spiritual pain in advanced cancer patients. *J Pain Symptom Manage*, 41, 986–994.

Denollet J. (1998). Personality and risk of cancer in men with coronary heart disease. *Psychological Medicine*, 28(4), 991–995.

Denollet J. (2005). DS14: standard assessment of negative affectivity, social inhibition, and Type D personality. *Psychosom Med*, 67, 89–97.

Denollet J., Kupper N. (2007). Type-D personality, depression, and cardiac prognosis: Cortisol dysregulation as a mediating mechanism. *Journal of Psychosomatic Research*, 62(6), 607–609.

Denollet J., Sys S. U., Stroobant N. et al. (1996). Personality as independent predictor of long-term mortality in patients with coronary heart disease. *Lancet,* 347, 417–421.

De Pablos R. M., Herrera A. J., Espinosa-Oliva A. M., et al. (2014). Chronic stress enhances microglia activation and exacerbates death of nigral dopaminergic neurons under conditions of inflammation. *Journal of Neuroinflammation*, 11, 1–18.

Depke M., Fusch G., Domanska G. et al. (2008). Hypermetabolic syndrome as a consequence of repeated psychological stress in mice. *Endocrinology*, 149(6), 2714–2723.

Depression guideline panel. (1993). Clinical practice guideline № 5. Depression in Primary Care: Vol. 2. *Detection and diagnosis*. Rockville: US Dept. of Health and Human Services. Agency for Health Care Policy and Research publication, 93–0551.

Derogatis L. R., Abeloff M. D., Melisaratos N. (1979). Psychological coping mechanisms and survival time in metastatic breast cancer. *JAMA*, 242(14), 1504–1508.

Derzhavina A. A. (2008). *Kak ya pobedila rak. Dnevnik isceleniya*. Krylov: Cifrovaya kniga.

Deshaies-Gendron D. (1701). *Recherches sur la nature et la guerison des cancers*. Paris: Laurent d'Haury.

Desyatnikov V. F., Sorokina T. T. (1981). *Skrytaya depressiya v praktike vrachej*. Minsk: Vyshejshaya shkola.

Deutsch F. (1933). Der gesunde und der kranke Korper in psychoanalytischer Betrachtung. *Int Z Psychoanal*, 19, 130–146.

Deveci A., Aydemir O., Taskin O. et al. (2007). Serum BDNF levels in suicide attempters related to psychosocial stressors: a comparative study with depression. *Neuropsychobiology*, 56(2-3), 93–97.

Devine E. C., Westlake S. K. (1995). The effects of psychoeducational care provided to adults with cancer: meta-analysis of 116 studies. *Oncology Nursing Forum*, 22(9), 1369–1381.

Dhabhar F. S., Saul A. N., Daugherty C. et al. (2010). Short-term stress enhances cellular immunity and increases early resistance to squamous cell carcinoma. *Brain Behav Immun*, 24(1), 127–137.

Dhabhar F. S., Saul A. N., Holmes T. H. et al. (2012). High-anxious individuals show increased chronic stress burden, decreased protective immunity, and increased cancer progression in a mouse model of squamous cell carcinoma. *PLoS One*, 7(4), e33069.

Dhillon V. S., Dhillon I. K. (1998). Chromosome aberrations and sister chromatid exchange studies in patients with prostate cancer possible evidence of chromosome instability. *Cancer Genetics*, 100, 143–147.

Dige U. (2000). *[Cancer miracles – in the physician's and the patient's perspective.]* Aarhus: Hovedland (in Danish).

Dilman V. M. (1986). *Bolshie biologicheskie chasy. V vedenie v integralnuyu medicinu*. Moscow: Znanie.

Dilts R. R. (2006). *Sleight of Mouth: The Magic of Conversational Belief Change*. Capitola: Meta Publications.

Dimitroglou E., Zafiropoulou M., Messini-Nikolaki N. et al. (2003). DNA damage in a human population affected by chronic psychogenic stress. *International Journal of Hygiene and Environmental Health*, 206(1), 39–44.

Dirksen S. R. (1995). Search for meaning in long-term cancer survivors. *J Adv Nurs*, 21(4), 628–633.

Diterikhs M. N. (1904). Istericheskie opuholi grudnoj zhelezy. *Rus hirurg arhiv*, 5, 800–819.

DKSU: Derzhavniy komitet statistiki Ukrayini. Retrieved 02.08.2014 from: http://www.ukrstat.gov.ua/.

Dmitriev A. Ostrov dolgoj zhizni. *Vokrug sveta*, 3 marta 2014. Retrieved 24.08.2015 from: http://www.vokrugsveta.ru/article/198633/.

Dobos G. J., Voiss P., Schwidde I. et al. (2012). Integrative oncology for breast cancer patients: introduction of an expert-based model. *BMC cancer*, 12(1), 1–12.

Doongaji D. R., Apte J. S., Dutt M. R. et al. (1985). Measurement of psycho-social stress in relationship to an illness (a controlled study of 100 cases of malignancy). *Journal of Postgraduate Medicine*, 31, 73–79.

Dourado de Souza C., deSouza B. C., deCastro S. D. et al. (2018). Association between life events after diagnosis of breast cancer and metastasis. *Ciência & Saúde Coletiva*, 23(2), 471–479.

Dowlati Y., Herrmann N., Swardfager W. et al. (2010). A meta-analysis of cytokines in major depression. *Biol Psychiatry*, 67(5), 446–457.

Doyen J. B. (1816). *Dissertation sur le cancer, considéré comme une maladie du système nerveux*. Thèse de doctorat de médecine. Paris: Didot jeune.

Dubskiy S. V., Kupriyanova I. E., Chojnzonov E. L., Balackaya L. N. (2008). Psihologicheskaya reabilitaciya i ocenka kachestva zhizni bolnyh rakom shitovidnoj zhelezy. *Sibirskiy Onkologicheskiy Zhurnal*, 4, 17–21.

Dudnichenko A. S., Dyshlevaya L. N., Dyshlevoj A.Y. (2003). O vazhnosti ocenki psihicheskogo sostoyaniya onkologicheskih bolnyh i chlenov ih semej. *Problemy Medicinskoj Nauki i Obrazovaniya*, 3, 34–37.

Duijts S. F., Zeegers M. P., Borne B. V. (2003). The association between stressful life events and breast cancer risk: a meta-analysis. *Int J Cancer*, 107(6), 1023–1029.

Duijts S. F., Faber M. M., Oldenburg H. S. et al. (2011). Effectiveness of behavioral techniques and physical exercise on psychosocial functioning and health-related quality of life in breast cancer patients and survivors—a meta-analysis. *Psycho-Oncology*, 20(2), 115–126.

Dukkha. (2013). Access to Insight (Legacy Edn), 5 November 2013. Retrieved 02.10.2015 from: http://www.accesstoinsight.org/ptf/dhamma/sacca/sacca1/dukkha.html.

Dunbar H. (1954). *Emotions and bodily changes; a survey of literature on psychosomatic inter-relationships 1910–1953*. New York: Columbia University Press.

Dunigan J. T., Carr B. I., Steel J. L. (2007). Posttraumatic growth, immunity and survival in patients with hepatoma. *Dig Dis Sci*, 9, 2452–2459.

Dunn H. L. (1961). *High-level wellness*. Thorofare, NJ: Charles B. Slack.

Dyer A. R. (2011). The need for a new" new medical model": a bio-psychosocial-spiritual model. *Southern Medical Journal*, 104(4), 297-298.

Dziegiel P., Podhorska-Okolow M., Zabel M. (2008). Melatonin: adjuvant therapy of malignant tumors. *Medical Science Monitor*, 14(5), RA64–RA70.

Edelman S., Kidman A. D. (1997). Mind and Cancer: Is There a Relationship?—A Review of Evidence. *Australian Psychologist*, 32(2), 79–85.

Edwards A., Pang N., Shiu V., Chan C. (2010). The understanding of spirituality and the potential role of spiritual care in end-of-life and palliative care: a meta-study of qualitative research. *Palliative Medicine*, 24(8), 753–770.

Egbert E. (1980). Concept of wellness. *Journal of Psychiatric Nursing and Mental Health Services*, 9–13.

Egikyan M. A. (2014). Onkologicheskoe zabolevanie v kontekste psihogennyh faktorov. *Vestnik Kostromskogo gosudarstvennogo universiteta im. N. A. Nekrasova. Seriya Gumanitarnye nauki*, 20, 4.

Ehrentheil O. F. (1956). Malignant tumors in psychotic patients: I. Studies of incidence. *AMA Archives of Neurology & Psychiatry*, 76(5), 529–535.

Eidemiller E. G. (1999). *Psihologiya i psihoterapiya semyi*. Saint Petersburg: Piter.

Einstein A., Murphy J., Sullivan J. W. N. (1930). Science and God. A German Dialogue. *The Forum*, June, 373–379.

Ekdahl C. T., Claasen J. H., Bonde S. et al. (2003). Inflammation is detrimental for neurogenesis in adult brain. *Proc Natl Acad Sci USA*, 100(23), 13632–13627.

Elenkov I. J., Chrousos G. P. (2002). Stress hormones, proinflammatory and antiinflammatory cytokines, and autoimmunity. *Ann N Y Acad Sci*, 966, 290–303.

Elias A. C. A., Ricci M. D., Rodriguez L. H. D. et al. (2015). The biopsychosocial spiritual model applied to the treatment of women with breast cancer, through RIME intervention (relaxation, mental images, spirituality). *Complementary Therapies in Clinical Practice*, 21(1), 1–6.

Elkins G., Fisher W., Johnson A. (2010). Mind-body therapies in integrative oncology. *Current Treatment Options in Oncology*, 11(3-4), 128–140.

Elzinga B. M., Schmahl C. G., Vermetten E. et al. (2003). Higher cortisol levels following exposure to traumatic reminders in abuse-related PTSD. *Neuropsychopharmacology*, 28, 1656–1665.

Engel G. L. (1968). A life setting conducive to illness: the giving-up—given-up complex. *Annals of Internal Medicine*, 69(2), 293–300.

Engel G. L. (1971). Sudden and rapid death during psychological stress: folklore or folk wisdom? *Annals of Internal Medicine*, 74(5), 771–783.

Engel G. L. (1977). The need for a new medical model: a challenge for biomedicine. *Science*, 196(4286), 129–136.

Engel G. L., Schmale A. H. (1967). Psychoanalytic theory of somatic disorder: Conversion, specifity and the disease onset situation. *J Amer Psychoanal Assoc*, (15), 344–365.

Engelman S. R., Craddick R. (1984). The Symbolic Relationship of Breast Cancer Patients to Their Cancer, Cure, Physician, and Themselves. *Psychother Psychosom*, 41, 68–76.

Engert V., Plessow F., Miller R. et al. (2014). Cortisol increase in empathic stress is modulated by emotional closeness and observation modality. *Psychoneuroendocrinology*, 45, 192–201.

Enlow M., Egeland B., Carlson E. et al. (2014). Mother-infant attachment and the intergenerational transmission of posttraumatic stress disorder. *Development and Psychopathology*, 26(01), 41–65.

Entringer S., Buss C., Wadhwa P. D. (2010). Prenatal stress and developmental programming of human health and disease risk: concepts and integration of empirical findings. *Current Opinion in Endocrinology, Diabetes, and Obesity*, 17(6), 507–516.

Entringer S., Epel E. S., Kumsta R. et al. (2011). Stress exposure in intrauterine life is associated with shorter telomere length in young adulthood. *Proc Natl Acad Sci USA*, 108(33), E513–518.

Entringer S., Wüst S., Kumsta R. et al. (2008). Prenatal psychosocial stress exposure is associated with insulin resistance in young adults. *Am J Obstet Gynecol*, 199(5), 498, e1–7.

Epel E. S., Blackburn E. H., Lin J. et al. (2004). Accelerated telomere shortening in response to life stress. *Proc Natl Acad Sci USA*, 101(49), 17312–17315.

Epel E. S., Lin J., Wilhelm F. H. et al. (2006). Cell aging in relation to stress arousal and cardiovascular disease risk factors. *Psychoneuroendocrinology*, 31(3), 277–287.

Epping-Jordan J. E., Compas B. E., Howell D. C. (1994). Predictors of cancer progression in young adult men and women: avoidance, intrusive thoughts, and psychological symptoms. *Health Psychology*, 13(6), 539–547.

Epstein A. (1989). *Mind, Fantasy, and Healing: One woman's journey from conflict and illness to wholeness and health*. New York: Delacorte.

Ernst E. (2001). *The Desktop Guide to Complementary and Alternative Medicine: An Evidence-Based Approach*. London: Mosby.

Eschwege P., Dumas F., Blanchet P. et al. (1995). Haematogenous dissemination of prostatic epithelial cells during radical prostatectomy. *Lancet*, 346(8989), 1528–1530.

Eskelinen M., Ollonen, P. (2010). Life stress and losses and deficit in adulthood as breast cancer risk factor: a prospective case–control study in Kuopio, Finland. *in vivo*, 24(6), 899–904.

Esserman L. J., Thompson I. M. Jr, Reid B. (2013). Overdiagnosis and overtreatment in cancer: an opportunity for improvement. *JAMA*, 310(8), 797–798.

Essex M. J., Boyce W. T., Hertzman C. et al. (2013). Epigenetic vestiges of early developmental adversity: childhood stress exposure and DNA methylation in adolescence. *Child Dev*, 84, 58–75.

Esterling B. A., Antoni M. H., Kumar M., Schneiderman N. (1990). Emotional repression, stress disclosure responses, and Epstein-Barr viral capsid antigen titers. *Psychosom Med*, 52(4), 397–410.

Esterling B. A., Kiecolt-Glaser J., Bodnar J., Glaser R. (1994). Chronic stress, social support and persistent alterations in the natural killer cell response to cytokines in older adults. *Health Psychol*, 13, 291–299.

Eusebio S. E., Torrado M. (2017). Attachment and Emotional Regulation in Breast Cancer. *Journal of Psychosomatic Research*, 97, 148.

Evans D. L., Leserman J., Perkins D. O. et al. (1995). Stress-associated reductions of cytotoxic T lymphocytes and natural killer cells in asymptomatic HIV infection. *Am J Psychiatry*, 152(4), 543–550.

Evans E. (1926). *A Psychological Study of Cancer*. New York: Dodd, Meadand Co.

Evans N. J., Baldwin J. A., Gath D. (1974). The incidence of cancer among in patients with affective disorders. *Brith J Psychiat*, 124(5), 518–525.

Everly G. S. Jr., Rosenfeld R., Allen R. J. et al. (1981). *The Nature and Treatment of the Stress Response. A Practical Guide for Clinicians*. New York: Springer.

Everson S. A., Goldberg D. E., Kaplan G. A. et al. (1996). Hopelessness and risk of mortality and incidence of myocardial infarction and cancer. *Psychosomatic Medicine*, 58(2), 113–121.

Everson T. C., Cole W. H. (1966). *Spontaneous Regression of Cancer*. Philadelphia, PA: W. B. Saunders.

Ewing J. (1940). *Neoplastic Diseases*. Philadelphia, PA: W. B. Saunders.

Eysenck H. J. (2000). *Smoking, Health and Personality*. Piscataway, NJ: Transaction Publishers.

Fagundes C. P., Diamond L. M., Allen K. P. (2012). Adolescent attachment insecurity and parasympathetic functioning predict future loss adjustment. *Personality and Social Psychology Bulletin*, 38(6), 821–832.

Fagundes C. P, Glaser R., Malarkey W. B., Kiecolt-Glaser J. K. (2013). Childhood adversity and herpesvirus latency in breast cancer survivors. *Health Psychol*, 32(3), 337–344.

Fagundes C. P., Bennett J. M., Alfano C. M. et al. (2012a). Social support and socioeconomic status interact to predict Epstein-Barr virus latency in women awaiting diagnosis or newly diagnosed with breast cancer. *Health Psychol*, 31(1), 11–19.

Fagundes C. P., Glaser R., Johnson S. L. et al. (2012b). Basal cell carcinoma: stressful life events and the tumor environment. *Arch Gen Psychiatry*, 69, 618–626.

Fairbank J. A, Putnam F. W., Harris W. W. (2007). The prevalence and impact of child traumatic stress. In: Friedman M. J., Keane T. M., Resick P. A. (eds), *Handbook of PTSD*. New York: Guilford Press, 229–251.

Falus A., Marton I., Borbényi E. et al. (2011). A challenging epigenetic message: telomerase activity is associated with complex changes in lifestyle. *Cell Biology International*, 35(11), 1079–1083.

Fan R. L., Zheng S. H., Wu Z. S. (1997). [Study on the relationship between lung cancer at preclinic stage and psycho-social factor. A case-control study]. *Zhonghua Liu Xing Bing Xue Za Zhi (Chinese Journal of Blood Diseases)*, 18(5), 289–292 (in Chinese).

Fang C. Y., Egleston B. L., Ridge J. A. et al. (2014). Psychosocial functioning and vascular endothelial growth factor in patients with head and neck cancer. *Head & Neck*, 36(8), 1113–1119.

Fang C. Y., Miller S. M., Bovbjerg D. H. et al. (2008). Perceived stress is associated with impaired T-cell response to HPV16 in women with cervical dysplasia. *Annals of Behavioral Medicine*, 35(1), 87–96.

Fang C. Y., Reibel D. K., Longacre M. L. et al. (2010). Enhanced psychosocial well-being following participation in a mindfulness-based stress reduction program is associated with increased natural killer cell activity. *J Altern Complement Med*, 16, 531–538.

Fang F., Fall K., Mittleman M. A. et al. (2012). Suicide and cardiovascular death after a cancer diagnosis. *New England Journal of Medicine*, 366(14), 1310–1318.

Fang F., Fall K., Sparén P. et al. (2011). Risk of infection-related cancers after the loss of a child: a follow-up study in Sweden. *Cancer Research*, 71(1), 116–122.

Farber M. L. (1968). *Theory of suicide*. New York: Funk & Wagnalls.

Fauver R. (2011). *The healing wisdom within: A preliminary experimental trial of Psycho-Spiritual Integrative Therapy for people with cancer*. Palo Alto: Institute of Transpersonal Psychology.

Fawzy F. I. (1995). A short-term psychoeducational intervention for patients newly diagnosed with cancer. *Supportive Care in Cancer*, 3(4), 235–238.

Fawzy F. I., Fawzy N. W., Hyun C. S. et al. (1993). Malignant melanoma: effects of an early structured psychiatric intervention, coping and affective state on recurrence and survival 6 years later. *Arch Gen Psychiat*, 50, 681–689.

Fawzy F. I., Kemeny M. E., Fawzy N. W. et al. (1990). A structured psychiatric intervention for cancer patients. *Arch Gen Psychiat*, 47, 729–735.

Fazel M., Salimibejestan H., Farahmand K., Smaeili M. (2016). [Presentation of posttraumatic growth model in cancer patients: a grounded theory]. *Culture of Counseling and Psychotherapy Journal*, 8(29), 79–105 (in Persian).

Feasibility Study: Therapeutic Targeting of Stress Factors in Ovarian Cancer Patients. (2012). ClinicalTrials.gov Identifier: NCT01504126. January 3. Retrieved 11.02.2016 from: https://clinicaltrials.gov/ct2/show/NCT01504126.

Fedorov S. P. (1928). *Klinicheskie lekcii po hirurgii*. Moscow, Leningrad: GIZ, VMA RKKA.

Feeney J., Ryan S. (1994). Attachment style and affect regulation: Relafionships with health behavior and family experiences with illness in a student sample. *Health Psychology*, 13, 334–345.

Feher S., Maly R. C. (1999). Coping with breast cancer in later life: the role of religious faith. *Psycho-Oncology*, 8(5), 408–416.

Feinberg A. P., Tycko B. (2004). The history of cancer epigenetics. *Nat Rev Cancer*, 4(2), 143–153.

Feinberg A. P., Vogelstein B. (1983). Hypomethylation distinguishes of ras genes of same human cancer from their normal counterparts. *Nature*, 301, 89—92.

Feinberg A. P., Ohlsson R., Henikoff S. (2006). The epigenetic progenitor origin of human cancer. *Nature reviews genetics*, 7(1), 21–33.

Feinstein D., Church D. (2010). Modulating gene expression through psychotherapy: The contribution of noninvasive somatic interventions. *Review of General Psychology*, 14(4), 283–295.

Feldenkrais M. (2009). *Awareness Through Movement: Easy-to-Do Health Exercises to Improve Your Posture, Vision, Imagination, and Personal Awareness*. San Francisco, CA: HarperOne.

Feldman L. A., Gotlib H. (1993). Social dysfunction. In: Costello G. (ed.), *Symptoms of depression*. New York: Willey, 85–164.

Felitti V. J., Anda R. F., Nordenberg D. et al. (1998). Relationship of childhood abuse and household dysfunction to many of the leading causes of death in adults. The Adverse Childhood Experiences (ACE) Study. *Am J Prev Med*, 14, 245–258.

Feng R., Rampon C., Tang Y. P. et al. (2001). Deficient neurogenesis in forebrain-specific presenilin-1 knockout mice is associated with reduced clearance of hippocampal memory traces. *Neuron*, 32, 911–926.

Feng Z., Liu L., Zhang C. et al. (2012). Chronic restraint stress attenuates p53 function and promotes tumorigenesis. *Proc Natl Acad Sci USA*, 109, 7013–7018.

Fentiman I. S., Tirelli U., Monfardini S. et al. (1990). Cancer in the elderly: Why so badly treated? *Lancet*, 335(8698), 1020–1022

Ferenczi S. (1908). Psychoanalysis and education. In: *Final contributions to the problems and methods of psycho-analysis*. Maresfield, 280–290.

Ferrell B. R., Smith S. L., Juarez G., Melancon C. (2003). Meaning of illness and spirituality in ovarian cancer survivors. *Oncol Nurs Forum*, 30(2), 249–257.

Fidler I. J. (1995). Modulation of the organ microenvironment for treatment of cancer metastasis. *J Natl Cancer Inst*, 87(21),1588–1592.

Figer A., Kreitler S., Kreitler M. et al. (2002). Personality dispositions of colon cancer patients. *Gastrointestinal Oncology*, 4, 81–92

Figueiredo H. F., Ulrich-Lai Y. M., Choi D. C., Herman J. P. (2007). Estrogen potentiates adrenocortical responses to stress in female rats. *Am J Physiol Endocrinol Metab*, 292(4), E1173–E1182.

Filipp S. H. (1992). Could it be worse? The diagnosis of cancer as a prototype of traumatic life events. In: L. Montada et al., (eds), *Life crises and experiences of loss in adulthood*, 23–56.

Filippova N. V., Barylnik Yu. B., Deeva M. A., Sobakina O. Yu. (2015). Duhovnaya destabilizaciya sovremennogo obshestva kak prediktor psihicheskih rasstrojstv u detej. *Psihiatriya*, 501, 1202–1212.

Finagentova N. V. (2010). *Psihologicheskie resursy v profilaktike recidivov pri onkologicheskih zabolevaniyah*. Avtoref. diss. kand. psihol. nauk. Saint Petersburg: Gos. Ped. Med. Akad.

Fincham F. D. Forgiveness, family relationships and health. In L. Toussaint et al. (eds), *Forgiveness and Health*. New York: Springer, 2015, 255–270.

Finlay-Jones R., Brown G. W. (1981). Types of stressful life event and the onset of anxiety and depressive disorders. *Psychological Medicine*, 11(4), 803–815.

Fischman H. K., Pero R. W., Kelly D. D. (1996). Psychogenic stress induces chromosomal and DNA damage. *Int J Neurosci*, 84(1–4), 219–227.

Fisun E. (2010). Sistemnyj podhod v psihologicheskoj rabote s onkopacientami i chlenami ih semej. *Obshestvo semejnyh psihoterapevtov i konsultantov*. Retrieved 02.01.2015 from: http://supporter.ru/biblioteka/hronich/fisun.doc.

Flint M. S., Baum A., Chambers W. H., Jenkins F. J. (2007). Induction of DNA damage, alteration of DNA repair and transcriptional activation by stress hormones. *Psychoneuroendocrinology*, 32(5), 470–479.

Flint M. S., Baum A., Episcopo B. et al. (2013). Chronic exposure to stress hormones promotes transformation and tumorigenicity of 3T3 mouse fibroblasts. *Stress*, 16(1), 114–121.

Flory N., Lang E. (2008). Practical hypnotic interventions during invasive cancer diagnosis and treatment. *Hematology/Oncology Clinics of North America*, 22(4), 709–725.

Forgeard M. J., Haigh E. A., Beck A. T. et al. (2011). Beyond depression: Toward a process-based approach to research, diagnosis, and treatment. *Clinical Psychology: Science and Practice*, 18(4), 275–299.

Foster T. (2011). Adverse life events proximal to adult suicide: a synthesis of findings from psychological autopsy studies. *Archives of Suicide Research*, 15(1), 1–15.

Fox B. H., Ragland D. R., Brand R. J., Rosenman R. H. (1987). Type A behavior and cancer mortality. Theoretical considerations and preliminary data. *Ann N Y Acad Sci*, 496, 620–627.

Fox C. M, Harper A. P, Hyner G. C., Lyle R. M. (1994). Loneliness, emotional repression, marital quality, and major life events in women who develop breast cancer. *J Community Health*, 19(6), 467–482.

Frankl V. (1984). *Man's Search for Meaning: An Introduction to Logotherapy*. New York: Touchstone Books.

Frankl V. (1991). *Die Psychotherapie in der Praxis*. Munchen: Piper Verlag.

Frankl V. (1992). Meaning in industrial society. *International Forum for Logotherapy*, 15, 66–70.

Frankl V. (2016). *Logotherapy and Existential Analysis: Proceedings of the Viktor Frankl Institute*. Vienna: Springer.

Franklin T. B., Russig H., Weiss I. C., et al. (2010). Epigenetic transmission of the impact of early stress across generations. *Biological 3sychiatry*, 68(5), 408–415.

Frenck R. W. Jr, Blackburn E. H., Shannon K. M. (1998). The rate of telomere sequence loss in human leukocytes varies with age. *Proc Natl Acad Sci USA*, 95(10), 5607–5610.

Freud A. (1937). *The Ego and the mechanisms of defense*. London: Hogarth Press and Institute of Psycho-Analysis.

Freud S. (1920). *General Introduction to Psychoanalysis*. New York: Horace Liveright.

Freud S. (1953). Psychical (or mental) treatment. In: *Complete Psychological Works of Sigmund Freud*. Standard Edition, Vol. 7. London: Hogarth Press, 281–302.

Freud S. (1990). *Complete Psychological Works of Sigmund Freud*. Standard Edition. J. Strachey (ed.). New York: W. W. Norton & Company.

Freyberger H. (1977). Supportive psychotherapeutic techniques in primary and secondary alexithymia. *Psychother Psychosom*, (28), 337–343.

Fridman M. V., Kupriyan S. V., Dugin A. V. (2002). Analiz smertelnyh oslozhnenij, svyazannyh s rostom i metastazirovaniem zlokachestvennoj opuholej. *Belorus med zhurnal*, 2, 58–62.

Friedman A. (1970). Hostility and clinical improvement in depressed patients. *Arch of General Psychiatry*, 23, 524–537.

Friedman L. C., Romero C., Elledge R. et al. (2007). Attribution of blame, self-forgiving attitude and psychological adjustment in women with breast cancer. *J Behav Med*, 30(4), 351–357.

Friedman M., Rosenman, R. H. (1959). Association of specific overt behavior pattern with blood and cardiovascular findings: blood cholesterol level, blood clotting time, incidence of arcus senilis, and clinical coronary artery disease. *Journal of the American Medical Association*, 169(12), 1286–1296.

Frodl T., Reinhold E., Koutsouleris N. et al. (2010). Interaction of childhood stress with hippocampus and prefrontal cortex volume reduction in major depression. *Journal of psychiatric research*, 44(13), 799–807.

Frolkis V. V. (1991). Stress-vozrast-sindrom. *Fiziol. Zhurn*, 3, 3–10.

Fromm E. (1990). *Man for Himself: An Inquiry Into the Psychology of Ethics*. New York: Holt Paperbacks.

Fromm E. (2016). *Der Wille zum Leben: The Will to Live*. Amazon Media EU.

Fukunishi I. (1998). Japanese consultation-liaison psychiatry in the areas of organ transplantation and cancer care. *Psychiatric Times*, 15, 48–49.

Fuligni A. J., Telzer E. H., Bower J. et al. (2009). A preliminary study of daily interpersonal stress and C-reactive protein levels among adolescents from Latin American and European backgrounds. *Psychosom Med*, 71(3), 329–333.

Fuller-Thomson E., Brennenstuhl S. (2009). Making a link between childhood physical abuse and cancer. *Cancer*, 115(14), 3341–3350.

Funkenstein D. H., King S. H., Drolette M. E. (1957). *Mastery of Stress*. Cambridge, MA: Harvard University Press.

Fusu M. N. (2013). Mehanizm vliyaniya osobennostej vzaimodejstviya s materyu na vozniknovenie psihosomaticheskih rasstrojstv vo vzroslom vozraste. *Mezhdunarodnyj Zhurnal Eksperimentalnogo Obrazovaniya*, 3, 61–62.

Futterman A. D., Kemeny M. E., Shapiro D., Fahey J. L. (1994). Immunological and physiological changes associated with induced positive and negative mood. *Psychosom Med*, 56(6), 499–511.

Gall T. L., Cornblat M. W. (2002). Breast cancer survivors give voice: A qualitative analysis of spiritual factors in long-term adjustment. *Psycho-Oncology*, 11, 524–535.

Gana K., Broc G., Saada Y. et al. (2016). Subjective wellbeing and longevity: Findings from a 22-year cohort study. *Journal of Psychosomatic Research*, 85, 28–34.

Gangemi R., Paleari L., Orengo A. M. et al. (2009). Cancer stem cells: a new paradigm for understanding tumor growth and progression and drug resistance. *Curr Med Chem*, 16(14), 1688–703.

Ganz P. A., Habel L. A., Weltzien E. K. et al. (2011). Examining the influence of beta blockers and ACE inhibitors on the risk for breast cancer recurrence: results from the LACE cohort. *Breast Cancer Research and Treatment*, 129(2), 549–556.

Gapp K., Jawaid A., Sarkies P. et al. (2014). Implication of sperm RNAs in transgenerational inheritance of the effects of early trauma in mice. *Nature Neuroscience,* 17(5), 667–669.

Garanyan N. G., Kholmogorova A. B., Yudeeva T. Y. (2003). Vrazhdebnost kak lichnostnyj faktor depressii i trevogi. V: Psihologiya: sovremennye napravleniya mezhdisciplinarnyh issledovanij. *Mat. nauchnoj konf.,* 8 oktyabrya 2002 g. Moscow: Institut psihologii RAN, 100–114.

Garbuzov V. I. (1999). *Koncepciya instinktov i psihosomaticheskaya patologiya. (Nadnozologicheskaya diagnostika i terapiya psihosomaticheskih zabolevaniy i nevrozov).* Saint Petersburg: Sotis.

García-Campayo J., Puebla-Guedea M., Labarga A. et al. (2018). Epigenetic response to mindfulness in peripheral blood leukocytes involves genes linked to common human diseases. *Mindfulness,* 9(4), 1146–1159.

Garkavi L. H., Kvakina E. B., Ukolova M. A. (1990). *Adaptacionnye reakcii i rezistentnost organizma.* Rostov na Donu: Izdatelstvo Rostovskogo universiteta.

Garkavi L. H., Kvakina E. B., Kuzmenko T. S., Shihlyarova A. I. (1998). *Antistressornye reakcii i aktivacionnaya terapiya.* Moscow: Imedis.

Garrett J. E, Wellman C. L. (2009). Chronic Stress Effects on Dendritic Morphology in Medial Prefrontal Cortex: Sex Differences and Estrogen Dependence. *Neuroscience,* 162(1), 195–207.

Garrido P. (2014). Aging and stress: past hypotheses, present approaches and perspectives. *Aging and Disease,* 2(1), 80–99.

Garssen B. (2004). Psychological factors and cancer development: evidence after 30 years of research. *Clinical Psychology Review,* 24(3), 315–338.

Garssen B. (2007). Repression: finding our way in the maze of concepts. *J Behav Med,* 30(6), 471–481.

Gatch W. D., Culbertson C. G. (1952). Theories on the treatment of breast cancer and observations on its natural course. *Annals of Surgery,* 135(6), 775–781.

Gattoni S., Kirschmeier P., Weinstein I. et al. (1982). Cellular Moloney murine sarcoma (c-mos) sequences are hypermethylated and transcriptionally silent in normal and transformed rodent cells. *Molec Cell Biol,* 1, 42—51.

Gawler I. (1984). *You Can Conquer Cancer: A New Way of Living.* South Yarra: Michelle Anderson Publishing.

Gehde E., Baltrusch H. J. (1990). Early experience and development of cancer in later life: implications for psychoneuroimmunologic research. *International Journal of Neuroscience,* 51(3-4), 257–260.

Geyer S. (1991). Life events prior to manifestation of breast cancer: a limited prospective study covering eight years before diagnosis. *J Psychosom Res,* 35, 355–363.

Giaconia R. M., Reinherz H. Z., Silverman A. B. et al. (1995). Traumas and posttraumatic stress disorder in a community population of older adolescents. *J Am Acad Child Adolesc Psychiatry,* 34(10), 1369–1380.

Gidron Y., Ronson A. (2008). Psychosocial factors, biological mediators, and cancer prognosis: a new look at an old story. *Curr Opin Oncol,* 20(4), 386–392.

Gidron Y., Russ K., Tissarchondou H., Warner J. (2006). The relation between psychological factors and DNA-damage: a critical review. *Biological Psychology,* 72(3), 291–304.

Giese-Davis J., Collie K., Rancourt K. M. et al. (2011). Decrease in depression symptoms is associated with longer survival in patients with metastatic breast cancer: a secondary analysis. *J Clin Oncol,* 29, 413–420.

Giese-Davis J., Sephton S. E., Abercrombie H. C. et al. (2004). Repression and high anxiety are associated with aberrant diurnal cortisol rhythms in women with metastatic breast cancer. *Health Psychol,* 23(6), 645–650.

Gil S., Gilbar O. (2001). Hopelessness Among Cancer Patients. *Journal of Psychosocial Oncology,* 19(1), 21 – 33.

Gilbreath B., Benson P. G. (2004). The contribution of supervisor behaviour to employee psychological well-being. *Work & Stress*, 18(3), 255–266.

Gindikin V. Y. (2000). *Somatogennye i somatoformnye psihicheskie rasstrojstva (klinika, differencialnaya diagnostika, lechenie). Spravochnik.* Moscow: Triada-H.

Giraldi T., Perissin L., Zorzet S. et al. (1994). Metastasis and neuroendocrine system in stressed mice. *International Journal of Neuroscience*, 74(1-4), 265–278.

Glaser R., Kiecolt-Glaser J. K. (1994). Stress-associated immune modulation and its implications for reactivation of latent herpesviruses. In: Glaser R., Jones J. (eds), *Human Herpesvirus Infections*. New York: Dekker, 245–270.

Glaser R., Kiecolt-Glaser J. K., Speicher C. E., Holliday J. E. (1985). Stress, loneliness, and changes in herpesvirus latency. *Journal of Behavioral Medicine*, 8(3), 249–260.

Glaser R., Pearl D., Kiecolt-Glaser J., Malarkey W. (1994). Plasma cortisol levels and reactivation of latent Epstein-Barr virus in response to examination stress. *Psychoneuroendocrinology*, 19, 765–772.

Glaser R., Lafuse W. P., Bonneau R. H. et al. (1993). Stress-associated modulation of proto-oncogene expression in human peripheral blood leukocytes. *Behav Neurosci*, 107(3), 525–529.

Glaser R., Pearson G., Bonneau R. et al. (1993a). Stress and the memory T-cell response to the Epstein-Barr virus in healthy medical students. *Health Psychol*, 112, 435–442.

Glaser R., Thorn B. E., Tarr K. L. et al. (1985). Effects of stress on methyltransferase synthesis: An important DNA repair enzyme. *Health Psychol*, 4, 403–412.

Gleave M. E., Elhilali M., Fradet Y. et al. (1998). Interferon gamma-1b compared with placebo in metastatic renal-cell carcinoma. *New England Journal of Medicine*, 338(18), 1265–1271.

Gluckman P. D., Hanson M. A. (2004). Living with the past: Evolution, development, and patterns of disease. *Science*, 305, 1733–1736.

Gnezdilov A. V. (1996). *Psihologicheskie aspekty onkologii v usloviyah hospisa.* Avtor. diss. d-ra med. nauk. Saint Petersburg: NIPI im. V. M. Bekhtereva.

Gnezdilov A. V. (2002). *Psihologiya i psihoterapiya poter. Posobie po palliativnoj medicine dlya vrachej, psihologov i vseh interesuyushihsya problemoj.* Saint Petersburg: Izdatelstvo Rech.

Goble F. G. (1980). *The Third Force: The Psychology of Abraham Maslow.* New York: Pocket Books.

Godbout J. P., Glaser R. (2006). Stress-induced immune dysregulation: implications for wound healing, infectious disease and cancer. *J Neuroimmune Pharmacol*, 1(4), 421–427.

Gold P. W., Goodwin F. K., Chrousos G. P. (1988). Clinical and biochemical manifestations of depression. Relation to the neurobiology of stress (2). *N Engl J Med*, 319, 413–420.

Goldbacher E. M., Matthews K. A. (2007). Are psychological characteristics related to risk of the metabolic syndrome? A review of the literature. *Ann Behav Med*, 34(3), 240–252.

Goldberg R. B. (2009). Cytokine and cytokine-like inflammation markers, endothelial dysfunction, and imbalanced coagulation in development of diabetes and its complications. *J Clin Endocrinol Metab*, 94(9), 3171–3182.

Goldney R. D. (1981). Parental loss and reported childhood stress in young women who attempt suicide. *Acta Psychiatrica Scandinavica*, 64(1), 34–49.

Gonyea J. G., Paris R., de Saxe Zerden L. (2008). Adult daughters and aging mothers: The role of guilt in the experience of caregiver burden. *Aging and Mental Health*, 12, 559–567.

Goodkin K., Antoni M. H., Blaney P. H. (1986). Stress and hopelessness in the promotion of cervical intraepithelial neoplasia to invasive squamous cell carcinoma of the cervix. *J Psychosom Res*, 30, 67–76.

Goodwin J. S., Zhang D. D., Ostir G. V. (2004). Effect of depression on diagnosis, treatment, and survival of older women with breast cancer. *Journal of the American Geriatrics Society*, 52(1), 106–111.

Gorbunova V. N., Imyanitov E. N. (2007). *Genetika i kancerogenez. Metodicheskoe posobie.* Saint Petersburg: GPMA.

Gorevaya A. N., Samundzhan Y. M., Guslitser L. N. (1974). Endokrinologicheskiye avspekty raka molochnoy zhelezy. V: *Materialy plenuma problemnoy komissii MZ SSSR po epidemiologii raka molochnoy zhelezy.* Tallin, 75–80.

Gorman G. (1997). Unconscious Memory—False or Fact. *European Journal of Clinical Hypnosis,* 4(3), 146–153.

Gostev A. A. (2007). O problemah stanovleniya religiozno orientirovannogo psihologicheskogo znaniya. Psihologiya. *Zhurnal Vysshej Shkoly Ekonomiki,* 4(4), 35–45.

Gotlieb W. H., Saumet J., Beauchamp M. C. et al. (2008). In vitro metformin anti-neoplastic activity in epithelial ovarian cancer. *Gynecol Oncol,* 110(2), 246–250.

Gouin J. P., Hantsoo L. V., Kiecolt-Glaser J. K. (2011). Stress, negative emotions, and inflammation. In: J. T Caccioppo & J. Decety (eds), *Handbook of Social Neurosciences.* New York: John Wiley and Sons, 814–829.

Gouin J. P., Glaser R., Malarkey W. B. et al. (2012). Chronic stress, daily stressors, and circulating inflammatory markers. *Health Psychology,* 31, 264–268.

Graham J. E., Ramirez A., Love S. et al. (2002). Stressful life experiences and risk of relapse of breast cancer: observational cohort study. *BMJ,* 324(7351), 1420–1423.

Graham J. E., Glaser R., Loving T. J. et al. (2009). Cognitive word use during marital conflict and increases in proinflammatory cytokines. *Health Psychology,* 28, 621–630.

Graham S., Furr S., Flowers C., Burke M. T. (2001). Research and Theory: Religion and spirituality in coping with stress. *Counseling and Values,* 46, 2–13.

Granovskaya R. M. (1988). *Elementy prakticheskoj psihologii.* Leningrad: Izdatelstvo Leningradskogo universiteta.

Granovskaya R. M. (2007). *Psikhologicheskaya zashchita.* Saint Petersburg: Rech'.

Grassi L., Molinari S. (1986). Family affective climate during the childhood of adult cancer patients. *Journal of Psychosocial Oncology,* 4, 53–62.

Grassi L., Malacarne P., Maestri A., Ramelli E. (1997). Depression, psychosocial variables and occurrence of life events among patients with cancer. *Journal of Affective Disorders,* 44(1), 21–30.

Grassi L., Sabato S., Rossi E. et al. (2005). Use of the diagnostic criteria for psychosomatic research in oncology. *Psychotherapy and psychosomatics,* 74(2), 100–107.

Graves P. L., Mead L. A., Pearson T. A. (1986). The Rorschach Interaction Scale as a potential predictor of cancer. *Psychosomatic Medicine,* 48(8), 549–563.

Greaves M. (2005). In utero origins of childhood leukaemia. *Early Hum Dev,* 81, 123–129.

Greaves M. (2006). Infection, immune responses and the aetiology of childhood leukaemia. *Nat Rev Cancer,* 6, 193–203.

Grebennikov L. R. (1994). *Mehanizmy psihologicheskoj zashity: genezis, funkcionirovanie, diagnostika.* Avtorefyu diss. kand. psihol. nauk. Moskva.

Green A. I., Austin C. P. (1993). Psychopathology of pancreatic cancer. A psychobiologic probe. *Psychosomatics,* 34(3), 208–221.

Green B. L., Epstein S. A., Krupnick J. L., Rowland J. H. (1997). Trauma and medical illness: assessing trauma-related disorders. In: J. P. Wilson, T. M. Keane (eds), *Assessing Psychological Trauma and PTSD.* New York: Guilford Press, 160–191.

Green B. L., Krupnick J. L., Rowland J. H. et al. (2000). Trauma history as a predictor of psychologic symptoms in women with breast cancer. *J Clin Oncol,* 18, 1084–1093.

Green B. L., Rowland J. H., Krupnick J. L. et al. (1998). Prevalence of posttraumatic stress disorder in women with breast cancer. *Psychosomatics,* 9, 102–111.

Greenberg R. P., Bornstein R. F. (1988). The Dependent Personality: I. Risk for Physical Disorders. *Journal of Personality Disorders,* 2(2), 126–135.

Greene W. A. (1966). The psychological setting of the development of leukemia and lymphoma. *Ann N Y Acad Sci,* 21, 125(3), 794–801.

Greene W. A., Miller G. (1958). Psychological factors and reticuloendothelial disease. IV. Observations on a group of children and adolescents with leukemia: an interpretation of disease development in terms of the mother-child unit. *Psychosom Med*, 20(2), 124–44.

Greene W. A., Swisher S. N. (1969). Psychological and somatic variables associated with the development and course of monozygotic twins discordant for leukemia. *Ann NY Acad Sci*, 164, 394–408.

Greer S., Morris T. (1975). Psychological attributes of women who develop breast cancer: A controlled study. *Journal of Psychosomatic Research*, 19(2), 147–153.

Greer S., Watson M. (1985). Towards a psychobiological model of cancer: psychological considerations. *Soc Sci Med*, 20(8), 773–777.

Greer S., Morris T., Pettingale K. W. (1979). Psychological response to breast cancer: Effect on outcome. *Lancet*, 13, 785–787.

Greer S., Morris T., Pettingale K. W. et al. (1990). Psychological response to breast cancer and 15-year outcome. *Lancet*, 335, 49–50.

Greisinger A. J., Lorimor R. J., Aday L. A. et al. (1997). Terminally ill cancer patients: their most important concerns. *Cancer Practice*, 5, 147–154.

Gritsevich T. D., Chernykh I. D. (2009). Osobennosti lichnosti zhenshin, stradayushih onkozabolevaniyami, i ih udovletvorennost brakom. *Psihoterapiya i Klinicheskaya Psihologiya* (Minsk), 1, 11–14

Grinker R. R. (1966). Psychosomatic aspects of the cancer problem. *Annals of the New York Academy of Sciences*, 125(3), 876–882.

Grinshpoon A., Barchana M., Ponizovsky A. et al. (2005). Cancer in schizophrenia: is the risk higher or lower? *Schizophrenia Research*, 73(2), 333–341.

Grishechkina I. A. (2011). Psihologicheskie faktory i gastroezofagealnaya reflyuksnaya bolezn. *Omskiy Nauchnyj Vestnik*, 1, 104.

Groenvold M., Petersen M. A., Idler E. et al. (2007). Psychological distress and fatigue predicted recurrence and survival in primary breast cancer patients. *Breast Cancer Research and Treatment*, 105(2), 209–219.

Grof S. (1985). *Beyond the Brain: Birth, Death, and Transendence in Psychotherapy* (Suny Series in Transpersonal & Humanistic Psychology). New York: State University of New York Press.

Grof S. (1996). *Realms of the Human Unconscious: Observations from LSD Research* (Condor Books). London: Souvenir Press.

Grof S. (2000). *Psychology of the Future: Lessons from Modern Consciousness Research* (Suny Series in Transpersonal and Humanistic Psychology). New York: State University of New York Press.

Grof S., Grof C. (1989). *Spiritual Emergency: When Personal Transformation Becomes a Crisis* (New Consciousness Readers). London: TarcherPerigee.

Grof S., Halifax J. (1978). *The Human Encounter with Death*. New York: Plume.

Gross A. L., Gallo J. J., Eaton W. W. (2010). Depression and cancer risk: 24 years of follow-up of the Baltimore Epidemiologic Catchment Area sample. *Cancer Causes Control*, 21, 191–199.

Grossarth-Maticek R. (1980). Psychosocial predictors of cancer and internal diseases. An overview. *Psychother Psychosom*, 33(3), 122–128.

Grossarth-Maticek R., Eysenck H. J. (1991). Creative novation behaviour therapy as a prophylactic treatment for cancer and coronary heart disease: Part I--Description of treatment. *Behav Res Ther*, 29(1), 1–16.

Grossarth-Maticek R., Bastiaans J., Kanazir D. T. (1985). Psychosocial factors as strong predictors of mortality from cancer, ischaemic heart disease and stroke: the Yugoslav prospective study. *J Psychosom Res*, 29(2), 167–176.

Grossarth-Maticek R., Eysenck H. J., Barrett P. (1993). Prediction of cancer and coronary heart disease as a function of method of questionnaire administration. *Psychol Rep*, 73(3 Pt 1), 943–959.

Grossarth-Maticek R., Eysenck H. J., Boyle G. J. (1994). An empirical study of the diathesis-stress theory of disease. *International Journal of Stress Management*, 1(1), 3–18.

Grossarth-Maticek R., Eysenck H. J., Vetter H. (1988). Personality type, smoking habit and their interaction as predictors of cancer and coronary heart disease. *Personality and Individual Differences*, 9(2), 479–495.

Grossarth-Maticek R., Siegrist J., Vetter H. (1982). Interpersonal repression as a predictor of cancer. *Social Science & Medicine*, 16(4), 493–498.

Grunebaum M. F., Galfalvy H. C., Mortenson L. Y. et al. (2010). Attachment and social adjustment: relationships to suicide attempt and major depressive episode in a prospective study. *Journal of Affective Disorders*, 123(1), 123–130.

Gruzelier J. H. (2002). A review of the impact of hypnosis, relaxation, guided imagery and individual differences on aspects of immunity and health. *Stress*, 5(2), 147–163.

Grytli H. H., Fagerland M. W., Fosså S. D., Taskén K. A. (2014). Association between use of β-blockers and prostate cancer-specific survival: a cohort study of 3561 prostate cancer patients with high-risk or metastatic disease. *European Urology*, 65(3), 635–641.

Gunst D. C., Kaatsch P., Goldbeck L. (2016). Seeing the good in the bad: which factors are associated with posttraumatic growth in long-term survivors of adolescent cancer? *Supportive Care in Cancer*, 24(11), 4607–4615.

Guo G., Sun X., Chen C. et al. (2013). Whole-genome and whole-exome sequencing of bladder cancer identifies frequent alterations in genes involved in sister chromatid cohesion and segregation. *Nat Genet*, 45(12), 1459–1463.

Gurskaya T. B., Ivanova O. B. (2013). Issledovanie emocionalnoj sfery pacientov v kontekste vnutrennej kartiny bolezni v onkoklinike. *Ukrayinskiy Naukovo-Medichniy Molodizhniy Zhurnal*, (2), 51–54.

Gurvich I. N. (2000). Teoreticheskie modeli, empiricheskie issledovaniya i ih prakticheskoe prilozhenie v zarubezhnoj psihologii zdorovya. V: *Psihologiya zdorovya*. Pod red. G. S. Nikiforova. Saint Petersburg: Izd-vo S.-Peterburgskogo un-ta, 89–127.

Gusev V. (2014). *Sredstvo ot bolezney*. IP Strelbickiy.

Gusev V. (2015). *Kurs lekciy psihoterapiya v rabote s psihosomatikoj. Institut gruppovoj i semejnoj psihologii i psihoterapii: publikacii.* Retrieved 05.08.2015 from: http://www.igisp.ru/.

Guseva L. Y. (1969). *Smertnost i prichiny smerti bolnyh shizofreniej*. Avtoref. dis. kand. med. nauk. Moscow: NII Psikhiatrii.

Guzińska K., Dziedziul J., Rudnik A. (2014). Psychologiczne uwarunkowania jakości życia pacjentek poddanych radioterapii w odniesieniu do stopnia zaawansowania choroby i wieku. *Psychoonkologia*, 2, 51–58.

Haetskiy I. K. (1965). Vliyanie gipotalamo-gipofizarnyh narushenij, vyzyvaemyh postoyannym osvesheniem, na razvitie inducirovannyh opuholej molochnyh zhelez u krys. *Voprosy Eksperimentalnoj Onkologii*, 1, 87–89.

Hagnell O. (1966). The premorbid personality of persons who develop cancer in a total population investigated in 1947 and 1957. *Ann NY Acad Sci*, 125, 846–855.

Hahn R. C., Petitti D. B. (1988). Minnesota Multiphasic Personality Inventory-rated depression and the incidence of breast cancer. *Cancer*, 61, 845–848.

Hajszan T., Dow A., Warner-Schmidt J. L. et al. (2009). Remodeling of hippocampal spine synapses in the rat learned helplessness model of depression. *Biol Psychiatry*, 65(5), 392–400.

Hall J. H., Fincham F. D. (2005). Self–forgiveness: The stepchild of forgiveness research. *Journal of social and clinical psychology*, 24(5), 621–637.

Hamama-Raz Y., Solomon Z. (2006). Psychological adjustment of melanoma survivors: The contribution of hardiness, attachment, and cognitive appraisal. *Journal of Individual Differences*, 27, 172–182.

Hamer R. G. (2000). *Summary of the New Medicine*. Malaga: Amici di Dirk.

Hampton M. R., Frombach I. (2000). Women's experience of traumatic stress in cancer treatment. *Health Care Int*, 21, 67–76.

Hanahan D., Weinberg R. A. (2000). The hallmarks of cancer. *Cell*, 100(1), 57–70.

Hanna E. A. (1990). The relationship between false self compliance and the motivation to become a professional helper. Part I: *Smith College studies in social work*, 60(2), 169–184; Part II: 60(3), 263–281.

Hansen M. J. (2002). Forgiveness as an educational intervention goal for persons at the end of life. *Dissertation Abstracts International*, 63(1224), 4A.

Hanssen L. M., Schutte N. S., Malouff J. M., Epel E. S. (2017). The relationship between childhood psychosocial stressor level and telomere length: a meta-analysis. *Health Psychology Research*, 5(1), 6378–6378.

Hara M. R., Kovacs J. J., Whalen E. J. et al. (2011). A stress response pathway regulates DNA damage through [bgr] 2-adrenoreceptors and [bgr]-arrestin-1. *Nature*, 477(7364), 349–353.

Harburg E., Julius M., Kaciroti N. et al. (2003). Expressive/Suppressive anger-coping responses, gender, and types of mortality: a 17-year follow-up (Tecumer, Michigan,1971-1988). *Psychosomatic medicine*, 65, 588–597.

Haritonov S. V. (2013). Nespecificheskie faktory suicidalnogo riska. *Tyumenskiy Medicinskiy Zhurnal*, 15(1), 30–31.

Harman D. (1957). Aging: a theory based on free radical and radiation chemistry. *J. Gerontol*, 2, 298–300.

Harris A. H., Thoresen C. E. (2005). Forgiveness, unforgiveness, health and disease. In E. L. Worthington, Jr (ed.), *Handbook of forgiveness*. New York: Brunner-Routledge, 321–334.

Harris G. A. (2005). Early childhood emotional trauma: an important factor in the aetiology of cancer and other diseases. *European Journal of Clinical Hypnosis*, 7(2), 2–10.

Harris R. E., Kasbari S., Farrar W. B. (1999). Prospective study of nonsteroidal anti-inflammatory drugs and breast cancer. *Oncol Rep*, 6(1), 71–73.

Harris T., Brown G. W., Bifulco A. (1986). Loss of parent in childhood and adult psychiatric disorder: the role of lack of adequate parental care. *Psychological medicine*, 16(03), 641–659.

Hasegawa H., Saiki I. (2002). Psychosocial stress augments tumor development through beta-adrenergic activation in mice. *Jpn J Cancer Res*, 93(7), 729–735.

Hassan S., Karpova Y., Baiz D. et al. (2013). Behavioral stress accelerates prostate cancer development in mice. *The Journal of Clinical Investigation*, 123(2), 874–886.

Hatala A. R. (2013). Towards a Biopsychosocial-Spiritual Approach in Health Psychology: Exploring Theoretical Orientations and Future Directions. *Journal of Spirituality in Mental Health*, 15(4), 256–276.

Haug T. T., Mykletun A., Dahl A. A. (2004). The association between anxiety, depression, and somatic symptoms in a large population: the HUNT-II study. *Psychosom Med*, 66(6), 845–851.

Haustova E. A. (2008). Psihosomaticheskiy podhod k boleznyam civilizacii (na primere metabolicheskogo sindroma H). *Gazeta Novosti Mediciny i Farmacii, vypusk Nevrologiya i Psihiatriya*, 243.

Havlik R. J., Vukasin A. P., Ariyan S. (1992). The impact of stress on the clinical presentation of melanoma. *Plastic and Reconstructive Surgery*, 90(1), 57–61.

Hay L. (1984). *You Can Heal Your Life. Heal Your Body*. Carlsbad, CA: Hay House.

Hay L. (1991). *The Power Is Within You*. Carlsbad, CA: Hay House.

Heim C., Newport D. J., Mletzko T. et al. (2008). The link between childhood trauma and depression: insights from HPA axis studies in humans. *Psychoneuroendocrinology*, 33(6), 693–710.

Heinroth J. C. A. (1818). Lehrbuch der Störungen des Seelenlebens oder der Seelenstörungen und ihrer Behandlung. Zwey Theile. Leipzig: Vogel.

Heinzelmann M., Gill J. (2013). Epigenetic mechanisms shape the biological response to trauma and risk for PTSD: a critical review. *Nursing Research and Practice*, 1–10.

Helgeson V. S., Snyder P., Seltman H. (2004). Psychological and physical adjustment to breast cancer over four years: Identifying distinct trajectories of change. *Health Psychology*, 23, 3–15.

Helgesson O., Cabrera C., Lapidus L. et al. (2003). Self-reported stress levels predict subsequent breast cancer in a cohort of Swedish women. *Eur J Cancer Prevent*, 12, 377–381.

Hendrix H. (2007). *Getting the Love You Want: A Guide for Couples*. New York: Henry Holt & Co.

Henn F. A., Vollmayr B. (2005). Stress models of depression: forming genetically vulnerable strains. *Neurosci Biobehav Rev*, 29(4-5), 799–804.

Hepburn Ferrer S. H. (2003). *Audrey Hepburn, An Elegant Spirit: A Son Remembers*. New York: Atria.

Herbert T. B., Cohen S. (1993). Stress and immunity in humans: a meta-analytic review. *Psychosom Med*, 55(4), 364–379.

Hermelink K., Voigt V., Kaste J. et al. (2015). Elucidating Pretreatment Cognitive Impairment in Breast Cancer Patients: The Impact of Cancer-Related Post-Traumatic Stress. *Journal of the National Cancer Institute*, 107(7), djv099.

Hermes G. L., Delgado B., Tretiakova M. et al. (2009). Social isolation dysregulates endocrine and behavioral stress while increasing malignant burden of spontaneous mammary tumors. *Proc Natl Acad Sci USA*, 106, 22393–22398.

Hertzman C. (1999). The biological embedding of early experience and its effects on health in adulthood. *Ann N Y Acad Sci*, 896, 85–95

Hewitt G., Jurk D., Marques F. D. et al. (2012). Telomeres are favoured targets of a persistent DNA damage response in ageing and stress-induced senescence. *Nature Communications*, 3, 708.

Heyn H., Sayols S., Moutinho C., Esteller M. (2014). Linkage of DNA Methylation Quantitative Trait Loci to Human Cancer Risk. *Cell Reports*, 7(2), 331–338.

Hickey B. E., Francis D., Lehman M. H. (2006). Sequencing of chemotherapy and radiation therapy for early breast cancer. *The Cochrane Database of Systematic Reviews,* Issue 4, CD005212.

Hinnen C., Ranchor A., Sandeman R. et al. (2008). Course of distress in breast cancer patients, their partners, and matched control couples. *Ann Behav Med*, 36, 141–148.

Hirai I., Kimura W., Ozawa K. et al. (2002). Perineural invasion in pancreatic cancer. *Pancreas*, 24(1), 15–25.

Hiroto D. S. (1974). Locus of control and learned helplessness. *Journal of Experimental Psychology*, 102(2), 187–193.

Hirsch J. K., Webb J. R., Jeglic E. L. (2012). Forgiveness as a moderator of the association between anger expression and suicidal behaviour. *Mental Health, Religion & Culture*, 15, 279–300.

Hirschberg C., O'Regan B. (1993). *Spontaneous Remission: An Annotated Bibliography*. Petaluma: IONS. Retrieved 12.05.2014 from: http://www.noetic.org/library/publication-bibliographies/spontaneous-remission-annotated-bibliography.

Hirshberg C., Barasch M. I. (1995). *Remarkable Recovery: What Extraordinary Healings Tell Us About Getting Well and Staying Well.* New York: Riverhead.

Hjelle L. A., Ziegler D. J. (1992). *Personality theories: Basic assumptions, research, and applications* (3rd edn). New York: Mcgraw-Hill Book Company.

Ho Y. C., Wang S. (2010). Adult neurogenesis is reduced in the dorsal hippocampus of rats displaying learned helplessness behavior. *Neuroscience*, 171(1), 153–161.

Hoffer A. (1994). Schizophrenia: an evolutionary defence against severe stress. *Journal of Orthomolecular Medicine*, 9, 205–205.

Hoffer A. (1998). *Vitamin B3 and Schizophrenia: Discovery, Recovery, Controversy*. Kingston (Ontario): Quarry Press.

Hoffer A., Foster H. D. (2000). Why Schizophrenics Smoke but Have a Lower Incidence of Lung Cancer: Implications for the Treatment of Both Disorder. *Journal of Orthomolecular Medicine*, 15(3), 141–144.

Holborn K. (2018). *Audrey Hepburn: An Audrey Hepburn Biography*. Independently published.

Holland J. C., Bultz B. D. (2007). The NCCN guideline for distress management: a case for making distress the sixth vital sign. *Journal of the National Comprehensive Cancer Network*, 5(1), 3–7.

Holland J. C., Rowland J. H. (1989). *Handbook of Psychooncology: Psychological Care of the Patient with Cancer*. New York: Oxford Press.

Holmberg C. (2014). No one sees the fear: becoming diseased before becoming ill-being diagnosed with breast cancer. *Cancer Nurs*, 37(3), 175–183.

Holt-Lunstad J., Smith T. B., Layton J. B. (2010). Social relationships and mortality risk: a meta-analytic review. *PLoS Med*, 7, e1000316.

Hong S. H., Christian D., Trinh E. et al. (2015). Prenatal stress increases neuroblastoma tumorigenesis in TH-MYCN mice model. *Cancer Research*, 75(15 Supplement), 3291–3291.

Horney K. (1992). *Our Inner Conflicts: A Constructive Theory of Neurosis*. New York: W. W. Norton & Company.

Horney K. (1994). *The neurotic personality of our time*. New York: W. W. Norton & Company.

Horowitz M. J. (1997). *Stress response syndromes* (3rd edn). Northvale, NJ: Jason Aronson.

Hsu T.-S. (2010). *Reborn at the End of the Road: Dr. Hsu Spiritual Prescriptions for Healing Cancer*. Taibei: Tien-Sheng Hsu Pub.

Huang T., Poole E. M., Okereke O. I. et al. (2015). Depression and risk of epithelial ovarian cancer: results from two large prospective cohort studies. *Gynecologic Oncology*, 139(3), 481–486.

Huang X., Wang M. L., Jinng J. (2004). Influence of cesarean section on children's neuropsychological development [J]. *Foreign Medical Sciences Section of Maternal and Child Health*, 1, 001.

Huggan R. E. (1968). Neuroticism and anxiety among women with cancer. *J Psychosom Res*, 12(3), 215–221.

Hughes J. W., Watkins L., Blumenthal J. A. et al. (2004). Depression and anxiety symptoms are related to increased 24-hour urinary norepinephrine excretion among healthy middle-aged women. *J Psychosom Res*, 57(4), 353–358.

Huis E. M., Vingerhoets A. J., Denollet J. (2011). Attachment style and self-esteem: The mediating role of Type D personality. *Personality and Individual Differences*, 50(7), 1099–1103.

Hung Y. J., Hsieh C. H., Chen Y. J. et al. Insulin sensitivity, proinflammatory markers and adiponectin in young males with different subtypes of depressive disorder. *Clin Endocrinol* (Oxf.), 67(5), 784–789.

Hurny C., Adler R. (1991). Psycho-onkologische Forschung. In: F. Meerwein (Hrsg.), *Einführung in die Psycho-Onkologie*. Bern: Huber, 15–57

Hunter R. G. (2012). Epigenetic effects of stress and corticosteroids in the brain. *Frontiers in Cellular Neuroscience*, 6, 18.

Hutchison E. D. (2008). *Dimensions of human behavior: Person and environment* (3rd edn). Thousand Oaks, CA: Sage Publications.

Hutschnecker A. A. (1983). *The Will to Live*. New York: Simon & Schuster.

Hutton S. K. (1912). *Among the Eskimos of Labrador*. London: Seeley.

Hyland M. E., Alkhalaf A. M., Whalley B. (2013). Beating and insulting children as a risk for adult cancer, cardiac disease and asthma. *Journal of Behavioral Medicine*, 36(6), 632–640.

Ignatova T. N., Kukekov V. G., Laywell E. D. et al. (2002). Human cortical glial tumors contain neural stem-like cells expressing astroglial and neuronal markers in vitro. *Glia*, 39(3), 193–206.

Igumnov S. A., Grigorieva I. V. (2014). Psihoterapiya v kompleksnoj reabilitacii pacientov, operirovannyh po povodu onkologicheskih zabolevanij. *Teoriya i Praktika Psihoterapii*, 1(1), 34–40.

Ikemi Y., Nakagawa S., Nakagawa T., Sugita M. (1975). Psychosomatic consideration on cancer patients who have made a narrow escape from death. *Dynamische Psychiatrie*, 8(2), 77–92.

Ilyin I. (2006). O stradanii. V: *O polze stradaniy i lishenij*. Sost. A. Baranov. Moscow: OBRAZ, 21–24.

Imperato A., Angelucci L., Casolini P. et al. (1992). Repeated stressful experiences differently affect limbic dopamine release during and following stress. *Brain Res*, 577(2), 194–199.

Imyanitov E. N. (2010). Skrining dlya lic s nasledstvennoj predraspolozhennostyu k raku. *Prakticheskaya Onkologiya*, 11(2), 102–109.

Infante J. R., Torres-Avisbal M., Pinel P. et al. (2001). Catecholamine levels in practitioners of the transcendental meditation technique. *Physiol Behav*, 72(1–2), 141–146.

Ingram R., Tranary L., Odom M., Berry L., Nelson T. (2007). Cognitive, affective and social mechanisms in depression risk: cognition, hostility and copying style. *Cognition and Cmotion*, 21(1), 78–94.

Inoue A., Kawakami N., Ishizaki M. et al. (2009). Three job stress models/concepts and oxidative DNA damage in a sample of workers in Japan. *J Psychosom Res*, 66, 329–334.

Inozemtsev F. K. (1845). Ob istochnike i obraze proishozhdeniya istinnogo raka. *Zap po Chasti Vracheb Nauk*, kn. 3.

Ioannidou-Mouzaka L., Mantonakis J., Toufexi H. et al. (1986). [Is prolonged psychological stress an etiological factor in breast cancer?]. *J Gynecol Obstet Biol Reprod* (Paris), 15(8), 1049–1053 (in French).

Irie M., Asami S., Nagata S. et al. (2001). Psychosocial factors as a potential trigger of oxidative DNA damage in human leukocytes. *Jpn J Cancer Res*, 92(3), 367–376.

Irie M., Asami S., Nagata S., et al. (2002). Psychological mediation of a type of oxidative DNA damage, 8-hydroxydeoxyguanosine, in peripheral blood leukocytes of non-smoking and non-drinking workers. *Psychotherapy and Psychosomatics*, 71(2), 90–96.

Irwin M. R., Daniels M., Risch S. C. et al. (1988). Plasma cortisol and natural killer cell activity during bereavement. *Biol Psychiatry*, 24(2),173–178.

Irwin M. R., Cole S. W. (2011). Reciprocal regulation of the neural and innate immune systems. *Nat Rev Immunol*, 11, 625–632.

Irwin M. R., Olmstead R., Breen E. C. et al. (2014). Tai chi, cellular inflammation, and transcriptome dynamics in breast cancer survivors with insomnia: a randomized controlled trial. *Journal of the National Cancer Institute*. Monographs, 2014(50), 295–301.

Isaev D. N. (2000). *Psihosomaticheskie rasstrojstva u detey*. Saint Petersburg: Piter.

Isaeva E. R. (2009). *Koping-povedenie i psihologicheskaya zashita lichnosti v usloviyah zdorovya i bolezni*. Saint Petersburg: SPbGU.

Ivashkina M. G. (1998). *Psihologicheskie osobennosti lichnosti onkologicheskih bolnyh*. Avtoref. diss. kand. psihol. nauk. Moscow: Institut Cheloveka.

Ivashkina M. G. (2010). Opyt psihokorrekcionnogo i psihoreabilitacionnogo soprovozhdeniya lichnosti v usloviyah onkologicheskogo zabolevaniya. *Lechebnoe Delo*, 3, 49–54.

Ivonin A. A., Ciceroshin M. N., Kutsenko D. O. et al. (2008). Osobennosti narusheniy processov mezhkorkovoj i korkovo-podkorkovoj integracii pri razlichnyh klinicheskih proyavleniyah nevroticheskoj depressii. *Fiziologiya Cheloveka*, 34(6), 10–22.

Iwamitsu Y., Shimoda K., Abe H., Okawa M. (2005). Anxiety, emotional suppression, and psychological distress before and after breast cancer diagnosis. *Psychosomatics*, 46(1), 19–24.

Iyengar U., Kim S., Martinez S. et al. (2014). Unresolved trauma in mothers: intergenerational effects and the role of reorganization. *Frontiers in Psychology*, 5, 966.

Jacobs G. D. (2001). Clinical applications of the relaxation response and Mind-body interventions. *The Journal of Alternative and Complementary Medicine*, 7, S93-S101.

Jacobs J. R., Bovasso G. B. (2000). Early and chronic stress and their relation to breast cancer. *Psychological Medicine*, 30(03), 669-678.

Jacobs T. J., Charles E. (1980). Life events and the occurrence of cancer in children. *Psychosom Med*, 42(1), 11–24.

Jacobs T. L., Epel E. S., Lin J. et al. (2011). Intensive meditation training, immune cell telomerase activity, and psychological mediators. *Psychoneuroendocrinology*, 36(5), 664–681.

Jacobsen E. (1962). *You Must Relax*. New York: McGraw-Hill Book Company.

Jacobsen P. B., Donovan K. A. (2011). Psychological co-morbidities of cancer. In: *Psychological co-morbidities of physical illness: a behavioral medicine perspective*. New York: Springer Science+Business Media, 163–206.

Jacobson E. (1932). Electrophysiology of mental activities. *The American Journal of Psychology*, 44, 677–694.

Jagannathan-Bogdan M., McDonnell M. E., Shin H. et al. (2011). Elevated proinflammatory cytokine production by a skewed T cell compartment requires monocytes and promotes inflammation in type 2 diabetes. *J Immunol*, 186, 1162–1172.

Jakovljevic G., Culic S., Benko M. et al. (2010). Parental type of personality, negative affectivity and family stressful events in children with cancer. *Psychiatr Danub*, 22(3), 436–440.

Jampolsky G. G. (1999). *Forgiveness: The Greatest Healer of All*. New York: Atria Books.

Janca A., Isaac M., Costa e Silva J. A. (1995). World Health Organization international study of somatoform disorders—background and rational. *Eur J Psychiatry*, 9, 373–378.

Jaremka L. M., Glaser R., Malarkey W. B., Kiecolt-Glaser J. K. (2013). Marital distress prospectively predicts poorer cellular immune function. *Psychoneuroendocrinology*, 38, 2713–2719.

Jaremka L. M., Fagundes C. P., Peng J. et al. (2013a). Loneliness promotes inflammation during acute stress. *Psychological Science*, 24,1089–1097.

Jayawickreme E., Blackie L. E. (2016). Exploring the Long-Term Benefits of Adversity: What Is Posttraumatic Wisdom?. In: E. Jayawickreme, L. E. R. Blackie, *Exploring the Psychological Benefits of Hardship*. Cham: Springer, 41–52.

Jemal A., Siegel R., Ward E. (2008). Cancer Statistics. *CA: a Cancer Journal for Clinicians*, 58, 71–96.

Jenkins F. J., Van Houten B., Bovbjerg D. H. (2014). Effects on DNA damage and/or repair processes as biological mechanisms linking psychological stress to cancer risk. *Journal of Applied Biobehavioral Research*, 19(1), 3–23.

Jenkins R. A., Pargament K. I. (1995). Religion and Spirituality as Resources for Coping with Cancer. *Journal of Psychosocial Oncology*, 13(1/2), 51–74.

Jensen M. R. (1987). Psychobiological factors predicting the course of breast cancer. *J Pers*, 55, 317–342.

Jessy T. (2011). Immunity over inability: The spontaneous regression of cancer. *Journal of Natural Science, Biology, and Medicine*, 2(1), 43–49.

Jevning R., Wilson A. F., Davidson J. M. (1978). Adrenocortical activity during meditation. *Hormones and Behavior*, 10(1), 54–60.

Jia L., Qian K. (2011). An evidence-based perspective of panax ginseng (Asian Ginseng) and panax quinquefolius (American Ginseng) as a preventing or supplementary therapy for cancer patients. In: W. C. Cho (ed.), *Evidence-based Anticancer Materia Medica*. Heidelberg: Springer Netherlands, 85–96.

Jia Y., Li F., Liu Y. F. et al. (2017). Depression and cancer risk: a systematic review and meta-analysis. *Public Health*, 149, 138–148.

Jim H. S., Andersen B. L. (2007). Meaning in life mediates the relationship between social and physical functioning and distress in cancer survivors. *British Journal of Health Psychology*, 12(3), 363–381.

Jim H. S., Purnell J. Q., Richardson S. A. et al. (2006). Measuring meaning in life following cancer. *Quality of Life Research*, 15(8), 1355–1371.

Jobs S. (2005). Commencement address to the graduates of Stanford University. June 12, 2005. Retrieved from: https://news.stanford.edu/2005/06/14/jobs-061505/.

Johansen C. (2010). Psychosocial Factors. In: J. C. Holland, W. S. Breitbart, P. B. Jacobsen (eds), *Psycho-Oncology*. Oxford: Oxford University Press, 57–62.

Johansson J. E., Adami H. O., Andersson S. O. et al. (1992). High 10-year survival rate in patients with early, untreated prostatic cancer. *JAMA*, 267(16), 2191–2196.

Johansson L., Guo X., Duberstein P. R et al. (2014). Midlife personality and risk of Alzheimer disease and distress: A 38-year follow-up. *Neurology*, 83(17), 1538–1544.

Johnstone S. E., Baylin S. B. (2010). Stress and the epigenetic landscape: a link to the pathobiology of human diseases? *Nature Reviews Genetics*, 11(11), 806–812.

Jones E. (1911). *Cancer - Its Causes, Symptoms and Treatment*. Boston: Therapeutic Publishing Company, Inc.

Jones H. P., Aldridge B., Boss-Williams K., Weiss J. M. (2017). A role for B cells in facilitating defense against an NK cell-sensitive lung metastatic tumor is revealed by stress. *Journal of Neuroimmunology*, 313, 99–108.

Jones W. H. S. (1923). *Hippocrates*. Vol. I–IV. London: William Heinemann.

Jørgensen A. (2013). Oxidatively generated DNA/RNA damage in psychological stress states. *Danish Medical Journal*, 60(7), B4685–B4685.

Joyce A., Etty-Leal J., Zazryn T., Hamilton A. (2010). Exploring a mindfulness meditation program on the mental health of upper primary children: A pilot study. *Advances in School Mental Health Promotion*, 3(2), 17–25.

Joyce P. D. (2015). *The efficacy of mindfulness as a complementary cancer therapy*. Doctoral dissertation, Elon University.

Jung C. G. (1966). *Collected Works: The Practice of Psychotherapy, vol. XVI*. New York: Pantheon, Bollingen Series.

Jung C. G. (1972). *Two Essays on Analytical Psychology*. Princeton, NJ: Princeton University Press.

Jung C. G. (1989). *Memories, Dreams, Reflections*. New York: Vintage; Reissue edn.

Jung C. G. (2015). *Letters of C. G. Jung*, Vol. 2; 1951–1961. G. Adler, J. Aniela (eds). Abingdon-on-Thames: Routledge.

Juster R.-P., Sindi S., Marin M.-F. et al. (2011). A clinical allostatic load index is associated with burnout symptoms and hypocortisolemic profiles in healthy workers. *Psychoneuroendocrinology*, 36, 797–805.

Justice A. (1985). Review of the effects of stress on cancer in laboratory animals: Importance of time of stress application and type of tumor. *Psychological Bulletin*, 98(1), 108–138.

Kabat-Zinn J. (2005). *Wherever You Go, There You Are: Mindfulness Meditation in Everyday Life*. New York: Hachette Books.

Kafkalides A. (1980). *The knowledge of the womb: autopsychognosia with psychodelic drugs*. Corfu: Triclino Hause.

Kaliman P., Alvarez-Lopez M. J., Cosin-Tomas M. (2014). Rapid changes in histone deacetylases and inflammatory gene expression in expert meditators. *Psychoneuroendocrinology*, 40, 96–107.

Kalweit H. (1999). When insanity is a blessing: the message of shamanism. In: S. Grof, C. Grof (eds). *Spiritual Emergency: When Personal Transformation Becomes a Crisis*. New York: Tarcher/Putnam US, 77–99.

Kamali M., Panahi H., Gilani O., Azadikhah Haghighat A. et al. (2015). Predicting Post-traumatic Stress Disorder Severity from Emotional Intelligence and Coping Strategies in PTSD Patients. *Journal of Police Medicine*, 4(1), 39–48.

Kamen C., Scheiber C., Janelsins M. et al. (2017). Effects of childhood trauma exposure and cortisol levels on cognitive functioning among breast cancer survivors. *Child Abuse & Neglect*, 72, 163–171.

Kameneckiy D. A. (2001). *Nevrozologiya i psihoterapiya*. Moscow: Gelios ARV.

Kang D. H., Park N. J., McArdle T. (2012). Cancer-specific stress and mood disturbance: implications for symptom perception, quality of life, and immune response in women shortly after diagnosis of breast cancer. *ISRN Nursing*, 608039.

Kang D. H., Weaver M. T., Park N. J. et al. (2009). Significant impairment in immune recovery following cancer treatment. *Nursing Research*, 58(2), 105–114.

Kang H. J., Kim J. M., Lee J. Y. et al. (2013). BDNF promoter methylation and suicidal behavior in depressive patients. *Journal of Affective Disorders*, 151(2), 679–685.

Kang K. A., Zhang R., Kim G. Y. et al. (2012). Epigenetic changes induced by oxidative stress in colorectal cancer cells: methylation of tumor suppressor RUNX3. *Tumor Biology*, 33(2), 403–412.

Kangas M., Henry J. L., Bryant R. A. (2005). The relationship between acute stress disorder and posttraumatic stress disorder following cancer. *Journal of Consulting and Clinical Psychology*, 73(2), 360–364.

Kaplan G. A., Reynolds P. (1988). Depression and cancer mortality and morbidity: prospective evidence from the Alameda County Study. *J Behav Med*, 11, 1–13.

Karpenko L. A., Petrovskiy A. V., Yaroshevskiy M. G. (1998). *Kratkiy psihologicheskiy slovar*. Rostov-na-Donu: Feniks.

Karpinets T. V., Foy B. D. (2005). Tumorigenesis: the adaptation of mammalian cells to sustained stress environment by epigenetic alterations and succeeding matched mutations. *Carcinogenesis*, 26(8), 1323–1334.

Karpinskiy K. V. (2011). Dezintegraciya smysla zhizni kak predposylka krizisa v razvitii lichnosti. *Chelovek. Soobshestvo. Upravlenie*, 2, 4–16.

Karpinskiy K. V. (2011a). Bezduhovnyj smysl zhizni kak istochnik krizisa v razvitii lichnosti. *Psihologiya: Zhurnal Vysshej Shkoly Ekonomiki*, 8(1), 27–58.

Karvasarskiy B. D. (1990). *Nevrozy*. Moscow: Medicina.

Karvasarskiy B. D. (ed.) (2008). *Klinicheskaya psihologiya*. Saint Petersburg: Piter.

Karvasarskiy B. D., Prostomolov V. F. (1988). *Nevroticheskie rasstrojstva vnutrennih organov*. Kishinev: Shtiintsa.

Kashdan T. B., McKnight P. E. (2009). Origins of purpose in life: Refining our understanding of a life well lived. *Psychological Topics*, 18, 303–316.

Kashenkova M. M. (2009). Osobennosti psihologicheskogo statusa onkologicheskih bolnyh s aleksitimiej. *Uchenye Zapiski Rossijskogo Gosudarstvennogo Socialnogo Universiteta*, 2(7), 35–38.

Kasser T., Ryan R. M. (1993). A dark side of the American dream: Correlates of financial success as a central life aspiration. *Journal of Personality and Social Psychology*, 65, 410–422.

Kasser T., Ryan R. M. (1996). Further examining the American dream: Differential correlates of intrinsic and extrinsic goals. *Personality and Social Psychology Bulletin*, 22, 280–287.

Kassil G. N. (1983). *Vnutrennyaya sreda organizma*. Moscow: Nauka.

Kavetskiy R. E. (1955). Pro rol izmeneniy centralnoj nervnoj sistemy v patogeneze opuholevoj bolezni. *Vopr Onkol*, 1(6), 3–9.

Kavetskiy R. E. (1962). *Opuhol i organizm*. Kiev: Gosmedizdat USSR.

Kazdin A. E., French N. H., Unis A. S. et al. (1983). Hopelessness, depression, and suicidal intent among psychiatrically disturbed inpatient children. *Journal of Consulting and Clinical Psychology*, 51, 504–510.

Kehlet H. (1997). Multimodal approach to control postoperative pathophysiology and rehabilitation. *British Journal of Anaesthesia*, 78(5), 606–617.

Keinan-Boker L., Vin-Raviv N., Liphshitz I. et al. (2009). Cancer incidence in Israeli Jewish survivors of World War II. *Journal of the National Cancer Institute*, 101, 1489–1500.

Kekelidze Z. I. (2001). Principy okazaniya psihologo-psihiatricheskoj pomoshi pri chrezvychajnyh situaciyah. *Psihiatriya i Psihofarmakoterapiya*, 3(4), 123–125.

Kelly-Irving M., Lepage B., Dedieu D. et al. (2013). Childhood adversity as a risk for cancer: findings from the 1958 British birth cohort study. *BMC Public Health*, 13(1), 767.

Kelly-Irving M., Mabile L., Grosclaude P. et al. (2013a). The embodiment of adverse childhood experiences and cancer development: potential biological mechanisms and pathways across the life course. *International Journal of Public Health*, 58(1), 3–11.

Kelman H. (1969). Kairos: The auspicious moment. *The American Journal of Psychoanalysis*, 29(1), 59–83.

Kendler K. S., Karkowski-Shuman L. (1997). Stressful life events and genetic liability to major depression: genetic control of exposure to the environment? *Psychol Med*, 27, 539–547.

Kenkel W., Paredes J., Yee J. et al. (2012). Neuroendocrine and behavioural responses to exposure to an infant in male prairie voles. *Journal of Neuroendocrinology*, 24(6), 874–886.

Kennedy B., Valdimarsdóttir U., Sundström K. et al. (2014). Loss of a parent and the risk of cancer in early life: a nationwide cohort study. *Cancer Causes Control*, 25(4), 499–506.

Kent J., Coates T. J., Pelletier K. R., O'Regan B. (1989). Unexpected recoveries: Spontaneous remission and immune functioning. *Advances*, 6(2), 66–73.

Kenyon T. (2013). *Emotional Cancer*. Retrieved 24.07.2013 from: http://www.tomkenyon.com/emotionalcancer.

Kernberg O. F. (1993). *Severe Personality Disorders: Psychotherapeutic Strategies*. New Haven, CT: Yale University Press.

Kernberg O. F. (1999). Persönlichkeitsentwicklung und Trauma. In: *Persönlichkeitsstörungen— Theorie und Therapie (PTT)*, 3(1), 5–15.

Kerr D., Krishnan C., Pucak M. L., Carmen J. (2005). The immune system and neuropsychiatric diseases. *International Review of Psychiatry*, 17(6), 443–449.

Keshavan M. S., Kaneko Y. (2013). Secondary psychoses: an update. *World Psychiatry*, 12(1), 4–15.

Kessler R. C., Davis C. G., Kendler K. S. (1997). Childhood adversity and adult psychiatric disorder in the US National Comorbidity Survey. *Psychological Medicine*, 27, 1101–1119.

Key T. J., Appleby P. N., Reeves G. K. et al. (2003). Body mass index, serum sex hormones, and breast cancer risk in postmenopausal women. *J Natl Cancer Inst*, 95, 1218–1226.

Khan M. M. (1963). The concept of cumulative trauma. *The Psychoanalytic Study of the Child*, 18, 286–306.

Khansari N., Shakiba Y., Mahmoudi M. (2009). Chronic inflammation and oxidative stress as a major cause of age-related diseases and cancer. *Recent Pat Inflamm Allergy Drug Discov*, 3(1), 73–80.

Khasraw M., Posner J.B. (2010). Neurological complications of systemic cancer. *Lancet Neurol*, 9, 1214–1227.

Kholmogorova A. B., Garanyan N. G. (1999). Emocionalnye rasstrojstva i sovremennaya kultura. Na primere somatoformnyh, depressivnyh i trevozhnyh rasstrojstv. *Moskovskiy Psihoterapevticheskiy Zhurnal*, 2, 61–90.

Kholmogorova A. B., Garanyan N. G. (2008). Somatizaciya: sovremennye traktovki, psihologicheskie modeli i metody psihoterapii. Chast 1. *Sovremennaya Terapiya Psihicheskih Rasstrojstv*, (2), 31–35.

Kholmogorova A. B., Garanyan N. G. (2008a). Somatizaciya: sovremennye traktovki, psihologicheskie modeli i metody psihoterapii. Ch. 2. *Sovremennaya Terapiya Psihicheskih Rasstrojstv*, (3), 21–30.

Kholmogorova A. B., Garanyan N. G., Shajb P., Virshing M. (2011). Emocii i psihicheskoe zdorove v socialnom i semejnom kontekste (na modeli somatoformnyh rasstrojstv). *Medicinskaya Psihologiya v Rossii: elektron. nauch. zhurn,* 1. Retrieved 21.12.2014 from: http:// medpsy.ru.

Kiecolt-Glaser J. K., Glaser R. (2002). Depression and immune function: central pathways to morbidity and mortality. *Journal of Psychosomatic Research,* 53(4), 873–876.

Kiecolt-Glaser J. K., Newton T. L. (2001). Marriage and health: his and hers. *Psychological Bulletin,* 127(4), 472–503.

Kiecolt-Glaser J. K., Christian L., Preston H. et al. (2010). Stress, inflammation, and yoga practice. *Psychosomatic Medicine,* 72(2), 113–121.

Kiecolt-Glaser J. K., Glaser R., Cacioppo J. T. et al. (1997). Marital conflict in older adults: Endocrinological and immunological correlates. *Psychosomatic Medicine,* 59, 339–349.

Kiecolt-Glaser J. K., Glaser R., Cacioppo J. T. et al. (1998). Marital stress: immunologic, neuroendocrine, and autonomic correlates. *Ann N Y Acad Sci,* 840, 656–663.

Kiecolt-Glaser J. K., Loving T. J., Stowell J. R. et al. (2005). Hostile marital interactions, proinflammatory cytokine production, and wound healing. *Archives of General Psychiatry,* 62, 1377–1384

Kiecolt-Glaser J. K., Malarkey W. B., Chee M. et al. (1993). Negative behaviour during marital conflict is associated with immunological down-regulation. *Psychosomat Med,* 55, 395–409.

Kiecolt-Glaser J. K., Preacher K. J., MacCallum R. C. et al. (2003). Chronic stress and age-related increases in the proinflammatory cytokine interleukin-6. *Proc Natl Acad Sci USA,* 100, 9090–9095.

Kiecolt-Glaser J. K., Stephen R. E., Lipetz P. D. et al. (1985). Distress and DNA repair in human lymphocytes. *J Behav Med,* 8, 311–320.

Kielholz P. (1973). *Masked depression.* Berne, Stuttgart, Vienna: Huber.

Kierkegaard S. (1981). The Concept of Anxiety: A Simple Psychologically Orienting Deliberation on the Dogmatic Issue of Hereditary Sin (*Kierkegaard's Writings,* VIII). Princeton, NJ: Princeton University Press.

Kierkegaard S. (2013). *Fear and Trembling and The Sickness Unto Death.* Princeton, NJ: Princeton University Press.

Killebrew D., Shiramizu B. (2004). Pathogenesis of HIV-associated non-Hodgkin lymphoma. *Curr HIV Res,* 2, 215–221.

Kinney C. K., Rodgers D. M., Nash K. A., Bray C. O. (2003). Holistic healing for women with breast cancer through a mind, body, and spirit self-empowerment program. *J Holist Nurs,* 21(3), 260–279.

Kirby E. D., Friedman A. R., Covarrubias D. et al. (2012). Basolateral amygdala regulation of adult hippocampal neurogenesis and fear-related activation of newborn neurons. *Molecular Psychiatry,* 17(5), 527–536.

Kissane D. W. (2000). Psychospiritual and existential distress. *Australian Family Physician,* 29, 1022–1025.

Kissane D. W., Clarke D. M., Street A. F. (2001). Demoralization syndrome: a relevant psychiatric diagnosis for palliative care. *Journal of Palliative Care,* 17, 12–21.

Kissane D. W., Love A., Hatton A. et al. (2004). Effect of cognitive-existential therapy on survival in early-stage breast cancer. *Journal of Clinical Oncology,* 22, 4255–4260.

Kissane D. W., Wein S., Love A. et al. (2004a). The Demoralization Scale. A report of its development and preliminary validation. *J Palliat Care,* 20, 269–276.

Kissen D. M. (1966). The Significance of Personality in Lung Cancer. *Men. Ann. N.Y. Acad. Sci,* 125, 3, 820–826.

Kissen D. M., Eysenck H. J. (1962). Personality in male lung cancer patients. *Journal of Psychosomatic Research,* 6(2), 123–127.

Kissen D. M., Rao L., G. (1969). Steroid Excretion Patterns and Personality in Lung Cancer Patients. *Ann NY Acad Sci*, 164, 2, 476–482.

Kitaev-Smyk L. A. (1983). *Psihologiya stressa*. Moscow: Nauka.

Klopfer B. (1957). Psychological variables in human cancer. *Journal of Projective Techniques*, 21(4), 331–340.

Kneier A. W., Temoshok L. (1984). Repressive coping reactions in patients with malignant melanoma as compared to cardiovascular disease patients. *Journal of Psychosomatic Research*, 28(2), 145–155.

Knobf M. T. (2007). Psychosocial responses in breast cancer survivors. *Semin Oncol Nurs*, 23, 71–83.

Kobau R., Sniezek J., Zack M. M. et al. (2010). Well-being assessment: An evaluation of well-being scales for public health and population estimates of well-being among US adults. *Applied Psychology: Health and Well-Being*, 2(3), 272–297.

Kocic B., Filipovic S., Vrbic S. et al. (2015). Stressful life events and breast cancer risk: a hospital-based case-control study. *Age (years)*, 30(39), 8–13.

Kotsyubinskiy A. P., Shejnina N. S., Penchul N. A. (2013). Predvestniki psihicheskogo zabolevaniya. Soobshenie 1. Psihopatologicheskiy diatez. *Obozrenie psihiatrii i medicinskoj psihologii*, 3, 11–16.

Koenig H. G. (2012). Religion, spirituality, and health: The research and clinical implications. *ISRN Psychiatry*, 278730–278730.

Kohanov V. P., Krasnov V. N. (2008). *Psihiatriya katastrof i chrezvychajnyh situacij*. Moscow: Prakticheskaya medicina.

Kohls N. B., Sauer S., Offenbächer M., Giordano J. (2011). Spirituality—an overlooked predictor of placebo response and effects? *Phil Trans R Soc*, B, 366, 1838–1848.

Kohut H. (2000). Analysis of the Self: Systematic Approach to Treatment of Narcissistic Personality Disorders. Madison, CT: International Universities Press.

Koivumaa-Honkanen H., Honkanen R., Viinamaeki H. et al. (2001). Life satisfaction and suicide: a 20-year follow-up study. *American Journal of Psychiatry*, 158(3), 433–439.

Kolata G. (2009). Cancers Can Vanish Without Treatment, but How? *New York Times*, October 26.

Kolata G. (2016). It's Not Cancer: Doctors Reclassify a Thyroid Tumor. *New York Times*, April 14.

Koller M., Heitmann K., Kussmann J., Lorenz W. (1999). Symptom reporting in cancer patients II: Relations to social desirability, negative affect, and self-reported health behaviors. *Cancer*, 86, 1609–1620.

Kologrivova I. V., Suslova T. E., Koshelskaya O. A. et al. (2013). Vliyanie glyukozy i insulina na sekreciyu citokinov mononuklearami pericheskoj krovi in vitro. *Immunologiya*, 5, 267–270.

Kondo T., Oue N., Yoshida K., at al. (2004). Expression of POT1 is associated with tumor stage and telomere length in gastric carcinoma. *Cancer Research*, 64, 523–529.

Kondratiev M. Y., Ilyin V. A. (2007). *Azbuka socialnogo psihologa-praktika*. Moscow: PER SE.

Koneva O. B., Kostichenko I. V. (2004). Vliyanie emocionalnyh otkloneniy na vnutrennyuyu kartinu bolezni (na primere onkologicheskih bolnyh). *Zhurn. Yuzhno-Uralskogo Gos. Univ*, 3, 12–18.

Koopman C., Butler L. D., Classen C. et al. (2002). Traumatic stress symptoms among women with recently diagnosed primary breast cancer. *Journal of Traumatic Stress*, 15(4), 277–287.

Korablina E. P., Akindinova I. A., Bakanova A. A., Rodina A. M. (2001). *Iskusstvo isceleniya dushi: Etyudy o psihologicheskoj pomoshi. Posobie dlya prakticheskih psihologov*. Pod red. E. P. Korablinoy. Saint Petersburg: Izd-vo RGPU im. A. I. Gercena, 167–181.

Korkina M. V., Marilov V. V. (1998). Rol psihosomaticheskih ciklov v geneze psihosomaticheskih zabolevanij. *Zhurnal Nevrologii i Psihiatrii im. S. S. Korsakova*, 98(11), 30–32.

Kornblith A. B. (1998). Psychosocial adaptation of cancer survivors. In J. C. Holland (ed.), *Psycho-oncology*. New York and Oxford: Oxford University Press.

Kornblith A. B., Mirabeau-Beale K., Lee H. et al. (2010). Long-term adjustment of survivors of ovarian cancer treated for advanced-stage disease. *Journal of Psychosocial Oncology*, 28(5), 451–469.

Korneva E. A., Perekrest S. V. (2013). Vzaimodejstvie nervnoj i immunnoj sistem v norme i patologii. *Medicinskiy Akademicheskiy Zhurnal*, 13(3), 7–17.

Kornfield J. (1999). Obstacles and vicissitudes in spiritual practice. In: S. Grof, C. Grof (eds). *Spiritual Emergency: When Personal Transformation Becomes a Crisis*. New York: Tarcher/Putnam US, 137–171.

Korol L. I. (2005). Osobennosti mezhlichnostnyh otnosheniy v semyah s detmi s onkologicheskimi zabolevaniyami. *Onkologiya*, 7(4), 366–368.

Korolenko C. P., Dmitrieva N. V. (2010). *Lichnostnye rasstrojstva*. Saint Petersburg: Piter.

Korolkova A. V. (2005). *Slovar aforizmov russkih pisatelej*. Moscow: Rus. Yaz. Media.

Korotneva E. V., Varshavskiy A. V. (2007). Posttravmaticheskoe stressovoe rasstrojstvo u bolnyh gemoblastozami. *Medicinskiy Vestnik Bashkortostana*, 2(6), 48–52.

Korzhikov A. V. (1999). *Onkologiya dlya Homo Sapiens*. Moscow: AST, Astrel.

Kosenkov N. I. (1997). *Fiziologicheskie mehanizmy psihologicheskoj adaptacii pri psihosomaticheskoj patologii*. Dis. d-ra med. nauk. Saint Petersburg: VMedA.

Kotler T., Buzwell S., Romeo Y. Bowland J. (1994). Avoidant attachment as a risk factor for health. *British Journal of Medical Psychology*, 67, 237–245.

Koupil I., Plavinskaia S., Parfenova N. et al. (2009). Cancer mortality in women and men who survived the siege of Leningrad (1941-1944). *Int J Cancer*, 124(6), 1416–1421.

Koutrouli N., Anagnostopoulos F., Potamianos G. (2012). Posttraumatic stress disorder and posttraumatic growth in breast cancer patients: a systematic review. *Women & Health*, 52(5), 503–516.

Kovalenko I. L., Galyamina A. G., Smagin D. A. et al. (2014). Extended effect of chronic social defeat stress in childhood on behaviors in adulthood. *PloS one*, 9(3), e91762.

Kovalev V. V. (1979). *Psihiatriya detskogo vozrasta*. Moscow: Medicina.

Kovalev Y. V. (2004). Trevoga i depressiya: kliniko-fenomenologicheskie shodstva i razlichiya (analiticheskiy obzor). *Ros psihiatr zhurn*, 1, 45–49.

Kowal S. J. (1955). Emotions as a cause of cancer; 18th and 19th century contributions. *Psychoanal Rev*, 42(3), 217–227.

Kozhevnikova E. P. (1953). K voprosu o vliyanii vysshej nervnoj deyatelnosti na razvitie eksperimentalnyh opuholej. *Arhiv patologii*, 15(1), 22–27.

Kozhevnikova M. (2006). Infantilizm i zrelost v buddijskoj modeli filosofii obrazovaniya. V: Materialy konf. *Obrazovanie vzroslyh: problemy i perspektivy*. Institut obrazovaniya vzroslyh, RAO.

Kozlov V. A., Zhuravkin I. N., Cyrlova I. G., Petrov R. V. (1982). *Stvolovaya krovetvornaya kletka i immunnyj otvet*. Moscow: Nauka.

Kozlov V. V. (2015) Krizis lichnosti – stadii preodoleniya. *Website of V. V. Kozlov*. Retrieved 09.02.2015 from: http://zi-kozlov.ru/articles/1129-personalitycrisis.

Krasnushkin E. K. (1960). *O nekotorykh otnosheniyakh mezhdu dushevnymi i somaticheskimi boleznyami (izbrannyye trudy)*. Moscow: Medgiz, 427–445.

Krause E. D., Mendelson T., Lynch T. R. (2003). Childhood emotional invalidation and adult psychological distress: the mediating role of emotional inhibition. *Child Abuse Negl*, 27(2), 199–213.

Kravchun N. A. (2010). Insulinorezistentnost i kancerogenez. *Mezhdunarodnyj endokrinologicheskiy zhurnal*, 5(29).

Kravtsova N. A. (2009). Model patogennogo psihosomaticheskogo fenotipa. *Aktualnye problemy klinicheskoj i prikladnoj psihologii. Materialy pervoj mezhdunarodnoj nauchno-prakticheskoj konferencii.* Vladivostok, 100–105.

Kreisel T., Frank M. G., Licht T. et al. (2014). Dynamic microglial alterations underlie stress-induced depressive-like behavior and suppressed neurogenesis. *Molecular psychiatry*, 19(6), 699–709.

Kroenke C. H., Kubzansky L. D., Schernhammer E. S. et al. (2006). Social networks, social support, and survival after breast cancer diagnosis. *Journal of Clinical Oncology*, 24(7), 1105–1111.

Kryston T. B., Georgiev A. B., Pissis P., Georgakilas A. G. (2011). Role of oxidative stress and DNA damage in human carcinogenesis. *Mutation Research*, 711, 193–201.

Kuchler T., Bestmann B., Rappat S. et al. (2007). Impact of psychotherapeutic support for patients with gastrointestinal cancer undergoing surgery: 10-year survival results of a randomized trial. *Journal of Clinical Oncology*, 25(19), 2702–2708.

Kudielka B. M., Hellhammer D. H., Wust S. (2009). Why do we respond so differently? Reviewing determinants of human salivary cortisol response to a challenge. *Psychoneuroendocrinology*, 34, 2–18.

Kühn K. G. (1821-1833). *Galeni Opera omnia*, vol. V.

Kukina M. (2009). Issledovanie mehanizmov psihologicheskoj zashity u inkurabelnyh onkologicheskih bolnyh. *Sedmaya volna psihologii.* Pod red. V. V. Kozlova, N. A. Kachanovoy. Yaroslavl, Minsk.: MAPN, YarGU, 6.

Kulakov S. A. (2003). *Osnovy psihosomatiki.* Saint Petersburg: Rech.

Kulakov S. A. (2009). Bio-psiho-socio-duhovnaya i sinergeticheskaya model razvitiya psihosomaticheskih rasstrojstv: sistemnyj podhod. *Psihicheskoe Ядorovje*, 9, 66–71.

Kulakov S. A. (2009a). Biopsihosocioduhovnaya i sinergeticheskaya model razvitiya onkologicheskogo zabolevaniya: sistemnyj podhod. *Izvestiya RGPU im. A. I. Gercena*, 100, 124–131.

Kulmala J., von Bonsdorff M. B., Stenholm S. et al. (2013). Perceived stress symptoms in midlife predict disability in old age: a 28-year prospective cohort study. *J Gerontol A Biol Sci Med Sci*, 68(8), 984–991.

Kune G. A., Kune S., Watson L. F., Bahnson C. B. (1991). Personality as a risk factor in large bowel cancer: data from the Melbourne Colorectal Cancer Study. *Psychological Medicine*, 21(01), 29–41.

Kuper E. R., Korneva T. V. (2013). Socialno-psihologicheskaya determinaciya zdorovesberegayushego povedeniya zhenshin v kontekste rannego vyyavleniya raka molochnoj zhelezy. *Nauchnye issledovaniya vypusknikov fakulteta psihologii SPbGU.* Saint Petersburg: Izd-vo SPBU, 1, 133–140.

Kutsenko S. A. (2002). *Osnovy toksikologii.* Saint Petersburg: Foliant.

Kutter P. (1989). *Moderne Psychoanalyse: Eine Einführung in die Psychologie unbewusster Prozesse.* Stuttgart: Klett-Cotta.

Kuznetsov Y. *Novaya filosofiya raka. Ideoanaliz.* Retrieved 07.11.2014 from: http://ideo.ru/onco.html.

Kvetnansky R., Munco A., Palkovits M., Mikulaj L. (1975). Catecholamines in individual hypothalamic nuclei in stressed rats. In: *Catecholamines and stress.* Proc. Int. Symp. Bratislava: Pergamon, 39–40.

Kvikstad A., Vatten L. J., Tretli S. (1995). Widowhood and divorce in relation to overall survival among middle-aged Norwegian women with cancer. *Br J Cancer*, 71(6), 1343–1347.

Labonte B., Turecki G. (2011). The epigenetics of suicide: explaining the biological effect of early life environmental adversity. *Archives of Suicide Research*, 14(4), 291–310.

Labrie V., Pai S., Petronis A. (2012). Epigenetics of major psychosis: progress, problems and perspectives. *Trends in Genetics*, 28(9), 427–435.

Laconi E., Tomasi C., Curreli F. et al. (2000). Early exposure to restraint stress enhances chemical carcinogenesis in rat liver. *Cancer letters*, 161(2), 215–220.

Lahtz C., Pfeifer G. P. (2011). Epigenetic changes of DNA repair genes in cancer. *Journal of Molecular Cell Biology*, 3(1), 51–58.

Laing R. D. (1999). Transcendental Experience In Relation to Religion and Psychosis. In: S. Grof, C. Grof (eds). *Spiritual Emergency: When Personal Transformation Becomes a Crisis*. New York: Tarcher/Putnam US, 63–77.

Lake F. (1980). *Constricted Confusion: Exploration of a Pre- and Perinatal Paradigm*. London: Bridge Pastoral Foundation.

Lake J., Helgason C., Sarris J. (2012). Integrative Mental Health (IMH): paradigm, research, and clinical practice. *Explore: The Journal of Science and Healing*, 8(1), 50–57.

Lama Zopa Rinpoche (2001). *Ultimate Healing: The Power of Compassion*. Somerville, MA: Wisdom Publications.

Lambert L. (2014). Having Cancer Was The Best Thing That Happened to Me. Retrieved 03.04.2014 from: http://thoughtcatalog.com/leslie-lambert/.

Lamkin D. M., Sloan E. K., Patel A. J. et al. (2012). Chronic stress enhances progression of acute lymphoblastic leukemia via β-adrenergic signaling. *Brain Behav Immun*, 26(4), 635–641.

Landmark B. T., Strandmark M., Wahl A. K. (2001). Living with newly diagnosed breast cancer—the meaning of existential issues: a qualitative study of 10 women with newly diagnosed breast cancer, based on grounded theory. *Cancer nursing*, 24(3), 220–226.

Lang K., Drell T. L., Lindecke A. et al. (2004). Induction of a metastatogenic tumor cell type by neurotransmitters and its pharmacological inhibition by established drugs. *International Journal of Cancer*, 112(2), 231–238.

Langner C. A., Epel E. S., Matthews K. A. et al. (2012). Social hierarchy and depression: the role of emotion suppression. *J Psychol*, 146(4), 417–436.

Lansky S. B., Cairns N. U., Hassanein R. et al. (1978). Childhood cancer: Parental discord and divorce. *Pediatrics*, 62(2), 184–188.

Lapochkina N. P. (2007). Psihologicheskie osobennosti zhenshin s zabolevaniyami molochnoj zhelezy. *Vestnik Novyh Medicinskih Tehnologiy*, 14(2).

Laudenslager M. L. (1988). The psychobiology of loss: Lessons from humans and nonhuman primates. *Journal of Social Issues*, 44, 19–36.

Laudenslager M. L., Ryan S. M., Drugan R. C., et al. (1983). Coping and immunosuppression: inescapable but not escapable shock suppresses lymphocyte proliferation. *Science*, 221(4610), 568–570.

Laughlin T. (1999). *The psychology of cancer*. Los Angeles, CA: Panarion Press.

Lavin N. (1999). *Endocrinology*. Moscow: Praktika.

Lawler-Row K. A, Elliott J. (2009). The role of religious activity and spirituality in the health and well-being of older adults. *J Health Psychol*, 14, 43–52.

Lawler-Row K. A., Karremans J. C., Scott C. et al. (2008). Forgiveness, physiological reactivity and health: The role of anger. *International Journal of Psychophysiology*, 68, 51–58.

Lazarus R. S. (1966). *Psychological Stress and the Coping Process*. New York: McGraw-Hill Book.

Le C. P., Nowell C. J., Kim-Fuchs C. et al. (2016). Chronic stress in mice remodels lymph vasculature to promote tumour cell dissemination. *Nature Communications*, 7, 10634.

Lebanon N. (2015). Reconceptualizing Stress in Cancer Treatment. *News Releases of Norris Cotton Cancer Center*. Retrieved 13.05.2015 from: http://cancer.dartmouth.edu.

Ledesma D., Kumano H. (2009). Mindfulness-based stress reduction and cancer: a meta-analysis. *Psycho-Oncology*, 18(6), 571–579.

Lee M. S., Hwa J. H., Sung-Soo H. et al. (2001). Psychoneuroimmunological effects of Qi-therapy: Preliminary study on the changes of level of anxiety, mood, cortisol, and melatonin and cellular function of neutrophil and NK cells. *Stress and Health*, 17, 17–24.

Lee V., Cohen S., Edgar L. et al. (2006). Meaning-making intervention during breast or colorectal cancer treatment improves self-esteem, optimism, and self-efficacy. *Soc Sci Med*, 62(12), 3133–3145.

Lehrer S. (1980). Life change and gastric cancer. *Psychosomatic Medicine*, 42(5), 499–502.

Lehrer S. (1981). Life change and lung cancer. *Journal of Human Stress*, 7(4), 7–11.

Lehto U. S., Ojanen M., Väkevä A. et al. (2008). Noncancer life stresses in newly diagnosed cancer. *Support Care Cancer*, 16(11),1231–1241.

Lemaire V., Lamarque S., Le Moal M. et al. (2006). Postnatal stimulation of the pups counteracts prenatal stress-induced deficits in hippocampal neurogenesis. *Biol Psychiatry*, 59(9), 786–792.

Lemeshow S., Sorensen H. T., Phillips G. et al. (2011). β-Blockers and survival among Danish patients with malignant melanoma: a population-based cohort study. *Cancer Epidemiology and Prevention Biomarkers*, 20(10), 2273-2279.

Lemon J., Edelman S., Kidman A. D. (2004). Perceptions of the "Mind-Cancer" relationship by members of the public, cancer patients and oncologists. *J Psychosoc Oncol*, 21, 43–58.

Lengacher C. A., Reich R. R., Kip K. E. et al. (2014). Influence of mindfulness-based stress reduction (MBSR) on telomerase activity in women with breast cancer (BC). *Biological Research for Nursing*, 16(4), 438–447.

Lerner M. (1996). *Choices In Healing. Integrating The Best Of Conventional And Complementary Approaches To Cancer*. Cambridge: MIT Press.

LeShan L. (1977). *You Can Fight For Your Life: Emotional Factors in the Treatment of Cancer*. New York: M. Evans & Company.

LeShan L. (1989). *Cancer As a Turning Point: A Handbook for People with Cancer, Their Families, and Health Professionals*. New York: Plume.

LeShan L., Reznikoff M. (1960). A psychological factor apparently associated with neoplastic disease. *Journal of Abnormal and Social Psychology*, 60, 1, 439–440.

Lessard J. C., Moretti M. M. (1998). Suicidal ideation in an adolescent clinical sample: attachment patterns and clinical implications. *Journal of Adolescence*, 21, 383–395.

Leuckin L. (1998). Childhood attachment and loss experiences affect adult cardiovascular and cortisol function. *Psychosom Med*, 60, 765–772.

Leuckin L. (2000). Parental caring and loss during childhood and adult cortisol responses to stress. *Psychol Health*, 15, 841–851.

Levav I., Kohn R., Iscovich J. et al. (2000). Cancer incidence and survival following bereavement. *Am J Public Health*, 90(10), 1601–1607.

Levav I., Lipshitz I., Novikov I. et al. (2007). Cancer risk among parents and siblings of patients with schizophrenia. *The British Journal of Psychiatry*, 190(2), 156–161.

Levenson F. B. (1985). *The Causes and Prevention of Cancer*. Briarcliff Manor: Stein & Day.

Levenson F. B., Levenson M. D., Ventegodt S., Merrick J. (2009). Qualitative analysis of a case report series of 75 cancer patients treated with psychodynamic psychotherapy combined with therapeutic touch (clinical holistic medicine). *International Journal on Disability and Human Development*, 8(3), 287–310.

Levi-Belz Y., Gvion Y., Horesh N., Apter A. (2013). Attachment Patterns in Medically Serious Suicide Attempts: The Mediating Role of Self-Disclosure and Loneliness. *Suicide and Life-Threatening Behavior*, 43(5), 511–522.

Levine P. A., Frederick A. (1997). *Waking the Tiger: Healing Trauma*. Berkeley, CA: North Atlantic Books.

Levine S. (1989). *Who Dies?: An Investigation of Conscious Living and Conscious Dying*. New York: Anchor. Reissue edn.

Levitan A. A. (1991). The use of hypnosis with cancer patients. *Psychiatric Medicine*, 10(1), 119–131.

Levy S. M., Wise B. D. (1987). Psychosocial risk factors, natural immunity, and cancer progression: Implications for intervention. *Current Psychology*, 6(3), 229–243.

Levy S. M., Herberman R., Lippman M., d'Angelo T. (1987). Correlation of stress factors with sustained depression of natural killer cell activity and predicted prognosis in patients with breast cancer. *Journal of Clinical Oncology*, 5(3), 348–353.

Levy S. M., Lee J., Bagley C., Lippman M. (1988). Survival hazards analysis in first recurrent breast cancer patients: seven years follow up. *Psychosom Med*, 50, 520–528.

Levy S. M., Herberman R. B., Lippman M. et al. (1991). Immunological and psychosocial predictors of disease recurrence in patients with early-stage breast cancer. *Behav Med*, 17, 67–75.

Levy S. M., Herberman R. B., Maluish A. M. et al. (1985). Prognostic risk assessment in primary breast cancer by behavioral and immunological parameters. *Health Psychology*, 4(2), 99–113.

Levy S. M., Herberman R. B., Whiteside T. et al. (1990). Perceived social support and tumor estrogen/progesterone receptor status as predictors of natural killer call activity in breast cancer patients. *Psychosomat Med*, 52, 73–85.

Lewis N. D. C. (1936). *Research in dementia praecox*. Oxford: National Committee for Mental Hygiene.

Li G. Y., Yao K. T., Glaser R. (1989). Sister chromatid exchange and nasopharyngeal carcinoma. *Int J Cancer*, 43, 613–618.

Li J., Johansen C., Olsen J. (2003). Cancer survival in parents who lost a child: a nationwide study in Denmark. *British Journal of Cancer*, 88(11), 1698–1701.

Li J., Vestergaard M., Cnattingius S. et al. (2014). Mortality after parental death in childhood: a nationwide cohort study from three Nordic countries. *PLoS Med*, 11(7), e1001679.

Li J., Vestergaard M., Obel C. et al. (2012). Antenatal maternal bereavement and childhood cancer in the offspring: a population-based cohort study in 6 million children. *British Journal of Cancer*, 107(3), 544–548.

Li L., Li X., Zhou W., Messina J. (2013). Acute psychological stress results in the rapid development of insulin resistance. *J Endocrinol*, 217(2), 175–184.

Li P., Huang J., Wu H. et al. (2016). Impact of lifestyle and psychological stress on the development of early onset breast cancer. *Medicine*, 95, e5529.

Li S., Sun Y., Gao D. (2013). Role of the nervous system in cancer metastasis. *Oncology Letters*, 5(4), 1101–1111.

Liguori I., Russo G., Curcio F., et al. (2018). Oxidative stress, aging, and diseases. *Clinical interventions in aging*, 13, 757–772.

Lillberg K., Verkasalo P. K., Kaprio J. et al. (2002). A prospective study of life satisfaction, neuroticism and breast cancer risk (Finland). *Cancer Causes & Control*, 13(2), 191–198.

Lillberg K., Verkasalo P. K., Kaprio J. et al. (2003). Stressful life events and risk of breast cancer in 10,808 women: a cohort study. *Am J Epidemiol*, 157(5), 415–423.

Limandri B. J., Boyle D. W. (1978). Instilling hope. *The American Journal of Nursing*, 78(1), 79–80.

Lin H. R., Bauer-Wu S. M. (2003). Psycho-spiritual well-being in patients with advanced cancer: an integrative review of the literature. *J Adv Nurs*, 44(1), 69–80.

Lin J., Blalock J. A., Chen M. et al. (2015). Depressive symptoms and short telomere length are associated with increased mortality in bladder cancer patients. *Cancer Epidemiology Biomarkers & Prevention*, 24(2), 336–343.

Lin Y., Wang C., Zhong Y. et al. (2013). Striking life events associated with primary breast cancer susceptibility in women: a meta-analysis study. *J Exp Clin Cancer Res*, 32(1), 53.

Linde N. D. (2000). Psihologicheskaya teoriya shizofrenii. *Zhurnal Prakticheskogo Psihologa*, (3-4), 24–35.

Linde N. D. (2006). *Emocionalno-obraznaya terapiya. Teoriya i praktika*. Moscow: Izd-vo MosGU.

Lindgren M. E., Fagundes C. P., Alfano C. M. et al. (2013). Beta-blockers may reduce intrusive thoughts in newly diagnosed cancer patients. *Psycho-Oncology*, 22(8), 1889–1894.

Lindheim S. R., Legro R. S., Bernstein L. et al. (1992). Behavioral stress responses in premenopausal and postmenopausal women and the effects of estrogen. *American Journal of Obstetrics and Gynecology*, 167(6), 1831–1836.

Lipowski Z. J. (1968). Review of consultation psychiatry and psychosomatic medicine. *Psychosom Med*, 30, 395–422.

Lipton B. (2016). *The Biology of Belief: Unleashing the Power of Consciousness, Matter & Miracles*. Carlsbad: Hay House.

Lissoni P., Messina G., Parolini D. et al. (2008). A spiritual approach in the treatment of cancer: relation between faith score and response to chemotherapy in advanced non-small cell lung cancer patients. *In Vivo*, 22(5), 577–581.

Litvak M. E. (2004). *Komandovat ili podchinyatsya?* Rostov-na-Donu: Feniks.

Liu S. Y., Wrosch C., Miller G. E., Pruessner J. C. (2014). Self-esteem change and diurnal cortisol secretion in older adulthood. *Psychoneuroendocrinology*, 41, 111–120.

Liu X., Wu W. K., Yu L. et al. (2008). Epinephrine stimulates esophageal squamous-cell carcinoma cell proliferation via β-adrenoceptor-dependent transactivation of extracellular signal-regulated kinase/cyclooxygenase-2 pathway. *Journal of Cellular Biochemistry*, 105(1), 53–60.

Lloyd-Williams M., Friedman T. (2001). Depression in palliative care patients–a prospective study. *European Journal of Cancer Care*, 10(4), 270–274.

Locke S., Hornig-Rohan M. (1983). *Mind and Immunity: Behavioral Immunology*. New York: Praeger.

Loffler-Stastka H., Szerencsics M., Bluml V. (2009). Dissociation, trauma, affect regulation and personality in patients with a borderline personality organization. *Bulletin of the Menninger Clinic*, 73, 2, 81–98.

Loi M., Del Savio L., Stupka E. (2013). Social epigenetics and equality of opportunity. *Public Health Ethics*, 6(2), 142–153.

Lopez A. D., Mathers C. D. (2006). Measuring the global burden of disease and epidemiological transitions: 2002-2030. *Ann Trop Med Parasitol*, 100, 481–499.

López Ibor J. J. (1972). Masked Depressions. *Br J Psychiatry*, 120(556), 245–258.

López M., Aguirre J. M., Cuevas N. et al. (2003). Gene promoter hypermethylation in oral rinses of leukoplakia patients-a diagnostic and/or prognostic tool? *Eur J Cancer*, 39, 2306–2309.

Losiak W. (1989). [Defense reactions and coping with stress in patients with cancer]. *Przegl Lek*, 46(3), 334–337 (in Polish).

Lourie J. B. (1996). Cumulative Trauma: The Nonproblem Problem. *Transactional Analysis Journal*, 26, 4, 276–283.

Lowden B. (1998). The health consequences of disclosing bad news. *European Journal of Oncology Nursing*, 2(4), 225–230.

Lowe G., Greenman J., Lowe G. (1999). Pleasure, guilt and secretory immunoglobulin A. *Psychological reports*, 85(1), 339–340.

Lowen A. (2006). *Love, Sex, & Your Heart*. Alachua, FL: Bioenergetics Press.

Lu H., Ouyang W., Huang C. (2006). Inflammation, a key event in cancer development. *Mol Cancer Res*, 4, 221–233.

Luban-Plozza B., Pöldinger W., Kröger F. (2013). *Der psychosomatisch Kranke in der Praxis*. Berlin: Springer.

Lucassen P. J., Naninck E. F., van Goudoever J. B. et al. (2013). Perinatal programming of adult hippocampal structure and function; emerging roles of stress, nutrition and epigenetics. *Trends in Neurosciences*, 36(11), 621–631.

Lung F. W., Chen N. C., Shu B. C. (2007). Genetic pathway of major depressive disorder in shortening telomeric length. *Psychiatr Genet*, 17, 195–199.

Lutgendorf S. K., DeGeest K., Bender D. et al. (2012). Social influences on clinical outcomes of patients with ovarian cancer. *Journal of Clinical Oncology*, 30(23), 2885–2890.

Lutgendorf S. K., Degeest K., Dahmoush L. et al. (2011). Social isolation is associated with elevated tumor norepinephrine in ovarian carcinoma patients. *Brain Behav Immun*, 25, 250–255.

Lutgendorf S. K., DeGeest K., Sung C. Y. et al. (2009). Depression, social support, and beta-adrenergic transcription control in human ovarian cancer. *Brain Behav Immun*, 23(2), 176–183.

Lutgendorf S. K., Johnsen E. L., Cooper B. et al. (2002). Vascular endothelial growth factor and social support in patients with ovarian carcinoma. *Cancer*, 95(4), 808–815.

Lutgendorf S. K., Lamkin D. M., DeGeest K. et al. (2008). Depressed and anxious mood and T-cell cytokine expressing populations in ovarian cancer patients. *Brain Behav Immun*, 22(6), 890–900.

Lutgendorf S. K., Lamkin D. M., Jennings N. B. et al. (2008a). Biobehavioral influences on matrix metalloproteinase expression in ovarian carcinoma. *Clin Cancer Res*, 1, 14(21), 6839–6846.

Lutgendorf S. K., Sood A. K., Anderson B. et al. (2005). Social support, psychological distress, and natural killer cell activity in ovarian cancer. *J Clin Oncol*, 23(28), 7105–7113.

Lutz A., Greischar L. L., Rawlings N. B. et al. (2004). Long-term meditators self-induce high-amplitude gamma synchrony during mental practice. *Proc Natl Acad Sci USA*, 101(46), 16369–16373.

Lynch C. D., Sundaram R., Maisog J. M. et al. (2014). Preconception stress increases the risk of infertility: results from a couple-based prospective cohort study—the LIFE study. *Hum Reprod*, 29(5), 1067–1075.

Lyutova M. (2012). Understanding the process of forgiving the self. In: *Aktual'nyye problemy prikladnoy sotsial'noy psikhologii*. Proc. Int. Conf. Saint Petersburg: IUUE, 249–250.

Mabry P. L., Olster D. H., Morgan G. D., Abrams D. B. (2008). Interdisciplinarity and systems science to improve population health: A view from the NIH Office of Behavioral and Social Sciences Research. *American Journal of Preventive Medicine*, 35(2), Suppl., S211–S224.

MacKinnon D. P., Lockwood C. M., Hoffman J. M. et al. (2002). A comparison of methods to test mediation and other intervening variable effects. *Psychological Methods*, 7, 83–104.

MacNiven E., Younglai E. V. (1992). Chronic stress increases estrogen and other steroids in inseminated rats. *Physiology & Behavior*, 52(1), 159–162.

Maddi S. (1967). The Existential Neurosis. *Journal of Abnormal Psychology*, 72, 311–325.

Madeira S., Melo M., Porto J. et al. (2007). The diseases we cause: Iatrogenic illness in a department of internal medicine. *European Journal of Internal Medicine*, 18(5), 391–399.

Maggini C., Raballo A. (2004). Alexithymia and schizophrenic psychopathology. *Acta Biol Med*, 75, 40–49.

Maier K. J., Waldstein S. R., Synowski S. J. (2003). Relation of cognitive appraisal to cardiovascular reactivity, affect, and task engagement. *Ann Behav Med*, 26(1), 32–41.

Maier S. F., Seligman M. E. (1976). Learned helplessness: Theory and evidence. *Journal of Experimental Psychology: General*, 105(1), 3–46.

Main M. (1995). Recent studies in attachment. In: Goldberg S., Muir R., Kerr J. (eds), *Attachment theory: Social, developmental, and clinical perspectives*. Hillsdale, NJ: Analytic Press, 407–474.

Main M., Hesse E. (1992). Disorganized/disoriented infant behavior in the Strange Situation, lapses in the monitoring of reasoning and discourse during the parent's Adult Attachment Interview, and dissociative states. In: M. Ammaniti, D. Stern (eds), *Attaccamento e psicoanalisi*. Rome: Laterza, 86–140.

Mainous A. G. 3rd, Everett C. J., Diaz V. A. et al. (2011). Leukocyte telomere length and marital status among middle-aged adults. *Age and Ageing*, 40(1),73–78.

Mako C., Galek K., Poppito S. R. (2006). Spiritual pain among patients with advanced cancer in palliative care. *Journal of Palliative Medicine*, 9(5), 1106–1113.

Malarkey W. B., Kiecolt-Glaser J. K., Pearl D., Glaser R. (1994). Hostile behavior during marital conflict affects pituitary and adrenal hormones. *Psychosomatic Medicine*, 56, 41–51.

Malatesta C. Z., Jonas R., Izard C. E. (1987). The relation between low facial expressivity during emotional arousal and somatic symptoms. *British Journal of Medical Psychology*, 60(2), 169–180.

Malberg J. E., Duman R. S. (2003). Cell proliferation in adult hippocampus is decreased by inescapable stress: reversal by fluoxetine treatment. *Neuropsychopharmacology*, 28, 1562–1571.

Malgina G. B. (2003). Patogenez, profilaktika i korrekciya perinatalnyh oslozhneniy pri psihoemocionalnom stresse v period beremennosti. *Avtoref Diss dokt med Nauk*. Saint Petersburg: VMA.

Malik S. T., Naylor M. S., East N. et al. (1990). Cells secreting tumour necrosis factor show enhanced metastasis in nude mice. *Eur J Cancer*, 26(10), 1031–1034.

Malkina-Pykh I. (2005). *Psihologicheskaya pomosh v krizisnyh situaciyah*. Moscow: Eksmo.

Malkina-Pykh I. (2013). *Psihosomatika*. Moscow: Eksmo.

Mallette F. A., Calabrese V, Ilangumaran S., Ferbeyre G. (2010). SOCS1, a novel interaction partner of p53 controlling oncogene–induced senescence. *Aging*, 2(7), 445–452.

Maltby J., Macaskill A., Day L. (2001). Failure to forgive self and others: A replication and extension of the relationship between forgiveness, personality, social desirability, and general health. *Personality and Individual Differences*, 30, 881–885.

Mamardashvili M. K. (1990). *Kak ya ponimayu filosofiyu*. Moscow: Progress.

Mandal J. M., Ghosh R., Nair L. (1992). Early childhood experiences & life events of male cancer patients, psychosomatic patients & normal persons: A comparative study. *Social Science International*, 8, 44–49.

Mann J. J. (1998). The neurobiology of suicide. *Nature Medicine*, 4(1), 25–30.

Mantovani F. M., Mendes F. R. P. (2010). The quality of life of elderly's chronic disease sufferers: qualitative-quantitative research. *Online Brazilian Journal of Nursing*, 9(1).

Manzaneque J. M., Vera F. M., Ramos N. S. et al. (2011). Psychobiological modulation in anxious and depressed patients after a mindfulness meditation programme: A pilot study. *Stress and Health: Journal of the International Society for the Investigation of Stress*, 27(3), 216–222.

Marsden W. N. (2011). Stressor-induced NMDAR dysfunction as a unifying hypothesis for the aetiology, pathogenesis and co-morbidity of clinical depression. *Med Hypotheses*, 77(4), 508–528.

Marie J. C., Forgeard M. J., Haigh E. A. et al. (2011). Beyond Depression: Towards a Process-Based Approach to Research, Diagnosis, and Treatment. *Clin Psychol (New York)*, 18(4), 275–299.

Marilova T. Y. (2002). Psihologicheskie osobennosti onkologicheskih bolnyh. *Vestnik RONC im. N. N. Blohina RAMN*, 13(3), 47–51.

Marilova T. Y., Shestopalova I. M. (2008). Trevoga i depressiya kak suicidalnyj risk pri rake. *Vestnik RONC im. N. N. Blohina RAMN*, 19(4), 53–54.

Marincheva L. P., Zlokazova M. V., Soloviev A. G. (2012). Osobennosti etiopatogeneza psihosomaticheskih i somatoformnyh rasstrojstv. *Kazanskiy Medicinskiy Zhurnal*, 93(3), 465–468.

Markham J. A., Koenig J. I. (2011). Prenatal stress: role in psychotic and depressive diseases. *Psychopharmacology (Berl.)*, 214(1), 89–106.

Markolin C. (2007). German New Medicine® (GNM). The New Medical Paradigm. *EXPLORE!*, 16, 2.

Martova T. Y., Malygin E. N. (2002). Psihologicheskie osobennosti onkologicheskih bolnyh. *Vestn. RONC im. N. N. Blohina RAMN*, 3, 47–51.

Marty P., de M'uzan M. (1963). La "pensee operatoire." *Rev Franc Psychanal*, 27, Suppl., 345–356.

Mascaro N., Rosen D. H. (2005). Existential Meaning's Role in the Enhancement of Hope and Prevention of Depressive Symptoms. *Journal of Personality*, 73, (4), 985–1014.

Mascaro N., Rosen D. H. (2006). The role of existential meaning as a buffer against stress. *Journal of Humanistic Psychology*, 46(2), 168–190.

Maslow A. H. (1954). *Motivation and Personality*. New York: Harper.

Maslow A. H. (1959). Critique of Self-Actualisation. *Journal of Individual Psychology*, 15, 24–32.

Maslow A. H. (1967). Self-actualizing and Beyond. In: J. F. T. Bugental, *Challenges of Humanistic Psychology*. New York: McGraw-Hill, 118–132.

Maslow A. H. (1999). *Toward a Psychology of Being*. New York: Wiley.

Maslow A. H., Maslow B. G. (1993). *The Farther Reaches of Human Nature*. London: Penguin/Arkana.

Massie M. J. (2004). Prevalence of depression in patients with cancer. *J Natl Cancer Inst Monogr*, 32, 57–71.

Mastrovito R. C., Deguire K. S., Clarkin J. et al. (1979). Personality-characteristics of women with gynecological cancer. *Cancer Detection and Prevention*, 2(2), 281–287.

Maté G. (2003). *When the body says no. Understanding the stress-disease connection*. Hoboken, NJ: John Wiley & Sons.

Mathews H. L., Konley T., Kosik K. L. et al. (2011). Epigenetic patterns associated with the immune dysregulation that accompanies psychosocial distress. *Brain, Behavior, and Immunity*, 25(5), 830–839.

Matrenitsky V. L. (1989). Molekulyarnye mehanizmy vozrastnoj kompaktizacii hromatina. *Uspehi Sovrem. Biol*, 108, 3(6), 358–374.

Matrenitsky V. L. (1992). *Vozrastnye osobennosti desensitizacii serdca k adrenalinu*. Avtoref. diss. kand. med. nauk. Kiev: Institute of Gerontology.

Matsumoto K., Yobimoto K., Huong N. T. et al. (1999). Psychological stress-induced enhancement of brain lipid peroxidation via nitric oxide systems and its modulation by anxiolytic and anxiogenic drugs in mice. *Brain Res*, 839, 74–84.

Matthews S. G., Phillips D. I. (2010). Minireview: transgenerational inheritance of the stress response: a new frontier in stress research. *Endocrinology*, 151(1), 7–13.

Maunder R. G., Hunter J. J. (2001). Attachment and psychosomatic medicine: developmental contributions to stress and disease. *Psychosom Med*, 63(4), 556–67.

Mauss I. B., Tamir M., Anderson C. L., Savino N. S. (2011). Can seeking happiness make people unhappy? Paradoxical effects of valuing happiness. *Emotion*, 11(4), 807.

Mayer A. E., Weitemeyer W. U. (1967). Zur Frage krankheitsdependenter Neurotisierung. *Arch Psychiat Nervenkr*, 209, 21.

Mayes L. C., Swain J. E., Leckman J. F. (2005). Parental attachment systems: neural circuits, genes, and experiential contributions to parental engagement. *Clin Neurosci Res*, 4(5-6), 301–313.

McClelland D. C., Floor E., Davidson R. J., Saron C. (1980). Stressed power motivation, sympathetic activation, immune function, and illness. *Journal of Human Stress*, 6(2), 11–19.

McCraty R., Atkinson M., Tomasino D. (2003). *Modulation of DNA conformation by heart-focused intention*. HeartMath Research Center, Institute of HeartMath, Publication No. 03-008. Boulder Creek, CA, 2.

McCullough M. E., Orsulak P., Brandon A., Akers L. (2007). Rumination, fear, and cortisol: an in vivo study of interpersonal transgressions. *Health Psychol*, 26, 126–132.

McEwen B. S. (2000). Allostasis and allostatic load: implications for neuropsychopharmacology. *Neuropsychopharmacology*, 22(2), 108–124.

McEwen B. S. (2007). Physiology and neurobiology of stress and adaptation: central role of the brain. *Physiol Rev*, 87, 873–904.

McEwen B. S. (2012). The ever-changing brain: cellular and molecular mechanisms for the effects of stressful experiences. *Dev Neurobiol*, 72(6), 878–890.

McEwen B. S., Gianaros P. J. (2010). Central role of the brain in stress and adaptation: Links to socioeconomic status, health, and disease. *Ann N Y Acad Sci*, 1186, 190–222.

McGarvey E. L., Canterbury R. J., Koopman C. et al. (1998). Acute stress disorder following diagnosis of cancer. *International Journal of Rehabilitation and Health*, 4(1), 1–15.

McGinty E. E., Zhang Y., Guallar E. et al. (2012). Cancer incidence in a sample of Maryland residents with serious mental illness. *Psychiatric Services*, 63(7), 714–717.

McGowan P. O., Sasaki A., D'Alessio A. C. et al. (2009). Epigenetic regulation of the glucocorticoid receptor in human brain associates with childhood abuse. *Nat Neurosci*, 12(3), 342–348.

McGregor B. A., Antoni M. H., Boyers A. et al. (2004). Cognitive-behavioral stress management increased benefit finding and immune function among women with early-stage breast cancer. *J Psychosom Res*, 56(1), 1–8.

McIntosh L. J., Sapolsky R. M. (1996). Glucocorticoids may enhance oxygen radical-mediated neurotoxicity. *Neurotoxicology*, 17(3-4), 873–882.

McKenna M. C., Zevon M., Corn B., Rounds J. (1999). Psychosocial factors and the development of breast cancer: A meta-analysis. *Health Psychology*, 18, 520–531.

McWilliams L. A., Bailey S. J. (2010). Associations between adult attachment ratings and health conditions: Evidence from the National Comorbidity Survey Replication. *Health Psychology*, 9(4), 446–453.

Meares A. (1978). Regression of osteogenic sarcoma metastases associated with intensive meditation. *Medical Journal of Australia*, 2, 433.

Meares A. (1980). What can the cancer patient expect from intensive meditation? *Australian Family Physician*, 9(5), 322–325.

Meares A. (1980a). Remission of massive metastasis from undifferentiated carcinoma of the lung associated with intensive meditation. *J Am SOC Psychosom Dent Med*, 27, 40–41.

Medawar P., Medawar J. (1983). *Aristotle to zoos*. Cambridge, MA: Harvard University Press.

Meehl P. E. (1962). Schizotaxia, schizotypy, schizophrenia. *American Psychologist*, 17, 827–838.

Meeker A. K., Hicks J. L., Iacobuzio-Donahue C. A. et al. (2004). Telomere length abnormalities occur early in the initiation of epithelial carcinogenesis. *Clinical Cancer Research*, 10(10), 3317–3326.

Mehta D., Klengel T., Conneely K. N. et al. (2013). Childhood maltreatment is associated with distinct genomic and epigenetic profiles in posttraumatic stress disorder. *Proc Natl Acad Sci*, 110(20), 8302–7.

Meinardi M. T., Gietema J. A., Van Der Graaf W. T. A. et al. (2000). Cardiovascular morbidity in long-term survivors of metastatic testicular cancer. *Journal of Clinical Oncology*, 18(8), 1725–1732.

Melchenko N. I., Dejneka N. V. (2011). Psihosocialnye problemy onkologii kishechnika. *Materialy 11 Mezhdunarodnoj nauchno-prakticheskoj konferencii "Psihologiya i medicina: puti poiska optimalnogo vzaimodejstviya."* Ryazan, 19–29 aprelya, 232.

Melhem-Bertrandt A., Chavez-MacGregor M., Lei X. et al. (2011). Beta-blocker use is associated with improved relapse-free survival in patients with triple-negative breast cancer. *Journal of Clinical Oncology*, 29(19), 2645–2652.

Melikhova E. F. (1956). Vliyanie hronicheskoj funkcionalnoj nervnoj travmy na hod novoobrazovatelnogo processa v kozhe pri eksperimentalnom rake u belyh myshej. *Materialy po evolyucionnoj fiziologii*, 1, 201–212.

Mello A. A. F., Mello M. F. D., Carpenter L. L., Price L. H. (2003). Update on stress and depression: the role of the hypothalamic-pituitary-adrenal (HPA) axis. *Brazilian Journal of Psychiatry*, 25(4), 231–238.

Mendelevich V. D. (2001). *Klinicheskaya i medicinskaya psihologiya: prakticheskoe rukovodstvo*. Moscow: MEDpress-inform.

Mendelevich V. D. (2003). *Narkozavisimost i komorbidnye rasstrojstva povedeniya (psihologicheskie i psihopatologicheskie aspekty)*. Moscow: MEDpress-inform.

Mendelevich V. D., Solovieva S. L. (2002). *Nevrozologiya i psihosomaticheskaya medicina*. Moscow: MEDpress-inform.

Meneghetti A. (1977). *La Psychosomatica*. Rome: Psicologia Editrice.

Meneghetti A. (2010). The psychosomatics of cancer. *Journal of Chinese Clinical Medicine*, 5(7), 271–387.

Meneghetti A. (2011). Forms of "I" behaviour in situations of pathology. *Values and Meanings*, 2(11), 24–39.

Menninger K. (1956). *Man Against Himself*. Wilmington, DE: Mariner Books.

Meraviglia M. (2006). Effects of spirituality in breast cancer survivors. *Oncol Nurs Forum*, 33(1), E1–E7.

Metalsky G. I., Joiner T. E. (1992). Vulnerability to depressive symptomatology: A prospective test of the diathesis-stress and causal mediation components of the hopelessness theory of depression. *Journal of Personality and Social Psychology*, 63, 667–675.

Metcalfe C., Smith G. D., Macleod J., Hart C. (2007). The role of self-reported stress in the development of breast cancer and prostate cancer: a prospective cohort study of employed males and females with 30 years of follow-up. *Eur J Cancer*, 43(6), 1060–1065.

Meyer A. E., Weitemeyer W. (1967). On the problem of disease dependency of (imagined) aggressive behavior. Picture frustration test results in male patients with bronchial asthma, lung tuberculosis or heart defects of different duration of history. *Psyche*, 21(4), 266–282.

Meyer T. J., Mark M. M. (1995). Effects of psychosocial interventions with adult cancer patients: a meta-analysis of randomized experiments. *Health psychology*, 14(2), 101–108.

Mickelson K. D., Kessler R. C., Shaver P. R. (1997). Adult attachment in a nationally representative sample. *J Pers Soc Psychology*, 73, 1092–1106.

Mickley J., Carson V., Soeken L. (1995). Religion and adult mental health: State of the science in nursing. *Issues in Mental Health Nursing*, 16, 345–360.

Mifsud K. R., Gutièrrez-Mecinas M., Trollope A. F. et al. (2011). Epigenetic mechanisms in stress and adaptation. *Brain, Behavior, and Immunity*, 25(7), 1305–1315.

Mihajlov V. V. (2001). *Osnovy patologicheskoj fiziologii*. Moscow: Medicina.

Mikulincer M., Orbach I. (1995). Attachment styles and repressive defensiveness: the accessibility and architecture of affective memories. *Journal of Personality and Social Psychology*, 68(5), 917–925.

Mikulincer M., Florian V., Weller A. (1993). Attachment styles, coping strategies, and posttraumatic psychological distress: The impact of the Gulf War in Israel. *Journal of Personality and Social Psychology*, 64, 817–826.

Milam J. E. (2004). Posttraumatic growth among HIV/AIDS patients. *Journal of Applied Social Psychology*, 34, 2353–2376

Miller A. H., Maletic V., Raison C. L. (2009). Inflammation and its discontents: the role of cytokines in the pathophysiology of major depression. *Biol Psychiatry*, 65(9), 732–741.

Miller C. A., Sweatt J. D. (2007). Covalent modification of DNA regulates memory formation. *Neuron*, 53(6), 857–869.

Miller G. E., Chen E., Parker K. J. (2011). Psychological stress in childhood and susceptibility to the chronic diseases of aging: moving toward a model of behavioral and biological mechanisms. *Psychological Bulletin*, 137(6), 959–997.

Miller G. E., Cohen S., Ritchey A. K. (2002). Chronic psychological stress and the regulation of pro-inflammatory cytokines: a glucocorticoid-resistance model. *Health Psychol*, 21(6), 531–541.

Miller G. E., Chen E., Sze J. et al. (2008). A functional genomic fingerprint of chronic stress in humans: blunted glucocorticoid and increased NF-$\varkappa$B signaling. *Biological psychiatry*, 64(4), 266–272.

Miller G. E., Dopp J. M., Myers H. F. et al. (1999). Psychosocial predictors of natural killer cell mobilization during marital conflict. *Health Psychol*, 18, 262–227

Miller T. Q., Smith T. W., Turner C. W. et al. (1996). Meta-analytic review of research on hostility and physical health. *Psychological Bulletin*, 119, 322–348.

Miller T. R. (1977). Psychophysiologic aspects of cancer: the James Ewing lecture. *Cancer*, 39, 413–418.

Mills M. E., Sullivan K. (1999). The importance of information giving for patients newly diagnosed with cancer: a review of the literature. *Journal of Clinical Nursing*, 8(6), 631–642.

Milrud F. S. (1930). O roli psihicheskoj travmy v razvitii zlokachestvennyh novoobrazovanij. *Vest Hir i Pogr Oblastej*, 21, 61, 80–82.

Misyak S. A. (2002). Duhovnist yak skladova chastina reabilitaciyi onkologichnih hvorih. *Visnik Zaporizkogo Derzhavnogo Universitetu*, 1, 68–75.

Mitchell C., Hobcraft J., McLanahan S. S. et al. (2014). Social disadvantage, genetic sensitivity, and children's telomere length. *Proc Natl Acad Sci USA*, 111(16), 5944–5949.

Mitscherlich A. (1954). Zur psychoanalytischen Auffassung psychosomatischer Krankheitsentstehung. *Psyche*, 7(10), 561–578.

Mittal R., Pater A., Pater M. M. (1993). Multiple human papillomavirus type 16 glucocorticoid response elements functional for transformation, transient expression, and DNA-protein interactions. *J Virol*, 67(9), 5656–5659.

Mittleman M. A., Maclure M., Sherwood J. B. et al. (1995). Triggering of myocardial infarction onset by episodes of anger. *Circulation*, 92, 1720–1725.

Mlodik I. Y. (2014). Mazohizm kak sposob vyzhit, ili obogrevaya vselennuyu. Vzglyad psihoterapevta. V: *Devochka na share. Kogda stradanie stanovitsya obrazom zhizni*. Moscow: Genezis.

Moerman D. E., Jonas W. B. (2002). Deconstructing the placebo effect and finding the meaning response. *Annals of Internal Medicine*, 136(6), 471–476.

Mohr B. (2001). *The Cosmic Ordering Service: A Guide to Realizing Your Dreams*. Newburyport, MA: Hampton Roads Publishing.

Mohr B., Mohr M. (2012). *The Miracle of Self-Love: The Secret Key to Open All Doors*. London: Hay House.

Molichuk I. G. (2007). *Medicinskaya psihologiya (klinicheskaya psihologiya)*. Minsk: Vyshejshaya shkola.

Mols F., Holterhues C., Nijsten T., van de Poll-Franse L. (2010). Personality is associated with health status and impact of cancer among melanoma survivors. *Eur J Cancer*, 46, 573–580.

Mols F., Husson O., Roukema J. A., van de Poll-Franse L. V. (2013). Depressive symptoms are a risk factor for all-cause mortality: results from a prospective population-based study among 3,080 cancer survivors from the PROFILES registry. *Journal of Cancer Survivorship*, 7(3), 484–492.

Mols F., Denollet J., Kaptein A. A. et al. (2012). The association between Type D personality and illness perceptions in colorectal cancer survivors: a study from the population-based PROFILES registry. *J Psychosom Res*, 73(3), 232–239.

Mols F., Oerlemans S., Denollet J. et al. (2012). Type D personality is associated with increased comorbidity burden and health care utilization among 3080 cancer survivors. *Gen Hosp Psychiatry*, 34(4), 352–359.

Momen N. C., Olsen J., Gissler M. et al. (2013). Early life bereavement and childhood cancer: a nationwide follow-up study in two countries. *BMJ Open*, 3(5), e002864.

Monje M., Dietrich J. (2012). Cognitive side effects of cancer therapy demonstrate a functional role for adult neurogenesis. *Behavioural Brain Research*, 227(2), 376–379.

Montazeri A., Jarvandi S., Ebrahimi M. et al. (2004). The role of depression in the development of breast cancer: analysis of registry data from a single institute. *Asian Pacific Journal of Cancer Prevention*, 5, 316–319.

Montgomery G. H., David D., Winkel G. et al. (2002). The effectiveness of adjunctive hypnosis with surgical patients: a meta-analysis. *Anesth Analg*, 4, 1639–1645.

Montgomery M., McCrone S. H. (2010). Psychological distress associated with the diagnostic phase for suspected breast cancer: systematic review. *J Adv Nurs*, 66(11), 2372–2390.

Moore B. E., Fine B. D. (eds) (1990). *Psychoanalytic Terms and Concepts*. New Haven, CT and London: The American Psychoanalytic Association and Yale University Press.

Moorjani A. (2012). *Dying to Be Me: My Journey from Cancer, to Near Death, to True Healing*. Carlsbad: Hay House.

Moreno-Smith M., Lutgendorf S. K., Sood A. K. (2010). Impact of stress on cancer metastasis. *Future Oncology*, 6(12), 1863–1881.

Moreno-Smith M., Lu C., Shahzad M. M. et al. (2011). Dopamine blocks stress-mediated ovarian carcinoma growth. *Clin Cancer Res: An Official J Am Assoc Cancer Res* 17, 3649–3659.

Morev M. V., Shabunova A. A., Gulin K. A. (2010). *Socialno-ekonomicheskie i demograficheskie aspekty suicidalnogo povedeniya*. Vologda: ISERT RAN.

Morgan G., Ward R., Barton M. (2004). The contribution of cytotoxic chemotherapy to 5-year survival in adult malignancies. *Clinical Oncology*, 16(8), 549–560.

Moritz A. (2008). *Cancer is not a Disease – It's a Survival Mechanism*. Landrum, SC: Ener-chi.

Mormont M. C., Levi F. (1997). Circadian-system alterations during cancer processes: A review. *International Journal of Cancer*, 70, 241–247.

Moroz B. B., Deshevoy Y. B. (1999). Rol emocionalnogo stressa v razvitii somaticheskih narusheniy u likvidatorov avarii na Chernobylskoj atomnoj stancii, obluchennyh v diapazone malyh doz. *Radiac Biol. Radioekol*, 39(1), 97–105.

Morris T., Greer S. (1980). A 'Type C' for cancer? Low trait anxiety in the pathogenesis of breast cancer. *Cancer Detection Prevention*, 3, Abstract 102.

Morton P. M., Schafer M. H., Ferraro K. F. (2012). Does childhood misfortune increase cancer risk in adulthood?. *Journal of Aging and Health*, 24(6), 948–984.

Moscicki A. B., Shiboski S., Hills N. K. et al. (2004). Regression of low-grade squamous intra-epithelial lesions in young women. *The Lancet*, 364(9446), 1678–1683.

Moseley J. B., O'Malley K., Petersen N. J. et al. (2002). A controlled trial of arthroscopic surgery for osteoarthritis of the knee. *New England Journal of Medicine*, 347(2), 81–88.

Mosienko V. S. (2014). Vzglyad na sovremennoe sostoyanie i budushee onkologii. *Zdorov'ya Ukrayini*, 5, 38–39.

Moskvitina S. A. (2012). Osobennosti lichnosti bolnyh rakom molochnoj zhelezy. *Alma mater (Vestnik vysshej shkoly)*. Spec. vyp."Premiya Menegetti," 32–37.

Motenko J. S. (2012). *The Spiritual Quests of Cancer Patients*. Doctoral dissertation. Seattle, WA: Antioch University.

Muller R. T., Gragtmans K., Baker R. (2008). Childhood physical abuse, attachment and adult social support: Test of a mediational model. *Canadian Journal of Behavioural Science, ProQuest Psychology Journals*, 40(2), 80–89.

Muravyev V. N. (1992). Vnutrenniy put. *Voprosy filosofii*, 1, 109.

Murphy J. (1957). *How to Use Your Healing Power*. Los Angeles, CA: Willing Publishing.

Murphy J. (2008). *Maximize Your Potential through the Power of Your Subconscious Mind to Develop Self Confidence and Self Esteem*. Carlsbad: Hay House.

Murray S. A., Kendall M., Boyd K. et al. (2004). Exploring the spiritual needs of people dying of lung cancer or heart failure: a prospective qualitative interview study of patients and their carers. *Palliative Medicine*, 18(1), 39–45.

Musial F., Büssing A., Heusser P. et al. (2011). Mindfulness-based stress reduction for integrative cancer care: a summary of evidence. *Forsch Komplementmed*, 8(4), 192–202.

Myasishchev V. N. (1960). *Lichnost i nevrozy*. Leningrad: Izd-vo Leningradskogo un-ta.

Myers J. E., Sweeney T. J., Witmer J. M. (2000). The Wheel of Wellness counseling for wellness: A holistic model for treatment planning. *Journal of Counseling & Development*, 78, 251–266.

Nabiullina R. R., Tuhtarova I. V. (2003). *Mehanizmy psihologicheskoj zashity i sovladaniya so stressom (opredelenie, struktura, funkcii, vidy, psihoterapevticheskaya korrekciya).* Kazan: KGMA.

Nagaraja A. S., Sadaoui N. C., Lutgendorf S. K. et al. (2013). β-blockers: a new role in cancer chemotherapy? *Expert opinion on investigational drugs*, 22(11), 1359–1363.

Naidich J. B., Motta R. W. (2000). PTSD-related symptoms in women with breast cancer. *Journal of Psychotherapy in Independent Practice*, 1, 35–54

Nair L., Deb S., Mandal J. (1993). A study on repression-sensitization, personality characteristics and early childhood experiences of male cancer patients. *Journal of Personality and Clinical Studies*, 9, 87–94.

Nakagawa K., Kuriyama K. (1975). Effect of taurine on alteration in adrenal functions induced by stress. *The Japanese Journal of Pharmacology*, 25(6), 737–746.

Nakane T., Szentendrei T., Stern L. et al. (1990). Effects of IL-1 and cortisol on beta-adrenergic receptors, cell proliferation, and differentiation in cultured human A549 lung tumor cells. *J Immunol*, 45, 260–266.

Nakau M., Imanishi J., Imanishi J. et al. (2013). Spiritual Care of Cancer Patients by Integrated Medicine in Urban Green Space: A Pilot Study. *Explore: The Journal of Science and Healing*, 9(2), 87–90.

Nakaya N., Tsubono Y., Hosokawa T. et al. (2003). Personality and the Risk of Cancer. *J Natl Cancer Inst*, 95(11), 799–805.

Nakaya N., Tsubono Y., Nishino Y. et al. (2005). Personality and cancer survival: the Miyagi Cohort Study. *Br J Cancer*, 92, 2089–2094.

Nan K. J., Wei Y. C., Zhou F. L. et al. (2004). Effects of depression on parameters of cell-mediated immunity in patients with digestive tract cancers. *World J Gastroenterol*, 10(2), 268–272.

Naranjo C. (1994). *Character and Neurosis: An Integrative View.* Southlake, TX: Gateways/IDHHB, Inc.

Narayan P., Singh V. K., Agarwal S. S. et al. (2001). Immunomodulation by opioid peptidomimetic compound. *Neuroimmunomodulation*, (3), 134–40.

Nausheen B., Carr N. J., Peveler R. C. et al. (2010). Relationship between loneliness and proangiogenic cytokines in newly diagnosed tumors of colon and rectum. *Psychosomatic Medicine*, 72, 912–916.

NCCN—National Comprehensive Cancer Network. (2007). *Clinical practice guidelines in oncology: Distress management* (v.1.2008).

Neeman E., Ben-Eliyahu S. (2013). The perioperative period and promotion of cancer metastasis: New outlooks on mediating mechanisms and immune involvement. *Brain, Behavior, and Immunity*, 30(Suppl), S32.

Neigh G. N., Gillespie C. F., Nemeroff C. B. (2009). The neurobiological toll of child abuse and neglect. *Trauma Violence Abuse*, 10, 389–410.

Neimeyer R. A., Prigerson H. G., Davies B. (2002). Mourning and meaning. *American Behavioral Scientist*, 46(2), 235–251.

Nekrut T. V. (2015). Mazohizm i ego vzaimosvyaz s ogranichennymi vozmozhnostyami zdorovya subekta. *Science Time*, 6(18), 372 – 379.

Nelson B. (2014). *The Emotion Code: How to Release Your Trapped Emotions for Abundant Health, Love and Happiness.* Mesquite, TX: Wellness Unmasked Publishing.

Nelson J. D. (2015). *Cancer My Personal Story: Pulling the positives out of the negatives.* CreateSpace Independent Publishing Platform.

Nemtsev A. V. (2012). *Duhovnye smysly v zhiznennom mire lyudej, stradayushih depressivnymi rasstrojstvami.* Avtoref dis. kand. psihol. nauk. Tomsk: NITPU.

Nepomnyashchaya N. I. (1998). O psihologicheskom aspekte onkologicheskih zabolevanij. *Psihologicheskiy Zhurnal*, 19(4), 132–145.

Newton B. W. (1982). The Use of Hypnosis in the Treatment of Cancer Patients. *American Journal of Clinical Hypnosis*, 25(2-3), 105–107.

Ng C. G., Zainal N. Z. (2015). Prevalence of Depression in Cancer Patients: A Review on the Comparison Between Different Regions. *Malaysian Journal of Psychiatry*, 23(2), 90–113.

Nicholls W., Hulbert-Williams N., Bramwell R. (2014). The role of relationship attachment in psychological adjustment to cancer in patients and caregivers: a systematic review of the literature. *Psycho-Oncology*, 23(10), 1083–1095.

Nidich S., Mjasiri S., Nidich R. et al. (2011). Academic achievement and transcendental meditation: A study with at-risk urban middle school students. *Education*, 131(3), 556–564.

Niemi T., Jaaskelainen J. (1978). Cancer morbidity in depressive persons. *J Psychosom Res*, 22(1), 117–120.

Nieminen S. H., Sajaniemi N. (2016). Mindful awareness in early childhood education. *South African Journal of Childhood Education*, 6(1), 1–9.

Nietzsche F. (2009). *Twilight of the Idols, or How to Philosophize with a Hammer*. Oxford: Oxford University Press.

Nikiforov A. M. (1994). *Klinicheskie proyavleniya vozdejstviya faktorov krupnomasshtabnoj radiacionnoj katastrofy*. Dis. d-ra med. nauk. Saint Petersburg: VMEDA.

Nikiforov Y. E., Seethala R. R., Tallini G. et al. (2016). Nomenclature Revision for Encapsulated Follicular Variant of Papillary Thyroid Carcinoma. *JAMA Oncology*, 2(8), 1023–1029.

Nikitin Yu. P., Openko T. G., Simonova G. I. (2012). Metabolicheskiy sindrom i ego komponenty kak vozmozhnye modificiruemye faktory riska raka (literaturnyj obzor). *Sibirskiy Onkologicheskiy Zhurnal*, 2(50), 68–72.

Nilsson M. B., Armaiz-Pena G., Takahashi R. et al. (2007). Stress hormones regulate interleukin-6 expression by human ovarian carcinoma cells through a Src-dependent mechanism. *J Biol Chem*, 282(41), 29919–29926.

Novitskiy V. V., Goldberg E. D., Urazova O. I. (eds) (2009). *Patofiziologiya*. Moscow: GEOTAR-Media, 2 vol.

Novikova I. A., Soloviev A. G. (2001). *Psihologicheskie aspekty psihosomaticheskih zabolevanij. Metod. Rekomendacii*. Pod red. P. I. Sidorova. Arhangelsk: SGMU.

Nozue A. T., Ono S. (1991). Effects of catecholamine and serotonin in central nervous system in newborn mice with special reference to neural crest cells; presumptive evidence of neural crest origin. *Anatomischer Anzeiger*, 173(3), 147–153

Nunn T. (1822). *Cancer of the breast*. London: Churchill.

O'Brien S. M., Scott L. V., Dinan T. G. (2006). Antidepressant therapy and C-reactive protein levels. *Br J Psychiatry*, 88, 449–452.

Obukhov Y. L. (1997). Glubinno-psihologicheskiy podhod v psihoterapii psihosomaticheskih zabolevanij. *Shkola Zdorovya*, 3, 43–61.

O'Connor J. F., Stern L. O. (1967). Symptom Alternation: An Evaluation of the Theory. *Archives of General Psychiatry*, 16(4), 432–436.

O'Connor M. F., Schultze-Florey C. R., Irwin M. R. et al. (2014). Divergent gene expression responses to complicated grief and non-complicated grief. *Brain Behav Immun*, 37, 78–83.

O'Connor T. G., Ben-Shlomo Y., Heron J. et al. (2005). Prenatal anxiety predicts individual differences in cortisol in pre-adolescent children. *Biol Psychiatry*, 58, 211–217.

O'Donnell K. J., Brydon L., Wright C. E., Steptoe A. (2008). Self-esteem levels and cardiovascular and inflammatory responses to acute stress. *Brain Behav Immun*, 22(8), 1241–1247.

O'Donnell K. J., Glover V., Jenkins J. et al. (2013). Prenatal maternal mood is associated with altered diurnal cortisol in adolescence. *Psychoneuroendocrinology*, 38(9), 1630–1638.

O'Donnell L. (2014). *Cancer is My Teacher*. London: Quartet Books.

O'Donovan A., Lin J., Dhabhar F. S. et al. (2009). Pessimism correlates with leukocyte telomere shortness and elevated interleukin-6 in post-menopausal women. *Brain, Behavior, and Immunity*, 23(4), 446–449.

O'Donovan A., Sun B., Cole S. et al. (2011). Transcriptional control of monocyte gene expression in post-traumatic stress disorder. *Dis Markers*, 30, 123–132.

O'Donovan A., Tomiyama A. J., Lin J. et al. (2012). Stress appraisals and cellular aging: A key role for anticipatory threat in the relationship between psychological stress and telomere length. *Brain, Behavior, and Immunity*, 26(4), 573–579.

Oerlemans M. E., van den Akker M., Schuurman A. G. et al. (2007). A meta-analysis on depression and subsequent cancer risk. *Clin Pract Epidemiol Ment Health*, 3(29), 1–11.

Ogorenko V. V. (2011). Socialno-psihologicheskaya harakteristika i osobennosti rannih psihopatologicheskih narusheniy u bolnyh zlokachestvennymi opuholyami golovnogo mozga. *Ukrayinskiy Visnik Psihonevrologiyi*, (19)2, 59–62.

O'Hanlon B., Cade W. H. (1993). *A brief guide to brief therapy*. New York: W. W. Norton & Company.

Olsen M. H., Bidstrup P. E., Frederiksen K. et al. (2012). Loss of partner and breast cancer prognosis—a population-based study, Denmark, 1994-2010. *British Journal of Cancer*, 106(9), 1560–1563.

O'Regan B., Hirschberg C. (1993). *Spontaneous Remission. An Annotated Bibliography*. Sausalito, CA: Institute of Noetic Sciences.

Orgel E., Mittelman S. D. (2013). The Links Between Insulin Resistance, Diabetes, and Cancer. *Current Diabetes Reports*, 13(2), 213–222.

Orlov Y. M. (2005). *Obida*. Moscow: Slajding.

Ornish D., Lin J., Daubenmier J. et al. (2008). Increased telomerase activity and comprehensive lifestyle changes: a pilot study. *The Lancet Oncology*, 9(11), 1048–1057.

Ornish D., Magbanua M. J. M., Weidner G. et al. (2008a). Changes in prostate gene expression in men undergoing an intensive nutrition and lifestyle intervention. *Proc Natl Acad Sci USA*, 105(24), 8369–8374.

Orr S. P., Metzger L. J., Lasko N. B. et al. (2000). De novo conditioning in trauma-exposed individuals with and without posttraumatic stress disorder. *J Abnorm Psychol*, 109, 290–298.

Orsi A. J., McCorkle R., Tax A. et al. (1996). The relationship between depressive symptoms and immune status phenotypes in patients undergoing surgery for colorectal cancer. *Psycho-Oncology*, 5, 311–319.

Ortega y Gasset J. (1972). Thoughts on Technology. In: C. Mitcham, R. Mackey (eds), *Philosophy and Technology: Readings in the Philosophical Problems of Technology*. New York: Free, 290–313.

Orzechowski A., Ostaszewski P., Wilczak J. et al. (2002). Rats with a glucocorticoid-induced catabolic state show symptoms of oxidative stress and spleen atrophy: the effects of age and recovery. *J Vet Med A Physiol Pathol Clin Med*, 49, 256–263.

Osipova A. (2014). *Rak mozhno pobedit*. Moscow: AST.

Ospina M. B., Bond K., Karkhaneh M. et al. (2007). Meditation practices for health: state of the research. *Evid Rep Technol Assess (Full Rep)*, 155, 1–263.

Ott M. J., Norris R. L., Bauer-Wu S. M. (2006). Mindfulness Meditation for Oncology Patients: A Discussion and Critical Review. *Integrative Cancer Therapies*, 5(2), 98–108.

Ouspensky P. D. (1959). *The Fourth Way*. Abingdon-on-Thames: Routledge.

Ovsyannikov S. A., Tsygankov B. D. (2001). *Pogranichnaya psihiatriya i somaticheskaya patologiya: Kliniko-prakticheskoe rukovodstvo*. Moscow: Triada-Farm.

Pace T. W., Negi L. T., Adame D. D. et al. (2009). Effect of compassion meditation on neuroendocrine, innate immune and behavioral responses to psychosocial stress. *Psychoneuroendocrinology*, 4, 87–98.

Padun M. A. (2007). Rol detskoj travmy i kognitivno-lichnostnyh harakteristik v razvitii priznakov depressii u vzroslyh. *Vestnik Rossijskogo Gumanitarnogo Nauchnogo Fonda*, 188–197.

Padun M. A., Zagryazhskaya E. A. (2006). Bazisnye ubezhdeniya v strukture psihologicheskogo distressa. *Psihosomaticheskaya medicina. Sbornik tezisov 1 Mezhdunarodnogo kongressa.* Saint Petersburg, 143.

Paget J. (1870). *Surgical pathology.* London: Longman's Green.

Palermo-Neto J., de Oliveira M. C., Robespierre de S. W. (2003). Effects of physical and psychological stressors on behavior, macrophage activity, and Ehrlich tumor growth. *Brain Behav Immun,* 17, 43–54.

Palesh O., Butler L. D., Koopman C. et al. (2007). Stress history and breast cancer recurrence. *J Psychosom Res,* 63(3), 233–239.

Palm D., Lang K., Niggemann B. et al. (2006). The norepinephrine-driven metastasis development of PC-3 human prostate cancer cells in BALB/c nude mice is inhibited by β-blockers. *International Journal of Cancer,* 118(11), 2744–2749.

Papadatou D. (1983). *Psychosocial factors related to the onset of childhood cancer (stress, family, Greece).* Ph.D. thesis, University of Arizona.

Pargament K. I. (2002). Is Religion Nothing But…? Explaining Religion Versus Explaining Religion Away. *Psychological Inquiry,* 13, 239–244.

Parikh D., De Ieso P., Garvey G. et al. (2015). Post-traumatic stress disorder and post-traumatic growth in breast cancer patients--a systematic review. *Asian Pac J Cancer Prev,* 6(2), 641–646.

Paris B. (2001). *Audrey Hepburn.* New York: Berkley. Reissue edn.

Park C. L. (2008). Estimated longevity and changes in spirituality in the context of advanced congestive heart failure. *Palliative and Supportive Care,* 6(01), 3–11.

Parker J., Klein S. L., McClintock M. K. et al. (2004). Chronic stress accelerates ultraviolet-induced cutaneous carcinogenesis. *J Am Acad Dermatol,* 1, 919–922.

Parker P. A, Kudelka A., Basen-Engquist K. et al. (2006). The associations between knowledge, CA125 preoccupation, and distress in women with epithelial ovarian cancer. *Gynecol Oncol,* 100(3), 495–500.

Parker W. (1885). *Cancer. A Study of 397 Cases of Cancer of the Female Breast, with Clinical Observations.* New York and London: GP Putnam's Sons.

Partecke L. I., Speerforck S., Käding A. et al. (2016). Chronic stress increases experimental pancreatic cancer growth, reduces survival and can be antagonised by beta-adrenergic receptor blockade. *Pancreatology,* 16(3), 423–433.

Passchier J., Gaudswaard P., Orlebeke J. F., Verhage F. (1988). Migraine and defence mechanisms: Psychophysiological relationships in young females. *Social Science and Medicine,* 26, 343–350.

Pavlov I. P. (1966). *Essential Works of Pavlov.* M. Kaplan (ed.). New York: Bantam Books.

Payne L. (1991). *Restoring the Christian soul: Overcoming barriers to completion in Christ through healing prayer.* Grand Rapids, MI: Baker Books.

Pearce M. J., Coan A. D., Herndon J. E. 2nd et al. (2012). Unmet spiritual care needs impact emotional and spiritual well-being in advanced cancer patients. *Support Care Cancer,* 20, 2269–2276.

Pears K. C., Capaldi D. M. (2001). Intergenerational transmission of abuse: A two generational prospective study of an at-risk sample. *Child Abuse and Neglect,* 25, 1439–1461.

Peled R., Carmil D., Siboni-Samocha O., Shoham-Vardi I. (2008). Breast cancer, psychological distress and life events among young women. *BMC Cancer,* 8, 245.

Peller S. (1952). *Cancer in Man.* New York: International University Press.

Peller S., Stephenson C. S. (1941). Cancer in the mentally ill. *Public Health Reports (1896-1970),* 132–149.

Pelletier K. R. (2002). Mind as healer, mind as slayer: Mind body medicine comes of age. *Advances in Mind Body Medicine*, 18, 4–15.

Pendergrass E. P. (1961). Host resistance and other intangibles in the treatment of cancer. *American Journal of Roentgenology*, 85, 891–896.

Penedo F. J., Dahn J. R., Kinsinger D. et al. (2006). Anger suppression mediates the relationship between optimism and natural killer cell cytotoxicity in men treated for localized prostate cancer. *J Psychosom Res*, 60(4), 423–427.

Pennebaker J. W. (1999). The effects of traumatic disclosure on physical and mental health: The values of writing and talking about upsetting events. *Int J Emerg Ment Health*, 1, 9–18.

Penninx B. W., Guralnik J. M., Havlik R. J. et al. (1998). Chronically depressed mood and cancer risk in older persons. *Journal of the National Cancer Institute*, 90(24), 1888–1893.

Pereira D. B., Sannes T., Dodd S. M. et al. (2010). Life stress, negative mood states, and antibodies to heat shock protein 70 in endometrial cancer. *Brain, Behavior, and Immunity*, 24(2), 210–214.

Pernin G. M, Pierce I. R. (1959). Psychosomatic aspects of cancer. A review. *Psychosom Med*, 1, 397–421.

Perron L., Bairati I., Harel F., Meyer F. (2004). Antihypertensive drug use and the risk of prostate cancer (Canada). *Cancer Causes Control*, 5(6), 535–541.

Persky V. W., Kempthorne-Rawson J., Shekelle R. B. (1987). Personality and risk of cancer: 20-year follow-up of the Western Electric Study. *Psychosomatic Medicine*, 49(5), 435–449.

Pert C. B. (1999). *Molecules Of Emotion: The Science Behind Mind-Body Medicine*. New York: Simon & Schuster.

Peseschkian N. (1991). *Psychosomatik und Positive Psychotherapie*. Berlin, Heidelberg: Springer.

Pestereva E. V. (2011). *Osobennosti psihologicheskoj adaptacii k bolezni pacientov so zlokachestvennymi limfomami na razlichnyh etapah zabolevaniya*. Diss. kand. psihol. nauk. Saint Petersburg: SPGU.

Peterlik D., J Flor P., Uschold-Schmidt N. (2016). The emerging role of metabotropic glutamate receptors in the pathophysiology of chronic stress-related disorders. *Current Neuropharmacology*, 14(5), 514-539.

Peterson P. K., Chao C. C., Molitor T. et al. (1991). Stress and pathogenesis of infectious disease. *Rev Infect Dis*, 13, 710–720.

Petrov N. N. (1958). *Rukovodstvo po obshej onkologii*. Moscow: Medicina.

Petrova M. K. (1946). *O roli funkcionalno oslablennoj kory golovnogo mozga v vozniknovenii razlichnyh patologicheskih processov v organizme*. Moscow: Medgiz.

Pettingale K. (1984). Coping and cancer prognosis. *J Psychosom Res*, 28, 363–364.

Pettingale K., Greer S., Tee D. E. H. (1977). Serum Ig A and emotional expression in breast cancer patients. *J Psychosom Res*, 21, 395–399.

Pettingale K., Morris T., Greer S., Haybittle J. (1985). Mental attitudes to cancer: an additional prognostic factor. *Lancet*, 30, 750.

Phillips K. M., Antoni M. H., Lechner S. C. (2008). Stress management intervention reduces serum cortisol and increases relaxation uring treatment for non metastatic breast cancer. *Psychosom Med*, 70, 1044-1049.

Phillips L. J., Osborne J. W. (1989). Cancer patients' experiences of forgiveness therapy. *Canadian Journal of Counseling*, 23, 236–251.

Piazza J. R., Charles S. T., Sliwinski M. J. et al. (2013). Affective reactivity to daily stressors and long-term risk of reporting a chronic physical health condition. *Ann Behav Med*, 45(1), 110–120.

Picardi A., Battisti F., Tarsitani L. et al. (2007). Attachment security and immunity in healthy women. *Psychosom Med*, 69(1), 40–46.

Pickering G. W. (1974). *Creative Malady: Illness in the Lives and Minds of Charles Darwin, Florence Nightingale, Mary Baker Eddy, Sigmund Freud, Marcel Proust, and Elizabeth Barrett Browning*. Oxford: Oxford University Press.

Pierce B. L., Ballard-Barbash R., Bernstein L. et al. (2009). Elevated biomarkers of inflammation are associated with reduced survival among breast cancer patients. *J Clin Oncol*, 27, 3437–3444.

Pietrini P., Guazzelli M., Basso G. et al. (2000). Neural correlates of imaginal aggressive behavior assessed by positron emission tomography in healthy subjects. *American Journal of Psychiatry*, 157, 1772–1781.

Pilipenko G. N., Shamshikova O. A., Harina K. A. (2009). Aleksitimiya v strukture lichnosti i ee rol v processah psihicheskoj adaptacii. V: *Sociokulturnye problemy sovremennogo cheloveka*. Ch. II. Novosibirsk: NGPU, 137–145.

Pilyagina G. Y. (1999). Autoagressiya: biologicheskaya celesoobraznost ili psihologicheskiy vybor?. *Tavricheskiy Zhurnal Psihiatrii*, 3(3), 24–27.

Pilyagina G. Y. (2000). Magicheskie arhetipy i rituay v patogeneze nevroticheskih rasstrojstv i autoagressivnogo povedeniya. *Tavricheskiy Zhurnal Psihiatrii*, 4(4), 64–67.

Pilyagina G. Y. (2002). Mnogolikost samorazrusheniya (osobennosti patogeneza autodestruktivnyh ekvivalentov). *Tavricheskiy Zhurnal Psihiatrii*, 6(2), 52–56.

Pilyagina G. Y. (2003). Mehanizmy patologicheskogo prisposobleniya i detskaya travmatizaciya v suicidogeneze. *Ukrayinskiy Medichniy Chasopis*, 6, 49–56.

Pilyagina G. Y. (2003a). Primenenie kompleksnyh metodov diagnostiki pri autoagressivnyh proyavleniyah. *Tavricheskiy Zhurnal Psihiatrii*, 7(3), 76–82.

Pilyagina G. Y. (2003b). Principy neotlozhnoj psihoterapii autoagressivnogo povedeniya. *Tavricheskiy Zhurnal Psihiatrii*, 7(4), 42–46.

Pilyagina G. Y. (2004). *Autoagressivnoe povedenie: patogeneticheskie mehanizmy i kliniko-tipologicheskie aspekty diagnostiki i lecheniya*. Avtoref. dis. d-ra med. nauk. Kiev: ISSPN.

Pilyagina G. Y. (2013). Ponyatie kognitivno-emocionalnogo disbalansa (deficita) i eg o znachenie v patogeneze psihicheskoj patologii i samorazrushayushego povedeniya. *Zbirnik Naukovih Prac Spivrobitnikiv NMAPO im. P. L. Shupika*, 22(2), 257–267.

Pilyagina G. Y. (2013a). Osobennosti patogeneza ekvivalentnoj formy samorazrushayushego povedeniya. *Suicidologiya*, 4(3/12), 36–48.

Pilyagina G. Y., Dubrovskaya E. V. (2007). Narusheniya privyazannosti kak osnova formirovaniya psihopatologicheskih rasstrojstv v detskom i podrostkovom vozraste. *Mistectvo Likuvannya*, 6, 71–79.

Pinar B., Lara P. C., Lloret M. et al. (2007). Radiation-induced DNA damage as a predictor of long-term toxicity in locally advanced breast cancer patients treated with high-dose hyperfractionated radical radiotherapy. *Radiation Research*, 168(4), 415–422.

Pinquart M., Duberstein P. R. (2010). Associations of social networks with cancer mortality: a meta-analysis. *Crit Rev Oncol Hematol*, 75(2), 122–137.

Piontkovskaya O. V. (2013). Soderzhanie i effektivnost sistemy mediko-psihologicheskoj pomoshi v klinike detskoj onkologii. *Mezhdunarodnyj Medicinskiy Zhurnal*, 3, 5–13.

Pirl W. F. (2004). Evidence report on the occurrence, assessment, and treatment of depression in cancer patients. *J Natl Cancer Inst Monogr*, 32, 32–39.

Pirmohamed M., James S., Meakin S. et al. (2004). Adverse drug reactions as cause of admission to hospital: prospective analysis of 18 820 patients. *BMJ*, 329(7456), 15–19.

Pirogov N. I. (1854). O trudnosti raspoznavaniya hirurgicheskih boleznej. *Voenno-Med Zhurnal*, 64, 1, 11.

Pitman R. K., Sanders K. M., Zusman R. M. et al. (2002). Pilot study of secondary prevention of posttraumatic stress disorder with propranolol. *Biol Psychiatry*, 51(2), 189–192.

Pittenger C., Duman R. S. (2008). Stress, Depression, and Neuroplasticity: A Convergence of Mechanisms. *Neuropsychopharmacology*, 33, 88–109.

618   Vladislav Matrenitsky

Planck M. (1931). Interviews With Great Scientists. VI.—Max Planck. *The Observer*, 25 January, 17.

Plant D. T., Pawlby S., Pariante C. M. (2013). 53. Exposure to depression in utero predicts adulthood inflammation. *Brain, Behavior, and Immunity*, 32, e15.

Pleshchits S. G. (ed.) (2012). *Osnovy konfliktologii: uchebnoe posobie*. Saint Petersburg: SPbGUEF.

Plesko M. M., Richardson A. (1984). Age-related changes in unscheduled DNA synthesis by rat hepatocytes. *Biochemical and Biophysical Research Communications*, 118(3), 730–735.

Polischuk Y. I. (2010). Faktor duhovnosti v psihiatrii i psihoterapii. *Psihicheskoe Zdorovje*, 3, 57–61.

Pollock R. E., Lotzova E., Stanford S. D. (1991). Mechanism of surgical stress impairment of human perioperative natural killer cell cytotoxicity. *Arch Surg*, 126, 338–342.

Polozhiy B. S., Panchenko E. A., Posvyanskaya A. D., Fritlinskiy V. S. (2014). Klinicheskie i sociokulturalnye harakteristiki bolnyh s depressivnymi rasstrojstvami, sovershivshih pokushenie na samoubijstvo. *Suicidologiya*, 5(2), 42–47.

Ponizovsky A. M., Vitenberg E., Baumgarten-Katz I., Grinshpoon A. (2013). Attachment styles and affect regulation among outpatients with schizophrenia: relationships to symptomatology and emotional distress. *Psychology and Psychotherapy: Theory, Research and Practice*, 86(2), 164–182.

Popkov V. M., Chesnokova N. P., Barsukov V. Y., Seleznev T. D. (2012). Kancerogenez: obshaya harakteristika, etiologicheskie faktory. Rol svobodnyh radikalov v mehanizmah onkogennoj transformacii kletok i opuholevoj progressii. V: V. M. Popkov, N. P. Chesnokova, M. Y. Ledvanov. *Aktivaciya lipoperoksidacii kak vedushiy patogeneticheskiy faktor razvitiya tipovyh patologicheskih processov i zabolevaniy razlichnoj etiologii*. Moscow: Akademiya Estestvoznaniya.

Popkov V. M., Chernenkov Y. V., Protopopov A. A. et al. (2011). Faktory, vliyayushie na razvitie psihosomaticheskoj patologii. *Bulletin of Medical Internet Conferences*, 1(7).

Porter L. S., Mishel M., Neelon V. et al. (2003). Cortisol levels and responses to mammography screening in breast cancer survivors: a pilot study. *Psychosomatic Medicine*, 65(5), 842–848.

Pothiwala P., Jain S. K., Yaturu S. (2009). Metabolic syndrome and cancer. *Metabolic Syndrome and Related Disorders*, 7(4), 279–288.

Potischman N., Troisi R. (1999). In-utero and early life exposures in relation to risk of breast cancer. *Cancer Causes & Control*, 10(6), 561–573.

Powe D. G., Voss M. J., Zänker K. S. et al. (2010). Beta-blocker drug therapy reduces secondary cancer formation in breast cancer and improves cancer specific survival. *Oncotarget*, 1(7), 628–638.

Powell N. D., Tarr A. J., Sheridana J. F. (2013). Psychosocial stress and inflammation in cancer. *Brain, Behavior, and Immunity*, 30, S41–S47.

Powell N. D., Sloan E. K., Bailey M. T. et al. (2013a). Social stress up-regulates inflammatory gene expression in the leukocyte transcriptome via β-adrenergic induction of myelopoiesis. *Proc Natl Acad Sci USA*, 110(41),16574–16579.

Powers S. I., Pietromonaco P. R., Gunlicks M., Sayer A. (2006). Dating couples' attachment styles and patterns of cortisol reactivity and recovery in response to a relationship conflict. *J Pers Soc Psychol*, 90(4), 613–628.

Price M. A., Tennant C. C., Smith R. C. et al. (2001). The role of psychosocial factors in the development of breast carcinoma: Part I. The cancer prone personality. *Cancer*, 91(4), 679–685.

Prigerson H. G., Shear M. K., Bierhals A. J. et al. (1997). Case histories of complicated grief. *Omega*, 35, 9–24.

Prikhozhan A. M. (1998). Prichiny, profilaktika i preodolenie trevozhnosti. *Psihologicheskaya Nauka i Obrazovanie*, 2, 11–17.

Protheroe D., Turvey K., Horgan K. et al. (1999). Stressful life events and difficulties and onset of breast cancer: case-control study. *BMJ*, 319(7216), 1027–1030.

Provencal N., Suderman M. J., Guillemin C. et al. (2014). Association of childhood chronic physical aggression with a DNA methylation signature in adult human T cells. *PloS One*, 9(4), e89839.

Prussak A. V. (1956). U istokov russkoj onkologii. *Voprosy Onkologii*, 6, 763–766.

Przezdziecki A., Sherman K. A., Baillie A. et al. (2013). My changed body: breast cancer, body image, distress and self-compassion. *Psycho-Oncology*, 22(8), 1872–1879.

Psellos M. (1841). Πόνημα ιατρικόν άριστον δι ιάμβων. In: J. L. Ideler. *Physici et Medici Graeci Minores*. Berlin: 1. J.

Puchalski C. M. (2013). Integrating spirituality into patient care: an essential element of personcentered care. *Pol Arch Med Wewn*, 123(9), 491–497.

Puchalski C. M., McSkimming S. (2006). Creating healing environments. *Health Progress*, 30–35.

Puig A., Lee S. M., Goodwin L., Sherrard P. A. (2006). The efficacy of creative arts therapies to enhance emotional expression, spirituality, and psychological well-being of newly diagnosed Stage I and Stage II breast cancer patients: A preliminary study. *The Arts in Psychotherapy*, 33(3), 218–228.

Puig J., Englund M. M., Simpson J. A., Collins W. A. (2013). Predicting adult physical illness from infant attachment: A prospective longitudinal study. *Health Psychology*, 32(4), 409–417.

Puig M. A. (2012). *Reinventarse: Tu segunda oportunidad*. Barcelona: Plataforma Editorial, S. L.

Purnell J. Q., Andersen B. L., Wilmot J. P. (2009). Religious practice and spirituality in the psychological adjustment of survivors of breast cancer. *Counseling and Values*, 53, 165–185.

Puterman E., Epel E. S., O'Donovan A. et al. (2013). Anger Is Associated with Increased IL-6 Stress Reactivity in Women, But Only Among Those Low in Social Support. *Int J Behav Med*, 21(6), 936–945.

Pyter L. M., Pineros V., Galang J. A. et al. (2009). Peripheral tumors induce depressive-like behaviors and cytokine production and alter hypothalamic-pituitary-adrenal axis regulation. *PNAS*, 106(22), 9069–9074.

Quan N., Avitsur R., Stark J. L. et al. (2001). Social stress increases the susceptibility to endotoxic shock. *J Neuroimmunol*, 115(1–2), 36–45.

Radtke K. M., Ruf M., Gunter H. M. et al. (2011). Transgenerational impact of intimate partner violence on methylation in the promoter of the glucocorticoid receptor. *Translational Psychiatry*, 1(7), e21.

Ragland D. R., Brand R. J., Fox B. H. (1992). Type A/B behavior and cancer mortality: The confounding/mediating effect of covariates. *Psycho-Oncology*, 1, 25–33.

Ragozinskaya V. G. (2010). *Emocionalnye sostoyaniya i ih nejrofiziologicheskie korrelyaty u bolnyh psihosomaticheskimi zabolevaniyami*. Diss. kand. psihol. nauk. Saint Petersburg: Gos. universitet.

Rahe R. H., Meyer M., Smith M. et al. (1964). Social stress and illness onset. *Journal of Psychosomatic Research*, 8, 35–44.

Raison C. L., Miller A. H. (2003). Depression in cancer: new developments regarding diagnosis and treatment. *Biol Psychiatry*, 54, 283–294.

Raison C. L., Capuron L., Miller A. H. (2006). Cytokines sing the blues: inflammation and the pathogenesis of depression. *Trends Immunol*, 27(1), 24–31.

Rak (sbornik). (2014). *Opyt boryushihsya. Metodiki lechashih*. Moscow: AST.

Rakhimkulova A. V., Rozanov V. A. (2015). Perceived stress, anxiety, depression and risky behavior in adolescents. In: *Proc. of 22nd Multidisciplinary ISBS International Neuroscience and Biological Psychiatry "Stress and Behavior" Conference*. Saint Petersburg, Russia, May 16-19, 31–32.

Ramirez A., Craig T., Watson J. et al. (1989). Stress and relapse of breast cancer. *BMJ*, 298, 291–293.

Ramos C., Costa P. A., Rudnicki T. et al. (2018). The effectiveness of a group intervention to facilitate posttraumatic growth among women with breast cancer. *Psycho-oncology*, 27(1), 258–264.

Rancour-Laferriere D. (1996). *The Slave Soul of Russia: Moral Masochism and the Cult of Suffering*. New York: New York University Press.

Rangaraju S., Levey D. F., Nho K. et al. (2016). Mood, stress and longevity: convergence on ANK3. *Molecular Psychiatry*, 21, 1037–1049

Rank O. (2010). *The Trauma of Birth*. Eastford, CT: Martino Fine Books.

Rauscher G. H., Umaima A. A., Warnecke R. B. (2011). Abstract A91: Does psychosocial stress play a role in the etiology of aggressive breast cancer? A cross-sectional study. *Cancer Epidemiology Biomarkers & Prevention*, 20(10 Supplement), A91–A91.

Ravitch R. (2013). *Gimn zhizni. Istorii zhizni detej, pobedivshih rak*. E-book: Accent Graphics Communications.

Rawnsley M. M. (1994). Recurrence of cancer: A crisis of courage. *Cancer Nursing*, 17(4), 342–347.

Ray O. (2004). The Revolutionary Health Science of Psychoendoneuroimmunology: A New Paradigm for Understanding Health and Treating Illness. *Annals of the New York Academy of Sciences. Biobehavioral Stress Response: Protective and Damaging Effects*, 1032, 35–51.

Ray R. A. (2002). *Indestructible Truth: The Living Spirituality of Tibetan Buddhism* (World of Tibetan Buddhism, Vol. 1). Boulder, CO: Shambhala Publishers.

Read J., Bentall R. P., Fosse R. (2009). Time to abandon the bio-bio-bio model of psychosis: Exploring the epigenetic and psychological mechanisms by which adverse life events lead to psychotic symptoms. *Epidemiologia e Psichiatria Sociale*, 18(04), 299–310.

Rebalance Focus Action Group. (2005). A position paper: screening key indicators in cancer patients: pain as a fifth vital sign and emotional distress as a sixth vital sign. *Canadian Strategy for Cancer Control Bulletin*, 7(Suppl), 4.

Rehse B., Pukrop R. (2003). Effects of psychosocial interventions on quality of life in adult cancer patients: meta analysis of 37 published controlled outcome studies. *Patient Education and Counseling*, 50(2), 179–186.

Reich M., Lesur A., Perdrizet-Chevallier C. (2008). Depression, quality of life and breast cancer: a review of the literature. *Breast Cancer Research and Treatment*, 110(1), 9–17.

Reich W. (1980). *Character Analysis*. New York: Farrar, Straus and Giroux.

Reiche E. M., Morimoto H. K., Nunes S. M. (2005). Stress and depression-induced immune dysfunction: implications for the development and progression of cancer. *Int Rev Psychiatry*, 17(6), 515–527.

Reiche E. M., Nunes S. O., Morimoto H. K. (2004). Stress, depression, the immune system, and cancer. *Lancet Oncol*, 5(10), 617–625.

Reikovskiy J. (1979). *Eksperimentalnaya psihologiya emocij*. Moscow: Progress.

Rein G., Atkinson M., McCraty R. (1995). The Physiological and Psychological Effects of Compassion and Anger. *Journal of Advancement in Medicine*, 8(2), 87–105.

Reinhardt C., Nagel M. (2003). *Stress bei Hunden*. Bernau: Animal Learn.

Reiser M. D. (1966). Retrospects and prospects. *The Annals of the New York Academy of Sciences*, 125(3), 1028–1055.

Reite M., Harbeck R., Hoffman A. (1981). Altered cellular immune response following peer separation. *Life Science*, 29, 1133–1136.

Reker G., Wong P. (1988). Aging as an individual process: Toward a theory of personal meaning. In: J. E. Bitten, V. L. Bengston (eds), *Emergent theories of aging*. New York: Springer, 214–246.

Relier J. P. (2001). Influence of maternal stress on fetal behavior and brain development. *Biology of the Neonate*, 79(3), 168–171.

Remen R. N. (2008). Tending the spirit in cancer. *Integrative Oncology*, 18, 778–785.

Ren H., Collins V., Clarke S. J. et al. (2012). Epigenetic changes in response to tai chi practice: a pilot investigation of DNA methylation marks. *Evidence-Based Complementary and Alternative Medicine*, ID 841810.

Renz M., Mao S. M., Omlin A. et al. (2013). Spiritual experiences of transcendence in patients with advanced cancer. *American Journal of Hospice and Palliative Medicine*, 32(2), 178–188.

Reuter S., Gupta S. C., Chaturvedi M. M., Aggarwal B. B. (2010). Oxidative stress, inflammation, and cancer: how are they linked? *Free Radic Biol Med*, 49(11), 1603–1616.

Reynolds P., Hurley S., Torres M. et al. (2000). Use of coping strategies and breast cancer survival: results from the Black/White Cancer Survival Study. *Am J Epidemiol*, 152(10), 940–949.

Reznikov A. G., Pishak V. P., Nosenko N. D. et al. (2004). *Prenatal'nyy stress i neyroendokrinnaya patologiya*. Chernovtsy: Medakademiya.

Rice D. (1979). No lung cancer in schizophrenics. *Brit J Psychiat*, 134, 128.

Richardson J., Smith J. E., McCall G. et al. (2007). Hypnosis for nausea and vomiting in cancer chemotherapy: a systematic review of the research evidence. *European Journal of Cancer Care*, 16(5), 402–412.

Richlin V. A., Arevalo J. M., Zack J. A., Cole S. W. (2004). Stress-induced enhancement of NF-kappaB DNA-binding in the peripheral blood leukocyte pool: effects of lymphocyte redistribution. *Brain Behav Immun*, 18(3), 231–237.

Rief W. (2005). Somatoforme und dissoziative Storungen (Konversionsstorungen): Atiologie/Bedingungesanalyse. In: M. Perrez, U. Baumann, *Lehrbuh: Klinische Psychologie—Psychotherapie* (3 Auflage). Bern: Verlag Hans Huber-Hogrefe AG, 947–956.

Rieger M., Pirke K. M., Buske-Kirchbaum A., et al. (2004). Influence of stress during pregnancy on HPA activity and neonatal behavior. *Annals of the New York Academy of Sciences*, 1032(1), 228–230.

Riley V. (1975). Mouse mammary tumors: alteration of incidence as apparent function of stress. *Science*, 189(4201), 465–467.

Riley V. (1981). Psychoneuroendocrine influences on immunocompetence and neoplasia. *Science*, 212, 1100–1109.

Ringdal G. I. (1995). Correlates of hopelessness in cancer patients. *Journal of Psychosocial Oncology*, 13(3), 47–66.

Rintala P. E., Rukkala E., Pakkulainen H. T., Veikko V. J. (2002). Self experienced physical workload and risk of breast cancer. *Scandanavian J Work Environ Health*, 28(3), 158–162.

Ritter H. D., Antonova L., Mueller C. R. (2012). The unliganded glucocorticoid receptor positively regulates the tumor suppressor gene BRCA1 through GABP beta. *Molecular Cancer Research*, 10(4), 558–569.

River C. E. (2013). *British Legends: The Life and Legacy of Audrey Hepburn*. CreateSpace Independent Publishing Platform.

Rizzolatti G., Craighero L. (2004). The mirror-neuron system. *Annual Review of Neuroscience*, 27, 169–192.

Rodríguez-Carvajal R., García-Rubio C., Paniagua D. et al. (2016). Mindfulness Integrative Model (MIM): Cultivating positive states of mind towards oneself and the others through mindfulness and self-compassion. *Anales de Psicología/Annals of Psychology*, 32(3), 749–760.

Roe A., Siegelman M. (1963). A parent-child relations questionnaire. *Child Dev*, 34, 355–369.

Rogentine N. G. Jr, Van Kammen D. P., Fox B. H. et al. (1979). Psychological Factors in the Prognosis of Malignant Melanoma: A Prospective Study. *Psychosomatic Medicine*, 41(8), 647–655.

Rogers C. (1995). *On Becoming a Person: A Therapists View of Psychotherapy*. Wilmington, DE: Mariner Books.

Rogers C. (1995a). *A Way of Being*. Boston, MA: Houghton Mifflin.

Romani M., Pistillo M. P., Banelli B. (2015). Environmental Epigenetics: Crossroad between Public Health, Lifestyle, and Cancer Prevention. *BioMed Research International*, 587983.

Romens S. E., McDonald J., Svaren J., Pollak S. D. (2015). Associations between early life stress and gene methylation in children. *Child development*, 86(1), 303–309.

Romero C., Friedman L. C., Kalidas M. et al. (2006). Self-forgiveness, spirituality, and psychological adjustment in women with breast cancer. *Journal of Behavioral Medicine*, 29, 29–36.

Rosch P. J. (1979). Stress and cancer: A disease of adaptation? In: J. Tache (ed.), *Cancer, stress, and death*. New York: Springer, 187–212.

Rosch P. J. (1991). Job Stress: America's Leading Adult Health Problem. *USA Magazine*, May, 2.

Rosch P. J. (1996). Stress and cancer: Disorders of communication, control, and civilization. In: C. L. Cooper, (ed.), *Handbook of Stress, Medicine, and Health*. Boca Raton, FL: CRC Press, 27–60.

Rosch P. J. (2014). *Stress and Cancer*. The American Institute of Stress. Retrieved 22.08.2014 from: http://www.stress.org/stress-and-cancer/.

Rose D. P., Komninou D., Stephenson G. D. (2004). Obesity, adipocytokines, and insulin resistance in breast cancer. *Obesity Reviews*, 5(3), 153–165.

Rose L. (1954). Some aspects of paranormal healing. *British Medical Journal*, 2(4900), 1329–1332.

Rosen G., Kleinman A., Katon W. (1982). Somatization in family practice: a biopsychosocial approach. *Journal of Family Practice*, 14(3), 493–502.

Rosen T. J., Terry N. S., Leventhal H. (1982). The role of esteem and coping in responce to a threat communication. *Journal of Research in Personality*, 16, 90–107.

Rosenkranz M. A., Davidson R. J., MacCoon D. G. et al. (2013). A comparison of mindfulness-based stress reduction and an active control in modulation of neurogenic inflammation. *Brain, Behavior, and Immunity*, 27, 174–184.

Ross K. (2008). Mapping Pathways From Stress to Cancer Progression. *JNCI*, 100(13), 914–917.

Ross S. A., Dwyer J., Umar A. et al. (2008). Introduction: diet, epigenetic events and cancer prevention. *Nutrition reviews*, 66(suppl 1), S1–S6.

Rossi E. L. (2000). In search of a deep psychobiology of hypnosis: Visionary hypotheses for a new millennium. *American Journal of Clinical Hypnosis*, 42(3-4), 178–207.

Rotenberg V. S., Bondarenko S. M. (1989). *Mozg. Obuchenie. Zdorovye*. Moscow: Prosveschenie.

Roth K. A., Mefford I. M., Barchas J. D. (1982). Epinephrine, norepinephrine, dopamine and serotonin: differential effects of acute and chronic stress on regional brain amines. *Brain Research*, 239(2), 417–424.

Roth M., Abnet C. C., Hu N. et al. (2007). p16, MGMT, RARβ2, CLCLDN3 and MT1G gene methylation in esophageal squamous cell carcinoma and its precursor lesions. *Oncol Rep*, 15, 1591–1597.

Roth T. L., Zoladz P. R., Sweatt J. D., Diamond D. M. (2011). Epigenetic modification of hippocampal Bdnf DNA in adult rats in an animal model of post-traumatic stress disorder. *J Psychiatr Res*, 45(7), 919–926.

Roud P. C. (1989). Psychospiritual dimensions of extraordinary survival. *Journal of Humanistic Psychology*, 29(1), 59–83.

Rozanov V. A. (2004). Nejrobiologicheskie osnovy suicidalnogo povedeniya. *Vestn Biol Psihiatrii (el byull)*, 6, 20–30.

Rozanov V. A. (2012). Stress, epigenetika i psihicheskoe zdorove. *Ukrayinskiy Visnik Psihonevrologiyi*, 20(3), 219.

Rozanov V. A. (2014). Samoubijstva sredi detej i podrostkov chto proishodit i v chem prichina? *Suicidologiya*, 5, 4(17), 16–31.

Rozanov V. A. (2015). Stress-inducirovannye epigeneticheskie fenomeny-eshe odin veroyatnyj biologicheskiy faktor suicida. *Suicidologiya*, 6, 3(20), 3–19.

Rozanov V. A., Emyasheva Z. V., Biron B. V. (2011). Vliyanie travmy detskogo vozrasta na nakoplenie stressovyh sobytiy i formirovanie suicidalnyh tendenciy v techenie zhizni. *Ukrainskiy Medicinskiy Zhurnal*, 6(86), XI–XII.

Rozhkova O. D. (2015). *Sistemnyj podhod v psihologicheskoj rabote s onkopacientami i chlenami ih semej.* Obshestvo semejnyh psihoterapevtov i konsultantov. Retrieved 02.01.2015 from: http://supporter.ru/biblioteka/hronich/rogkova.doc.

Rozhkova O. D., Druzhkova E. A. (2003). Prenatalnyj sindrom, diagnostika i terapiya. *V: Opyt i problemy razvitiya tradicionnyh metodov diagnostiki i lecheniya v Rossii.* Moscow: FNKEC, 3, 36.

Rudnitskiy I. (1930). Psihicheskie perezhivaniya i rak. *Vestnik Hirurgii*, 21, (61), 83.

Rudoy Y. (2016). *Cancer: The Best Gift of My Life.* CreateSpace Independent Publishing Platform.

Rusina N. A. (2009). Telesnost psihosomaticheskogo bolnogo. *Psihologiya telesnosti: teoreticheskie i prakticheskie issledovaniya. Sbornik.* Penza: PGPU, 164–173.

Rusina N. A. (2010). Psihologicheskoe soprovozhdenie onkologicheskih bolnyh na raznyh etapah razvitiya bolezni i ee lecheniya. *Materialy Vserossijskoj nauchno-prakticheskoj konferencii "Psihologicheskoe soprovozhdenie lechebnogo processa."* Kursk.: KGMU, 271–281.

Rusina N. A. (2011). Psihologicheskie osnovy psihosomatiki (Psihoterapevticheskie misheni v rabote s pacientom psihosomaticheskoj kliniki). *Byulleten Medicinskih Internet-Konferencij*, 1(7), 20–23.

Rusina N. A. (2012). Psihologicheskiy status i adaptacionnye resursy onkologicheskih bolnyh. *Rossijskiy Mediko-Biologicheskiy Vestnik Imeni Akademika I. P. Pavlova*, 3, 116–123.

Rusina N. A., Moiseeva K. S. (2013). Kliniko-psihologicheskoe issledovanie pacientov, stradayushih rakom gortani. *Vestnik Yuzhno-Uralskogo Gosudarstvennogo Universiteta. Seriya: Psihologiya*, (1), 14–19.

Russek L. G., Schwartz G. E. (1997). Perceptions of Parental Caring Predict HealthStatus in Midlife: A 35-Year Follow-up of the Harvard Mastery of Stress Study. *Psychosomatic Medicine*, 59, 114–149.

Russo A., Autelitano M., Bisanti L. (2008). Metabolic syndrome and cancer risk. *European Journal of Cancer*, 44(2), 293–297.

Ryan R. M. (1995). Psychological needs and the facilitation of integrative processes. *Journal of Personality*, 63, 397–427.

Ryan R. M., Deci E. L. (2001). A Review of Research on Hedonic and Eudaimonic Well-Being. *Annual Review of Psychology*, 52: 141–166.

Sabbage S. (2016). *The Cancer Whisperer: How to let cancer heal your life.* London: Coronet.

Sachs G., Rasoul-Rockenschaub S., Aschauer H. et al. (1995). Lytic effector cell activity and major depressive disorder in patients with breast cancer: A prospective study. *J Neuroimmunol*, 59, 83–89.

Sadalskaya E. V., Nikolaeva V. V., Enikolopov S. N. (2001). Psihosomaticheskiy podhod v klinike vnutrennih boleznej. V: *Materialy konferencii, posvyashennoj 30-letiyu bolnicy Zavoda im. Lihacheva.* Moscow, 115.

Sadock B. J., Sadock V. A. (2007). *Kaplan and Sadock's Synopsis of Psychiatry*: Behavioral Sciences/Clinical Psychiatry. Philadelphia, PA: LWW.

Sagalakova O. A., Truevcev D. V., Sagalakov A. M. (2014). Psihologicheskie mehanizmy antivitalnoj nastroennosti lichnosti. *Universum: Psihologiya i obrazovanie*, 10(9). Retrieved 01.04.2015 from: http://7universum.com/ru/psy/archive/item/1637.

Saito-Nakaya K., Bidstrup P. E., Nakaya N. et al. (2012). Stress and survival after cancer: A prospective study of a Finnish population-based cohort. *Cancer Epidemiology*, 36(2), 230–235.

Salgado R., Junius S., Benoy I. et al. (2003). Circulating interleukin-6 predicts survival in patients with metastatic breast cancer. *Int J Cancer*, 103, 642–646.

Samundjan E. M. (1954). Vpliv funkcionalnogo oslablennya kori golovnogo mozgu na rist pereshepnih puhlin u mishej. *Med Zhurnal AN USSR*, 24, 10–14.

Sanchis-Gomar F., Garcia-Gimenez J. L., Perez-Quilis C. et al. (2012). Physical exercise as an epigenetic modulator: Eustress, the "positive stress" as an effector of gene expression. *The Journal of Strength & Conditioning Research*, 26(12), 3469–3472.

Sandomirskiy M. E. (2005). *Psihosomatika i telesnaya psihoterapiya: Prakticheskoe rukovodstvo.* Moscow: Klass.

Santarnecchi E., D'Arista S., Egiziano E., Gardi C., Petrosino R. et al. (2014). Interaction between Neuroanatomical and Psychological Changes after Mindfulness-Based Training. *PLoS ONE*, 9(10), e108359.

Santos-Reboucas C. B., Pimentel M. M. (2007). Implication of abnormal epigenetic patterns for human diseases. *Eur J Hum Genet*, 15(1), 10–17.

Sapolsky R. M., Donnelly T. M. (1985). Vulnerability to stress-induced tumor growth increases with age in rats: role of glucocorticoids. *Endocrinology*, 117(2), 662–666.

Sarkar D. K., Murugan S., Zhang C., Boyadjieva N. (2012). Regulation of cancer progression by β-endorphin neuron. *Cancer Res*, 72(4), 836–840.

Saskia F. A. Duijts S., Maurice P. A. et al. (2003). The association between stressful life events and breast cancer risk: A meta-analysis. *International Journal of Cancer*, 107(6), 1023–1029.

Sastry K. S., Karpova Y., Prokopovich S. et al. (2007). Epinephrine protects cancer cells from apoptosis via activation of cAMP-dependent protein kinase and BAD phosphorylation. *J Biol Chem*, 82, 14094–14100.

Saul A. N., Oberyszyn T. M., Daugherty C. et al. (2005). Chronic stress and susceptibility to skin cancer. *Journal of the National Cancer Institute*, 97(23), 1760–1767.

Scheffold K., Philipp R., Koranyi S. et al. (2018). Insecure attachment predicts depression and death anxiety in advanced cancer patients. *Palliative & Supportive Care*, 16(3), 308–316.

Scheflen A. E. (1951). Malignant tumors in the institutionalized psychotic population. *AMA Archives of Neurology & Psychiatry*, 66(2), 145–155.

Scherg H., Blohmke M. (1988). Associations between selected life events and cancer. *Behavioral Medicine*, 14(3), 119–124.

Scherg H., Cramer I., Blohmke M. (1981). Psychosocial factors and breast cancer: A critical reevaluation of established hypotheses. *Cancer Detection and Prevention*, 4, 165–171.

Schernhammer E. S., Hankinson S. E., Rosner B. et al. (2004). Job stress and breast cancer risk: the nurses' health study. *Am J Epidemiol*, 160(11), 1079–1086.

Schilder J. N., de Vries M. J., Goodkin K., Antoni M. (2004). Psychological changes preceding spontaneous remission of cancer. *Clinical Case Studies*, 3(4), 288–312.

Schlatter M. C, Cameron L. D. (2010). Emotional suppression tendencies as predictors of symptoms, mood, and coping appraisals during AC chemotherapy for breast cancer treatment. *Ann Behav Med*, 40(1), 15–29.

Schmale A. H. (1964). A genetic view of affects: With special reference to the genesis of helplessness and hopelessness. *The Psychoanalytic Study of the Child*, 19(1), 287–310.

Schmale A. H, Iker H. P. (1964). The affect of hopelessness in the development of cancer: Part 1: The prediction of uterine cervical cancer in women with atypical cytology. *Psychosom Med*, 26, 634–635.

Schmale A. H., Iker H. P. (1971). Hopelessness as a predictor of cervical cancer. *Social Science & Medicine*, 5(2), 95–100.

Schmidt M. E., Chang-Claude J., Vrieling A. et al. (2012). Fatigue and quality of life in breast cancer survivors: temporal courses and long-term pattern. *J Cancer Surviv*, 6(1), 11–19.

Schmidt S. D., Blank T. O., Bellizzi K. M., Park C. L. (2012). The relationship of coping strategies, social support, and attachment style with posttraumatic growth in cancer survivors. *Journal of Health Psychology*, 17(7), 1033–1040.

Schneider R. H., Nidich S. I., Salerno J. W. et al. (1998). Lower lipid peroxide levels in practitioners of the Transcendental Meditation program. *Psychosom Med*, 60(1), 38–41.

Schoemaker M. J., Jones M. E., Wright L. B. et al. (2016). Psychological stress, adverse life events and breast cancer incidence: a cohort investigation in 106,000 women in the United Kingdom. *Breast Cancer Research*, 18(1), 72.

Schofield T. J., Lee R. D., Merrick M. T. (2013). Safe, stable, nurturing relationships as a moderator of intergenerational continuity of child maltreatment: a meta-analysis. *J Adolesc Health*, 53, S32–S38.

Schore A. N. (2001). The effects of early relational trauma on right brain development, affect regulation, and infant mental health. *Infant Mental Health Journal*, 22, 201–269.

Schrepf A., Clevenger L., Christensen D. et al. (2013). Cortisol and inflammatory processes in ovarian cancer patients following primary treatment: relationships with depression, fatigue, and disability. *Brain, Behavior, and Immunity*, 30, S126–S134.

Schuller H. M., Al-Wadei H. A., Ullah M. F. Plummer H. K. III (2011). Regulation of pancreatic cancer by neuropsychological stress responses: a novel target for intervention. *Carcinogenesis*, 33(1), 191–196.

Schur M. (1955). Comments on the metapsychogy of somatisation. *The Psychoanalytic of the Child*, 10, 119–164.

Schwartz R., Geyer S. (1984). Social and psychological differences between cancer and noncancer patients: cause or consequence of the disease? *Psychother Psychosom*, 41, 195–199.

Schwarz R., Heim M. (2000). Psychosocial considerations about spontaneous remission of cancer. *Oncology Research and Treatment*, 23(5), 432–435.

Schweitzer A. (1957). Preface to *Cancer: Nature, Cause and Cure*, by Dr Alexander Berglas. Paris: Institut Pasteur.

Seawell A. H., Toussaint L. L., Cheadle A. C. (2014). Prospective associations between unforgiveness and physical health and positive mediating mechanisms in a nationally representative sample of older adults. *Psychol Health*, 29(4), 375–389.

Segerstrom S. C., Miller G. E. (2004). Psychological Stress and the Human Immune System: A Meta-Analytic Study of 30 Years of Inquiry. *Psychol Bull*, 130(4), 601–630.

Sehlen S., Hollenhorst H., Schymura B. et al. (2000). Radiotherapy: impact of quality of life and need for psychological care: results of a longitudinal study. *Onkologie*, 23(6), 565–570.

Selemon L. D., Rajkowska G., Goldmanrakic P. S. (1995). Abnormally high neuronal density in the schizophrenic cortex – a morphometric analysis of prefrontal area-9 and occipital area-17. *Arch Gen Psychiatry*, 52, 805–818.

Selhub E. M. (2002). Stress and distress in clinical practice: a mind-body approach. *Nutr Clin Care*, 5(4), 182–190.

Seligman M. E. P. (1975). *Helplessness: On depression, development, and death*. San Francisco, CA: Freeman.

Seligson D. B., Horvath S., Shi T. et al. (2005). Global histone modification patterns predict risk of prostate cancer recurrence. *Nature*, 435, 1262–1266.

Selye H. (1952). *The story of the adaptation syndrome: Told in the form of informal, illustrated lectures*. Montreal: Acta.

Selye H. (1975). *Stress Without Distress*. New York: Signet Publishing.

Semenov I. V. (2005). *Teoreticheskie voprosy etiologii, patofiziologii, patomorfologii i kulturologii duhovno-psihosomaticheskih boleznej. Traktat*. Barnaul: AGMU.

Semenov S. P. (2007). *Antropoptoz. Socialno obuslovlennaya samolikvidaciya cheloveka*. Saint Petersburg: ZAO TAT.

Semenovich A. V. (2002). *Nejropsihologicheskaya diagnostika i korrekciya v detskom vozraste: Uchebnoe posobie dlya vysshih uchebnyh zavedenij.* Moscow: Akademiya.

Senkov O. (2010). Epigenetika: perepisat kod zhizni. *Zdorovje*, January 2010. Retrieved 07.11.2011 from: http://zdr.ru.

Sephton S. E., Sapolsky R. M., Kraemer H. C., Spiegel D. (2000). Diurnal cortisol rhythm as a predictor of breast cancer survival. *J Natl Cancer Inst*, 92, 994–1000.

Sephton S. E., Dhabhar F. S., Keuroghlian A. S. et al. (2009). Depression, cortisol, and suppressed cell-mediated immunity in metastatic breast cancer. *Brain Behav Immun*, 3(8), 1148–1155.

Sephton S. E., Lush E., Dedert E. A. et al. (2013). Diurnal cortisol rhythm as a predictor of lung cancer survival. *Brain Behav Immun*, 30 Suppl, S163– S170.

Serebryanaya O. (2006). Ne-Lolita. *Oktyabr*, 1, 176–184.

Serova L. I., Maharjan S., Sabban E. L. (2005). Estrogen modifies stress response of catecholamine biosynthetic enzyme genes and cardiovascular system in ovariectomized female rats. *Neuroscience*, 32(2), 249–259.

Servan-Schreiber D. (2009). *Anticancer: A New Way of Life.* New York: Viking.

Seth R., Tai L. H., Falls T. et al. (2013). Surgical stress promotes the development of cancer metastases by a coagulation-dependent mechanism involving natural killer cells in a murine model. *Annals of surgery*, 258(1), 158–168.

Seybold K. S., Hill P. C., Neumann J. K., Chi D. S. (2001). Physiological and psychological correlates of forgiveness. *Journal of Psychology and Christianity*, 20, 250–259.

Shaffer J., Duszynski K., Thomas C. (1982). Family attitudes in youth as possible precursor of cancer among physicians. *J Behav Med*, 5, 143–163.

Shaffer J., Graves P., Swank R., Pearson T. (1987). Clustering of personality traits in youth and the subsequent development of cancer among physicians. *J Behav Med*, 10, 441–447.

Shand L. K., Cowlishaw S., Brooker J. E. et al. (2015). Correlates of post-traumatic stress symptoms and growth in cancer patients: A systematic review and meta-analysis. *Psycho-Oncology*, 24(6), 624–634.

Shansky R. M., Glavis-Bloom C., Lerman D. et al. (2004). Estrogen mediates sex differences in stress-induced prefrontal cortex dysfunction. *Molecular psychiatry*, 9(5), 531–538.

Shapiro D. (1990). *The Bodymind Workbook: Exploring How the Mind and the Body Work Together.* New York: Element Books.

Shapiro F. (2001). *Eye Movement Desensitization and Reprocessing (EMDR): Basic Principles, Protocols, and Procedures.* New York: The Guilford Press.

Shaposhnikov A. V. (1998). *Yatrogeniya. Terminologicheskiy analiz i konstruirovanie ponyatij.* Rostov-na-Donu: Kniga.

Sharma A., Sharp D. M., Walker L. G., Monson J. R. (2008). Patient personality predicts postoperative stay after colorectal cancer resection. *Colorectal Dis*, 10(2),151–156.

Sharma H., Datta P., Singh A. et al. (2008). Gene expression profiling in practitioners of Sudarshan Kriya. *J Psychosom Res*, 64(2), 213–218.

Shave D. W. (1974). Depression as a manifestation of unconscious guilt. *Journal of the American Academy of Psychoanalysis*, 2(4), 309–327.

Shaw A., Joseph S., Linley P. A. (2005). Religion, spirituality, and posttraumatic growth: A systematic review. *Mental Health, Religion & Culture*, 8(1), 1–11.

Shekelle R. B., Raynor W. J. Jr, Ostfeld A. M. et al. (1981). Psychological Depression and 17-Year Risk of Death from Cancer. *Psychosomatic medicine*, 43(2), 117–125.

Shelby R. A., Golden-Kreutz D. M., Andersen B. L. (2008). PTSD diagnoses, subsyndromal symptoms, and comorbidities contribute to impairments for breast cancer survivors. *Journal of traumatic stress*, 21(2), 165–172.

Shennan C., Payne S., Fenlon D. (2011). What is the evidence for the use of mindfulness-based interventions in cancer care? A review. *Psycho-Oncology*, 20(7), 681–697.

Shchepin V., Masyakin A. (2014). Struktura osnovnyh prichin letalnosti bolnyh shizofreniej v g. Moskve (2007-2013 gg.). *Ros Psihiatr Zhurn*, 3, 57–60.

Sheridan J. F., Dobbs C., Jung J. et al. (1998). Stress-induced neuroendocrine modulation of viral pathogenesis and immunity. *Ann N Y Acad Sci*, 840, 803–808.

Shevchenko Y., Velikanova L. (2014). Koncepciya mnogourovnevogo podhoda k psihoterapii psihosomaticheskih rasstrojstv. *Teoriya i Praktika Psihoterapii*, 2, 19–27.

Shevelenkova T. D., Fesenko P. P. (2005). Psihologicheskoe blagopoluchie lichnosti. *Psihologicheskaya Diagnostika*, 3, 95–129.

Shin L. M., Wright C. I., Cannistraro P. A. et al. (2005). A functional magnetic resonance imaging study of amygdala and medial prefrontal cortex responses to overtly presented fearful faces in posttraumatic stress disorder. *Arch Gen Psychiatry*, 62(3), 273–281.

Shively C. A., Register T. C., Grant K. A. et al. (2004). Effects of social status and moderate alcohol consumption on mammary gland and endometrium of surgically postmenopausal monkeys. *Menopause*, 11(4), 389–399.

Shmakova T. V., Baranskaya L. T., Klimusheva N. F. (2009). Vliyanie samoregulyacii i psihologicheskogo reabilitacionnogo potenciala na kachestvo zhizni u onkogematologicheskih bolnyh. *Psihologicheskiy Vestnik Uralskogo Gosudarstvennogo Universiteta*, 7, 147–163.

Shneidman E. S. (1998). *The Suicidal Mind*. Oxford: Oxford University Press.

Shonkoff J. P., Boyce W. T., McEwen B. S. (2009). Neuroscience, molecular biology, and the childhood roots of health disparities: Building a new framework for health promotion and disease prevention. *JAMA*, 301, 2252–2259.

Shoygu Y. S. (2007). *Psihologiya ekstremalnyh situaciy dlya spasatelej i pozharnyh*. Moscow: Smysl.

Shpak V. S., Makarov A. V., Sokur I. V., Mavrovskaya T. N. (2016). Izmenenie kachestva zhizni bolnyh rakom molochnoj zhelezy v techenie treh nedel posle mastektomii na fone cigun-treninga i v otdelnom sluchae metastaticheskogo raka molochnoj zhelezy na protyazhenii 9 mesyacev nablyudeniya i cigun-treninga. *Reabilitaciya ta Paliativna Medicina*, 1(3), 105.

Shtrakhova A. V., Kulikova E. V. (2012). Psihodinamicheskiy aspekt issledovaniya struktury lichnosti kak faktora riska psihosomaticheskih narushenij. Chast II (rezultaty klinicheskogo i eksperimentalnogo issledovaniya). *Vestnik Yuzhno-Uralskogo Gos Univ, Seriya Psihologiya*, 45(304), 88–99.

Shulsinger F., Kety S., Rosenthal D. et al. (1979). A family story of suicide. In: M. Schou & E. Stromgen (eds), *Origins, prevention and treatment of affective disorders*. New York: Academic Press, 277–278.

Shutcenberger A. A. (1990). Tyazhelobolnoj pacient (15-letniy opyt primeneniya psihodramy dlya lecheniya raka). *Voprosy Psihologii*, (5), 94–106.

Sidorov P. I., Novikova I. A. (2007). Sinergeticheskaya koncepciya formirovaniya psihosomaticheskih zabolevanij. *Socialnaya i Klinicheskaya Psihiatriya*, 17(3), 76–81.

Sidorov P. I., Novikova I. A. (2010). Psihosomaticheskie zabolevaniya: koncepcii, rasprostranennost, KZh, mediko-socialnaya pomosh bolnym. *Medicinskaya Psihologiya v Rossii: Elektronnyj Nauchnyj Zhurnal*. Retrieved 02.10.2014 from: http://medpsy.ru.

Sidorov P. I., Sovershaeva E. P. (2015). Sinergeticheskaya biopsihosocioduhovnaya koncepciya socialnoj epidemii onkologicheskih zabolevanij. *Ekologiya Cheloveka*, 4, 44–57.

Sidorova O. A. (2001). *Nejropsihologiya emocij*. Moscow: Nauka.

Siegel B. S. (1989). *Peace, Love and Healing: Bodymind Communication & the Path to Self-Healing: An Exploration*. New York: Harper & Row.

Siegel B. S. (1998). *Love, Medicine and Miracles: Lessons Learned about Self-Healing from a Surgeon's Experience with Exceptional Patients*. New York: William Morrow.

Siegman A. W., Townsend S. T., Blumenthal R. S. et al. (1998). Dimensions of anger and CHD in men and women: self-ratings versus spouse ratings. *Journal of Behavioral Medicine*, 21(4), 315–336.

Sim B. Y., Lee Y. W., Kim H., Kim S. H. (2015). Post-traumatic growth in stomach cancer survivors: Prevalence, correlates and relationship with health-related quality of life. *European Journal of Oncology Nursing*, 19(3), 230–236.

Simon W. E., Albrecht M., Trams G. et al. (1984). In vitro growth promotion of human mammary carcinoma cells by steroid hormones, tamoxifen, and prolactin. *Journal of the National Cancer Institute*, 73(2), 313–321.

Simonov P. V. (1987). *Motivirovannyj Mozg*. Moscow:Nauka.

Simonton O. C., Matthews-Simonton S., Creighton J. (1978). *Getting Well Again: A Step-By-Step Self-Help Guide to Overcoming Cancer for Patients and Their Families*. Los Angeles: J. P. Tarcher.

Simonton O. C., Henson R. M. (1992). *The Healing Journey*. New York: Bantam Books.

Simonton-Atchley S. (1993). The influence of psychological therapy on the immune system in patients with advanced cancer. *Dissertation Abstracts International*, 55, 128.

Sindelar W. F., Ketcham A. S. (1976). Regression of cancer following surgery. *NCIM*, 44, 81–84.

Sinelnikov V. (2012). *Vozlyubi bolezn svoyu. Kak stat zdorovym, poznav radost zhizni*. Moscow: Centrpoligraf.

Sinha A. K., Kumar S. (2014). Integrating spirituality into patient care: An essential element of modern healthcare system. *Indian Heart Journal*, 66(3), 395.

Sirota N. A., Moskovchenko D. V., Yaltonskaya A. V. (2014). Sovladayushee povedenie zhenshin s onkologicheskimi zabolevaniyami reproduktivnoj sistemy. *Medicinskaya Psihologiya v Rossii: Elektron Nauch zhurn*, 1(24), 10. Retrieved 15.12.2014 from: http://mprj.ru.

Sirotkina M. Y., Bergfeld A. Y. (2012). Uroven stressoustojchivosti kak korrelyat prodolzheniya onkologicheskogo zabolevaniya. V: *Budushee psihologii*. Materialy konferencii. Perm: PGNIU, 141–153.

Sivonova M., Zitnanova I., Hlincikova L. et al. (2004). Oxidative stress in university students during examinations. *Stress*, 7, 183–188.

Sklar L. S., Anisman H. (1980). Social stress influences tumor growth. *Psychosomatic Medicine*, 42(3), 347–365.

Skovoroda G. S. (1973). *Narkiss*. Povne zibrannya tvoriv u 2-h t. K.: Naukova dumka, T. 1, 154–200.

Slater G. R. (1982). *Regression of cancer as an instance of Gotthard Booth's concept of kairos*. Doctoral dissertation, Boston University.

Slavich G. M., O'Donovan A., Epel E. S., Kemeny M. E. (2010). Black sheep get the blues: a psychobiological model of social rejection and depression. *Neuroscience & Biobehavioral Reviews*, 35(1), 39–45.

Sloan E. K., Priceman S. J., Cox B. F. et al. (2010). The sympathetic nervous system induces a metastatic switch in primary breast cancer. *Cancer Research*, 70(18), 7042–7052.

Smirnov M. (2007). *Ne uhodi iz zhizni. Kak uderzhat ot greha samoubijstva?* Saint Petersburg: Satis.

Smith J. E., Richardson J., Hoffman C., Pilkington K. (2005). Mindfulness-Based Stress Reduction as supportive therapy in cancer care: systematic review. *J Adv Nurs*, 52(3), 315–327.

Smith S. K., Zimmerman S., Williams C. S. et al. (2011). Post-traumatic stress symptoms in long-term non-Hodgkin's lymphoma survivors: does time heal? *Journal of Clinical Oncology*, JCO–2011.

Smith W. R., Sebastian H. (1976). Emotional history and pathogenesis of cancer. *Journal of Clinical Psychology*, 32(4), 863–866.

Smulevich A. B. (1997). Psihosomaticheskie rasstrojstva. *Socialnaya i Klinicheskaya Psihiatriya*, 7(1), 5–18.

Smulevich A. B. (2007). *Depressii v obshej medicine: Rukovodstvo dlya vrachej*. Moscow: Med. inf. agenstvo

Smulevich A. B. (2011). *Psihicheskie rasstrojstva v klinicheskoj praktike*. Moscow: Medpress-inform.

Snow H. L. (1893). *Cancer and the cancer process*. London: J. & A. Churchill.

Snow H. L. (1893a). *A Treatise: Practical and Theoretic on Cancers and the Cancer Process*. London: J. & A. Churchill.

Sobel D. S. (2000). The cost-effectiveness of mind-body medicine interventions. *Prog Brain Res*, 122, 393–412.

Soczynska J. K., Kennedy S. H., Woldeyohannes H. O. et al. (2011). Mood disorders and obesity: understanding inflammation as a pathophysiological nexus. *Neuromolecular Med*, 13(2), 93–116.

Sokolova E. D., Berezin F. B., Barlas T. V. (1996). Emocionalnyj stress: psihologicheskie mehanizmy, klinicheskie proyavleniya, psihoterapiya. *MateriaMedica*, 1(9), 5–25.

Sokolova E. T., Sotnikova Y. A. (2006). Problema suicida: kliniko-psihologicheskiy rakurs. *Voprosy Psihologii*, 4, 103–115.

Sokolova G. B., Tsarkova M. Y. (1987). Znachenie opredeleniya obshih nespecificheskih adaptacionnyh reakciy organizma v klinike vnutrennih boleznej. *Estestvennye nauki—zdravoohraneniyu*. Tezisy dokl. konf. Perm, 37–38.

Soldatova O. G., Savchenkov Yu. I., Shilov S. N. (2007). Temperament cheloveka kak faktor, vliyayushiy na uroven zdorovya. *Fiziologiya Cheloveka*, 33(2), 76–80.

Solomon S. S., Odunusi O., Carrigan D. et al. (2010). TNF-alpha inhibits insulin action in liver and adipose tissue: A model of metabolic syndrome. *Horm Metab Res*, 42(2), 115–121.

Soloviev V. L. (1990). *Opravdanie dobra. Nravstvennaya filosofiya*. Soch. v 2-h t. Moscow: Mysl, 1, 47–548.

Solozhenkin V. V. (2003). *Psihologicheskie osnovy vrachebnoj deyatelnosti: Uchebnik dlya studentov vysshih uchebnyh zavedenij*. Moscow: Akad. Proyect.

Song C., Leonard B. E. (2000). *Fundamentals of Psychoneuroimmunology*. New York: John Wiley & Sons.

Song L., Zheng J., Li H. et al. (2009). Prenatal stress causes oxidative damage to mitochondrial DNA in hippocampus of offspring rats. *Neurochem Res*, 34(4), 739–745.

Sood A. K., Lutgendorf S. K. (2011). Stress Influences on Anoikis. *Cancer Prev Res (Phila)*, 4(4), 481–485.

Sood A. K., Bhatty R., Kamat A. A. et al. (2006). Stress hormone-mediated invasion of ovarian cancer cells. *Clin Cancer Res*, 12, 369–375.

Sorokina T. T., Evsegneev R. A. (1986). O psihosomaticheskom balansirovanii. *Zhurn Nevropatol i Psihiatr*, 1, 1730–1732.

Sotnikov V. A. (2014). *Kriterii psihologicheskoj adaptacii lichnosti zhenshiny k kriticheskoj zhiznennoj situacii onkologicheskogo zabolevaniya*. Diss. kand. psihol. nauk. Kursk: KGMU.

Soto A. M., Sonnenschein C. (2005). Emergentism as a default: cancer as a problem of tissue organization. *J Biosci*, 30(1), 103–118.

Southwick S. M., Paige S., Morgan C. A. 3rd et al. (1999). Neurotransmitter alterations in PTSD: catecholamines and serotonin. *Seminars in Clinical Neuropsychiatry*, 4(4), 242–248.

Specht J. A., King G. A., Willoughby C. et al. (2005). Issues and Insights: Spirituality: A coping mechanism in the lives of adults with congenital disabilities. *Counseling and Values*, 50, 51–62.

Spector L. G. (2010). Assessing parental contributions to childhood cancer risk. *Future Oncol*, 6(1), 5–7.

Spence D. (1979). Somato-psychic signs of cervical cancer. Read before the *87th Annual American Psychiatric Association Convention*, New York, Sept 1.

Speranskiy A. D. (1937). *Elementy postroeniya teorii mediciny*. Moscow-Leningrad: VIEM.

Spiegel D. (1991). A Psychosocial Intervention and Survival Time of Patients with Metastatic Breast Cancer. *Advances*, 7(3),10–19.

Spiegel D. (2001). Mind matters: Coping and cancer progression. *Journal of Psychosomatic Research*, 50(5), 287–290.

Spiegel D. (2012). Mind Matters in Cancer Survival. *Psycho–oncology*, 21(6), 588–593.

Spiegel D., Yalom I. D. (1978). A support group for dying patients. *Int J Group Psychother*, 28, 233–245.

Spiegel D., Kraemer H., Bloom J., Gottheil E. (1989). Effect of psychosocial treatment on survival of patients with metastatic breast cancer. *The Lancet*, 334(8668), 888–891.

Spivak L. I. (1988). Izmenennye sostoyaniya soznaniya u zdorovyh lyudej (postanovka voprosa, perspektivy issledovanij). *Fiziologiya Cheloveka*, 14(1), 138–147.

Spoletini I., Gianni W., Repetto L. et al. (2008). Depression and cancer: an unexplored and unresolved emergent issue in elderly patients. *Critical Reviews in Oncology/Hematology*, 65(2), 143–155.

Spoto D. (2007). *Enchantment: The Life of Audrey Hepburn*. New York: Three Rivers Press.

Srikumar R., Parthasarathy N. J., Manikandan S. et al. (2006). Effect of Triphala on oxidative stress and on cell-mediated immune response against noise stress in rats. *Mol Cell Biochem*, 283, 67–74.

Stahl S. M. (2012). Psychotherapy as an epigenetic 'drug': psychiatric therapeutics target symptoms linked to malfunctioning brain circuits with psychotherapy as well as with drugs. *Journal of Clinical Pharmacy and Therapeutics*, 37(3), 249–253.

Stark D., Kiely M., Smith A. et al. (2002). Anxiety disorders in cancer patients: their nature, associations, and relation to quality of life. *J Clin Oncol*, 20(14), 3137–3148.

Starostin O. A. (2013). Holisticheskiy podhod v diagnostike i psihoterapii somatoformnyh rasstrojstv. *Vestnik Psihoterapii*, 47, 23–29.

Starshenbaum G. V. (2005). *Suicidologiya i krizisnaya psihoterapiya*. Moscow: Kogito-Centr.

Starshenbaum G. V. (2015). *Psihosomatika i psihoterapiya. Iscelenie dushi i tela*. Rostov-na-Donu: Feniks.

Statham D. J., Heath A. C., Madden P. A. et al. (1998). Suicidal behavior: an epidemiological and genetic study. *Psychological Medicine*, 28, 839–855.

Steel J. L., Geller D. A., Gamblin T. C. et al. (2007). Depression, immunity, and survival in patients with hepatobiliary carcinoma. *J Clin Oncol*, 25, 2397–2405.

Stefanski V., Ben-Eliyahu S. (1996). Social confrontation and tumor metastasis in rats: defeat and beta-adrenergic mechanisms. *Physiol Behav*, 60(1), 277–282.

Stefansson V. (1960). *Cancer: Disease of Civilization?: An Anthropological and Historical Study*. New York: Hill and Wang.

Stein K. D., Syrjala K. L., Andrykowski M. A. (2008). Physical and psychological long-term and late effects of cancer. *Cancer*, 112(11 Suppl), 2577–2592.

Stellar J. E., John-Henderson N., Anderson C. L. et al. (2015). Positive affect and markers of inflammation: Discrete positive emotions predict lower levels of inflammatory cytokines. *Emotion*, 15(2), 129.

Stengrevics S., Sirois C., Schwartz C. E. et al. (1996). The prediction of cardiac surgery outcome based upon preoperative psychological factors. *Psychology and Health*, 11(4), 471–477.

Stepanchuk E., Zhirkov A., Yakovleva A. (2013). The Coping Strategies, Psychological Defense Mechanisms and Emotional Response to the Disease in Russian Patients with Chronic Leukemia. *Procedia—Social and Behavioral Sciences*, 86, 248–255.

Stepanenko A. A., Kavsan V. M. (2012). Immortalization and malignant transformation of Eukaryotic cells. *Cytology and Genetics*, 46(2), 96–129.

Stepanov N. S. (2007). *Gipnoz i rak. Opyt prakticheskogo primeneniya*. Rostov-na-Donu: Feniks.

Stepp S. D., Morse J. Q., Yaggi K. E. et al. (2008). The Role of Attachment Styles and Interpersonal Problems in Suicide-Related Behaviors. *Suicide and Life-Threatening Behavior*, 38(5), 592–607.

Steptoe A., Hamer M., Butcher L. et al. (2011). Educational attainment but not measures of current socioeconomic circumstances are associated with leukocyte telomere length in healthy older men and women. *Brain Behav Immun*, 25(7), 1292–1298.

Steptoe A., Phil D., Cropley M. et al. (2000). Job strain and anger expression predict early morning elevations in salivary cortisol. *Psychosom Med*, 62, 286–292.

Stewart D. E., Duff S., Wong F. et al. (2001). The views of ovarian cancer survivors on its cause, prevention, and recurrence. *Medscape Women's Health*, 6(5), 5.

Stewart F. W. (1952). Experiences in spontaneous regression of neoplastic disease in man. *Texas Reports on Biology and Medicine*, 10(1), 239–253.

Stommel M., Given B. A., Given C. W. (2002). Depression and functional status as predictors of death among cancer patients. *Cancer*, 94(10), 2719–2727.

Stone A. A. (1987). Event content in a daily survey is differentially associated with concurrent mood. *Journal of Personality and Social Psychology*, 52(1), 56–58.

Stone A. A., Mezzacappa E. S., Donatone B. A., Gonder M. (1999). Psychosocial stress and social support are associated with prostate-specific antigen levels in men: results from a community screening program. *Health Psychol*, 18(5), 482–486.

Stone H., Winkelman S. (1988). *Embracing Our Selves: Voice Dialogue Manual*. Springfield, CA: Nataraj Publishing.

Stone R. B., Silva J. (1992). *You the Healer: The World-Famous Silva Method on How to Heal Yourself and Others*. Novato, CA: H. J. Kramer.

Stowe R. P., Pierson D. L., Barrett A. D. (2001). Elevated stress hormone levels relate to Epstein-Barr virus reactivation in astronauts. *Psychosom Med*, 63(6), 891–895.

Stowe R. P., Peek M. K., Perez N. A. et al. (2010). Herpesvirus reactivation and socioeconomic position: a community-based study. *J Epidemiol Community Health*, 64(8), 666–671.

Strand J., Goulding A., Tidefors I. (2015). Attachment styles and symptoms in individuals with psychosis. *Nordic Journal of Psychiatry*, 69(1), 67–72.

Straub R., Harle P. (2005). Sympathetic neurotransmitters in joint inflammation. *Rheum Dis Clin N Am*, 31(1), 43–59.

Strauman T. J., Lemieux A. M., Coe C. L. (1993). Self-discrepancy and natural killer cell activity: Immunological consequences of negative self-evaluation. *Journal of Personality and Social Psychology*, 64, 1042–1052.

Strukov A. I., Esipova I. K., Kakturskiy L. V. et al. (1990). *Obshaya patologiya cheloveka: Rukovodstvo dlya vrachey*. V 2 tomah. Moscow: Medicina.

Strunecka A., Hynie S., Klenerova V. (2009). Role of Oxytocin/Oxytocin Receptor System in Regulation of Cell Growth and Neoplastic Processes. *Folia Biologica*, 55(5), 159–165.

Stuckelberger A. (2005). Spirituality, Religion and Health. *United Nations Geneva Panel Report: Spirituality, Religion and Social Health*. 58th World Health Assembly in Geneva. Retrieved 04.05.2015 from: http://reseau-crescendo.org/wp-content/uploads/2014/04/SPIRITUALITY.pdf.

Subnis U. B., Starkweather A. R., McCain N. L., Brown R. F. (2014). Psychosocial therapies for patients with cancer: A current review of interventions using psychoneuroimmunology-based outcome measures. *Integr Cancer Ther*, 13(2), 85–104.

Sudakov K. V. (2005). Individualnost emocionalnogo stressa. *Zhurnal Nevrologiya i Psihiatriya*, 2, 4–12.

Sudakov K. V. (2007). Teoriya funkcionalnyh sistem: postulaty i principy postroeniya organizma cheloveka v norme i pri patologii. *Patologicheskaya Fiziologiya i Eksperimentalnaya Terapiya*, 4, 2–11.

Sugano K. (2008). Multiple genetic and epigenetic changes involving many key regulatory factors occur in chronic gastritis, eventually leading to cancer. *Gastric Cancer: Pathogenesis, Screening, and Treatment. Gastrointestinal endoscopy clinics of North America*, 18(3), 513–522.

Suhail N., Bilal N., Hasan S. et al. (2015). Chronic unpredictable stress (CUS) enhances the carcinogenic potential of 7, 12-dimethylbenz (a) anthracene (DMBA) and accelerates the onset of tumor development in Swiss albino mice. *Cell Stress and Chaperones*, 20(6), 1023–1036.

Sulmasy D. (2002). A Biopsychosocial-Spiritual Model for the Care of Patients at the End of Life. *The Gerontologist*, 42, Special Issue III, 24–33.

Sumalla E. C., Ochoa C., Blanco I. (2009). Posttraumatic growth in cancer: reality or illusion? *Clin Psychol Rev*, 29(1), 24–33.

Sumin A. N., Rajh O. I., Sumina L. Y., Barbarash N. A. (2012). *Tip lichnosti D pri serdechno-sosudistyh zabolevaniyah: klinicheskoe znachenie, metodika vyyavleniya.* Kemerovo: KemGMA.

Sun Y., Campisi J., Higano C. et al. (2012). Treatment-induced damage to the tumor microenvironment promotes prostate cancer therapy resistance through WNT16B. *Nature medicine*, 18(9), 1359–1368.

Svalina S. S., Webb J. R. (2012). Forgiveness and health among people in outpatient physical therapy. *Disabil Rehabil*, 4(5), 383–392.

Svrakic D. M., Zorumski C. F., Svrakic N. M. et al. (2013). Risk architecture of schizophrenia: the role of epigenetics. *Current Opinion in Psychiatry*, 26(2), 188–195.

Svyadosh A. M. (1971). *Nevrozy i ih lechenie.* Moscow: Medicina.

Swan G. E., Carmelli D., Dame A. et al. (1991). The Rationality/Emotional Defensiveness Scale-I. Internal Structure and Stability. *Journal of Psychosomatic Research*, 35, 545–554.

Swanson J. M., Entringer S., Buss C., Wadhwa P. D. (2009). Developmental origins of health and disease: environmental exposures. *Semin Reprod Med*, 27(5), 391–402.

Syrian I. (1998). *Slova podvizhnicheskie.* Moscow: Izd. Sretenskogo monastyrya.

Szanto K., Shear M. K., Houck P. R. (2006). Indirect self-destructive behavior and overt suicidality in patients with complicated grief. *J Clin Psychiatry*, 67, 233–239.

Szlosarek P., Charles K. A., Balkwill F. R. (2006). Tumour necrosis factor-alpha as a tumour promoter. *Eur J Cancer*, 2(6), 745–750.

Szyf M., Weaver I. C., Champagne F. A. et al. (2005). Maternal programming of steroid receptor expression and phenotype through DNA methylation in the rat. *Front Neuroendocrinol*, 6, 139–162.

Tacon A. M. (1998). *Parent-child relations, attachment, and emotional control in the development of breast cancer: a dissertation in human development and family studies.* A dissertation for the degree of Ph.D. Lubbock, TX: Texas Tech University.

Tacon A. M. (2006). Developmental health contextualism: from attachment to mindfulness-based therapy in cancer. In: M. E. Abelian, *Trends in psychotherapy research*. New York: Nova Publishers, 1–32.

Tacon A. M. (2012). PTSD in the Context of Malignant Disease. In: Ovuga E. (ed.), *Post Traumatic Stress Disorders in a Global Context*. Rijeka: INTECH, 227–246.

Tao Y., Ruan J., Yeh S. H. et al. (2011). Rapid growth of a hepatocellular carcinoma and the driving mutations revealed by cell-population genetic analysis of whole-genome data. *Proc Natl Acad Sci USA*, 108(29), 12042–12047.

Tarabrina N. V. (2014). Posttravmaticheskiy stress u bol'nykh ugrozhayushchimi zhizni (onkologicheskimi) zabolevaniyami. *Konsul'tativnaya Psikhologiya i Psikhoterapiya*, 1, 40–63.

Tarabrina N. V., Gens G. P., Padun M. A. et al. (2008). Vzaimosvyaz psihologicheskih harakteristik posttravmaticheskogo stressa i immunologicheskih parametrov u bolnyh rakom molochnoj zhelezy. *Socialnaya i Klinicheskaya Psihiatriya*, 18(4), 22–28.

Tarabrina N. V., Vorona O. A., Kurchakova M. S. et al. (2010). *Onkopsihologiya: posttravmaticheskiy stress u bolnyh rakom molochnoj zhelezy.* Moscow: Institut psihologii RAN.

Tarnavskiy Y. B. (1990). *Pod maskoj telesnogo neduga (problemy psihosomatiki).* Moscow: Znanie.

Tarnovskaya N. N. (2014). Opyt garmonizacii lokusa kontrolya onkologicheskih bolnyh v hode psihologicheskogo soprovozhdeniya. *Istoricheskaya i Socialno-Obrazovatelnaya Mysl,* 5.

Tart C. (1987). *Waking Up: Overcoming the Obstacles to Human Potential.* Boulder, CO: Shambhala.

Tas F., Karalar U., Aliustaoglu M. et al. (2012). The major stressful life events and cancer: stress history and cancer. *Med Oncol,* 29(2), 1371–1377.

Taylor E. J. (2003). Spiritual needs of patients with cancer and family caregivers. *Cancer nursing,* 26(4), 260–266.

Taylor G. J. (1984). Alexithymia: concept, measurement and implications for treatment. *Am J Psychiat,* 141(6), 725–732.

Tedeschi R. G., Calhoun L. G. (1995). *Trauma and transformation: Growing in the aftermath of suffering.* Thousand Oaks, CA: Sage Publications.

Tedeschi R. G., Calhoun L. G. (2004). Posttraumatic growth: Conceptual foundations and empirical evidence. *Psychological Inquiry,* 15(1), 1–18.

Teicher M. (2002). Scars that will not heal: The neurobiology of child abuse. *Scientific American,* 286(3), 68–75.

Temoshok L. (1985). Biopsychosocial Studies on Cutaneous Malignant Melanoma: Psychosocial Factors Associated with Prognostic Indicators, Progression, Psychophysiology, and Tumor-Host Response. *Social Science and Medicine,* 20(8), 833–840.

Temoshok L. (1987). Personality, coping style, emotion and cancer: towards an integrative model. *Cancer Surveys,* 6(3), 545–567.

Temoshok L., Dreher H. (1993). *The Type C Connection - The Behavioral Link to Cancer and Your Health.* New York: Random House.

Tereshchuk E. I. (2012). Suicidalnoe povedenie kak krizis adaptacii. *ARS medica. Iskusstvo Mediciny: Psihoterapiya i Psihiatriya,* 1, 27–31.

Teunis M. A., Kavelaars A., Voest E. et al. (2002). Reduced tumor growth, experimental metastasis formation, and angiogenesis in rats with a hyperreactive dopaminergic system. *FASEB J,* 6(11), 1465–1467.

Teutsch J. M., Teutsch C. K. (1975). *From Here to Greater Happiness or How to Change Your Life for Good!* London: Price Stern Sloan.

Thaker P. H., Sood A. K. (2008). Neuroendocrine influences on cancer biology. *Seminars in Cancer Biology,* 3(18), 164–170.

Thaker P. H., Han L. Y., Kamat A. A. et al. (2006). Chronic stress promotes tumor growth and angiogenesis in a mouse model of ovarian carcinoma. *Nat Med,* 12(8), 939–944.

Thewes B., Butow P., Zachariae R. et al. (2011). Fear of cancer recurrence: a systematic literature review of self-report measures. *Psycho-Oncology,* 21(6), 571–587.

Thomas C. B., Duszynski K. R., Shaffer J. W. (1974). Closeness to Parents and the Family Constellation in a Prospective Study of Five Disease States: Suicide, Mental Illness, Malignant Tumor, Hypertension, and Coronary Heart Disease. *Johns Hopkins Medical Journal,* 134, 251–270.

Thomas C. B., Duszynski K. R., Shaffer J. W. (1979). Family attitudes reported in youth as potential predictors of cancer. *Psychosomatic Medicine,* 41(4), 287–302.

Thomas J. A., Badini M. (2011). The role of innate immunity in spontaneous regression of cancer. *Indian Journal of Cancer,* 48(2), 246–241.

Thomas R. M., Hotsenpiller G., Peterson D. A. (2007). Acute psychosocial stress reduces cell survival in adult hippocampal neurogenesis without altering proliferation. *The Journal of Neuroscience,* 27(11), 2734–2743.

Thomas S. P., Groer M., Davis M. et al. (2000). Anger and cancer: an analysis of the linkages. *Cancer Nurs,* 23(5), 344–349.

Thompson L. Y., Snyder C. R., Hoffman L. et al. (2005). Dispositional forgiveness of self, others, and situations. *Journal of Personality,* 73, 313–360.

Thoresen C. E., Harris A. H. S., Luskin F. (2000). Forgiveness and health: An unanswered question. In: M. E. McCullough, K. I. Pargament (eds). *Forgiveness: Theory, research, and practice*. New York: Guilford Press, 254–280.

Thornton L. M., Andersen B. L., Crespin T. R., Carson W. E. (2007). Individual trajectories in stress covary with immunity during recovery from cancer diagnosis and treatments. *Brain, Behavior, and Immunity*, 21, 185–194.

Thornton L. M., Andersen B. L., Schuler T. A. et al. (2009). A psychological intervention reduces inflammatory markers by alleviating depressive symptoms: secondary analysis of a randomized controlled trial. *Psychosom Med*, 71(7), 715–724.

Tiganov A. S., Vidmanova L. N., Platonova T. P., Suhovskiy A. A. (1986). *Maskirovannaya depressiya (klinika i diagnostika)*. Moscow: COLIUV.

Tigranyan R. A. (1988). *Stress i ego znachenie dlya organizma*. Moscow: Nauka.

Tijhuis M. A., Elshout J. R., Feskens E. J. et al. (2000). Prospective investigation of emotional control and cancer risk in men (the Zutphen Eldery Study) (the Netherlands). *Cancer Causes Control*, 11(7), 589–595.

Tiliopoulos N., Goodall K. (2009). The neglected link between adult attachment and schizotypal personality traits. *Personality and Individual Differences*, 47(4), 299–304.

Tillich P. (1964). *Theology of Culture*. Oxford: Oxford University Press

Tilvis R. S., Laitala V., Routasalo P. E., Pitkala K. H. (2011). Suffering from loneliness indicates significant mortality risk of older people. *J Aging Res*, 534781.

Tipping C. C. (2000). *Radical Forgiveness: Making Room for the Miracle*. Southlake, TX: Gateway.

Tjemsland L., Søreide J. A., Malt U. F. (1996). Traumatic distress symptoms in early breast cancer I: Acute response to diagnosis. *Psycho-Oncology*, 5(1), 1–8.

Tjemsland T., Soreide J. A., Matre R. et al. (1997). Preoperative psychological variables predict immunological status in patients with operable breast cancer. *Psycho-Oncology*, 6(4), 311–320.

Tkachenko G. A. (2008). Psihologicheskaya korrekciya krizisnogo sostoyaniya lichnosti zhenshin, stradayushih rakom molochnoj zhelezy. *Sibirskiy Psihol Zhurn*, 30, 97–101.

Tkachenko G. A., Shestopalova I. M. (2007). Osobennosti lichnosti bolnyh rakom molochnoj zhelezy v otdalennom periode. *Vestnik Psihoterapii*, 21(26), 66–78.

Tkachenko G. A., Vorotnikov I. K., Bujdenok Y. V. (2010). Rol psihoterapii v lechenii bolnyh rakom molochnoj zhelezy. *Vestnik RONC im. N. N. Blohina RAMN*, 21(3), 61 – 64.

Todarello O., Casamassima A., Marinaccio M. et al. (1997). Alexithymia, immunity and cervical intraepithelial neoplasia: replication. *Psychother Psychosom*, 66(4), 208–213.

Todarello O., La Pesa M. W., Zaka S. et al. (1989). Alexithymia and breast cancer. *Psychother Psychosom*, 51, 51–55.

Todorov I. N., Todorov G. I. (2003). *Stress, starenie i ih biohimicheskaya korrekciya*. Moscow: Nauka.

Tomei L. D., Kiecolt-Glaser J. K., Kennedy S., Glaser R. (1990). Psychological stress and phorbol ester inhibition of radiation-induced apoptosis in human PBLs. *Psychiatry Res*, 33, 59–71.

Tomich P. L., Helgeson V. S. (2006). Cognitive Adaptation Theory and Breast Cancer Recurrence: Are There Limits? *Journal of Consulting and Clinical Psychology*, 74(5), 980–987.

Tomiyama A. J., O'Donovan A., Lin J. et al. (2012). Does cellular aging relate to patterns of allostasis? An examination of basal and stress reactive HPA axis activity and telomere length. *Physiol Behav*, 106(1), 40–45.

Topolyanskiy V. D., Strukovskaya M. V. (1986). *Psihosomaticheskie rasstrojstva*. Moscow: Medicina.

Torrey E. F. (2006). Prostate cancer and schizophrenia. *Urology*, 68(6), 1280–1283.

Tosoian J. J., Trock B. J., Landis P. et al. (2011). Active surveillance program for prostate cancer: an update of the Johns Hopkins experience. *Journal of Clinical Oncology*, 29(16), 2185–2190.

Tottenham N., Hare T. A., Quinn B. T. et al. (2010). Prolonged institutional rearing is associated with atypically large amygdala volume and difficulties in emotion regulation. *Dev Sci*, 13(1), 4661.

Touitou Y., BogdanA., Levi F. et al. (1996). Disruption of the circadian patterns of serum cortisol in breast and ovarian cancer patients: relationships with tumour marker antigens. *British Journal of Cancer*, 74(8), 1248–1252.

Toussaint L., Owen A. D., Cheadle A. (2010). Forgiveness and reduced risk of cancer onset. *Poster presentation at the annual meeting of the Society for Behavioral Medicine.* Seattle, WA.

Toussaint L., Barry M., Bornfriend L., Markman M. (2014). Restore: the journey toward self-forgiveness: a randomized trial of patient education on self-forgiveness in cancer patients and caregivers. *J Health Care Chaplain*, 20(2), 54–74.

Traleg Kyabgon (2001). *The Essence of Buddhism: An Introduction to Its Philosophy and Practice.* Boulder, CO: Shambhala.

Tran E., Rouillon F., Loze J. Y. et al. (2009). Cancer mortality in patients with schizophrenia: an 11-year prospective cohort study. *Cancer*, 115(15), 3555–3562.

Troshin V. D. (2009). Problemy klinicheskoj preventologii. *Nevrologicheskiy Vestnik*, 41(4-S), 68–72.

Troshin V. D. (2009a). Duhovnaya dominanta i starenie organizma. *Byulleten Sibirskoj Mediciny*, (3), 2, 67–71.

Troshin V. D. (2011). Strategiya i taktika preventivnoj nevrologii. *Medicinskiy Almanah*, 1, 37–44.

Trudy 1-go Vseukrainskogo sezda hirurgov. (1927). Odessa, 15.09—19.09 1926 g. Prilozhenie k zhurnalu *Novyj Hirurgicheskiy Arhiv.* Dnepropetrovsk.

Trunov D. G. (2013). Prichinniy analiz suicidalnoj aktivnosti. *Vestnik Permskogo universiteta. Filosofiya. Psihologiya. Sociologiya*, 2(14), 121–127.

Tsankova N. M., Berton O., Renthal W. et al. (2006). Sustained hippocampal chromatin regulation in a mouse model of depression and antidepressant action. *Nat Neurosci*, 9(4), 519–525.

Tsuang M. T. (1983). Risk of suicide in the relatives of schizophrenics, manics, depressives and controls. *J Clin Psychol*, 44, 396–400.

Tsuchiya Y., Sawada S., Yoshioka I. et al. (2003). Increased surgical stress promotes tumor metastasis. *Surgery*, 133(5), 547–555.

Tuinman M. A. (2008). *Surviving testicular cancer: relationship aspects.* Doctoral dissertation. Groningen: University Press.

Tukaev R. D. (2003). Psihicheskaya travma i suicidalnoe povedenie. Analiticheskiy obzor literatury s 1986 po 2001 gody. *Socialnaya i Klinicheskaya Psihiatriya*, 1, 151–163.

Tukaev R. D. (2012). Triggernye mehanizmy biologicheskogo i psihicheskogo stressa v sootnesenii s diatez-stressovymi modelyami psihiatrii. *Socialnaya i Klinicheskaya Psihiatriya*, 22(2), 69–76.

Turkevich N. M. (1955). Znachenie tipologicheskih osobennostej nervnoj sistemy pri vozniknovenii i razvitii raka molochnoj zhelezy u myshej. *Voprosy Onkologii*, 1, 64–70.

Turnbull A. V., Rivier C. L. (1999). Regulation of the hypothalamic-pituitary-adrenal axis by cytokines: actions and mechanisms of action. *Physiol Rev*, 79(1), 1–71.

Tycko B. (2000). Epigenetic gene silencing in cancer. *J Clin Invest*, 105, 401–407.

Uchadze S. S. (2008). Dvojstvennaya priroda psihoduhovnogo krizisa lichnosti. *Vestnik Universiteta Rossijskoj Akademii Obrazovaniya*, 2008, 4(42), 114–122.

Uddin M., Aiello A. E., Wildman D. E. et al. (2010). Epigenetic and immune function profiles associated with posttraumatic stress disorder. *Proc Natl Acad Sci USA*, 107(20), 9470–9475.

Ukhtomskiy A. A. (2000). *Dominanta dushi: iz gumanitarnogo naslediya.* Rybinsk: Rybinskoye Podvor'ye.

Ukhtomskiy A. A. (2002). *Dominanta.* Saint Petersburg: Piter.

Ukolova M. A. (1963). Vliyanie razdrazheniya gipotalamusa na opuholevyj process. V: *Trudy VIII Mezhdunar. protivorakovogo kongressa.* Moscow, 488–490.

Umanskiy S. V., Semke V. Y. (2008). Psihoterapevticheskie strategii v kompleksnom lechenii onkologicheskih bolnyh. *Sibirskiy Vestnik Psihiatrii i Narkologi,* 4(51), 68–71.

Uriadnitskaya N. A. (1998). *Psihologicheskaya samoregulyaciya u detej s onkologicheskoj patologiej.* Avtoref diss kand psihol nauk. Moscow: MGU.

Uryvaev Y. V., Babenkov G. I. (1981). Psikhosomaticheskiye rasstroystva. Moscow: Znanie.

Vagin Y. R. (2003). *Tifoanaliz.* Perm: PONITsAA.

Vagin Y. R. (2011). Voprosyi fenomenologicheskoy suitsidologii. *Suitsidologiya,* 2(3/4), 3–17.

Vaillant G. E. (1974). Natural history of male psychological health, II: some antecedents of healthy adult adjustment. *Arch Gen Psychiatry,* 31, 15–22.

Vaillant G. E. (1977). *Adaptation to life.* Cambridge, MA: Harvard University Press.

Vaiva G., Ducrocq F., Jezequel K. et al. (2003). Immediate treatment with propranolol decreases posttraumatic stress disorder two months after trauma. *Biol Psychiatry,* 54(9), 947–949.

Valentine A. D., Meyers C. A. (2005). Neurobehavioral effects of interferon therapy. *Current Psychiatry Reports,* 7(5), 391–395.

Valenzuela F. O. (2014). *Psycho-Oncology, Hypnosis and Psychosomatic Healing in Cancer.* Bloomington, IN: Trafford Publishing.

Van Baalen D. C., de Vries M. J., Gondrie M. T. (1987). *Psycho-Social Correlates of Spontaneous' Regression in Cancer.* Rotterdam: Erasmus University.

Van der Kolk B. A. (ed.) (1987). *Psychological Trauma.* Washington, DC: APA Press.

Van der Ploeg H. M., Kleijn W. C., Mook J. et al. (1989). Rationality and antiemotionality as a risk factor for cancer: concept differentiation. *J Psychosom Res,* 33(2), 217–225.

Van Der Pompe G., Antoni M. H., Duivenvoorden H. J. et al. (2001). An exploratory study into the effect of group psychotherapy on cardiovascular and immunoreactivity to acute stress in breast cancer patients. *Psychotherapy and Psychosomatics,* 70(6), 307–318.

Vanderwerker L. C., Jacobs S. C., Parkes C. M., Prigerson H. G. (2006). An exploration of associations between separation anxiety in childhood and complicated grief in later life. *The Journal of Nervous and Mental Disease,* 194(2), 121–123.

Van IJzendoorn M. (1995). Adult attachment representations, parental responsiveness and infant attachment: A meta-analysis on the predictive validity of the adult attachment interview. *Psychological Bulletin,* 117, 387–403.

Van Voorhees E., Scarpa A. (2004). The effects of child maltreatment on the hypothalamic-pituitary-adrenal axis. *Trauma Violence Abuse,* 5(4), 333–352.

Varga A. Y., Hamitova I. Y. (2005). Teoriya semeynyih sistem Myurreya Bouena. *Zhurnal Prakticheskoy Psihologii i Psihoanaliza,* 4. Retrieved 07.03.2015 from: http://psyjournal.ru/.

Vasilenko T. D. (2011). Transformatsiya sotsialnoy identichnosti v situatsii onkologicheskogo zabolevaniya u zhenschin. *Uchenyie Zapiski. Elektronnyiy nauchnyiy zhurnal Kurskogo gosudarstvennogo universiteta,* 1(17). Retrieved 07.02.2015 from: http://cyberleninka.ru.

Vasilyuk F. E. (1984). *Psihologiya perezhivaniya.* Moscow: MGU.

Vasyutin A. (2011). *Spasenie est - ono v tebe! Rak kak psihosomatoz.* Rostov-na-Donu: Feniks.

Vayserman A. M. (2008). K epigeneticheskoy etiologii vozrast-zavisimyih zabolevaniy. *Uspehi Gerontologii,* 21(3), 477–479.

Vayserman A. M., Voytenko V. P., Mehova L. V. (2011). Epigeneticheskaya epidemiologiya vozrast-zavisimyih zabolevaniy. *Ontogenez,* 42(1), 1–21.

Velikanova L. P. (2006). Dinamicheskie sootnosheniya nevrozov i psihosomaticheskih rasstroystv (chast 2). *Sotsialnaya i Klinicheskaya Psihiatriya,* 16(1), 95–100.

Velikanova L. P., Shevchenko Y. S. (2005). Psihosomaticheskie rasstroystva: sovremennoe sostoyanie problemyi (chast 1). *Sotsialnaya i Klinicheskaya Psihiatriya*, 15(4), 79–91.

Velyaminov N. A. (1904). Isteriya v hirurgii. *Rus Hirurg Arhiv*, 5, 593–618.

Ventegodt S., Anderson N. J., Merrick J. (2003). Quality of life philosophy V. Seizing the meaning of life and becoming well again. *The Scientific World Journal*, 3, 1210–1229.

Ventegodt S., Merrick J., Andersen N. J. (2003a). Quality of life as medicine: a pilot study of patients with chronic illness and pain. *The Scientific World Journal*, 3, 520–532.

Ventegodt S., Hermansen D. T., Kandel I., Merrick J. (2005). Human development XX: A theory for accelerated, spontaneous existential healing (salutogenesis): "human adult metamorphosis". *Journal of Alternative Medicine Research*, 1(4), 465–474.

Ventegodt S., Kandel I., Neikrug S., Merrick J. (2005a). Clinical holistic medicine: the existential crisis--life crisis, stress, and burnout. *The Scientific World Journal*, 5, 300–312.

Ventegodt S., Kromann M., Andersen N. J., Merrick J. (2004). The life mission theory VI. A theory for the human character: healing with holistic medicine through recovery of character and purpose of life. *The Scientific World Journal*, 4, 859–880.

Ventegodt S., Morad M., Hyam E., Merrick J. (2004a). Clinical Holistic Medicine: Induction of Spontaneous Remission of Cancer by Recovery of the Human Character and the Purpose of Life (the Life Mission). *The Scientific World Journal*, 4, 362–377.

Ventegodt S., Endler P. C., Andersen N. J. et al. (2010). Therapeutic value of anti-cancer drugs: A critical analysis of Cochrane meta-analyses of the therapeutic value of chemotherapy for cancer. *J Altern Med Res*, 2(4), 371–384.

Ventegodt S., Flensborg-Madsen T., Andersen N. J. et al. (2004b). Clinical Holistic Medicine: A Pilot Study on HIV and Quality of Life and a Suggested Cure for HIV and AIDS. *The Scientific World Journal*, 4, 264–272

Ventegodt S., Solheim E., Saunte M. E. et al. (2004c). Clinical Holistic Medicine: Metastatic Cancer. *The Scientific World Journal*, 4, 913–935.

Ventura A., Kirsch D. G., McLaughlin M. E. et al. (2007). Restoration of p53 function leads to tumour regression in vivo. *Nature*, 445(7128), 661–665.

Verbitskiy A. A. (2013). *Entsiklopedicheskiy slovar po psihologii i pedagogike*. E-book. Retrieved 20.02.2016 from: http://psychology_pedagogy.academic.ru/19183/.

Vereina L. V., Prohorova L. V. (2012). PsihologichnI prichini viniknennya onkozahvoryuvan u zhInok. *Visnik Harkivskogo Natsionalnogo Universitetu imeni V. N. Karazina*. Seriya: Psihologiya, 49, 153–157.

Verhoeven J. E., Revesz D., Epel E. S. et al. (2014). Major depressive disorder and accelerated cellular aging: results from a large psychiatric cohort study. *Molecular Psychiatry*, 19(8), 895–901.

Verma R., Foster R. E., Horgan K. et al. (2016). Lymphocyte depletion and repopulation after chemotherapy for primary breast cancer. *Breast Cancer Research*, 18(1), 1–12.

Vespa A., Jacobsen P. B., Spazzafumo L., Balducci L. (2011). Evaluation of intrapsychic factors, coping styles, and spirituality of patients affected by tumors. *Psycho-Oncology*, 20(1), 5–11.

Vickberg S. M., Bovbjerg D. H., DuHamel K. N. et al. (2000). Intrusive thoughts and psychological distress among breast cancer survivors: global meaning as a possible protective factor. *Behav Med*, 25(4), 152–160.

Vihristyuk O. V., Miller L. V., Orlova E. V., Leskina E. A. (2010). Psihologicheskaya pomosch lyudyam, perezhivshim psihotravmiruyuschee sobyitie. *Elektronnyiy Zhurnal Psihologicheskaya Nauka i Obrazovanie*, 5. Retrieved 2.11.2015 from: http://psyjournals.ru/.

Viilma L. (2014). *V soglasii s soboy. Kniga gordosti i styida*. Moscow: AST.

Vinichuk N. V. (2012). Osobennosti predstavleniy psihosomaticheskih bolnyih o schaste. *Vestnik Vostochno-Sibirskoy Otkryitoy Akademii: el. zh. Psihologicheskie Issledovaniya*. Retrieved 04.07.2015 from: http://vsoa.esrae.ru/pdf/2013/8/736.pdf.

Vinogrodskiy B. (2014). *Traktat Zheltogo imperatora o vnutrennem.* V 2 chastyah. Moscow: Profit Stayl.

Visconti R., Grieco D. (2009). New insights on oxidative stress in cancer. *Curr Opin Drug Discov Devel,* 12(2), 240–245.

Visintainer M. A., Volpicelli J. R., Seligman M. E. P. (1982). Tumor rejection in rats after inescapable or escapable shock. *Science,* 6, 437–438.

Visser A., Garssen B., Vingerhoets A. (2010). Spirituality and well-being in cancer patients: a review. *Psycho-Oncology,* 19, 565–572.

Vodakova E. I., Serdyukova O. A. (1955). Izuchenie osobennostey rosta i razvitiya perevivaemyih opuholey u kriys razlichnogo vozrasta pri vyizyivanii u nih eksperimentalnogo nevroza. *Voprosyi Onkologii,* 1(3), 121–125.

Volden P. A., Conzen S. D. (2013). The influence of glucocorticoid signaling on tumor progression. *Brain, Behavior, and Immunity,* 30, S26–S31.

Volkov V. P. (2013). Prichinyi estestvennoy smerti pri shizofrenii. V: *Sovremennaya meditsina: aktualnyie voprosyi: sb st po mater XVII mezhdunar nauch-prakt konf* Novosibirsk: SibAK, 9–19.

Volodin B. Y. (2007). *Psihosomaticheskie vzaimootnosheniya i psihoterapevticheskaya korrektsiya u bolnyih rakom molochnoy zhelezyi i opuholevoy patologiey tela matki.* Avtoref. dis. d-ra med. nauk. Ryazan: RGMU.

Voloshin P. V., Shestopalova L. F., Podkoryitov V. S. (2004). Posttravmaticheskie stressovyie rasstroystva: problemyi lecheniya i profilaktiki. *Mezhdunarodnyiy Meditsinskiy Zhurnal,* 1, 33 – 37.

Vorobiev V. M. (1993). Psihicheskaya adaptatsiya kak problema meditsinskoy psihologii i psihiatrii. *ObozreniePpsihiatrii i Meditsinskoy psihologii im. V. M. Bekhtereva,* 2, 33–39.

Vorobiev V. V. (2008). Psihicheskoe sostoyanie kak prediktor razvitiya mastopatii u zhenschin. *Ukrainskiy Visnik Psihonevrologiyi,* 16(3), 50–55.

Vorona O. A. (2005). *Psihologicheskie posledstviya stressa u bolnyih rakom molochnoy zhelezyi.* Avtoref. dis. kand. psihol. nauk. Moscow: In-t psihologii RAN.

Voronov M. (2011). *Psihosomatika. Prakticheskoe rukovodstvo.* Kiev: Nika-Centr.

Wachholtz A. B., Pargament K. I. (2005). Is spirituality a critical ingredient of meditation? Comparing the effects of spiritual meditation, secular meditation, and relaxation on spiritual, psychological, cardiac, and pain outcomes. *Journal of Behavioral Medicine,* 8(4), 369–384.

Wager N., Fieldman G., Hussey T. (2003). The effect on ambulatory blood pressure of working under favourably and unfavourably perceived supervisors. *Occupational and Environmental Medicine,* 60(7), 468–474.

Wakai K., Kojima M., Nishio K. et al. (2007). Psychological attitudes and risk of breasl cancer in Japan: a prospective study. *Cancer Causes Control,* 8, 259–267.

Walker C. L., Ho S. M. (2012). Developmental reprogramming of cancer susceptibility. *Nature Reviews Cancer,* 12(7), 479–486.

Walker L. G., Walker M. B., Ogston K. et al. (1999). Psychological, clinical and pathological effects of relaxation training and guided imagery during primary chemotherapy. *British Journal of Cancer,* 80, 262–268.

Walker R., Tynan R., Beynon S., Nilsson M. (2013). 70. Chronic stress induces profound structural atrophy of astrocytes within the prefrontal cortex: An emerging story in glial remodeling in response to stress. *Brain, Behavior, and Immunity,* 32, e20–e21.

Walshe W. (1846). *The nature and treatment of cancer.* London: Taylor and Walton.

Wang A. W., Hoyt M. A. (2018). Benefit finding and diurnal cortisol after prostate cancer: The mediating role of positive affect. *Psycho-Oncology,* 27(4), 1200–1205.

Wang B., Katsube T., Begum N., Nenoi M. (2016). Revisiting the health effects of psychological stress—its influence on susceptibility to ionizing radiation: a mini-review. *Journal of Radiation Research,* 57(4), 325–335.

Wang J.-L. (2016). *Jeanne Louise Calment: world's oldest*. Retrieved 12.04.2016 from: http://anson.ucdavis.edu/~wang/calment.html.

Wang S.-M. *The Glory of Life*. Retrieved 17.01.2016 from: http://drhsu.seth101.com/glory-of-life/the-glory-of-life-si-mei/.

Ward M. J., Kessler D. B., Altman S. C. (1993). Infant-mother attachment in children with failure to thrive. *Infant Mental Health Journal*, 14, 208–20

Wasserman D. (2001). A stress-vulnerability model and the development of the suicidal process. In: D. Wasserman (ed.), *Suicide, an unnecessary death*. London: Martin Dunitz, 13–27.

Waters S. F., West T. V., Mendes W. B. (2014). Stress Contagion Physiological Covariation Between Mothers and Infants. *Psychological Science*, 25(4), 934–942.

Watkins J. L., Thaker P. H., Nick A. M. et al. (2015). Clinical impact of selective and nonselective beta-blockers on survival in patients with ovarian cancer. *Cancer*, 121(19), 3444–3451.

Watson M., Haviland J. S., Greer S. et al. (1999). Influence of psychological response on survival in breast cancer: a population-based cohort study. *The Lancet*, 354(9187), 1331–1336.

Watson P., Milliron J., Morris R., Hood R. (1994). Religion and rationality: II.Comparative analysis of rational-emotive and intrinsically religious irrationalities. *Journal of Psychology and Christianity*, 13, 373–384.

Watson T. (1871). *Lectures on the Principles and Practice of Physic*. London: Jon W. Parker.

Watters E. (2006). DNA Is Not Destiny: The New Science of Epigenetics. *Discover*, November 22.

Wayment H. A., Vierthaler J. (2002). Attachment style and bereavement reactions. *Journal of Loss &Trauma*, 7(2), 129–149.

Weaver I. C. (2007). Epigenetic programming by maternal behavior and pharmacological intervention. Nature versus nurture: let's call the whole thing off. *Epigenetics*, 2(1), 22–28.

Weaver I. C., Cervoni N., Champagne F. A. et al. (2004). Epigenetic programming by maternal behavior. *Nature Neuroscience*, 7, 847–854.

Webster A. (2008). Resiliency: Creating a new now. In: Proc. conf. *Spirituality and Healing in Medicine: The Resiliency Factor*. Boston, MA.

Weil A. (2000). *Spontaneous Healing: How to Discover and Embrace Your Body's Natural Ability to Maintain and Heal Itself*. New York: Ballantine Books.

Weinstock C. (1977). Recent progress in cancer psychobiology and psychiatry. *Journal of the American Society of Psychosomatic Dentistry & Medicine*, 24(1), 4–14.

Weinstock C. (1983). Psychosomatic elements in 18 consecutive cancer regressions positively not due to somatic therapy. *Journal of the American Society of Psychosomatic Dentistry & Medicine*, 30, 151–155.

Weisman A. D., Worden J. W. (1977). The existential plight in cancer: significance of the first 100 days. *Int J Psychiatry Med*, 7(1), 1–15.

Weitzman S. A., Gordon L. I. (1990). Inflammation and cancer: role of phagocyte-generated oxidants in carcinogenesis. *Blood*, 76, 655–663.

Weizsäcker V. V. (1940). *Der Gestaltkreis (Theorie der Einheit von Wahrnehmen und Bewegen)*. Leipzig: Thieme.

Welch H. G., Black W. C. (1997). Using autopsy series to estimate the disease "reservoir" for ductal carcinoma in situ of the breast: how much more breast cancer can we find? *Ann Intern Med*, 127(11), 1023–1028.

Welwood J. (2000). *Toward a psychology of awakening: Buddhism, psychotherapy, and the path of personal and spiritual transformation*. Boston, MA: Shambhala.

Wendling C. A. (2016). Adverse childhood experiences, breast cancer, and psychotherapy. *Psycho-Oncologie*, 10(3), 221–226.

Wenner M., Kawamura N., Ishikawa T. (2000). Reward linked to increased natural killer cell activity in rats. *Neuroimmuno Modulation*, 7, 1–5.

Wentzensen I., Mirabello L., Pfeiffer R. M., Savage S. A. (2011). The association of telomere length and cancer: a meta-analysis. *Cancer Epidemiology Biomarkers & Prevention*, 20(6), 1238–1250.

West P. M. (1954). *Psychological Variables in Human Cancer.* Oakland, CA: University of California Press, 1–16.

Westgate C. (1996). Spiritual wellness and depression. *Journal of Counseling & Development*, 75, 26–35.

White V. M., English D. R., Coates H. et al. (2007). Is cancer risk associated with anger control and negative affect? Findings from a prospective cohort study. *Psychosomatic Medicine*, 69, 667–674.

White W. A. (1929). The social significance of mental disease. *Archives of Neurology & Psychiatry*, 22(5), 873–900.

WHO (World Health Organization). Review of the Constitution..., 1997, EB 10 1/7, 2.

Wiart Y. (2014). *Stress et Cancer, quand notre attachement nous joue des tours.* Louvain-la-Neuve: De Boeck.

Widom C. S., Czaja S. J., Kozakowski S. S., Chauhan P. (2017). Does adult attachment style mediate the relationship between childhood maltreatment and mental and physical health outcomes?. *Child Abuse & Neglect*, 76, 533–545.

Willcox S. J., Stewart B. W., Sitas F. (2011). What factors do cancer patients believe contribute to the development of their cancer? (New South Wales, Australia). *Cancer Causes Control*, 22(11), 1503–1511.

Willeit P., Willeit J., Mayr A. et al. (2010). Telomere length and risk of incident cancer and cancer mortality. *JAMA*, 304(1), 69–75.

Williams L., O'Connor R. C., Howard S. et al. (2008). Type D personality mechanisms of effect: the role of health-related behaviour and social support. *Journal of Psychosomatic Research*, 64(1), 63–69.

Wingenfeld K., Whooley M. A., Neylan T. C. et al. (2015). Effect of current and lifetime posttraumatic stress disorder on 24-h urinary catecholamines and cortisol: Results from the Mind Your Heart Study. *Psychoneuroendocrinology*, 52, 83–91.

Wingert P. (2009). Breaking: Health Author Suzanne Somers Mostly Wrong About Science. *Medicine. Newsweek*, 23.10.2009. Retrieved 09.08.2015 from: http://europe.newsweek.com.

Winnicott D. W. (1953). Psychoses and Child Care. *British Journal of Medical Psychology*, 26(1), 68–74.

Winnicott D. W. (1965). Ego distortion in terms of true and false self. In: D. Winnicott, *The maturational processes and the facilitating environment.* London: Hogarth Press, 140–152.

Winnicott D. W. (1994). *Talking To Parents.* Boston, MA: Da Capo Press.

Winokur A., Maislin G., Phillips J. L., Amsterdam J. D. (1988). Insulin resistance after oral glucose tolerance testing in patients with major depression. *Am J Psychiatry*, 145(3), 315–330.

Wirsching M., Hoffmann F., Stierlin H. et al. (1985). Prebioptic psychological characteristics of breast cancer patients. *Psychother Psychosom*, 43(2), 69–76.

Witek-Janusek L., Gabram S., Mathews H. L. (2007). Psychologic stress, reduced NK cell activity, and cytokine dysregulation in women experiencing diagnostic breast biopsy. *Psychoneuroendocrinology*, 32(1), 22–35.

Wittchen H. U., Jacobi, F. (2005). Size and burden of mental disorders in Europe—a critical review and appraisal of 27 studies. *European Neuropsychopharmacology*, 15(4), 357–376.

Witek-Janusek L., Albuquerque K., Chroniak K. R. et al. (2008). Effect of mindfulness based stress reduction on immune function, quality of life and coping in women newly diagnosed with early stage breast cancer. *Brain Behav Immun*, 22, 969–981.

Witvliet C. V. O., Ludwig T. E., Vander Laan K. L. (2001). Granting forgiveness or harboring grudges: implications for emotion, physiology, and health. *Psychological Science*, 121, 117–123.

Wohleb E. S., Hanke M. L., Corona A. W. et al. (2011). Beta-Adrenergic receptor antagonism prevents anxiety-like behavior and microglial reactivity induced by repeated social defeat. *J Neurosci*, 31, 6277–6288.

Wolford C. C., McConoughey S. J., Jalgaonkar S. P. et al. (2013). Transcription factor ATF3 links host adaptive response to breast cancer metastasis. *The Journal of clinical investigation*, 123(7), 2893–2906.

Wolkowitz O. M., Mellon S. H., Epel E. S. et al. (2011). Leukocyte telomere length in major depression: correlations with chronicity, inflammation and oxidative stress-preliminary findings. *PloS One*, 6(3), e17837.

Wolman B. (1975). Principles of International Psychotherapy. *Psychotherapy: Theory, Research and Practice*, 12, 149–159.

Wong P. T. (1998). Spirituality, meaning, and successful aging. In: P. T. P. Wong & P. Fry (eds), *The human quest for meaning: A handbook of psychological research and clinical applications*. Mahwah, NJ: Lawrence Erlbaum, 359–394.

Wong P. T. (1998a). Implicit theories of meaningful life and the development of the personal meaning profile. In: P. T. P. Wong & P. S. Fry (eds), *The human quest for meaning: A handbook of psychological research and clinical applications*. Mahway, NJ: Lawrence Erlbaum, 111–140.

Worthington E. L. Jr (2013). *Moving forward: Six steps to forgiving yourself and breaking free from the past*. Colorado Springs, CO: WaterBrook/Multnomah.

Worthington E. L. Jr, Witvliet C. V. O., Lerner A. J., Scherer M. (2005). Forgiveness in health research and medical practice. *Explore (NY)*, 1(3), 169–176.

Worthington E. L. Jr, Witvliet C. V. O., Pietrini P., Miller A. J. (2007). Forgiveness, health, and well-being: A review of evidence for emotional versus decisional forgiveness, dispositional forgivingness, and reduced unforgiveness. *Journal of Behavioral Medicine*, 30(4), 291–302.

Wright J., Briggs S., Behringer J. (2005). Attachment and the body in suicidal adolescents: A pilot study. *Clinical Child Psychology and Psychiatry*, 10, 477–491.

Wrona D., Trojniar W. (2003). Chronic electrical stimulation of the lateral hypothalamus increases natural Killer cell cytotoxicity in rats. *J Neuroimmunol*, 14(1–2), 20–29.

Wrye H. (1979). The crisis of cancer: Intervention perspectives. *Journal writing with women with breast cancer, Read before the 87th American Psychiatric Association Convention*, New York.

Wu L., Holbrook C., Zaborina O. et al. (2003). Pseudomonas aeruginosa expresses a lethal virulence determinant, the PA-I lectin/adhesin, in the intestinal tract of a stressed host: the role of epithelia cell contact and molecules of the Quorum Sensing Signaling System. *Annals of Surgery*, 238(5), 754–764.

Wu S. M., Andersen B. L. (2011). *Prevalence of mood and anxiety disorders in cancer patients: A systematic review and meta-analysis*. Columbus, OH: The Ohio State University.

Wu W., Chaudhuri S., Brickley D. R. et al. (2004). Microarray analysis reveals glucocorticoid-regulated survival genes that are associated with inhibition of apoptosis in breast epithelial cells. *Cancer Res*, 64, 1757–1764.

Wu W., Yamaura T., Murakami K. et al. (1999). Involvement of TNF-α in enhancement of invasion and metastasis of colon 26–L5 carcinoma cells in mice by social isolation stress. *Oncol Res*, 11, 461–469.

Wu X., Liu B. J., Ji S. et al. (2015). Social defeat stress promotes tumor growth and angiogenesis by upregulating vascular endothelial growth factor/extracellular signal-regulated kinase/matrix metalloproteinase signaling in a mouse model of lung carcinoma. *Molecular Medicine Reports*, 12(1), 1405–1412.

Wu Y., Zhou B. P. (2009). Inflammation: a driving force speeds cancer metastasis. *Cell Cycle*, 8(20), 3267–3273.

Wu Y., Sarkissyan M., Vadgama J. V. (2015). Epigenetics in breast and prostate cancer. In: M. Verma (ed.), *Cancer Epigenetics: Risk Assessment, Diagnosis, Treatment, and Prognosis*. New York: Humana Press, 425–466.

Xia Y., Tong G., Feng R. et al. (2014). Psychosocial and Behavioral Interventions and Cancer Patient Survival Again: Hints of an Adjusted Meta-Analysis. *Integr Cancer Ther*, 13, 301–309.

Xu Z., Taylor J. A. (2014). Genome-wide age-related DNA methylation changes in blood and other tissues relate to histone modification, expression and cancer. *Carcinogenesis*, 35(2), 356–364.

Yatskevich K. V. (2007). *Rak - ne prigovor, a samyj sereznyj povod izmenitsya*. Moscow: Izdatelstvo Alekseya Varaksina.

Yalom I. (1980). *Existential psychotherapy*. New York: Basic Books.

Yam D., Fink A., Mashiah A., BenHur E. (1996). Hyperinsulinemia in colon, stomach and breast cancer patients. *Cancer Lett*, 104, 129–132.

Yamaguchi K., Takagi Y., Aoki S. et al. (2000). Significant detection of circulating cancer cells in the blood by reverse transcriptase-polymerase chain reaction during colorectal cancer resection. *Ann Surg*, 232(1), 58–65.

Yang E. V., Kim S. J., Donovan E. L. et al. (2009). Norepinephrine upregulates VEGF, IL-8, and IL-6 expression in human melanoma tumor cell lines: implications for stress-related enhancement of tumor progression. *Brain, Behavior, and Immunity*, 23(2), 267–275.

Yang E. V., Sood A. K., Chen M. et al. (2006). Norepinephrine up-regulates the expression of vascular endothelial growth factor, matrix metalloproteinase (MMP)-2, and MMP-9 in nasopharyngeal carcinoma tumor cells. *Cancer Research*, 66(21), 10357–10364.

Yang W., Staps T., Hijmans E. (2012). Going through a Dark Night. *Studies in Spirituality*, 22, 311–339.

Yehuda R. (2001). Biology of posttraumatic stress disorder. *J Clin Psychiatry*, 62, Suppl 17, 41–46.

Yehuda R., LeDoux J. (2007). Response variation following trauma: a translational neuroscience approach to understanding PTSD. *Neuron,* 56(1), 19–32.

Yehuda R., Daskalakis N. P, Desarnaud F. et al. (2013). Epigenetic biomarkers as predictors and correlates of symptom improvement following psychotherapy in combat veterans with PTSD. *Front Psychiatry*, 4, 118.

Yongey Mingyur Rinpoche, Swanson E. (2008). *The Joy of Living: Unlocking the Secret and Science of Happiness*. New York: Harmony.

Young W. S., Lightman S. L. (1992). Chronic stress elevates enkephalin expression in the rat paraventricular and supraoptic nuclei. *Brain Res Mol Brain Res*, 13, 111–117.

Yu O., Lee M., Koposov R. et al. (2012). Differential patterns of whole-genome DNA methylation in institutionalized children and children raised by their biological parents. *Developmental Psychopathology*, 24(1), 143–155.

Yu T., Tsai H. L., Hwang M. L. (2003). Suppressing tumor progression of in vitro prostate cancer cells by emitted psychosomatic power through Zen meditation. *The American Journal of Chinese Medicine*, 31(03), 499–507.

Yuryeva L. N. (2006). *Klinicheskaya suicidologiya*. Dnepropetrovsk: Porogi.

Yurmin E. A. (1954). Vpliv centralnoyi nervnoyi sistemi na rist i rozvitok pereshepnoyi puhlini Broun-Pirs. *Med zhurnal AN USSR*, 24, 3, 28–31.

Zabora J., Brintzenhofeszoc K., Curbow B. et al. (2001). The prevalence of psychological distress by cancer site. *Psycho-Oncology*, 10(1), 19–28.

Zahl P. H., Mæhlen J., Welch H. G. (2008). The natural history of invasive breast cancers detected by screening mammography. *Archives of Internal Medicine*, 168(21), 2311–2316.

Zaidan H., Leshem M., Gaisler-Salomon I. (2013). Prereproductive stress to female rats alters corticotropin releasing factor type 1 expression in ova and behavior and brain corticotropin releasing factor type 1 expression in offspring. *Biological Psychiatry,* 74(9), 680–687.

Zakharov A. I. (1982). Psihoterapiya nevrozov u detej i podrostkov. Leningrad: Meditsina.

Zalevskiy G. V., Zalevskiy V. G., Kuzmina Yu. V. (2009). Antropologicheskaya psihologiya: biopsihosocionoeticheskaya model razvitiya lichnosti i ee zdorovya. *Sibirskiy Psihologicheskiy Zhurnal*, 33, 99–103.

Zalmanov A. S. (1997). *Glubinnaya medicina. Tajnaya mudrost chelovecheskogo organizma*. Moscow: Ripol Klassik.

Zamora E. R., Yi J., Akter J. et al. (2017). 'Having cancer was awful but also something good came out': Post-traumatic growth among adult survivors of pediatric and adolescent cancer. *European Journal of Oncology Nursing*, 28, 21–27.

Zannas A. S., Wiechmann T., Gassen N. C., Binder E. B. (2016). Gene-Stress-Epigenetic Regulation of FKBP5: Clinical and Translational Implications. *Neuropsychopharmacology*, 41(1), 261–274.

Zannas A. S., Arloth J., Carrillo-Roa T. et al. (2015). Lifetime stress accelerates epigenetic aging in an urban, African American cohort: relevance of glucocorticoid signaling. *Genome Biology*, 16(1), 1–12.

Zebrack B. J., Yi J., Petersen L., Ganz P. A. (2008). The impact of cancer and quality of life for long-term survivors. *Psycho-Oncology*, 17(9), 891–900.

Zeng H., Irwin M. L., Lu L. et al. (2012). Physical activity and breast cancer survival: an epigenetic link through reduced methylation of a tumor suppressor gene L3MBTL1. *Breast Cancer Research and Treatment*, 133(1), 127–135.

Zeng Y., Luo T., Xie H. et al. (2014). Health benefits of qigong or tai chi for cancer patients: a systematic review and meta-analyses. *Complementary Therapies in Medicine*, 22(1), 173–186.

Zglinicki T. von (2002). Oxidative stress shortens telomeres. *Trends Biochem Sci*, 27(7), 339–344.

Zhang C., Sarkar D. K. (2012). β-endorphin neuron transplantation: a possible novel therapy for cancer prevention. *Oncoimmunology*, 1(4), 552–554.

Zhang X., Odom D. T., Koo S. H. et al. (2005). Genome-wide analysis of cAMP-response element binding protein occupancy, phosphorylation, and target gene activation in human tissues. *Proc Natl Acad Sci USA*, 102, 4459–4464.

Zhao Q., Yang Y., Liang X. et al. (2014). The clinicopathological significance of neurogenesis in breast cancer. *BMC Cancer*, 14(1), 484.

Zhao W. Q., Chen H., Quon M. J., Alkon D. L. (2004). Insulin and the insulin receptor in experimental models of learning and memory. *Eur J Pharmacol*, 490(1–3), 7181.

Zhao X. Y., Malloy P. J., Krishnan A. V. et al. (2000). Glucocorticoids can promote androgen-independent growth of prostate cancer cells through a mutated androgen receptor. *Nature Medicine*, 6(6), 703–706.

Zhou F. L., Zhang W. G., Wei Y. C. et al. (2005). Impact of comorbid anxiety and depression on quality of life and cellular immunity changes in patients with digestive tract cancers. *World Journal of Gastroenterology*, 11(15), 2313–2318.

Zika S., Chamberlain K. (1992). On the relation between meaning in life and psychological well-being. *British Journal of Psychology*, 83, 133–145.

Zilber L. A. (1948). *Osnovy immuniteta*. Moscow: Medgiz.

Zonderman A. B., Costa P. T. Jr, McCrae R. R. (1989). Depression as a risk for cancer morbidity and mortality in a nationally representative sample. *JAMA*, 62, 1191–1195.

Zorrilla E. P., Luborsky L., McKay J. R. et al. (2001). The relationship of depression and stressors to immunological assays: a meta-analytic review. *Brain Behav Immun*, 15(3), 199–226.

Zorzet S., Perissin L., Rapozzi V. et al. (1998). Restraint stress reduces the antitumor efficacy of cyclophosphamide in tumor-bearing mice. *Brain Behav Immun*, 2(1), 23–33.

Zotov G. (2014). Umer do sta let - sam durak! Istoriya kitajskogo goroda dolgozhitelej. *Ezhenedelnik Argumenty i Fakty*, 17, April 23.

Zovkic I. B., Meadows J. P., Kaas G. A., Sweatt J. D. (2013). Interindividual Variability in Stress Susceptibility: A Role for Epigenetic Mechanisms in PTSD. *Front Psychiatry*, 4, 60.

Zubarev P. N., Bryusov P. G. (2017). *Klinicheskaya onkologiya.* Moscow: Litres.

Zubova E. Y. (2012). Tuberkulez legkih v psihiatricheskih stacionarah. *Vestnik Tambovskogo Universiteta. Seriya: Estestvennye i Tehnicheskie Nauki*, 17(1), 256–262.

Zur Hausen H. (1991). Viruses in human cancers. *Science*, 254, 1167–1173.

About the Author

Vladislav Matrenitsky M.D., Ph.D., is the founder and head of the Center for Psychotherapy, Psychosomatics and Psycho-oncology Expio, the first specialized organization for psychosocial cancer care in Ukraine. He graduated from Odessa State Medical University (Ukraine) and qualified as a General Practitioner in 1986. In 1992, Vladislav completed a postgraduate course at the Institute of Gerontology Academy of Medical Science of USSR (Kiev), and was awarded a Ph.D. in the physiology and molecular biology of stress in ageing. After that, he worked as a Research Fellow in the same Institute and published in the field of gerontology.

Later on, Vladislav came to the understanding that the real secrets of life, illnesses, aging, and death lie not only on the physical but also on the spiritual level. Being disappointed in pharmacy-oriented medicine, he started learning ancient and modern spiritual knowledge and healing traditions.

Vladislav studied Psychotherapy at Kiev's State Academy of Postgraduate Medical Education, and then was qualified as a Transpersonal Psychotherapist by the European Transpersonal Association (EUROTAS). Psychosomatic medicine and psycho-oncology became his main area of practice. Since 2002, Dr. Matrenitsky has given many workshops and private sessions throughout European countries, and also presented his work at a number of European and World conferences and congresses on Transpersonal psychology and psychotherapy.

His book, Carcinogenic Mind, was initially published in 2007 in Ukraine and was greeted warmly as the first manual on psycho-oncology in the country. Dr. Matrenitsky is a co-founder of the European Transpersonal Psychology Association (ETPA) and a member of the International Psycho-Oncology Society (IPOS). Currently he holds a private practice, treating patients in his Center in Kiev and online, develops the transpersonal psycho-oncology and gives lectures and workshops worldwide. For more information, please visit www.anticancer.help.

Appendix

ANTICANCER

An online transpersonal psycho-oncology treatment program by Dr. Vladislav Matrenitsky

Integrative psychobiosocial-spiritual therapy
Rehabilitation of cancer patients
Prevention of cancer onset and recurrence

Years of practice and research in the fields of psychosomatic medicine, psycho-oncology, molecular biology, gerontology, and transpersonal psychotherapy have helped me to formulate my own understanding of oncological diseases, which is reflected in this book.

How are these ideas put into practice? Through my development of a specialized stream of psychotherapy—transpersonal psycho-oncology.

Traditional psycho-oncology concentrates mainly on correcting personality and psychopathological disorders, which arise as a result of disease. Transpersonal psycho-oncology, in contrast, is aimed at psychotherapy addressing the true causes of the disease—the psycho-spiritual life crisis resulting from untreated psycho-traumatic events and intrapersonal conflicts. It actively involves the mind, subconscious, and spiritual potential of the patient in activating the natural healing resources of the body.

I do not treat cancer as a physical disease—I help the person reconstruct the mind and heal the soul. Being harmonized, they restore the body's control over the anti-cancer forces, so it starts to fight disease more effectively. My program does not reject conventional medical treatment, but instead makes it much more effective and eliminates many side effects and complications.

The objectives of my therapy program are as follows:

— Terminate the factors that exacerbate the disease and block the treatment: depression, helplessness, and hopelessness.

— Neutralize the main causes of cancer development: oncodominant, existential and spiritual crisis, and loss of will to live.

– Deactivate the basic predisposition to cancer: disorders of attachment to parents and childhood traumas, as well as the resulting distortions in perception of oneself and the outside world.

– Eliminate the chronic oncogenic distress that has arisen due to unresolved conflicts and psychic traumas during adulthood.

– Transform the post-traumatic stress, that feeds the tumor process, into post-traumatic growth that mobilizes the suppressed healing resources of the body.

– Cure the psychic traumas caused by a diagnosis, operation, or disability.

– Help examine the patient's personality and its role in the origin of the disease.

– Jointly with the patient develop a strategy for movement toward life, and the disposal of the consequences of illness.

– Recreate and strengthen the will to live, which activates the immune system and other protective systems of the body.

– Change the patient's attitude toward the disease—from passivity and surrender to life-affirming activity.

– Awaken and maximize the patient's psychophysical potential for restoration and preservation of health.

– Eliminate the psychosocial factors that lead to the relapse of the disease.

– Help the patient to learn how to accept and respect him/herself and the world.

– Reduce fear of uncertainty about the future.

An integrative approach means approaching a person as a whole system, where the body, energy, mind, and spirituality are equal partners. Therefore, work with the patient needs to be carried out at the corresponding four levels of his/her being.

I use methods of classical and transpersonal psychotherapy, hypnotherapy, sensorimotor psychosynthesis by Vladimir Kucherenko, the Simontons' system, symbolic modeling by David Grove, some ancient trance techniques of working with the subconscious, and methods I have developed myself.

I work with patients who have completed or in the process of a course of medical treatment and/or who do not have side effects, such as "chemobrain," that violate the functioning of consciousness. Also eligible are patients under the active surveillance program at an early stage of the cancer. The patient should have stable enough mental, physical, and energetic states to be able to work effectively for about 1.5 hrs during the session and practice at home. I also help to prevent cancer in those who are in a precancerous state or in the cancer risk group.

In adition, I offer lectures on psychosomatics and psycho-oncology, and the teaching program "Sound-based stress reduction," in workshop format. Many research studies have showed that harmonious sounds can relieve stress and anxiety, induce relaxation and analgesia, and even destroy cancer cells. Using the technique of overtone throat singing as the instrument of trance induction, it is possible to reach a deep meditative state that can activate our dormant healing potential.

Practicing overtone sounds calms the mind, broadens the awareness, helps in the attainment of a transpersonal experience, and leads to the restoration of harmony in affected organs.

For more information and to book appointments visit the website www.anticancer.help.

Dear Reader,

Thank you for purchasing and reading this book. I hope that it gave you a new vision of cancer disease and perhaps even added at value and quality to your everyday life. If so, it would be really nice if you could share this book with your friends and family by posting to Facebook, Twitter or any other social network.

My FB page can be found at www.fb.me/carcinogenic.mind.book.
If you enjoyed this book and found some benefit in reading this, I'd like to hear from you and hope that you could take some time to post a review on Amazon and/or Goodreads.com. Your feedback and support will help this author to greatly improve his writing craft for future projects and make this book even better.

You can usually find the link to Amazon review page as following: www.amazon.com/review/review-your-purchases/.

I want you to know that your review is very important and so, if you'd like to leave a feedback, all you have to do is log in your Amazon and Goodreads accounts and post the text.

I wish you prosperity and good health!

Dr. Vladislav Matrenitsky

Made in the USA
Coppell, TX
08 August 2021